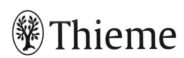

Top 3 Differentials in Neuroradiology

A Case Review

William T. O'Brien Sr., DO
Program Director, Diagnostic Radiology Residency
David Grant USAF Medical Center
Travis Air Force Base, California

Former Chairman, Department of Radiology
Wilford Hall USAF Ambulatory Surgical Center
Joint Base San Antonio-Lackland, Texas

Associate Clinical Professor
Department of Radiology
University of California, Davis School of Medicine
Sacramento, California

Thieme
New York • Stuttgart • Delhi • Rio de Janeiro

Executive Editor: William Lamsback
Managing Editor: J. Owen Zurhellen IV
Assistant Managing Editor: Heather Allen
International Production Director: Andreas Schabert
Senior Vice President, Editorial and E-Product
  Development: Cornelia Schulze
International Marketing Director: Fiona Henderson
International Sales Director: Louisa Turrell
Director of Sales, North America: Mike Roseman
Senior Vice President and Chief Operating
  Officer: Sarah Vanderbilt
President: Brian D. Scanlan

Library of Congress Cataloging-in-Publication Data

O'Brien, William T., author.
  Top 3 differentials in neuroradiology : a case review /
William T. O'Brien.
     p. ; cm.
  Top three differentials in neuroradiology
  Includes bibliographical references.
  ISBN 978-1-60406-723-1 (pbk. : alk. paper) –
  ISBN 978-1-60406-724-8 (e-book)
  I. Title. II. Title: Top three differentials in neuroradiology.
  [DNLM: 1. Diagnosis, Differential–Case Reports. 2. Neuro-
radiography–Case Reports. 3. Central Nervous System–radiogra-
phy–Case Reports. 4. Central Nervous System Diseases–
radiography–Case Reports. WL 141.5.N47]
  RC71.5
  616.07'5–dc23
                                                2014026028

© 2015 Thieme Medical Publishers, Inc.

Thieme Publishers New York
333 Seventh Avenue, New York, NY 10001 USA, 1-800-782-3488
customerservice@thieme.com

Thieme Publishers Stuttgart
Rüdigerstrasse 14, 70469 Stuttgart, Germany,
+49 [0]711 8931 421
customerservice@thieme.de

Thieme Publishers Delhi
A-12, Second Floor, Sector-2, NOIDA-201301, Uttar Pradesh, India,
+91 120 45 566 00
customerservice@thieme.in

Thieme Publishers Rio, Thieme Publicações Ltda.
Argentina Building 16th floor, Ala A, 228 Praia do Botafogo Rio de
Janeiro 22250-040 Brazil, +55 21 3736-3631

Printed in India by Replika Press Pvt. Ltd.

5 4 3 2 1

ISBN 978-1-60406-723-1

Also available as an e-book:
eISBN 978-1-60406-724-8

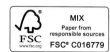

Dedicated in memory of

Robert L. Meals, DO

12 March 1928–9 June 2005

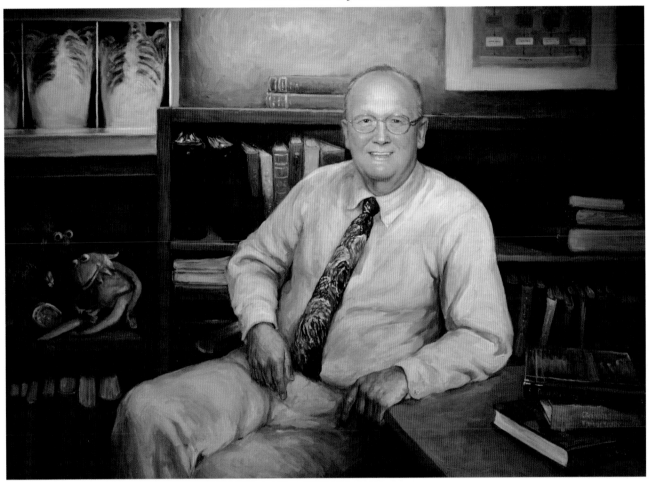

© *Susan Schary 2005*

For decades, Dr. Meals inspired thousands of students while serving as Academic Chairman of the
Department of Radiology, Philadelphia College of Osteopathic Medicine, Philadelphia, Pennsylvania.
Dr. Meals was more than an instructor; he was a mentor and a true friend.
To those who chose to pursue a career in radiology, he will always be a legend.
He is sorely missed but will never be forgotten.

Contents

Foreword

Unique!

That is the best word to describe *Top 3 Differentials in Neuroradiology* by William T. O'Brien—unique in its approach to the clinical practice of neuro-imaging, and unique in its approach to education in this rapidly expanding subspecialty. The traditional clinical practice of a neurologist, neurosurgeon, orthopedic surgeon—any physician ordering a neuro-imaging examination—is to evaluate the patient's history in conjunction with signs and symptoms, come to a probable conclusion, and then request an imaging study to confirm or deny that clinical conclusion.

The clinical practice of a radiologist initially requires the recognition of a combination of findings on an imaging study within the stated clinical context. This is followed by the iterative comparison of these findings to examples from diagnostic categories, including masses, demyelinating diseases, ischemia, infection, degenerative disease, etc. This iterative process may be mental or actually require comparison with published examples. The result is a differential diagnosis that may vary in specificity and depth. One might list the top three possible diagnoses, or one could list the most likely with that which is the most dangerous and thus must be excluded, along with one that would be easy to exclude with more studies.

How do we traditionally educate a reader of neuro-imaging studies? We usually ensure that the novice reader has seen examples from the various diagnostic categories with which we deal, and has learned how diseases within each category differ from those in other categories. The organization of our books and our teaching sessions is typically based upon such categories: Neoplasms, Congenital Disease, Infections, etc. However, what happens when the imager is confronted with an "unknown," a finding that does not fit easily into one of the categories to which he or she has become so accustomed? Unfortunately, even though the imager has learned the appearances of the majority of entities within a given category of disease, the finding does not tell the imager to which category it belongs! So, the imager must now search the categorically based textbooks for a "look alike," which is very time-consuming and may not even be successful.

Dr. O'Brien's approach to both the clinical practice and the education of neuro-imaging is quite unique amongst the textbooks I have seen over many years as a neuroradiologist. He has divided this book into three sections: Brain, Head and Neck, and Spine. Within each section, he concentrates on the most apparent imaging finding(s) within the presenting clinical context, and gives the "Top 3" potential diagnoses for that appearance (that "gamut"), including entities that may well derive from multiple diagnostic categories. For some appearances, he even includes some uncommon but potentially important considerations ("Additional Diagnostic Considerations"), thus providing more than just three possibilities for cases with more nonspecific findings. He finishes each case with clinical and imaging "Pearls," which provide quick differentiating features. He also provides some selected references for more in-depth reading on the topic.

Some imaging appearances within each section are unique, without differential diagnoses and not having a Top 3; they are called "Aunt Minnies." Dr. O'Brien considers a number of these to be fundamental to the knowledge base of the student, so they are presented at the end of each section. Each has an extensive discussion regarding pathophysiology and characteristic imaging appearances, along with selected references, similar to that found with the cases having Top 3 differential possibilities.

How did Dr. O'Brien validate his Top 3 choices with so many varied appearances in diverse clinical contexts? By doing extensive research as to the most common diagnoses for a given finding; by consulting with many radiologists who subspecialize in neuroradiology, head and neck radiology, and spinal radiology; and by incorporating entities that tend to be favorites in general and subspecialty board examinations.

How will this book change how we practice and teach neuro-imaging? It is vital that neuro-imagers have ingrained in their brain the basic categories of neuropathology, so that they can be sure that they cover all potential disease categories when confronted with an unknown case. However, O'Brien's approach can easily be superimposed on that basic knowledge of disease organization. It is fast, accurate, and removes the potential that the reader will be slowed down, trying to ensure that all categories are covered. This approach provides a way to be "complete" in developing differential diagnoses rapidly and accurately.

I found reading this book to be a joy. One can approach it by playing the student, viewing each image as an unknown, determining what the most prominent finding is, and then giving one's own Top 3. Frankly, this is a book not just for the resident or fellow, but one that will give any academic faculty member a positive learning experience, just like the one that I had!

Richard E. Latchaw, MD
Professor of Radiology
Neuroradiology Section
University of California, Davis Medical Center
Sacramento, California

Preface

It is a distinct pleasure to present *Top 3 Differentials in Neuroradiology: A Case Review*. Developing a neuroradiology version of the original "Top 3" book, *Top 3 Differentials in Radiology*, had been an aspiration of mine since its publication in 2010. This subspecialty version is primarily designed for senior radiology residents, neuroradiology fellows, and staff radiologists preparing for the neuroradiology portion of initial and recertification board examinations; however, it may also prove useful for clinicians and surgeons who routinely utilize neuroimaging.

This book is organized into three main sections: brain, head and neck, and spine imaging; and further divided into subsections based upon anatomic region or pattern of imaging abnormality. Each section begins with a series of unknown differential-based cases and ends with "Roentgen Classics," which are cases with imaging findings characteristic of a single diagnosis.

On the first page of each case, readers are presented with images from an unknown case, along with a clinical history and an image legend. The images are meant to illustrate a key imaging finding, which is the basis for the subsequent case discussion. The second page lists the key imaging finding, from which a list of differentials is broken down into the Top 3, along with "additional diagnostic considerations." The discussion section of each case provides a brief review of important imaging and clinical manifestations for all entities on the list of differentials, making this a high-yield reference for board preparation. Imaging pearls are provided at the end of each case to allow for a quick review of key points. The final diagnosis is provided for each case; however, it is by no means the focus of this review book. In fact, many illustrative cases have a final diagnosis that would not be considered in the Top 3 for the particular gamut. Instead, the primary aim of the book is to generate and have an understanding of a reasonable list of gamut-based differentials rather than to obtain the "correct" answer.

As with the earlier *Top 3 Differentials in Radiology*, it is important to realize that the differentials and discussions are based on the key finding or gamut and not necessarily the illustrative cases that are shown. This is by design, because I felt it would be more high-yield to base the differentials and discussions on the overall gamut/key finding rather than the illustrative case presented. Having an understanding of gamut-based differentials will allow one to subsequently tailor the list of differentials for any case that is shown within the gamut, whereas basing the differentials on the selected images would be more limited in terms of future utility.

Given the vast, evolving field of neuroimaging, this book is not meant to be a comprehensive reference book; rather, it is meant to serve as a high-yield review for board preparation, as well as a quick reference for clinical practice. With these intentions in mind, the selection and ordering of differentials for each gamut were based upon a combination of the most likely diagnoses to be encountered in a board setting, as well as clinical practice. Some "additional diagnostic considerations" were selected over others (which may actually be more common) in order to provide the opportunity to discuss as many diagnostic entities as possible throughout the book.

I sincerely hope that you find this Top 3 case-based approach enjoyable and useful, and I wish you all the best in your future endeavors.

Acknowledgments

This book would not have been possible without the contributions of numerous colleagues and mentors. First and foremost, I am forever indebted to the faculty of David Grant USAF Medical Center, the University of California–Davis, and Oakland Children's Hospital, where I completed my radiology residency training, as well as the University of Cincinnati and Cincinnati Children's Hospital Medical Center, where I completed my neuroradiology fellowships. The dedicated staff at these institutions afforded me their time and expertise during my years of training and have had a profound impact on my career. Their influence is what inspires me to remain in academics in the hopes of having a similar impact on the next generation of radiologists.

Several colleagues contributed to the content of this book through images and case material, some of which was included in the original "Top 3" book, *Top 3 Differentials in Radiology*. Their contributions have greatly enhanced the final manuscript. The contributors are listed at the end of the image legend for each case in which they were involved. I cannot possibly thank them enough for their significant contributions to this book. Although there are far too many to name individually, I would like to especially thank Paul M. Sherman, MD, who not only authored portions of the neuroimaging sections in the original "Top 3" book, but also served as my neuroradiology mentor during residency and has been one of my neuroradiology partners in San Antonio for the past 4 years.

Lastly, I would like to thank my family for their continuous love and support, as well as the sacrifices they made during completion of this project. I have been blessed with a wonderful wife, Annie; two sons, Patrick and Liam; and a daughter, Shannon. Annie and I have been together for nearly two decades, and we could not be more proud of our three incredible children. I am grateful beyond words for the joy that they bring into my life each and every day.

Section I

Brain

Case 1

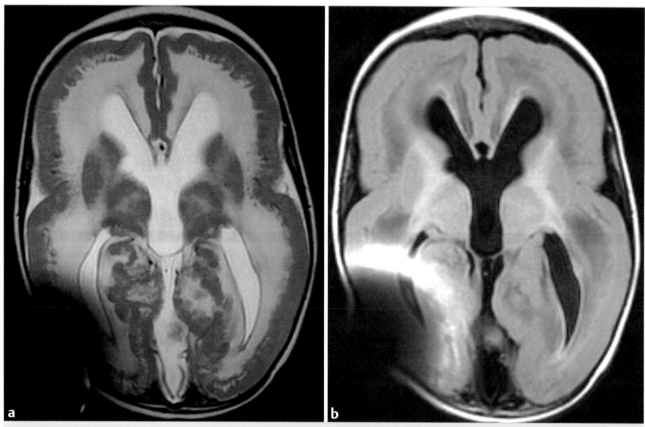

Fig. 1.1 Axial T2 **(a)** and T1 **(b)** images demonstrate a "figure 8" appearance of the brain with a thickened cortex and absence of the normal gyral and sulcal pattern. The inner surface of the cortex has an irregular "cobblestone" appearance. Diffuse abnormal signal intensity is identified throughout the brain parenchyma. Susceptibility artifact from a shunt catheter is noted overlying the right occipital and posterior temporal lobes.

■ Clinical Presentation

An infant boy with seizures, weakness, and failure to meet developmental milestones (▶ Fig. 1.1)

■ **Key Imaging Finding**

Agyria

■ **Top 3 Differential Diagnoses**

• **Type 1 lissencephaly.** Type 1 or classic lissencephaly is a congenital neuronal migration disorder that results in a smooth appearance of the brain secondary to absence of the normal gyral and sulcal pattern. There may be diffuse involvement (agyria) or focal involvement (pachygyria) of the cerebral cortex. Diffuse involvement results in a "figure 8" appearance of the brain with vertically oriented Sylvian fissures and absence of the normal gyral and sulcal pattern. On pathologic evaluation, there is a thickened, smooth four-layer cortex with a thin ribbon of subcortical band heterotopia, rather than a normal six-layer cortex. Type 1 lissencephaly may be associated with cytomegalovirus (CMV) infection, Miller-Dieker syndrome, and cerebellar hypoplasia. With CMV infection, periventricular and intraparenchymal calcifications are noted. Patients with Miller-Dieker syndrome demonstrate midline septal calcifications, microcephaly, and characteristic dysmorphic facial features.

• **Type 2 lissencephaly.** Type 2 or cobblestone lissencephaly is characterized by overmigration of neurons, severe disorganization of the gray matter, underdevelopment of gyri and sulci, and diffuse white matter hypomyelination. The disorganized gray matter results in an irregular, "cobblestone" appearance of the cortex. There is an association with congenital muscular dystrophies, including Walker-Warburg syndrome, Fukuyama congenital muscular dystrophy, and to a lesser degree, muscle-eye-brain disease. Patients present early in life with severe muscular weakness, eye abnormalities, developmental delay or mental retardation, and complications of associated brain malformations. Patients with Walker-Warburg often have characteristic findings, including occipital cephaloceles, cerebellar and brain stem hypoplasia, and kinking of the brain stem with a classic "striking cobra" appearance on sagittal sequences. Hydrocephalus is present in the vast majority of cases.

• **Band heterotopia.** Gray matter heterotopia refers to collections of disorganized neurons in abnormal locations. It results from premature arrest of normal neuronal migration. Neurons migrate from the ependymal surface of the lateral ventricles to the peripheral cortex, and then undergo organization into a normal six-layer cortex. If arrest occurs at any point during migration, heterotopias occur. Heterotopia may be classified as nodular (most common), which most often occurs along the margins of the lateral ventricles, or band, which is located within the subcortical or deep white matter. When diffuse and subcortical in location, band heterotopia may mimic lissencephaly. Patients typically present with seizures, developmental delay, and spasticity.

■ **Additional Differential Diagnoses**

• **Prematurity.** Prior to ~26 weeks gestation, the fetal brain normally appears lissencephalic due to lack of gyral and sulcal development. After 26 weeks gestation, the gyral and sulcal pattern gradually progresses until its relatively normal appearance at term. Therefore, lissencephaly should not be diagnosed until after 26 weeks gestation. When uncertain, a follow-up examination may be helpful to evaluate for interval gyral and sulcal formation.

■ **Diagnosis**

Type 2 cobblestone lissencephaly in a patient with Walker-Warburg syndrome

✓ **Pearls**

• The premature infant brain normally appears lissencephalic prior to 26 weeks gestation.
• Lissencephaly is a neuronal migration disorder with absence of normal gyri/sulci and a thickened cortex.

• Type 1 lissencephaly is smooth and may be associated with CMV, Miller-Dieker, and cerebellar hypoplasia.
• Type 2 lissencephaly has a "cobblestone" appearance and is associated with congenital muscular dystrophies.

Suggested Readings

Barkovich AJ, Chuang SH, Norman D. MR of neuronal migration anomalies. Am J Roentgenol 1988; 150: 179–187

Ghai S, Fong KW, Toi A, Chitayat D, Pantazi S, Blaser S. Prenatal US and MR imaging findings of lissencephaly: review of fetal cerebral sulcal development. Radiographics 2006; 26: 389–405

Case 2

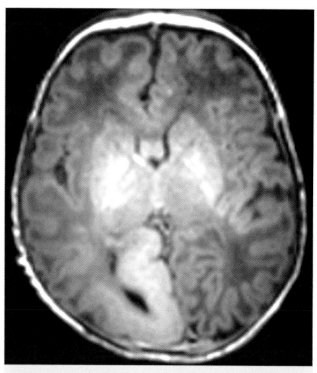

Fig. 2.1 Axial T1 image demonstrates abnormal cortical thickening and absence of the normal gyri and sulci within the right occipital lobe. Abnormal cortical and subcortical signal intensity is noted involving the right occipital and temporal lobes.

■ **Clinical Presentation**

A 2-day-old boy with seizures and spasms (▶ Fig. 2.1)

■ Key Imaging Finding

Cortical malformation

■ Top 3 Differential Diagnoses

- **Pachygyria.** Pachygyria is an incomplete or focal form of lissencephaly. As with lissencephaly, there is both abnormal neuronal migration and failure to form the normal six-layer cortex. Instead, a four-layer cortex is most commonly seen pathologically. Imaging findings are characterized by short, broad gyri with a lack of sulcation in the involved segments. Symptoms depend upon the extent and location of parenchymal involvement. Patients may present with seizures, developmental delay, mental retardation, and/or spasticity.
- **Polymicrogyria.** Polymicrogyria is a neuronal migration abnormality characterized by abnormal distribution of neurons along the cortical surface. Multiple, small gyri replace the normal organized gyral and sulcal pattern. It is thought to result from laminar necrosis of neurons after they reach the cortical surface. It is commonly seen in association with cytomegalovirus (CMV) infection. Para-Sylvian locations are commonly involved. The polymicrogyria pattern is best depicted on magnetic resonance imaging (MRI). Abnormal signal is commonly seen in the subjacent white matter. Clinically, patients present with seizures, developmental delay, mental

retardation, and, occasionally, hemiparesis. Polymicrogyria may be associated with various syndromes, including Aicardi (callosal anomalies, infantile spasms, and retinal lesions) and Zellweger (cerebrohepatorenal) syndromes.
- **Hemimegalencephaly.** Hemimegalencephaly is a hamartomatous overgrowth of all or a portion of one cerebral hemisphere with associated neuronal migration abnormalities of varying severity. It is thought to occur as a result of an insult during neuronal migration. The ipsilateral hemisphere and ventricle are enlarged. Affected gyri are thickened and may show a primitive lissencephalic appearance with shallow or absent sulci. There is often abnormal attenuation (computed tomography) and signal intensity (MRI) within the subjacent white matter. Calcifications are not uncommon. Clinically, the patient may present with seizures, developmental delay, mental retardation, and/or hemiplegia. Syndromes associated with hemimegalencephaly include neurofibromatosis type 1, Klippel-Trenaunay-Weber syndrome, tuberous sclerosis, and Proteus syndrome.

■ Additional Differential Diagnoses

- **Subcortical band heterotopia.** Gray matter heterotopia refers to collections of disorganized neurons in abnormal locations due to premature arrest of normal migration. Neurons migrate from the ependymal surface of the lateral ventricles to the peripheral cortex, and then undergo organization into a normal six-layer cortex. If arrest occurs at any point during migration, heterotopias occur. Heterotopia may be classified as nodular, which most often occurs along the margins of the lateral ventricles, or band-type, which occurs within the subcortical or deep white matter. Patients typically present with seizures, developmental delay, and spasticity.
- **Schizencephaly.** Schizencephaly is a congenital malformation characterized by gray matter–lined clefts extending from the

pial surface to the ventricle. The clefts are typically para-Sylvian in location and lined by polymicrogyric gray matter. In Type I (closed-lip) schizencephaly, the gray matter linings are apposed with a small ventricular dimple of cerebrospinal fluid (CSF) extending into the cleft. Type II (open-lip) schizencephaly consists of a large CSF-filled space between the gray matter linings. Schizencephaly may be bilateral and associated with septooptic dysplasia. Clinical manifestations depend upon the severity of the lesion. Patients with type I are often almost normal in terms of development, but may have seizures and hemiparesis. Type II patients usually demonstrate mental retardation, seizures, hypotonia, spasticity, inability to walk or speak, and blindness.

■ Diagnosis

Pachygyria

✓ Pearls

- Pachygyria is a form of focal lissencephaly with a thickened, four-layer cortex (instead of the normal six layers).
- With polymicrogyria, small gyri replace the normal, organized gyral pattern; it is associated with CMV.
- Heterotopia (nodular or band) refers to collections of disorganized neurons in abnormal locations.

Suggested Readings

Barkovich AJ, Chuang SH, Norman D. MR of neuronal migration anomalies. Am J Roentgenol 1988; 150: 179–187

Broumandi DD, Hayward UM, Benzian JM, Gonzalez I, Nelson MD. Best cases from the AFIP: hemimegalencephaly. Radiographics 2004; 24: 843–848

Hayashi N, Tsutsumi Y, Barkovich AJ. Morphological features and associated anomalies of schizencephaly in the clinical population: detailed analysis of MR images. Neuroradiology 2002; 44: 418–427

Case 3

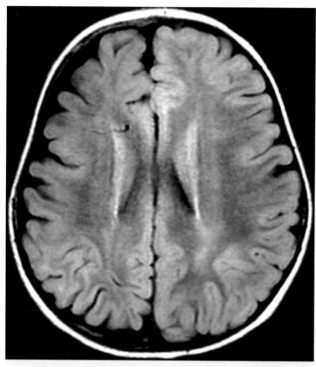

Fig. 3.1 Axial fluid-attenuated inversion recovery (FLAIR) MR image demonstrates asymmetry of the cerebral hemispheres with the right smaller than the left and associated prominence of the sulci on the right. An enlarged medullary vein is seen along the anterior margin of the right lateral ventricle. Hazy, periatrial white matter signal intensity corresponds to regions of terminal myelination.

■ Clinical Presentation

A 2-year-old girl with developmental delay (▶ Fig. 3.1)

▨ Key Imaging Finding

Asymmetry of cerebral hemispheres

▨ Top 3 Differential Diagnoses

- **Normal variant.** Slight variation in size of an entire cerebral hemisphere, one or more lobes, or individual sulci is not uncommon, occurring in ~10% of normal cases. Parenchymal morphology, attenuation, and signal intensity should otherwise be normal and are useful discriminators from pathologic causes of parenchymal volume loss. Patients are often neurologically and developmentally intact for age.
- **Encephalomalacia.** Encephalomalacia refers to parenchymal volume loss as a result of some form of insult. Hypoxic-ischemic injury is the most common cause of encephalomalacia, followed by trauma and infectious or inflammatory processes. Ischemic injury typically follows a vascular distribution. During the acute phase of injury, there is often focal edema and swelling. In the chronic stage, there is volume loss with surrounding gliosis. In the setting of an asymmetric small cerebral hemisphere, a large

territory infarct (middle cerebral artery) is the most likely cause of encephalomalacia.
- **Sturge-Weber syndrome (SWS; encephalotrigeminal angiomatosis).** SWS is a sporadic phakomatosis thought to result from abnormal development of venous drainage. It is characterized by a cutaneous port-wine stain (usually in the V1 distribution of the trigeminal nerve) and pial angiomatosis overlying the ipsilateral cerebral hemisphere. Venous drainage is diverted through enlarged medullary and subependymal veins. Hemiatrophy results, likely from venous hypertension. Magnetic resonance imaging (MRI) shows cerebral atrophy, abnormal leptomeningeal enhancement, and increased enhancement within a hypertrophied ipsilateral choroid plexus. The involved hemisphere may demonstrate abnormal signal, cortical enhancement, and cortical calcifications in a "tram track" configuration.

▨ Additional Differential Diagnoses

- **Dyke-Davidoff-Mason syndrome (DDMS).** DDMS refers to compensatory enlargement of the ipsilateral calvarium, paranasal sinuses, and mastoid air cells secondary to underdevelopment or atrophy of the underlying cerebral hemisphere. The most common causes of ipsilateral cerebral atrophy include a large-territory ischemic insult at a young age or SWS. Symptoms are related to the causative process.
- **Hemimegalencephaly.** Hemimegalencephaly is a hamartomatous overgrowth of all or a portion of one cerebral hemisphere with associated neuronal migration abnormalities. It is thought to result from an insult during neuronal migration. The ipsilateral hemisphere and ventricle are enlarged. Affected gyri are thickened and may show a lissencepahlic appearance with shallow or absent sulci. There is often abnormal attenuation (computed tomography) and signal intensity (MRI) within the white matter of the ipsilateral hemisphere.

Calcifications are not uncommon. Clinically, patients may present with seizures, developmental delay, mental retardation, and hemiplegia. Associated syndromes include neurofibromatosis type 1, Klippel-Trenaunay-Weber syndrome, tuberous sclerosis, and Proteus syndrome.
- **Rasmussen encephalitis.** Rasmussen encephalitis is a rare, progressive, inflammatory neurological disorder of unknown origin. A viral or postviral autoimmune etiology has been postulated. Patients present in childhood with persistent, relentless, focal motor seizures (epilepsia partialis continua), hemiplegia, and cognitive deficits. Early on, MRI demonstrates abnormal edema and increased T2 signal within the involved hemisphere. Chronically, findings are more characteristic with abnormal signal, asymmetric atrophy, and decreased perfusion and metabolism on the affected side. Treatment consists of functional hemispherectomy.

▨ Diagnosis

Sturge-Weber syndrome

✓ Pearls

- Encephalomalacia refers to parenchymal volume loss from some form of insult; ischemia is most common.
- SWS is characterized by seizures, cutaneous port-wine stain, and pial angiomatosis of the ipsilateral hemisphere.

- Hemimegalencephaly is a hamartomatous overgrowth of all or part of one cerebral hemisphere.

Suggested Readings

Shapiro R, Galloway SJ, Shapiro MD. Minimal asymmetry of the brain: a normal variant. Am J Roentgenol 1986; 147: 753–756

Sener RN, Jinkins JR. MR of craniocerebral hemiatrophy. Clin Imaging 1992; 16: 93–97

Case 4

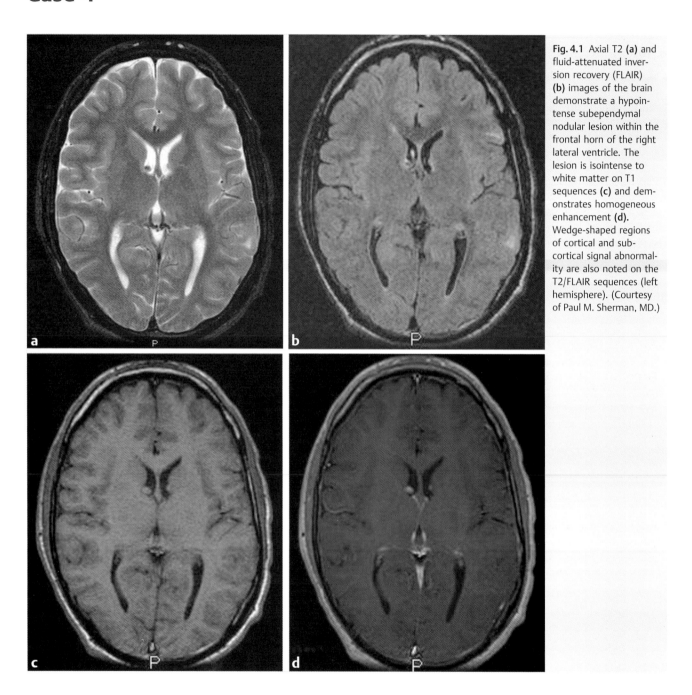

Fig. 4.1 Axial T2 **(a)** and fluid-attenuated inversion recovery (FLAIR) **(b)** images of the brain demonstrate a hypointense subependymal nodular lesion within the frontal horn of the right lateral ventricle. The lesion is isointense to white matter on T1 sequences **(c)** and demonstrates homogeneous enhancement **(d)**. Wedge-shaped regions of cortical and subcortical signal abnormality are also noted on the T2/FLAIR sequences (left hemisphere). (Courtesy of Paul M. Sherman, MD.)

■ **Clinical Presentation**

An adolescent with seizures (▶ Fig. 4.1)

■ Key Imaging Finding

Subependymal nodules

■ Top 3 Differential Diagnoses

- **Tuberous sclerosis (TS).** TS is a neurocutaneous syndrome that results from gene mutations affecting chromosomes 9q34.3 (hamartin) and 16p13.3 (tuberin). Two-thirds of cases occur sporadically, whereas the remaining occur in an autosomal dominant fashion with variable penetrance. The classic triad consists of facial angiofibromas, mental retardation, and seizures, but it is only seen in approximately one-third of cases. Central nervous system (CNS) manifestations include cortical/subcortical tubers, white matter lesions that occur in a radial pattern along paths of neuronal migration, subependymal nodules, and subependymal giant cell astrocytomas (SEGAs). The cortical/subcortical tubers are composed of disorganized glial tissue and heterotopic neuronal elements. They present as triangular regions of cortical and subcortical signal abnormality that may calcify and occasionally demonstrate enhancement. Subependymal nodules have variable T1 and T2 signal intensity and commonly enhance. They demonstrate gradient echo susceptibility (hypointensity) when calcified; the majority are calcified by 20 years of age. SEGAs are low-grade tumors that occur in ~10 to 15% of cases. They are located at the foramen of Monro, enlarge over time, and enhance. Interval growth is the best sign to distinguish SEGAs from dominant subependymal nodules. Treatment is typically geared toward cerebrospinal fluid diversion. Common abnormalities associated with TS include retinal hamartomas, cardiac rhabdomyomas, renal cysts and angiomyolipomas, pulmonary lymphangioleiomyomatosis, subungual fibromas, and skin lesions, such as "ash-leaf spots" and shagreen patches.

- **Heterotopic gray matter.** Heterotopic gray matter results from arrest or disruption of normal neuronal migration from the subependymal region to the overlying cortex. It is thought to occur secondary to some form of fetal insult during development. Heterotopia may be nodular or bandlike. Subependymal heterotopic gray matter is isointense to gray matter on all magnetic resonance (MR) sequences, does not enhance, and does not calcify. Patients often present with seizures and developmental delay. Mild cases, however, may be asymptomatic.

- **TORCH infection.** The TORCH infections consist of toxoplasmosis, rubella, cytomegalovirus (CMV), and herpes simplex virus. CMV is the most common TORCH infection to result in subependymal and periventricular calcifications, mimicking tuberous sclerosis on computed tomography (CT). Toxoplasmosis also causes intracranial calcifications; however, the distribution is more random with less propensity for the periventricular region. Common associated findings include microcephaly and neuronal migration abnormalities, including polymicrogyria and pachygyria. Patients commonly suffer from mental retardation, seizures, and hearing loss.

■ Additional Differential Diagnoses

- **Metastatic disease.** Subependymal metastatic disease may result from primary CNS neoplasms or hematogenous spread from extracranial malignancies. Primary CNS neoplasms prone to subependymal spread include glioblastoma multiforme, medulloblastoma, ependymoma, primary CNS lymphoma, germ cell neoplasms, pineal cell neoplasms, and choroid plexus tumors. Extracranial metastases from multiple primary sites may involve the subependymal surfaces and choroid plexus, particularly breast carcinoma.

■ Diagnosis

Tuberous sclerosis

✓ Pearls

- TS results in subependymal nodules, which calcify and demonstrate enhancement.
- Heterotopic gray matter is due to an insult in utero and follows gray matter signal on all MR sequences.
- CMV is the most common TORCH infection to cause subependymal/periventricular calcifications.
- Metastases from primary CNS or extracranial malignancies may present as subependymal nodules.

Suggested Readings

Barkovich AJ, Chuang SH, Norman D. MR of neuronal migration anomalies. Am J Roentgenol 1988; 150: 179–187

Braffman BH, Bilaniuk LT, Naidich TP et al. MR imaging of tuberous sclerosis: pathogenesis of this phakomatosis, use of gadopentetate dimeglumine, and literature review. Radiology 1992; 183: 227–238

Fink KR, Thapa MM, Ishak GE, Pruthi S. Neuroimaging of pediatric central nervous system cytomegalovirus infection. Radiographics 2010; 30: 1779–1796

Case 5

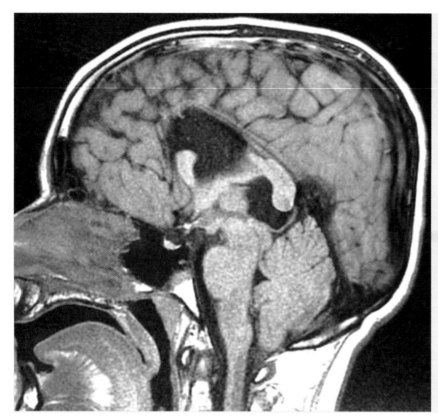

Fig. 5.1 Sagittal T1 magnetic resonance image shows a defect involving the anterior body of the corpus callosum with adjacent porencephaly that communicates with the lateral ventricle. The genu, posterior body, splenium, and rostrum are present. Additional findings include signal abnormality in the region of the hypothalamus, enlargement of the posterior third ventricle, and a small posterior fossa with mild tonsillar ectopia.

■ Clinical Presentation

A 16-year-old boy with difficulties in school (► Fig. 5.1)

▨ Key Imaging Finding

Callosal abnormality

■ Top 3 Differential Diagnoses

- **Agenesis/hypogenesis of the corpus callosum (ACC).** Normal development of the corpus callosum occurs from anterior to posterior with formation of the genu first, followed by the body and splenium. The rostrum is located along the inferior margin of the genu and is the last portion to form. Imaging findings with complete agenesis include absence of the corpus callosum and lack of visualization of the cingulate gyrus due to failure of rotation. As a result, the third ventricle is elevated between the lateral ventricles, which are parallel in configuration on axial images. There is colpocephaly with dilatation of the atria and occipital horns of the lateral ventricles. The white matter tracts that would cross through the corpus callosum instead align along the medial margin of the lateral ventricles and run in an anterior-posterior direction. These tracts are referred to as Probst bundles. On coronal sequences, the frontal horns of the lateral ventricles demonstrate a "long-horn" configuration secondary to indentation medially by the Probst bundles and absence of the genu. The gyri of the medial cerebral hemispheres extend to the margin of the third ventricle with a radial configuration. ACC is nearly always associated with additional anomalies. With hypogenesis of the corpus callosum, portions of the body, splenium, and rostrum are absent. Absence of the rostrum is a key feature in distinguishing hypogenesis (rostrum absent) from an encephaloclastic process in which the rostrum is typically present. Pericallosal lipomas are often seen in the setting of abnormal callosal development.

- **Callosal injury/encephaloclastic process.** The majority of encephaloclastic injuries are from surgical interventions, usually associated with resection of a mass within the third ventricle or suprasellar region. Trauma and hemorrhage are less common causes of callosal destruction. Imaging findings include absence of the callosum in the region of injury, whereas the remaining portions of the callosum are intact. Presence of the rostrum excludes hypogenesis.

- **Holoprosencephaly.** Holoprosencephaly is a spectrum of anomalies characterized by failure of the forebrain to separate into two distinct hemispheres. There are three variants: alobar, semilobar, and lobar, all of which have complete or partial absence of the falx and septum pellucidum. In the alobar form (most severe), there is a large dorsal interhemispheric cyst (monoventricle), and the remaining cerebral parenchyma is fused and flattened anteriorly. Thalami are also fused. The corpus callosum, anterior falx, interhemispheric fissure, and Sylvian fissures are absent. Associated craniofacial abnormalities include hypotelorism and cleft palate. In the semilobar variant, the posterior portions of the callosum are usually present, whereas anterior portions, including the rostrum, are absent. In the least severe lobar variant, the corpus callosum may appear normal or demonstrate partial absence of the genu. Holoprosencephaly is the one congenital anomaly in which the genu may be absent whereas the body and splenium are present.

■ Additional Differential Diagnoses

- **Volume loss.** The volume of the corpus callosum is related to the volume of white matter within the supratentorial brain. Prior to myelination, the corpus callosum normally appears thin. As myelination progresses, it obtains its more typical volume and appearance. With severe supratentorial parenchymal injury, all or portions of the corpus callosum demonstrate atrophy, because the callosal volume is dependent upon the white matter fibers forming the tracts. Severe hydrocephalus may produce similar findings secondary to pressure-related changes or encephalomalacia of the corpus callosum.

▨ Diagnosis

Callosal injury/encephaloclastic process (postsurgical)

✓ Pearls

- With ACC or hypogenesis, all or a portion of the corpus callosum is absent, including the rostrum, which is last to form.
- Callosal injury is most often postsurgical, followed by trauma and hemorrhage.
- Holoprosencephaly is the one congenital anomaly where the genu may be absent and the splenium present.

Suggested Readings

Battal B, Kocaoglu M, Akgun V, Bulakbasi N, Tayfun C. Corpus callosum: normal imaging appearance, variants and pathologic conditions. J Med Imaging Radiat Oncol 2010; 54: 541–549

Sztriha L. Spectrum of corpus callosum agenesis. Pediatr Neurol 2005; 32: 94–101

Case 6

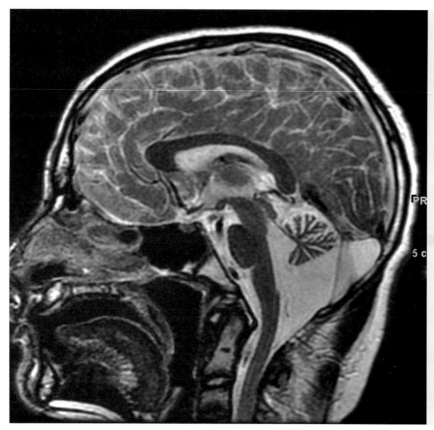

Fig. 6.1 Sagittal T2 image demonstrates significantly decreased volume of the cerebellar vermis with prominence of the sulci. The brain stem appears normal in size and morphology.

■ Clinical Presentation

A 20-year-old man with chronic ataxia and progressive neurological decline (▶ Fig. 6.1)

■ Key Imaging Finding

Cerebellar atrophy/volume loss

■ Top 3 Acquired Differential Diagnoses

- **Alcohol abuse.** Alcohol abuse results in progressive cerebellar degeneration. Alcohol is neurotoxic, causing cerebellar and cortical (frontal lobe predominant) degeneration, as well as peripheral polyneuropathies. There is disproportionate involvement of the superior vermis and cerebellum compared with the cerebral hemispheres. Associated findings may include Wernicke encephalopathy, which presents as abnormal T2 hyperintensity within the periaqueductal gray matter, mammillary bodies, medial thalamus, and hypothalamus; and less commonly Marchiafava-Bignami disease, which results in abnormal signal intensity within the corpus callosum.
- **Anticonvulsant therapy.** Both seizures and long-term anticonvulsant therapy may produce irreversible cerebellar degeneration with disproportionate cerebellar atrophy. Patients present with ataxia, nystagmus, and peripheral neuropathies. Phenytoin is the most common drug therapy, and its use may also result in diffuse calvarial thickening.
- **Paraneoplastic syndrome.** Cerebellar degeneration may occur as a result of a paraneoplastic syndrome. Breast and lung cancer are by far the most common primary neoplasms. Less common associated malignancies include gastrointestinal and genitourinary neoplasms, Hodgkin lymphoma, and neuroblastoma. The cerebellar degeneration is thought to result from autoantibodies to Purkinje fibers or a cytotoxic process associated with T cells. The paraneoplastic cerebellar degeneration often precedes the diagnosis of a primary tumor.

■ Top 3 Sporadic or Inherited Differential Diagnoses

- **Sporadic olivopontocerebellar atrophy (sOPCA).** sOPCA, also referred to as multisystem atrophy, is a neurodegenerative disorder of unknown etiology that typically presents in adulthood. Cross-sectional imaging demonstrates atrophy of the ventral pons and midbrain with enlargement of the fourth ventricle and widening of the superior and middle cerebellar peduncles. There is hemispheric greater than vermian cerebellar atrophy, as well as less pronounced cerebral atrophy, which most preferentially involves the frontal and parietal lobes. Cruciform-like T2 hyperintensity in the base of the pons gives the characteristic "hot cross bun" sign. Abnormal signal intensity is also seen in the middle cerebellar peduncles and dorsolateral putamen. Patients present with parkinsonian features, ataxia, dysarthria, and autonomic dysfunction.
- **Ataxia telangiectasia (AT).** AT is an autosomal recessive complex that results in spinocerebellar degeneration, ocular and cutaneous telangiectases, radiation sensitivity, immunodeficiencies, and increased risk of neoplasms. Patients often present as toddlers with signs of ataxia. The neurological decline is progressive. Cross-sectional imaging demonstrates cerebellar atrophy with enlargement of the cerebellar sulci and compensatory enlargement of the fourth ventricle. There is also atrophy of the dentate nuclei. Intracranial telangiectases may result in scattered foci of gradient echo susceptibility secondary to microhemorrhages. Occasionally, associated supratentorial white matter demyelination or dysmyelination may be seen.
- **Friedreich ataxia.** Also known as spinocerebellar ataxia, Friedreich ataxia typically presents in the second decade of life and has both autosomal dominant and recessive forms. Cross-sectional imaging demonstrates mild atrophy of the vermis and paravermian structures, a small medulla, and significant atrophy of the spinal cord. The dorsal cord has a flattened appearance. Clinically, patients often present with lower extremity ataxia, upper extremity tremors, and kyphoscoliosis.

■ Diagnosis

Ataxia telangiectasia

✓ Pearls

- Alcohol, anticonvulsant therapy, and paraneoplastic syndromes are secondary causes of cerebellar atrophy.
- sOPCA results in cerebellar and brain stem atrophy; pontine hyperintensity is referred to as "hot cross bun" sign.
- AT presents with spinocerebellar degeneration, telangiectases, immunodeficiencies, and risk of neoplasms.

Suggested Readings

Fischbein NJ, Dillon WP, Barkovich AJ. Teaching Atlas of Brain Imaging. New York, NY: Thieme, 1999

Huang YP, Tuason MY, Wu T, Plaitakis A. MRI and CT features of cerebellar degeneration. J Formos Med Assoc 1993; 92: 494–508

Case 7

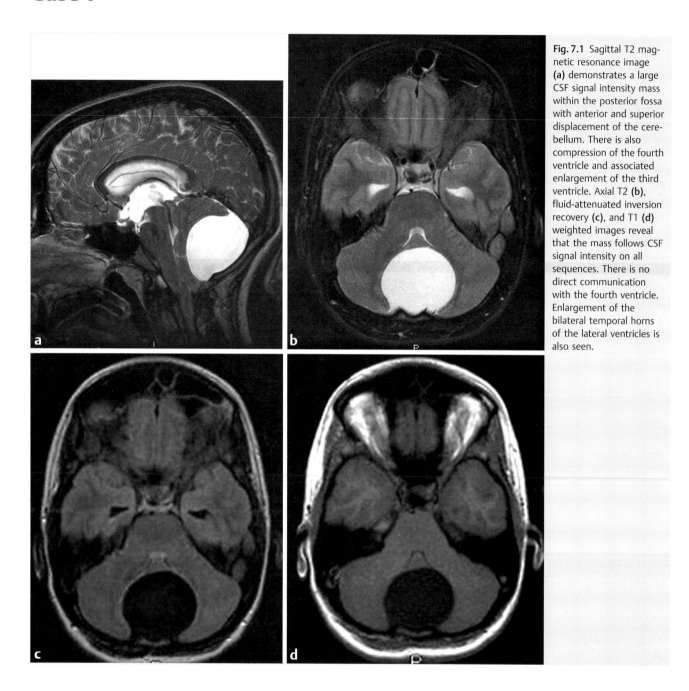

Fig. 7.1 Sagittal T2 magnetic resonance image **(a)** demonstrates a large CSF signal intensity mass within the posterior fossa with anterior and superior displacement of the cerebellum. There is also compression of the fourth ventricle and associated enlargement of the third ventricle. Axial T2 **(b)**, fluid-attenuated inversion recovery **(c)**, and T1 **(d)** weighted images reveal that the mass follows CSF signal intensity on all sequences. There is no direct communication with the fourth ventricle. Enlargement of the bilateral temporal horns of the lateral ventricles is also seen.

■ **Clinical Presentation**

Adolescent boy with headaches (▶ Fig. 7.1)

▓ Key Imaging Finding

Posterior fossa cerebrospinal fluid (CSF) collection

■ Top 3 Differential Diagnoses

- **Mega cisterna magna.** A mega cisterna magna is a common normal variant in which the CSF-filled cisterna magna posterior to the cerebellum is prominent. It can usually be differentiated from an arachnoid cyst or Dandy-Walker malformation by the normal appearance and size of the posterior fossa, normal cerebellar vermis and fourth ventricle, minimal to no mass effect, and the presence of internal vessels and the falx cerebelli.
- **Arachnoid cyst.** Arachnoid cysts are developmental CSF-filled spaces within the arachnoid. Although typically asymptomatic and discovered incidentally, they may exert local mass effect. The majority are supratentorial within the middle cranial fossa or along the convexities. Common infratentorial locations include the cerebellopontine angle and cistern magna. When located within the posterior fossa, they may be large enough to compress the fourth ventricle or cerebral aqueduct, resulting in obstructive hydrocephalus. Arachnoid cysts follow CSF fluid signal on all magnetic resonance imaging pulse sequences; occasionally, they may have slight increased signal intensity on proton density due to stasis of

CSF. Mass effect is evident by displacement of vessels and the falx cerebelli around the arachnoid cyst and scalloping of overlying cortex.
- **Dandy-Walker continuum.** Dandy-Walker malformation is a developmental abnormality that results from a defect in the cerebellar vermis and fourth ventricle during embryogenesis. The malformation consists of an enlarged posterior fossa, partial or complete absence of the cerebellar vermis, hypoplasia of the cerebellar hemispheres, and a dilated fourth ventricle that is in direct communication with a posterior CSF-filled fluid collection. The enlarged posterior fossa results in superior displacement of the torcula above the lambdoid sutures (torcular-lambdoid inversion). Dandy-Walker malformation is associated with additional central nervous system anomalies, including corpus callosal agenesis or hypogenesis and neuronal migration abnormalities. The Dandy-Walker variant is characterized by vermian hypoplasia and an enlarged fourth ventricle that communicates with a prominent cistern magna posteriorly; the posterior fossa is typically normal in size.

▓ Additional Differential Diagnoses

- **Joubert syndrome (vermian hypoplasia).** Joubert syndrome is an uncommon posterior fossa malformation characterized by a dysplastic and hypoplastic cerebellar vermis, as well as malformations of various nuclei and tracts. Patients present with neonatal hyperpnea, apnea, and mental retardation. Imaging findings include a dysplastic and hypoplastic cerebellar vermis (more pronounced superiorly), a bulbous fourth

ventricle that has a characteristic "bat wing" configuration, and a "molar tooth" appearance of the midbrain secondary to a narrow, deep interpeduncular cistern and elongated superior cerebellar peduncles that are parallel with each other. Posterior fossa CSF collections may be seen but are not a typical manifestation of Joubert syndrome.

▓ Diagnosis

Arachnoid cyst

✓ Pearls

- Mega cisterna magna is a normal variant with a normal-sized posterior fossa and normal cerebellar vermis.
- Arachnoid cysts follow CSF signal on all pulse sequences and exert local mass effect.
- Joubert syndrome results in a "bat wing" configuration of the fourth ventricle and "molar tooth" midbrain.

- Dandy-Walker malformation refers to vermian hypoplasia and a posterior fossa CSF collection communicating with the fourth ventricle.

Suggested Readings

Barkovich AJ, Kjos BO, Norman D, Edwards MS. Revised classification of posterior fossa cysts and cystlike malformations based on the results of multiplanar MR imaging. Am J Roentgenol 1989; 153: 1289–1300

O'Brien WT, Palka PS et al. Pediatric neuroimaging. In: Quattromani F, et al. Pediatric Imaging: Rapid-fire Questions and Answers. New York, NY: Thieme, 2007

Ten Donkelaar HJ, Lammens M. Development of the human cerebellum and its disorders. Clin Perinatol 2009; 36: 513–530

Case 8

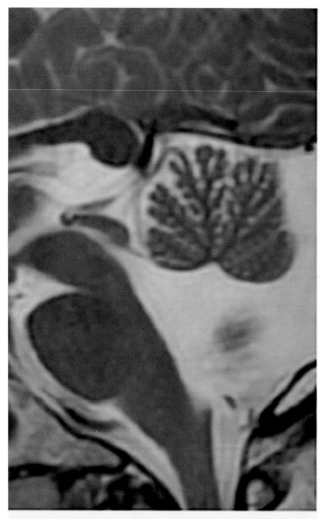

Fig. 8.1 Sagittal T2 image demonstrates hypoplasia of the inferior cerebellar vermis and an enlarged fourth ventricle that communicates with a retrocerebellar CSF collection. The posterior fossa was enlarged with torcular-lambdoid inversion (not shown).

▦ Clinical Presentation

A young adult woman with headache and history of mild developmental delay as a child (▶ Fig. 8.1)

■ Key Imaging Finding

Vermian hypoplasia

■ Top 3 Differential Diagnoses

- **Dandy-Walker malformation (DWM) or variant (DWV).** DWM is a developmental abnormality that results from a defect in the cerebellar vermis and fourth ventricle during embryogenesis. Imaging findings include an enlarged posterior fossa, partial or complete absence of the cerebellar vermis, hypoplasia of the cerebellar hemispheres, and a dilated fourth ventricle that is in direct communication with a posterior cerebrospinal fluid (CSF)-filled fluid collection. The enlarged posterior fossa results in superior displacement of the torcula above the lambdoid sutures (lambdoid-torcular inversion). The DWV is a less severe anomaly characterized by a relatively normal-sized posterior fossa with inferior vermian hypoplasia. The fourth ventricle is enlarged and communicates with the cistern magna posteriorly, which is prominent. In general, the DWM has more severe clinical manifestations because it is often associated with additional central nervous system anomalies, including corpus callosal agenesis or hypogenesis and neuronal migration abnormalities. The clinical manifestations of DWV are more variable and less severe, typically ranging from normal to relatively mild developmental delay and neurological deficits. The presence of additional abnormalities often determines the clinical course.
- **Joubert syndrome.** Joubert syndrome is a rare form of congenital vermian hypoplasia that presents early in life and is characterized clinically by ataxia, apnea or hyperpnea, hypotonia, and developmental delay or mental retardation. The majority of cases occur sporadically, although autosomal patterns have also been observed. Cross-sectional imaging demonstrates a dysplastic and hypoplastic cerebellar vermis with a midline cleft (best seen on coronal sequences or reformats). The small vermis results in an enlarged fourth ventricle in a "bat wing" configuration. The superior cerebellar peduncles are elongated, enlarged, and parallel with one another. This configuration, combined with a hypoplastic midbrain, results in the characteristic "molar tooth" appearance on axial images. Although once considered to be pathognomonic of Joubert syndrome, the molar tooth sign may be seen with additional syndromes. Unlike DWM, the posterior fossa is normal in size, and posterior fossa CSF collections are not a typical manifestation of Joubert syndrome.
- **Rhombencephalosynapsis.** Rhombencephalosynapsis is an uncommon developmental anomaly characterized by fusion or failure of segmentation of the cerebellar hemispheres. The cerebellar vermis is either absent or significantly hypoplastic. The abnormal cerebellar configuration results in a transverse orientation of the cerebellar folia and posterior pointing of the fourth ventricle, which assumes a "keyhole" configuration. There is typically fusion of the superior cerebellar peduncles and dentate nuclei as well. Associated supratentorial anomalies are variable and include fused thalami, fornices, and colliculi; absence of the septum pellucidum; aqueductal stenosis with hydrocephalus; callosal and anterior commissure dysgenesis; and neuronal migrational abnormalities. Facial defects have also been reported. Prognosis is related to the presence and severity of supratentorial abnormalities.

■ Diagnosis

Dandy-Walker malformation

✓ Pearls

- DWM refers to vermian hypoplasia and a posterior fossa CSF collection communicating with the fourth ventricle.
- Joubert syndrome is characterized by vermian hypoplasia with a "molar tooth" configuration of the midbrain.
- Rhombencephalosynapsis is congenital fusion of the cerebellar hemispheres with vermian aplasia/hypoplasia.

Suggested Readings

Kendall B, Kingsley D, Lambert SR, Taylor D, Finn P. Joubert syndrome: a clinico-radiological study. Neuroradiology 1990; 31: 502–506

Patel S, Barkovich AJ. Analysis and classification of cerebellar malformations. Am J Neuroradiol 2002; 23: 1074–1087

Case 9

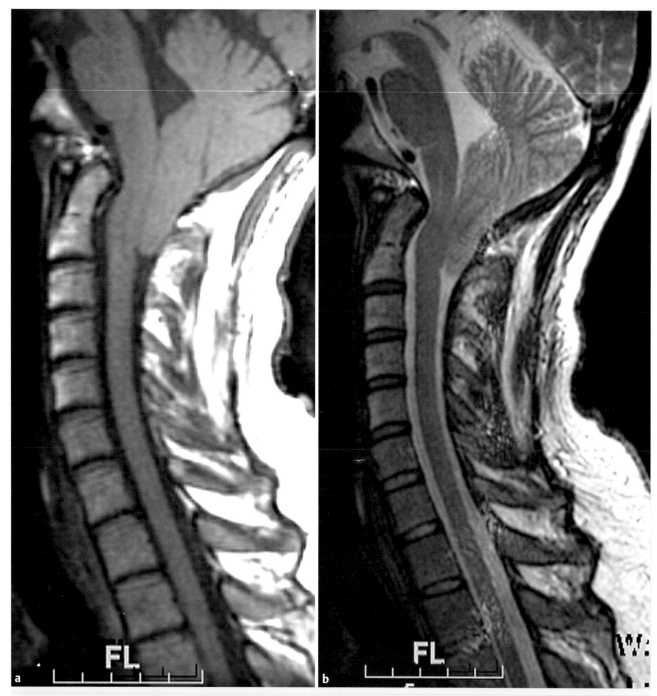

Fig. 9.1 Sagittal T1 **(a)** and T2 **(b)** images of the cervical spine demonstrate significant cerebellar tonsillar herniation below the foramen magnum with "peg-like" tonsils. The posterior fossa is small and there is mass effect upon the brain stem. No syrinx is identified.

▪ Clinical Presentation

A 34-year-old man with headaches and vertigo (▶ Fig. 9.1)

▨ Key Imaging Finding

Tonsillar ectopia

▨ Top 3 Differential Diagnoses

- **Chiari malformations.** Type I and II Chiari malformations, although separate and very distinct entities, both demonstrate a small posterior fossa with caudal protrusion of "peg-shaped" cerebellar tonsils below foramen magnum ≥ 5 mm. The degree of tonsillar ectopia and crowding at the craniocervical junction is typically greater in Chiari II malformations. Chiari I malformations are associated with osseous abnormalities of the skull base and cervical spine, such as Klippel-Feil syndrome, and syringohydromyelia of the cord. Patients with Chiari I typically do not have additional central nervous system anomalies or malformations. Approximately half of Chiari I patients are asymptomatic, whereas the remaining may have headache or symptoms associated with brain stem compression or syringohydromyelia. Chiari II malformations are associated with a lumbosacral myelomeningocele (open neural tube defect) and additional intracranial anomalies. Intracranial imaging findings include tonsillar ectopia, cervicomedullary kinking, compressed and elongated fourth ventricle, a beaked tectum, "towering" cerebellum protruding cranially through the incisura, enlarged massa intermedia, low-lying torcula, and a Lückenschädel or lacunar skull (bony dysplasia that lasts up until 6 months of age). Dysgenesis of the corpus callosum is seen in 90% of cases. Hydrocephalus is present in nearly all cases (~98%). Chiari III malformations are exceedingly rare and consist of low occipital and/or high cervical cephaloceles with intracranial findings of Chiari II malformations and upper cervical spine dysraphism.
- **Intracranial hypotension.** Intracranial hypotension results in "sagging" of the brain and inferior tonsillar displacement. Etiologies include iatrogenia (postsurgical or procedural, such as lumbar puncture), trauma, violent coughing or strenuous exercise, spontaneous dural tear, ruptured arachnoid diverticulum, severe dehydration, and, rarely, disc protrusion with dural injury. Reduced intracranial pressure results in brain descent. Tonsillar ectopia is seen in up to 75% of cases. Additional findings include diffuse thickened, fluid-attenuated inversion recovery hyperintense, enhancing dura, and subdural fluid collections, typically hygromas. There is a sagging midbrain (below dorsum sella) and a "fat midbrain sign" (elongated appearance of the midbrain and pons). Radionuclide cisternography or computed tomography myelography can be used to search for the site of cerebrospinal fluid leakage if blood patch therapy fails.
- **Ependymoma.** Ependymoma is the third most common posterior fossa tumor in children (after medulloblastoma and juvenile pilocytic astrocytoma [JPA]) and arises from the ependymal cells of the fourth ventricle. It is a soft, pliable tumor that may extend through the fourth ventricular outlet foramina into the cerebellopontine angle or foramen magnum. Extension through the foramen magnum may mimic cerebellar tonsillar ectopia. Calcification is seen in ~50% of cases; cysts and hemorrhage are less common. The mass is heterogeneous and typically iso- or hyperintense on T2 sequences with heterogeneous enhancement. Patients often present with headache, vomiting, and/or ataxia. Peak incidence is in the first decade of life.

▨ Additional Differential Diagnoses

- **Posterior fossa mass.** Any primary or secondary posterior fossa mass may cause tonsillar herniation secondary to local mass effect. Common causes in children include medulloblastoma and JPA; common lesions in adults include infarction, metastases, hemangioblastoma, vascular malformations, and hypertensive hemorrhage.

▨ Diagnosis

Chiari I malformation

✓ Pearls

- Chiari I is characterized by tonsillar ectopia, skull-base/cervical spine malformations, and syrinx.
- Chiari II is characterized by tonsillar ectopia, myelomeningocele, and multiple intracranial abnormalities.
- Ependymoma extension through the foramen magnum may mimic tonsillar ectopia.
- A posterior fossa mass or "sagging" from intracranial hypotension may result in tonsillar ectopia.

Suggested Readings

Fishman RA, Dillon WP. Dural enhancement and cerebral displacement secondary to intracranial hypotension. Neurology 1993; 43: 609–611

Koeller KK, Sandberg GD Armed Forces Institute of Pathology. From the archives of the AFIP. Cerebral intraventricular neoplasms: radiologic-pathologic correlation. Radiographics 2002; 22: 1473–1505

Milhorat TH, Chou MW, Trinidad EM et al. Chiari I malformation redefined: clinical and radiographic findings for 364 symptomatic patients. Neurosurgery 1999; 44: 1005–1017

Case 10

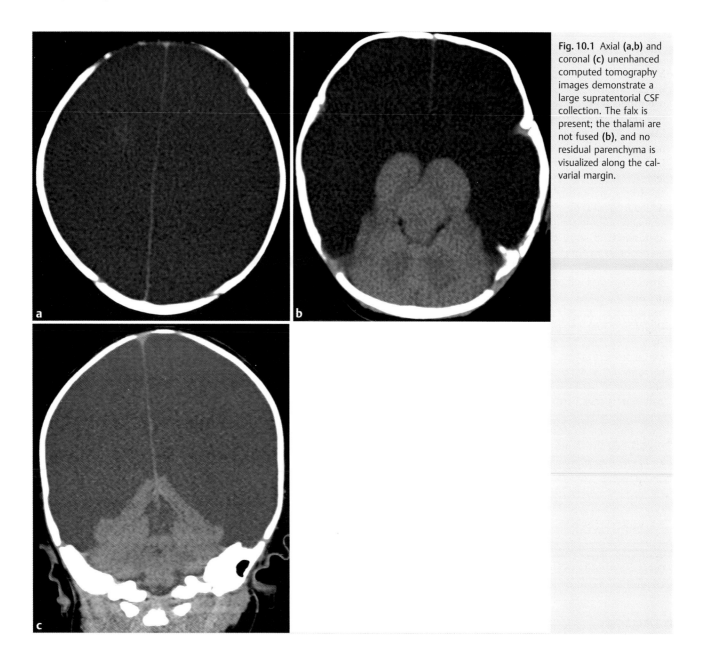

Fig. 10.1 Axial (**a,b**) and coronal (**c**) unenhanced computed tomography images demonstrate a large supratentorial CSF collection. The falx is present; the thalami are not fused (**b**), and no residual parenchyma is visualized along the calvarial margin.

■ **Clinical Presentation**

A 7-week-old adopted girl with failure to thrive and developmental delay (► Fig. 10.1)

▓ Key Imaging Finding

Supratentorial cerebrospinal fluid (CSF) collection

■ Top 3 Differential Diagnoses

- **Massive hydrocephalus.** Hydrocephalus refers to ventriculomegaly with increased volume of CSF due to obstruction, overproduction, or decreased resorption. In the newborn, this results in macrocephaly because the sutures are open. Massive hydrocephalus displaces and compresses the brain parenchyma along the peripheral calvarial margin, mimicking hydranencephaly or holoprosencephaly. Key distinguishing features include a thin mantle of cortex along the inner calvarial margin and the presence of the falx, respectively. Aqueductal stenosis is a common cause of massive hydrocephalus. Additional causes include obstructing masses, such as posterior fossa, pineal gland, tectal plate, and intraventricular neoplasms. Transependymal flow of CSF is seen in cases of acute uncompensated hydrocephalus. Causes of nonobstructive communicating hydrocephalus include a history of prior meningitis or ventriculitis, as well as prior subarachnoid hemorrhage.

- **Hydranencephaly.** Hydranencephaly is characterized by liquefactive necrosis of the supratentorial brain parenchyma in the anterior (internal carotid artery) circulation secondary to some form of in utero insult. There is sparing of the parenchyma in the posterior (posterior cerebral artery and cerebellar branch vessels) circulation. Most cases are thought to result from an ischemic, traumatic, or toxic insult between ~20 and 27 weeks gestation. Key distinguishing features include the presence of the falx cerebri; intact thalami, brain stem, cerebellum, and typically portions of the posterior occipital and parietal lobes; and absence of a cortical mantle around a large supratentorial CSF-filled cavity. Neonates commonly present with macrocrania and neurological function limited to the brain stem; death typically occurs in infancy or early childhood.

- **Alobar holoprosencephaly.** Holoprosencephaly is a spectrum of congenital forebrain malformations characterized as alobar, semilobar, and lobar variants. The alobar form is most severe and is characterized by a large, dorsal interhemispheric cyst and fusion of the thalami and remaining brain parenchyma, which is flattened anteriorly. The corpus callosum, anterior falx, interhemispheric fissure, and Sylvian fissures are absent. Associated craniofacial abnormalities include hypotelorism, fused metopic suture, and cleft palate. Semilobar and lobar variants are less severe forms with varying degrees of defective separation of the anterior and central brain structures, as well as complete or partial absence of the falx. An azygous anterior cerebral artery is commonly seen.

■ Additional Differential Diagnoses

- **Agenesis of the corpus callosum (ACC) with midline interhemispheric cyst.** ACC may be associated with midline interhemispheric cysts in addition to elevation of the third ventricle. The cysts may represent a diverticulum of the lateral ventricle (type I) or multiple interhemispheric cysts (type II). Ventriculomegaly is commonly seen. The interhemispheric cysts result in lateral displacement of the brain parenchyma. One-half to three-fourths of cases of ACC have additional central nervous system malformations.

- **Bilateral open-lip schizencephaly.** Type II (open-lip) schizencephaly consists of a large CSF-filled cleft that is lined by polymicrogyric gray matter. The abnormality may be bilateral in up to half of cases and may be associated with septo-optic dysplasia. Differentiating features include gray matter–lined clefts and an intact falx. Heterotopia or cortical dysplasia may be associated findings. Patients often present with seizures and varying degrees of developmental delay and/or motor deficits.

■ Diagnosis

Hydranencephaly

✓ Pearls

- Massive hydrocephalus in a neonate is commonly due to obstruction; a thin peripheral cortical mantle is seen.
- Hydranencephaly is liquefactive necrosis in the anterior circulation; falx is present with no cortical mantle.
- Alobar holoprosencephaly results in a large dorsal monoventricle with fused parenchyma anteriorly.

Suggested Readings

Dublin AB, French BN. Diagnostic image evaluation of hydranencephaly and pictorially similar entities, with emphasis on computed tomography. Radiology 1980; 137: 81–91

Oh KY, Kennedy AM, Frias AE, Jr, Byrne JL. Fetal schizencephaly: pre- and postnatal imaging with a review of the clinical manifestations. Radiographics 2005; 25: 647–657

Case 11

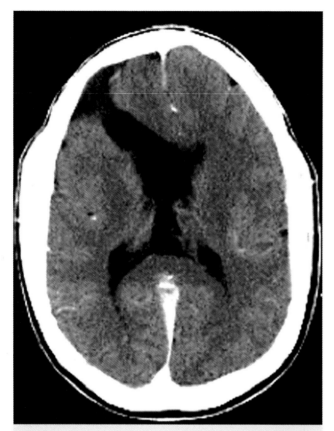

Fig. 11.1 Contrast-enhanced axial computed tomography image through the lateral ventricles demonstrates a gray matter–lined CSF cleft that communicates with the frontal horn of the right lateral ventricle. There is also absence of the septum pellucidum.

■ Clinical Presentation

An adolescent with seizures (▶ Fig. 11.1)

▣ Key Imaging Finding

Cerebrospinal fluid (CSF) collection communicating with ventricle

▣ Top 3 Differential Diagnoses

- **Schizencephaly.** Schizencephaly is a congenital malformation characterized by parenchymal clefts that extend from the pial surface to the lateral ventricles. The clefts are lined by dysplastic (usually polymicrogyric) gray matter and often parasylvian in location. In type I (closed-lip) schizencephaly, the gray matter linings are apposed, making the malformation less conspicuous. Along the ventricular aspect of the cleft, there is often a "dimple" with CSF extending from the ventricle into the opening of the cleft. Type II (open-lip) schizencephaly is characterized by a large CSF-filled cleft lined by dysplastic gray matter. Approximately 50% of cases of schizencephaly are bilateral; when bilateral, the open-lip variant is more common. Clinical manifestations depend upon the severity of the defect, as well as the presence of additional malformations. Patients with type I schizencephaly are often almost normal in terms of development, but may have seizures and hemiparesis. Patients with type II schizencephaly usually have significant neurological deficits, especially if bilateral, including mental retardation, seizures, paresis, mutism, and/or blindness. Both variants may be associated with septo-optic dysplasia. Heterotopia or cortical dysplasia may be associated findings.
- **Porencephalic cyst.** Porencephalic cysts are CSF-filled cavities that are lined by gliotic white matter and typically communicate with the ventricles and/or subarachnoid space. In many cases, the communication with the ventricles or subarachnoid space may be occult. Porencephalic cysts may be congenital secondary to a perinatal insult after brain development or acquired from a postnatal insult in childhood or young adulthood. Common acquired causes include infarct, infection, and trauma. Familial porencephaly has been described but is rare. The cysts vary significantly in size from relatively small to

quite large and may be unilateral or bilateral. In general, congenital cysts are smooth with little surrounding gliosis, whereas acquired cysts tend to have irregular walls and more pronounced gliosis. The adjacent ventricle is typically enlarged due to volume loss. Occasionally, the cysts may enlarge due to a ball-valve type communication with the ventricle or adhesions. Superficial cysts may remodel the overlying calvarium, similar to arachnoid cysts. When symptomatic, treatment includes resection or fenestration of the cysts. Patients with porencephaly often present with spastic hemiplegia and seizures. Severe neurological deficits may be seen with large or multiple regions of porencephaly. Porencephaly has been described in association with various syndromes, as well as amygdala-hippocampal atrophy, which may be related to seizure activity.
- **Encephalomalacia.** Parenchymal injury results in volume loss with encephalomalacia and compensatory dilatation of the ventricles and adjacent sulci. Common causes of encephalomalacia include arterial infarct, primary intracranial hemorrhage, and hemorrhagic venous infarct. The region of encephalomalacia approaches CSF attenuation (computed tomography) and signal (magnetic resonance imaging) and is lined by gliotic white matter, similar to porencephalic cysts. The morphology depends upon the location, size, and type of parenchymal injury. Occasionally, it may appear cystic. Arterial infarcts are typically wedge-shaped. On MR imaging, the gliotic parenchyma along the border of encephalomalacia is increased in T2 and fluid-attenuated inversion recovery signal intensity. Hemosiderin staining may be seen along the margin of encephalomalacia on gradient echo or susceptibility-weighted imaging.

▣ Diagnosis

Schizencephaly (type II, open-lip)

✓ Pearls

- Schizencephaly results in CSF clefts lined by dysplastic gray matter; it is due to an intrauterine insult.
- Schizencephaly is associated with neural migration abnormalities and septo-optic dysplasia.

- Porencephalic cysts are often caused by a perinatal insult and are lined by dysplastic white matter.
- Encephalomalacia results in volume loss from prior parenchymal injury; arterial infarct is the most common cause.

Suggested Readings

Denis D, Chateil JF, Brun M et al. Schizencephaly: clinical and imaging features in 30 infantile cases. Brain Dev 2000; 22: 475–483

Van Tassel P, Curé JK. Nonneoplastic intracranial cysts and cystic lesions. Semin Ultrasound CT MR 1995; 16: 186–211

Case 12

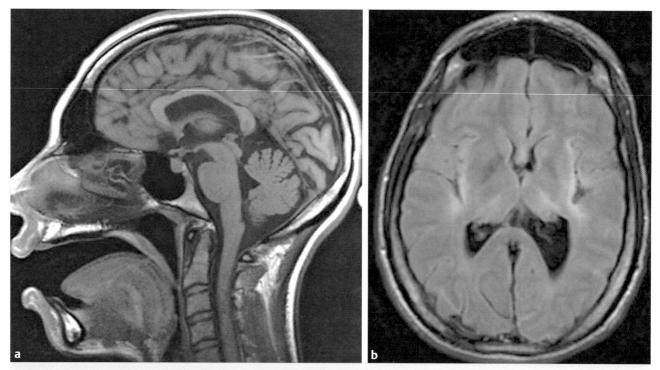

Fig. 12.1 Sagittal T1 magnetic resonance image **(a)** demonstrates microcephaly with a decreased craniofacial ratio. Axial fluid-attenuated inversion recovery image **(b)** reveals abnormal signal intensity involving the thalami, as well as abnormal signal intensity and encephalomalacia within the bilateral insular cortex and subcortical white matter.

■ **Clinical Presentation**

A young adult with severe mental retardation (▶ Fig. 12.1)

▩ Key Imaging Finding

Microcephaly

▩ Top 3 Differential Diagnoses

- **Primary microcephaly.** Microcephaly is defined as a small head in relation to facial structures (decreased craniofacial ratio), usually at least 3 standard deviations below the mean. The growth of the calvarium is dependent upon the growth of the underlying brain parenchyma. Growth of facial structures, however, occurs independently. Primary microcephaly is a genetic defect in which the brain parenchyma appears grossly normal but is small and demonstrates a simplified gyral pattern. There may be associated neuronal migration abnormalities, holoprosencephaly, or cortical malformations. White matter abnormalities, when present, consist of diffuse hypomyelination. Affected patients suffer from severe mental retardation and seizures in some cases.
- **Hypoxic-ischemic encephalopathy (HIE).** The pattern of HIE depends upon both the cause and severity of the insult. In both premature and full-term infants, severe HIE affects the areas of the brain that are most metabolically active, including the deep and superficial gray matter, brain stem, and cerebellum. Mild to moderate HIE results in periventricular leukomalacia in premature babies and watershed distribution infarcts in full-term neonates. With severe injury, parenchymal atrophy and encephalomalacia results in secondary microcephaly. Clinically, neurological deficits are related to the extent of injury.
- **TORCH infection.** The TORCH infections consist of toxoplasmosis, rubella, cytomegalovirus (CMV), and herpes simplex virus. The severity of deficits in the setting of TORCH infections is dependent more upon the timing of the insult, rather than the causative organism. Early insults often lead to congenital malformations, whereas those that occur later result in destruction of formed structures. Cytomegalovirus (CMV) is the most common TORCH infection. Typical imaging findings with CMV include microcephaly, ventriculomegaly, cortical malformations, and parenchymal calcifications with a characteristic periventricular distribution. Toxoplasmosis is transmitted after consumption of undercooked meats or exposure to cat feces. The primary parenchymal findings are microcephaly, ventriculomegaly, and parenchymal calcifications with a more random distribution compared with CMV. Affected patients have significant neurological disabilities.

▩ Additional Differential Diagnoses

- **Nonaccidental trauma (NAT).** Neurological injury from NAT is a leading cause of death. The majority of abused children are infants < 1 year old, and many have chronic illnesses or developmental abnormalities. The type of intracranial injury depends upon the form of abuse. With "shaken baby" syndrome, children most often have subdural hemorrhages over the cerebral convexities, extending into the interhemispheric fissure, and along the tentorium. More importantly, these patients often have diffuse ischemic injury. With direct trauma to the skull, fractures, extraaxial hemorrhages, and coup–contracoup injuries are common. Caution should be used in trying to date extraaxial hemorrhages based upon signal intensity.
- **Fetal alcohol syndrome.** Both the amount of alcohol and the timing of the insult in terms of development determine the overall neurological deficits. Affected individuals often demonstrate parenchymal injury and characteristic facial features. As with other fetal insults, earlier injury often results in congenital defects, whereas later injury often results in destruction of formed structures. The most common parenchymal findings include microcephaly, callosal anomalies, neuronal migration abnormalities, and cerebellar hypoplasia. Common facial deformities include short palpebral fissures, smooth philantrum, thin upper lip, upturned nose, and flat midface. Clinically, patients often have significant developmental and cognitive deficits.

▩ Diagnosis

Microcephaly secondary to neonatal ischemia

✓ Pearls

- Primary microcephaly is a genetic defect with a decreased craniofacial ratio and a simplified gyral pattern.
- Secondary microcephaly refers to a decreased craniofacial ratio due to some form of parenchymal insult.
- Common causes of secondary microcephaly include hypoxic-ischemic, infectious, traumatic, and toxic insults.

Suggested Readings

Chao CP, Zaleski CG, Patton AC. Neonatal hypoxic-ischemic encephalopathy: multimodality imaging findings. Radiographics 2006; 26 Suppl 1: S159–S172

Custer DA, Vezina LG, Vaught DR et al. Neurodevelopmental and neuroimaging correlates in nonsyndromal microcephalic children. J Dev Behav Pediatr 2000; 21: 12–18

Case 13

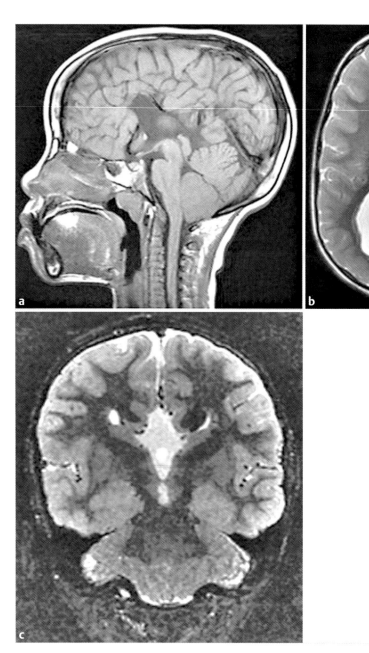

Fig. 13.1 Sagittal T1 magnetic resonance image **(a)** demonstrates absence of the corpus callosum with a high-riding third ventricle and extension of the medial cerebral hemisphere gyri to the ventricular margin in a radial configuration. Axial T2 image **(b)** shows a parallel configuration of the lateral ventricles with colpocephaly. Nodular foci of gray matter are visualized along the sub-ependymal surfaces of the ventricles, consistent with heterotopia. Coronal T2 image **(c)** reveals a "longhorn" configuration of the frontal horns of the lateral ventricles secondary to medial indentation by white matter fibers (Probst bundles). The third ventricle is elevated in the midline.

▦ Clinical Presentation

A 6-year-old boy with seizure disorder and developmental delay (▸ Fig. 13.1)

▨ Key Imaging Finding

Absence of the corpus callosum

▪ Diagnosis

Agenesis of the corpus callosum. The corpus callosum consists of compact white matter tracts that allow for communication between the cerebral hemispheres. It normally forms between 8 and 20 weeks gestation and is associated with development of the limbic system, which includes the cingulate gyrus and hippocampal formations. Normal development occurs anterior to posterior with formation of the genu first, followed by the body and splenium. The rostrum is located along the inferior margin of the genu and is the last portion of the corpus callosum to form. The presence or absence of the rostrum is important in distinguishing partial absence of the corpus callosum (rostrum absent) from an encephaloclastic process involving the corpus callosum (rostrum present unless in location of insult).

Complete agenesis of the corpus callosum is the most severe form of callosal malformation. On computed tomography (CT) or magnetic resonance imaging (MRI), the corpus callosum is absent. As a result, there is elevation of the third ventricle between the lateral ventricles, which are parallel in configuration on axial images. The white matter tracts that would form the corpus callosum instead align along the medial margin of the lateral ventricles and run in an anterior-posterior direction. These tracts are referred to as Probst bundles. The Probst bundles indent the superomedial margin of the frontal horns of the lateral ventricles on coronal sequences, resulting in a "long-horn" or "steer-horn" appearance. The lack of tight white matter tracts along the margin of the lateral ventricles results in dilatation of the atria and occipital horns of the lateral ventricles, known as colpocephaly.

ACC is associated with hypoplasia and failure of rotation of the cingulate gyrus, as well as absence of the cingulate sulcus. As a result, the gyri of the medial cerebral hemispheres extend to the margin of the elevated third ventricle and maintain a radial configuration. Compensatory hypertrophy of the commissures may occur and should not be mistaken for remnants of the absent corpus callosum. ACC may be associated with interhemispheric cysts. The cysts are classified as ventricular diverticula (type 1) or interhemispheric cysts that do not communicate with the ventricles (type 2). Type 2 cysts have an increased association with neuronal migrational abnormalities. Care must be taken not to mistake the elevated third ventricle for an interhemispheric cyst. The presence of a midline lipoma in the setting of ACC is variable.

Numerous syndromes and malformations are associated with ACC, including Aicardi syndrome (ACC, infantile spasms, and chorioretinopathy), Chiari II malformation, and Dandy-Walker malformation, to name a few. Most patients suffer from varying degrees of mental retardation, developmental delay, and seizures.

✓ Pearls

- The corpus callosum allows for communication between hemispheres and is an integral part of the limbic system.
- The corpus callosum forms anterior to posterior (genu, body, splenium), followed by the rostrum.
- Ventricular findings with ACC include parallel lateral ventricles, colpocephaly, and "steer-horn" frontal horns.
- Absence of the corpus callosum results in a high-riding third ventricle with or without interhemispheric cysts.

Suggested Readings

Atlas SW, Zimmerman RA, Bilaniuk LT et al. Corpus callosum and limbic system: neuroanatomic MR evaluation of developmental anomalies. Radiology 1986; 160: 355–362

Barkovich AJ, Simon EM, Walsh CA. Callosal agenesis with cyst: a better understanding and new classification. Neurology 2001; 56: 220–227

Sztriha L. Spectrum of corpus callosum agenesis. Pediatr Neurol 2005; 32: 94–101

Case 14

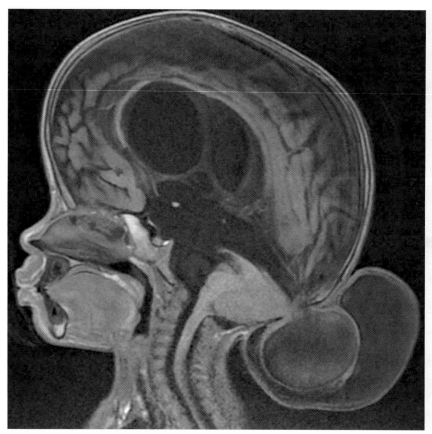

Fig. 14.1 Sagittal T1 image demonstrates a large mass containing cerebrospinal fluid, meninges, and parenchymal tissue extending through an occipital bone defect. The protruding mass has a "cyst within a cyst" appearance. The cerebellum and brain stem are posteriorly displaced with compression of the fourth ventricle, resulting in marked hydrocephalus.

■ Clinical Presentation

A 20-month-old boy recently adopted with enlarged head, scalp mass, and developmental delay (▶ Fig. 14.1)

▨ Key Imaging Finding

Intracranial contents extending through a posterior calvarial defect

▨ Diagnosis

Occipital cephalocele. Cephaloceles are neural tube defects characterized by herniation of intracranial contents through a calvarial defect. Occipital cephaloceles are the most common in Europe and Western countries, accounting for > 75% of cases. Cephaloceles may be subclassified based upon their contents. Meningoceles are composed of herniated meninges, whereas encephaloceles contain both meninges and dysplastic parenchymal tissue. Prognosis is primarily based upon the amount and specific portion of parenchymal tissue within the defect, as well as the severity of additional central nervous system malformations, if present.

Occipital cephaloceles may occur sporadically or in association with syndromes and malformations, such as Meckel-Gruber syndrome, Walker-Warburg syndrome, and Chiari III malformation. They may also be seen in association with Dandy-Walker malformation, which consists of an enlarged posterior fossa, aplastic or hypoplastic cerebellar vermis, and enlarged fourth ventricle that communicates with a retrocerebellar cerebrospinal fluid collection. Meckel-Gruber syndrome is an autosomal disorder characterized by an occipital cephalocele, polycystic kidneys, and polydactyly. Walker-Warburg syndrome consists of cobblestone (type 2) lissencephaly, an occipital encephalocele, cerebellar and brain stem hypoplasia, and kinking of the brain stem, resulting in the classic "striking cobra" appearance on sagittal sequences. Chiari III malformations are exceedingly rare and consist of low occipital and/or high cervical cephaloceles that involve the opisthion, as well as intracranial findings of Chiari II malformations and upper cervical dysraphism.

Most occipital cephaloceles are diagnosed in utero by ultrasound in the setting of elevated levels of alpha-fetoprotein. They are characterized as low or high based upon whether or not there is involvement of the foramen magnum (involved with low occipital cephaloceles). Low occipital encephaloceles most often contain portions of the cerebellum. When large, the brain stem may also extend through the defect. High occipital encephaloceles may contain portions of the cerebellum and/or supratentorial brain parenchyma. The involved portions of the brain parenchyma are typically dysplastic and nonfunctional, which accounts for their heterogeneous signal intensity on magnetic resonance imaging (MRI). Often times, the herniated meninges and parenchyma result in a "cyst within a cyst" appearance, seen both on ultrasound and MRI. In the preoperative workup of these patients, it is critical to identify the venous anatomy, as inadvertent resection of involved or anomalous dural venous sinuses can be devastating. This is best evaluated on MR angiography.

An atretic cephalocele typically presents as a small scalp mass in the parietal or upper occipital region. Identification of a small calvarial defect associated with the scalp lesion is key to making the diagnosis. A persistent falcine sinus is commonly seen in association with these types of cephaloceles.

✓ Pearls

- Cephaloceles are neural tube defects that may be subclassified as meningoceles or encephaloceles.
- Occipital cephaloceles are the most common form in Europe and Western countries.
- Parenchyma within the defect is typically dysplastic and nonfunctional; identification of venous structures is critical.

- Occipital cephaloceles may be associated with Meckel-Gruber syndrome, Walker-Warburg syndrome, and Chiari III malformations.

Suggested Reading

Martínez-Lage JF, Poza M, Sola J et al. The child with a cephalocele: etiology, neuroimaging, and outcome. Childs Nerv Syst 1996; 12: 540–550

Case 15

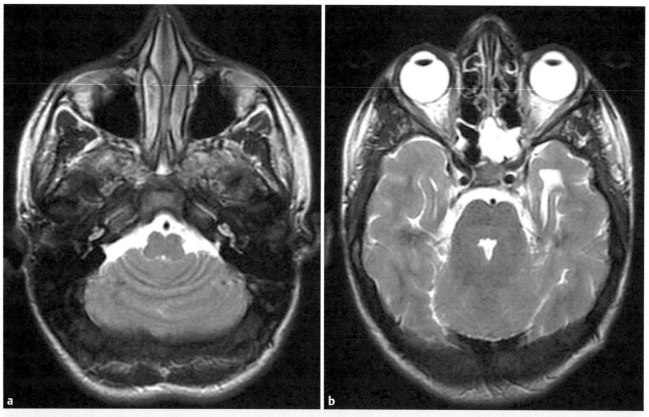

Fig. 15.1 (a,b) Axial T2 images demonstrate absence of the cerebellar vermis with fusion or failure of segmentation of the cerebellar hemispheres.

■ Clinical Presentation

A 15-year-old girl with long-standing gait instability and cognitive deficits (▶ Fig. 15.1)

■ Key Imaging Finding

Absent vermis with fused cerebellar hemispheres

■ Diagnosis

Rhombencephalosynapsis. Rhombencephalosynapsis is an uncommon developmental anomaly that results in fusion or failure of segmentation of the cerebellar hemispheres. The cerebellar vermis is either absent or significantly hypoplastic. The anomaly results in a transverse orientation of the cerebellar folia and posterior pointing of the fourth ventricle, which assumes a "keyhole" configuration. More often than not, there is fusion of the superior cerebellar peduncles and dentate nuclei as well. Associated supratentorial anomalies are variable and include fused thalami, fornices, and colliculi; absence of the septum pellucidum; aqueductal stenosis with hydrocephalus; callosal and anterior commissure dysgenesis; and neuronal migrational abnormalities. Facial defects have also been reported.

The precise cause of rhombencephalosynapsis remains unknown. Patients usually present early in life with ataxia and/or developmental delay. Prognosis and neurological deficits vary widely and are generally related to the presence and severity of additional supratentorial abnormalities. Mimics of rhombencephalosynapsis include findings associated with chronic overshunting, Chiari II malformations, and Joubert syndrome; the key distinction is that these entities result in approximation rather than fusion of the cerebellar hemispheres.

✓ Pearls

- Rhombencephalosynapsis is congenital fusion or failure of segmentation of the cerebellar hemispheres.
- More often than not, there is also fusion of the superior cerebellar peduncles and dentate nuclei.
- There is transverse orientation of the cerebellar folia and a "keyhole" configuration of the fourth ventricle.
- Mimics of rhombencephalosynapsis include overshunting, Chiari II malformations, and Joubert syndrome.

Suggested Readings

Toelle SP, Yalcinkaya C, Kocer N et al. Rhombencephalosynapsis: clinical findings and neuroimaging in 9 children. Neuropediatrics 2002; 33: 209–214

Truwit CL, Barkovich AJ, Shanahan R, Maroldo TV. MR imaging of rhombencephalosynapsis: report of three cases and review of the literature. Am J Neuroradiol 1991; 12: 957–965

Case 16

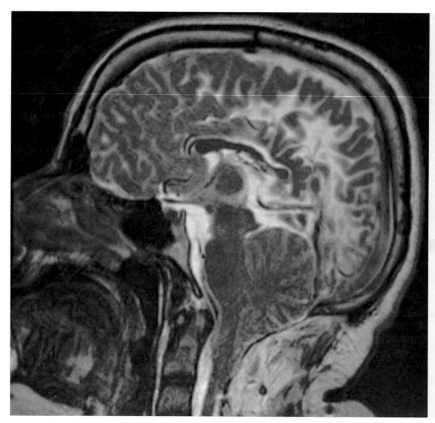

Fig. 16.1 Sagittal T2 magnetic resonance image demonstrates cerebellar tonsillar herniation through the foramen magnum with effacement of cerebrospinal fluid at the craniocervical junction, cervicomedullary kinking, a "beaked" tectum, enlarged massa intermedia, low-lying torcula, hypoplasia and partial agenesis of the corpus callosum (absent rostrum), and stenogyria.

■ Clinical Presentation

A young adult with long-standing neurological issues (▶ Fig. 16.1)

▦ Key Imaging Finding

Tonsillar ectopia with intracranial malformations

■ Diagnosis

Chiari II malformation. Chiari II is a complex malformation affecting the brain, skull, and spine. It is caused by failure of neural tube closure and is associated with folate deficiency. Nearly 100% of patients present with a lumbosacral myelomeningocele, which is classified as an open spinal dysraphism. Preoperative imaging of the neural tube defect demonstrates fetal elongation of the cord with the neural placode and meninges extending posteriorly through a spinal dysraphism. There is no overlying skin covering; hence, it is an open defect. The spinal cord is tethered within the defect.

Imaging of the skull demonstrates a small posterior fossa with a normal-sized cerebellum. The cerebellar tonsils are inferiorly displaced through the foramen magnum, wrap around the medulla, and demonstrate a pointed configuration. Inferior displacement of the brain stem/medulla results in kinking at the cervicomedullary junction secondary to anchoring of the upper cervical cord by ligamentous attachments, as well as "beaking" of the tectum. The fourth ventricle becomes elongated and inferiorly displaced. Stenosis at the craniocervical junction leads to obstructive hydrocephalus in ~80% of patients. Upward extension of the superior aspect of the cerebellum through a widened tentorial incisura is referred to as a towering cerebellum. The combination of a small posterior fossa and tonsillar herniation results in a low-lying torcula.

Additional findings include a fenestrated falx with interdigitation of gyri, an enlarged massa intermedia, and dilatation of the atria and occipital horns of the lateral ventricles, referred to as colpocephaly. The gyri may be narrowed and spaced closely together, which is referred to as stenogyria. Lückenchädel is a membranous bony dysplasia that is seen early in life in association with a myelomeningocele and is characterized by regions of bony thinning. It typically resolves by 6 months of age. Complete or partial agenesis of the corpus callosum and neuronal migrational anomalies are commonly associated with Chiari II malformations.

Many patients are identified prenatally by ultrasound after elevated alpha-fetoprotein levels are detected. Characteristic ultrasound findings include the presence of a lumbosacral myelomeningocele, as well as a lemon-shaped head and a banana-shaped cerebellum.

✓ Pearls

- Chiari II malformation affects the brain, skull, and spine; nearly 100% have a lumbosacral myelomeningocele.
- Posterior fossa is small with tonsillar ectopia, cervicomedullary kinking, "beaked" tectum, and low-lying torcula.

- Hydrocephalus, callosal dysgenesis, and neuronal migrational anomalies are commonly seen with Chiari II.
- Fetal ultrasound findings include a myelomeningocele, a lemon-shaped head, and a banana-shaped cerebellum.

Suggested Reading

Wolpert SM, Anderson M, Scott RM, Kwan ES, Runge VM. Chiari II malformation: MR imaging evaluation. Am J Roentgenol 1987; 149: 1033–1042

Case 17

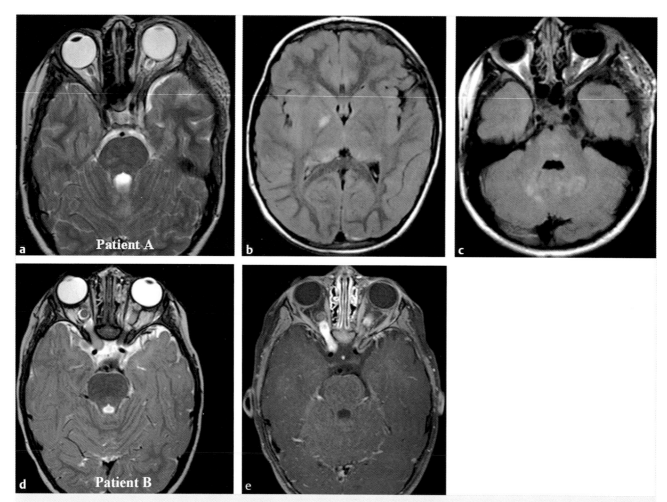

Fig. 17.1 Patient A: Axial T2 magnetic resonance image **(a)** demonstrates left sphenoid wing dysplasia, enlargement and elongation of the left optic nerve with kinking, and a soft-tissue mass overlying the left orbit and temporal bone with intraorbital extension. Axial fluid-attenuated inversion recovery (FLAIR) images **(b,c)** show similar findings with additional regions of signal abnormality involving the basal ganglia, thalami, brain stem, and dentate nuclei. Patient B: Axial T2 **(d)** and T1 postcontrast with fat suppression **(e)** images reveal bilateral optic nerve enlargement and enhancement.

■ Clinical Presentation

Patient A: A 9-year-old boy with skin lesions; Patient B: A 2-year-old girl with skin lesions and visual loss (► Fig. 17.1)

Key Imaging Finding

Bilateral optic pathway gliomas (OPGs), parenchymal signal abnormality, bony dysplasia, and subcutaneous mass

Diagnosis

Neurofibromatosis type 1 (NF1). NF1, also known as von Recklinghausen disease, is the most common of the neurocutaneous syndromes. It may occur sporadically or be inherited in an autosomal dominant fashion. The genetic defect affects chromosome 17q12 and results in decreased production of neurofibromin, which acts as a tumor suppressor. The disease affects the brain, skull, orbits, spine, musculoskeletal system, and skin/integumentary system. Diagnostic criteria for NF1 include the presence of two or more of the following: first-degree relative with NF1, six or more café-au-lait spots, two or more neurofibromas (NFs) or one plexiform NF, OPG, bony dysplasia, axillary or inguinal freckling, and two or more Lisch nodules.

Central nervous system (CNS) manifestations include characteristic NF "spots" and low-grade neoplasms. The NF spots are regions of signal abnormality involving the basal ganglia, thalami, dentate nuclei, cerebellar peduncles, optic radiations, and brain stem. They are thought to represent regions of myelin vacuolization. The lesions are hyperintense on T2 and typically iso- to mildly hyperintense on T1 images. There may be apparent but not true mass effect, especially with lesions located within the thalami, cerebellar peduncles, and brain stem. However, there should be no enhancement; the presence of enhancement suggests development of a low-grade glioma. The lesions may wax and wane for the first decade of life and then regress in both size and signal abnormality.

The most common CNS neoplasms associated with NF1 are low-grade OPGs. Bilateral optic nerve gliomas are pathognomonic for NF1. Although low grade, the lesions may extend to the optic chiasm and along the optic radiations. Vision loss and interval change in size are the most important considerations in terms of management. Enhancement characteristics are variable and do not impact treatment decisions. Low-grade cerebellar, brain stem, tectal plate, and basal ganglia gliomas are also common in the setting of NF1. Obstructive hydrocephalus may result from a tectal plate or brain stem glioma or as a result of aqueductal stenosis, which has an increased incidence in patients with NF1.

In addition to OPG, orbital findings include sphenoid wing dysplasia with associated pulsatile exophthalmos, buphthalmos (globe enlargement), and intraorbital extension of a plexiform NF (PNF). Vascular abnormalities include regions of stenosis, moyamoya, and aneurysm formation. These are best visualized on magnetic resonance angiography studies.

Spinal manifestations of NF1 include multiple bilateral NFs with extension through and expansion of the neuroformina. NFs are more likely than schwannomas to demonstrate the "target sign," which refers to peripheral increased and central decreased T2 signal intensity. Large retroperitoneal PNFs are prone to malignant degeneration, which is best characterized by interval growth. Additional spinal manifestations include kyphoscoliosis, dural ectasia with posterior vertebral body scalloping, and lateral thoracic meningoceles. Rarely, intramedullary lesions, typically low-grade astrocytomas, may present in patients with NF1.

Extra CNS and spinal manifestations include cutaneous NFs, café-au-lait spots, extremity long-bone pseudoarthroses and bowing deformities, "ribbon" ribs, and hypertrophy or overgrowth of all or a portion of a limb. NF1 is associated with an increased incidence of several tumors, including pheochromocytoma, medullary thyroid carcinoma, gastrointestinal stromal tumors, melanoma, Wilms tumor, leukemia, and lymphoma.

✓ Pearls

- NF1 is the most common neurocutaneous syndrome and results from a genetic defect affecting chromosome 17.
- Patients are prone to low-grade neoplasms; bilateral optic pathway gliomas are pathognomonic of NF1.
- NF1 "spots" are thought to represent myelin vacuolization; they wax and wane in the first decade then regress.

Suggested Readings

DiMario FJ, Jr, Ramsby G. Magnetic resonance imaging lesion analysis in neurofibromatosis type 1. Arch Neurol 1998; 55: 500–505

Egelhoff JC, Bates DJ, Ross JS, Rothner AD, Cohen BH. Spinal MR findings in neurofibromatosis types 1 and 2. Am J Neuroradiol 1992; 13: 1071–1077

Rodriguez D, Young Poussaint T. Neuroimaging findings in neurofibromatosis type 1 and 2. Neuroimaging Clin N Am 2004; 14: 149–170, vii

Case 18

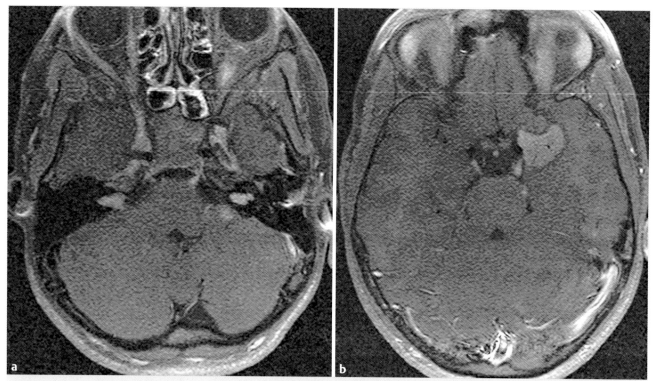

Fig. 18.1 Axial T1 postcontrast magnetic resonance images with fat suppression demonstrate bilateral extraaxial enhancing masses within and expanding the internal auditory canals, cavernous sinuses, along the anterolateral left cerebellar hemisphere (**a**), and within the left middle cranial fossa (**b**). The left middle cranial fossa mass demonstrates a broad dural base. There is also abnormal enhancement of the cisternal segments of numerous bilateral cranial nerves (**a,b**).

▓ Clinical Presentation

A 9-year-old boy with hearing loss and multiple cranial nerve deficits (▶ Fig. 18.1)

▓ Key Imaging Finding

Numerous enhancing extraaxial masses, including bilateral vestibular schwannomas

▓ Diagnosis

Neurofibromatosis type 2 (NF2). NF2 results from a genetic defect affecting chromosome 22q12, resulting in multiple intracranial and spinal schwannomas and meningiomas, as well as ependymomas within the brain stem and spinal cord. Approximately 50% of cases have a positive family history, whereas the remainder are sporadic. NF2 is 10-fold less common than NF1, which is the most common of the phakomatoses. In NF2, cutaneous lesions occur less frequently than with NF1 and tend to be fewer in number and less conspicuous.

Patients most often present in adolescence or young adulthood with hearing loss related to bilateral vestibular schwannomas, which are pathognomonic for NF2. Schwannomas may be composed of two tissue types, Antoni A and B. Antoni A tissue is densely packed with darker signal on T2 images, whereas Antoni B tissue is loosely packed with brighter signal on T2 images. The border of a vestibular schwannoma usually makes an acute angle with the petrous temporal bone. There is typically widening of the internal auditory canal and flaring of the porus acousticus. The lesions often demonstrate avid enhancement. Cystic change and hemorrhage may occur; calcification is uncommon. In the setting of NF2, multiple cranial nerve schwannomas may be seen with the trigeminal nerve being the second most commonly involved.

Intracranial meningiomas in adults are common, especially in middle-aged women. Meningioma in a child, however, should at least raise the consideration of NF2, especially when multiple and in the absence of prior craniospinal radiation (another cause of multiple meningiomas). Meningiomas occur along the dural surfaces or within the ventricles, most commonly within the atria of the lateral ventricles. They may be circumscribed or plaque-like with a broad dural base. On noncontrast computed tomography, meningiomas are often iso- to hyperdense compared with brain parenchyma and commonly have regions of calcification. There may be hyperostosis along the adjacent bone. The enhancement pattern is homogenous with a dural tail.

Ependymomas occur most commonly in the cord (cervical more often than thoracic), followed by the brain stem. They present as a central lesion with relatively uniform cord enlargement, although exophytic components are not uncommon. The lesions typically span three to four vertebral segments. Enhancement is seen but varies from intense and homogeneous to nodular and heterogeneous. Hemorrhage and intratumoral cysts are more common compared with spinal astrocytomas. A hemosiderin cap may be seen along the margins of the tumor.

The majority of schwannomas affecting the spine present as well-circumscribed, enhancing, intradural, and extramedullary lesions (75% of cases). Less common presentations include lesions with both intra- and extradural components (classic dumbbell lesions) or isolated extradural lesions. Most schwannomas are iso- or hyperintense to cord signal. Cystic change and hemorrhage may be seen; calcification is rare. Lesions may enlarge the neural foramina and/or result in posterior vertebral body scalloping.

Meningiomas are the second most common intradural extramedullary spinal masses (after schwannomas). Greater than 90% of lesions are intradural, whereas the remainder present as both intra- and extradural (dumbbell lesion), purely extradural, or rarely paraspinous or intraosseous lesions. They occur most frequently within the thoracic spine. Meningiomas are isointense to cord on T1 and iso- to hyperintense on T2 images. Calcification is less common than with intracranial meningiomas, occurring only in about 5% of cases. They are typically round and may have a broad dural base. The lesions intensely enhance and may demonstrate a dural tail, although this feature also occurs less frequently than with intracranial meningiomas.

✓ Pearls

- NF2 results from a defect of chromosome 22; bilateral vestibular schwannomas are pathognomonic.
- NF2 is characterized by multiple cranial and spinal schwannomas, meningiomas, and ependymomas.

- Patients often present with hearing loss related to vestibular schwannomas or cranial nerve deficits.

Suggested Readings

Aoki S, Barkovich AJ, Nishimura K et al. Neurofibromatosis types 1 and 2: cranial MR findings. Radiology 1989; 172: 527–534

Patronas NJ, Courcoutsakis N, Bromley CM, Katzman GL, MacCollin M, Parry DM. Intramedullary and spinal canal tumors in patients with neurofibromatosis 2: MR imaging findings and correlation with genotype. Radiology 2001; 218: 434–442

Case 19

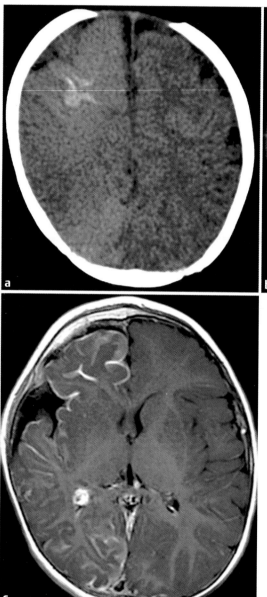

Fig. 19.1 Axial computed tomography image **(a)** reveals increased attenuation throughout the right cerebral hemisphere with right frontal lobe cortical calcifications in a "tram track" configuration. Axial T2 image **(b)** demonstrates volume loss within the right cerebral hemisphere with decreased signal intensity within the subcortical white matter. Axial T1 postcontrast image **(c)** shows abnormal leptomeningeal enhancement overlying the right cerebral hemisphere, as well as prominent enhancement within a hypertrophied ipsilateral choroid plexus. Image C also demonstrates calvarial thickening overlying the right frontal lobe.

■ Clinical Presentation

A 3-year-old boy with seizures (▶ Fig. 19.1)

▦ Key Imaging Finding

"Tram-track" calcifications, pial angiomatosis, and cerebral parenchymal atrophy

▦ Diagnosis

Sturge-Weber syndrome (SWS). SWS, also known as encephalotrigeminal angiomatosis, is a sporadic neurocutaneous disorder. It is characterized by a cutaneous facial angioma (port-wine stain or nevus plexus flammeus) that is associated with ipsilateral pial angiomatosis and seizures. The port-wine stain typically occurs in the ophthalmic distribution, followed by the maxillary distribution, of the trigeminal nerve (cranial nerve [CN] V). Rarely, the pial angiomatosis may be bilateral or contralateral to the facial angioma. Clinically, patients present with seizures (most common), hemiplegia, visual disturbances, and/or developmental delay.

The primary cause of the central nervous system malformation is failure to form normal cortical venous drainage in the involved portion(s) of the brain with either development or persistence of a leptomeningeal vascular plexus. Although any portion of the brain may be involved, the occipital and parietal lobes are most frequently involved. The overlying vascular plexus consists of thin-walled, dilated veins and capillaries. There is also an increase in the number and size of collateral medullary and subependymal veins on the affected side. The increased flow leads to hypertrophy and increased enhancement of the ipsilateral choroid plexus. Venous congestion results in underlying chronic venous ischemia and hypoxic parenchymal injury.

Imaging findings parallel the pathophysiology of the malformation. Enhanced studies reveal leptomeningeal enhancement of the pial angiomatosis, enhancement of the enlarged ipsilateral collateral medullary and subependymal veins, and hypertrophy and increased enhancement of the ipsilateral choroid plexus. Chronic venous ischemia underlying the angiomatosis results in parenchymal atrophy, decreased subcortical T2 signal intensity, and "tram-track" cortical calcifications. Late findings include compensatory ipsilateral calvarial thickening and enlargement of the paranasal sinuses (Dyke-Davidoff-Mason syndrome) as a result of underlying parenchymal volume loss. Orbital findings include choroidal angiomas, which may lead to glaucoma.

✓ Pearls

- SWS is characterized by a facial angioma, pial angiomatosis, cortical atrophy, and seizures.
- Imaging findings include cortical "tram track" calcifications, atrophy, and leptomeningeal enhancement.
- Increased collateral deep venous drainage results in increase size and enhancement of the choroid plexus.

Suggested Readings

Akpinar E. The tram-track sign: cortical calcifications. Radiology 2004; 231: 515–516

Smirniotopoulos JG, Murphy FM. The phakomatoses. Am J Neuroradiol 1992; 13: 725–746

Case 20

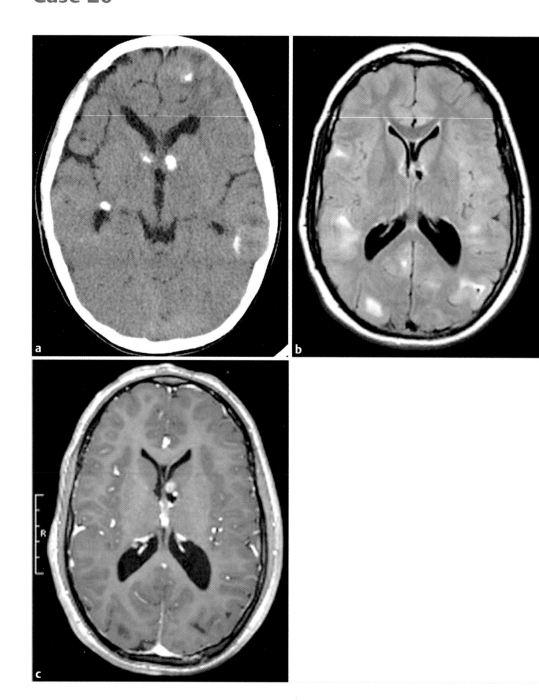

Fig. 20.1 Axial computed tomography image (a) demonstrates calcified subependymal lesions, regions of decreased cortical and subcortical attenuation, and regions of subcortical calcification. Axial fluid-attenuated inversion recovery image (b) shows multifocal wedge-shaped regions of increased cortical and subcortical signal intensity. Small focus of decreased subcortical signal intensity within the posterior left temporal lobe represents a small calcification. A small subependymal nodule is faintly seen within the frontal horn of the left lateral ventricles. Axial T1 postcontrast image (c) at the same level as image B reveals enhancement of the left frontal horn subependymal nodule.

■ **Clinical Presentation**

An adolescent boy with chronic seizures (▶ Fig. 20.1)

■ Key Imaging Finding

Partially calcified subependymal nodules and regions of cortical/subcortical signal abnormality

■ Diagnosis

Tuberous sclerosis (TS). TS, also known as Bourneville-Pringle syndrome, may occur sporadically or in an autosomal dominant fashion with variable penetrance. It is caused by gene mutations affecting hamartin (chromosome 9q34.3) and tuberin (chromosome 16p13.3). The classic clinical triad consists of facial angiofibromas, mental retardation, and seizures; however, all three components of the triad are only seen in ~30% of cases.

Central nervous system (CNS) manifestations include cortical/subcortical tubers, white matter lesions, subependymal nodules (98% of cases), and subependymal giant cell astrocytomas (SEGAs). Cortical/subcortical tubers and white matter lesions occur in the vast majority (95%) of cases. They are composed of a combination of disorganized glial tissue and heterotopic neuronal elements. A tuber is typically triangular in shape with its base along the cortical/subcortical junction and its tip pointing medially. Prior to myelination, tubers may appear hyperintense on T1 sequences. After myelination, tubers are typically T2 hyperintense unless calcified. Enhancement of tubers is relatively uncommon, occurring in ~10% of cases. The white matter lesions of TS occur in a radial distribution, extending from the ventricular margin to the overlying cortical/subcortical tuber. The radial pattern supports a component of abnormal neuronal migration.

At a young age, subependymal nodules demonstrate variable T1 and T2 signal intensity; however, they do not follow gray matter signal on all sequences as is seen with nodular heterotopia, which is one of the main differential considerations in a child with seizures and subependymal lesions. Many of the lesions will enhance. Nearly all subependymal nodules calcify by age 20, at which point they with demonstrate gradient echo susceptibility (hypointensity).

SEGAs are low-grade (World Health Organization grade I) tumors that result from degeneration of subependymal nodules in the region of the foramina of Monro. They occur in ~10 to 15% of patients with TS. Interval growth of a subependymal lesion is the most specific and reliable finding to suggest development of an SEGA. Enhancement is not a distinguishing factor because both subependymal nodules and SEGAs may enhance. Treatment of SEGA is typically geared toward cerebrospinal fluid diversion in the setting of obstruction, rather than resection of the lesions.

Additional manifestations of TS include retinal hamartomas, cardiac rhabdomyomas, renal cysts and angiomyolipomas, pulmonary lymphangioleiomyomatosis, subungual fibromas, and skin lesions, such as "ash-leaf spots" and shagreen patches.

✓ Pearls

- The classic triad of facial angiofibromas, mental retardation, and seizures is seen in ≅30% of cases.
- CNS manifestations of TS include cortical/subcortical tubers, white matter lesions, and subependymal nodules.

- SEGAs occur in ≅10 to 15% of cases; interval growth of a subependymal nodule is the most specific sign.

Suggested Reading

Braffman BH, Bilaniuk LT, Naidich TP et al. MR imaging of tuberous sclerosis: pathogenesis of this phakomatosis, use of gadopentetate dimeglumine, and literature review. Radiology 1992; 183: 227–238

Case 21

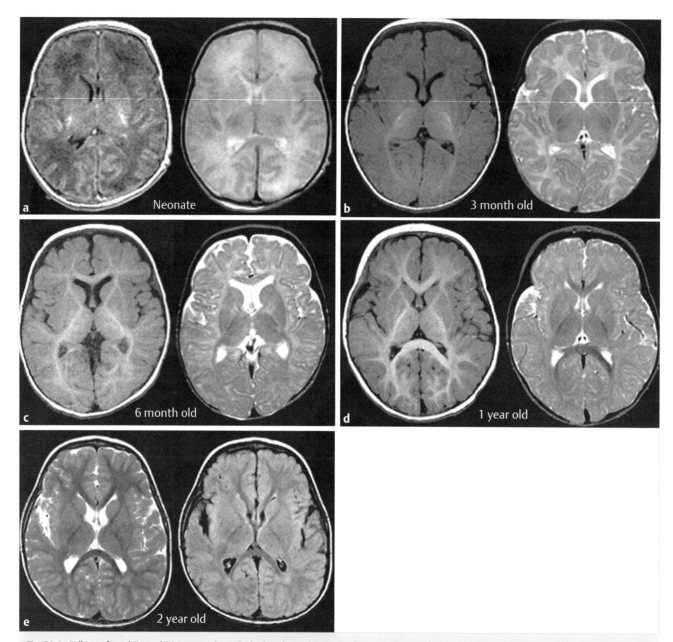

Fig. 21.1 Collage of axial T1 and T2 images through the basal ganglia, deep white matter, and thalami at various stages of the first year of life **(a–d)** demonstrate varying degrees of progressive white matter myelination, characterized by increased T1 and decreased T2 signal intensity. Regions of myelination are depicted earlier on T1 sequences. The neonatal T1 image **(a)** reveals myelination within the posterior limb of the internal capsules and ventral lateral thalami. At 3 months of age **(b)**, myelination on T1 extends into the anterior limb of the internal capsules and has progressed along optic pathways. By 6 months of age **(c)**, the internal capsules, genu of the corpus callosum, much of the deep white matter, and portions of the subcortical white matter are myelinated on T1. T1 signal intensity at 1 year of age **(d)** is similar to an adult brain. Axial T2 and fluid-attenuated inversion recovery images in a 2-year-old **(e)** show white matter signal intensity similar to that of an adult brain.

▩ Clinical Presentation

Children of various ages with noncontributory clinical findings (▶ Fig. 21.1)

■ **Key Imaging Finding**

Appropriate myelination for age

■ **Diagnosis**

Patterns of myelination. From infancy through the first few years of life, white matter tracts become myelinated in a fairly predictable pattern, although there is a spectrum of normal variation. Magnetic resonance imaging (MRI) provides a means of determining whether patterns and progression of myelination in a particular patient are normal, delayed, or abnormal. To make this determination, however, one must be familiar with the general patterns and age-specific milestones of myelination on different MR sequences.

T1- and T2-weighted sequences remain the primary sequences to evaluate patterns of myelination. Diffusion tensor imaging allows for assessment of myelination based upon the inherent directionality of anisotropy within myelinated white matter but has not yet become widely used in most imaging centers. T2 fluid-attenuated inversion recovery is substandard in assessment of unmyelinated white matter; therefore, its use is generally not recommended until the final stages of myelination (usually 18 to 24 months of age).

Myelination follows a predictable pattern in both distribution and age of onset. Additionally, myelination patterns mirror functional developmental milestones seen clinically. In general, myelination progresses from caudal to rostral, posterior to anterior, and centrally to peripherally. Visual and motor pathways myelinate earlier than association pathways, which correlates to relatively early progression of infants' visual and motor function.

In an infant brain with limited myelination, the gray-white matter differentiation is reversed from that of an adult. At birth, the white matter is hypointense on T1 and hyperintense on T2 sequences compared with gray matter. As specific regions are myelinated, they become hyperintense on T1 and hypointense on T2 compared with gray matter. Myelin-associated signal changes are seen earlier on T1 sequences; therefore, T1 sequences are most useful in the first year of development. In the second year of life, T2 sequences better depict the patterns of normal myelination. Even though the brain parenchyma eventually demonstrates a similar MR appearance to that of an adult (12 months of age on T1; 24 months of age on T2), myelination continues throughout childhood.

On T1 sequences in a neonate, myelination may be seen as regions of hyperintense signal in the medulla, dorsal pons, midbrain, brachium pontis, cerebellar peduncles, cerebral peduncles, ventral lateral thalami, posterior limbs of the internal capsules, corticospinal tracts, and within the optic nerve and portions of the visual pathways. At around 3 months of age, myelination is seen in the anterior limb of the internal capsules and cerebellum and continues in the optic pathways. The splenium of the corpus callosum begins to myelinate by 4 months of age and extends to the genu by 6 months of age. Subcortical white matter myelination begins around 3 months of age and typically involves the subcortical U-fibers by 7 months of age. Myelination of the subcortical regions of the frontal and temporal lobes progresses more slowly than other portions of the brain. By 12 months of age, the brain has a similar appearance to that of an adult on T1 sequences.

Myelination on T2 sequences follows a similar pattern to T1 but at later stages. In the neonate, decreased signal associated with myelination is seen in the medulla, dorsal pons, cerebellar peduncles, midbrain, and ventral lateral thalami. By 2 months of age, myelination involves the brachium pontis, posterior limb of the internal capsule, and corticospinal tracts. At 4 months of age, myelination is seen in the optic nerves and portions of the optic pathways. Myelination of the corpus callosum is noted in the splenium at 6 months of age and extends to the genu by 8 months of age, along with the anterior limb of the internal capsule. The ventral pons shows myelination at 6 months of age; the cerebellum is myelinated between 12 and 18 months of age. Central hemispheric white matter myelination is seen at 7 months posteriorly and 11 months anteriorly. Subcortical myelination is noted posteriorly by 15 months and anteriorly at 24 months. By 24 months of age, the brain has a similar appearance to that of an adult on T2 sequences.

✓ **Pearls**

- Myelination follows a predictable pattern in both distribution and age of onset.
- Myelination progresses from caudal to rostral, posterior to anterior, and centrally to peripherally.
- Myelination patterns are best depicted on T1 sequences in the first year of life and T2 during the second year.

Suggested Reading

Welker KM, Patton A. Assessment of normal myelination with magnetic resonance imaging. Semin Neurol 2012; 32: 15–28

Case 22

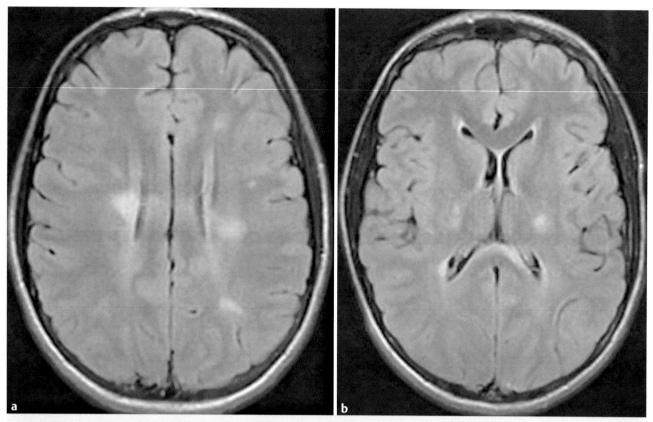

Fig. 22.1 Axial fluid-attenuated inversion recovery (FLAIR) images demonstrate numerous ovoid hyperintense periventricular lesions oriented perpendicular to the lateral ventricles **(a)**. Abnormal increased FLAIR signal intensity is also noted within the posterior limbs of the internal capsules, posterior aspect of the lentiform nuclei, and along the inner margin of the splenium of the corpus callosum **(b)**.

■ Clinical Presentation

A young adult woman with visual changes and transient numbness of the upper extremities (► Fig. 22.1)

▨ Key Imaging Finding

Multifocal regions of periventricular signal abnormality

▨ Top 3 Differential Diagnoses

- **Microvascular ischemic disease (MID).** MID is common in middle-aged and elderly individuals. It may be advanced for age with hypertension, diabetes, and hyperlipidemia. Magnetic resonance imaging (MRI) demonstrates asymmetric white matter T2 hyperintensities without enhancement, except for subacute infarcts that may enhance. White matter involvement may be patchy or confluent. Lacunar infarcts demonstrate signal intensity similar to cerebrospinal fluid with surrounding gliosis; common locations include the basal ganglia, thalami, deep white matter, and brain stem.
- **Demyelinating disease.** Multiple sclerosis (MS) demonstrates perpendicular periventricular T2 hyperintensities with perivenular extension ("Dawson fingers"). Lesions are bilateral and often involve the corpus callosum, cerebellum, and cerebellar peduncles. There is enhancement and possible restricted diffusion during active demyelination. Plaques may occasionally be masslike or tumefactive. Optic neuritis is commonly seen. Clinically, MS has a relapsing, remitting course. Acute disseminated encephalomyelitis is a monophasic process affecting children and young adults following a viral infection or vaccination. It is similar in appearance to MS but is more likely to be confluent and involve gray matter structures. Both processes may involve the brain stem and spinal cord.
- **Infectious/inflammatory.** Lyme disease and sarcoid are systemic processes that may involve the central nervous system (CNS). Lyme disease is a tick-borne illness caused by the spirochete *Borrelia burgdorferi*. It occurs in northern climates during warm months. White matter lesions simulate MS; however, patients also have a viral-like illness or rash. Enhancement is variable. Cranial nerve (CN; especially CN VII) and meningeal involvement is common. Sarcoid is a granulomatous disease that is most common in young African Americans. Symptomatic CNS involvement occurs in about 5% of patients. It preferentially involves the basal cisterns. Meningeal, CN, infundibular, and perivascular infiltration and enhancement are the most common patterns. Parenchymal lesions occur in about 30% of cases.

▨ Additional Differential Diagnoses

- **Vasculopathy.** Vasculitis results in inflammatory infiltration of arterial walls. Causative etiologies include autoimmune, infection or granulomatous disease, radiation, and drugs. MRI demonstrates bilateral regions of superficial and deep gray and white matter signal abnormality. Gradient echo imaging may reveal hemorrhage, which is common in vasculitis. Patchy enhancement may be seen. Angiography is often necessary to visualize characteristic alternating regions of stenosis and dilatation because MR angiography and computed tomography (CT) angiography are less sensitive. Biopsy is diagnostic. Patients with migraine headaches are also prone to white matter lesions, thought to be secondary to a form of vasculopathy.
- **CADASIL.** Cerebral autosomal dominant arteriopathy with subcortical infarcts and leukoencephalopathy results from a defect of chromosome 19. Arteriopathy of the small penetrating vessels results in multiple infarcts, transient ischemic attacks, and migraines in young to middle-aged adults. Ischemic changes are most notable in the deep gray and white matter. Subcortical involvement of the anterior temporal lobes is highly characteristic.
- **Susac syndrome.** Susac syndrome is a rare autoimmune microangiopathy that results in encephalopathy, hearing loss, and retinal artery occlusions. It presents in young to middle-aged adults and is more common in women. Although typically self-limiting over the span of a few years, deficits may be permanent. MRI demonstrates multiple round lesions involving the periventricular white matter, corpus callosum (midsubstance), deep gray and white matter, and brain stem. Enhancement and restricted diffusion may be seen.

▨ Diagnosis

Demyelinating disease (multiple sclerosis)

✓ Pearls

- Demyelinating lesions affect the periventricular white matter, corpus callosum, posterior fossa, and brain stem.
- MID results in patchy or confluent white matter lesions; it may be advanced for age with co-morbid conditions.
- Lyme disease and sarcoid may occasionally result in CNS involvement; lesions mimic demyelinating plaques.

Suggested Readings

Cross AH, Trotter JL, Lyons J. B cells and antibodies in CNS demyelinating disease. J Neuroimmunol 2001; 112: 1–14

Hildenbrand P, Craven DE, Jones R, Nemeskal P. Lyme neuroborreliosis: manifestations of a rapidly emerging zoonosis. Am J Neuroradiol 2009; 30: 1079–1087

Pomper MG, Miller TJ, Stone JH, Tidmore WC, Hellmann DB. CNS vasculitis in autoimmune disease: MR imaging findings and correlation with angiography. Am J Neuroradiol 1999; 20: 75–85

Case 23

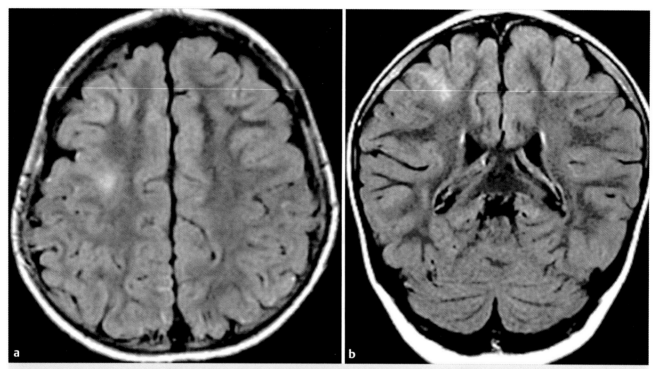

Fig. 23.1 Axial **(a)** and coronal **(b)** FLAIR images demonstrate a focal region of ill-defined increased signal intensity involving the right frontal cortex and subcortical white matter with blurring of the gray-white matter junction.

▨ Clinical Presentation

A 6-year-old girl with seizures (▸ Fig. 23.1)

■ Key Imaging Finding

Solitary region of cortical/subcortical signal abnormality in a child with seizures

■ Top 3 Differential Diagnoses

- **Cortical dysplasia.** Focal cortical dysplasia (FCD) is a neuronal migrational disorder characterized by abnormal cortical development secondary to some form of insult. There are two distinct subtypes: type 1 in which there is abnormal cortical development without abnormal neurons, and type 2 in which there is both abnormal cortical development and dysmorphic neurons. Taylor dysplasia is a subset of type 2 that contains characteristic balloon cells on pathologic examination. On magnetic resonance imaging (MRI), cortical dysplasia presents with focal abnormal increased T2/fluid-attenuated inversion recovery (FLAIR) signal intensity involving the cortex and subcortical white matter with blurring of the gray-white matter junction. The signal abnormality is commonly wedge-shaped with tapered signal pointing toward the ventricles. The overlying cortex may be thickened. Regions of increased cortical signal intensity on heavily T1-weighted sequences are fairly characteristic and helpful in distinguishing from neoplasms.
- **Gliosis.** Gliosis refers to nonspecific astrocyte proliferation and scar formation in response to some form of insult. It typically involves the subcortical and periventricular white matter. Common causes include hypoxemia/ischemia, infectious or inflammatory processes, trauma, vasculitis, demyeli-

nating disease, and neurodegenerative disorders. On MRI, gliosis presents as regions of increased T2/FLAIR signal. Enhancement may occasionally be seen, especially in the setting of active demyelination or subacute infarct. On follow-up studies, regions of gliosis are typically stable, although progression may be seen if causative factors persist.
- **Low-grade neoplasm.** Low-grade neoplasms may cause seizures, especially when cortically based. Gliomas are most common and present as fairly well-circumscribed regions of increased T2/FLAIR signal abnormality involving the gray or white matter. Enhancement is absent or minimal when low grade. Oligodendrogliomas are less common. They are typically centered within the white matter with extension to the cortex and have a higher incidence of calcification (~75 to 90%). Additional epileptogenic tumors include ganglioglioma (most common), dysembryoplastic neuroepithelial tumor (DNET), and pleomorphic xanthoastrocytoma (PXA). These are most often seen in the temporal lobes in younger patients, are cortically based, and have overlapping imaging characteristics; most demonstrate signal abnormality with no or minimal surrounding edema. Enhancement and cystic changes are variable but most common with ganglioglioma and PXA. DNET is associated with regions of cortical dysplasia.

■ Additional Differential Diagnoses

- **Encephalitis.** Encephalitis refers to focal parenchymal infection due to hematogenous or direct spread of infectious and inflammatory cells. With direct spread, the infection is often focal, whereas hematogenous spread often results in multifocal regions of involvement. Patients typically present with seizures, headaches, and focal neurological deficits. MRI shows ill-defined regions of increased T2 and decreased T1 signal intensity. Enhancement, if any, is usually ill-defined or linear. The presence of meningeal enhancement is more suggestive of infection, although some cortically based tumors

may also result in focal meningeal enhancement. Restricted diffusion may be seen acutely.
- **Seizure edema.** Seizures result in focal increased cerebral perfusion and disruption of the blood–brain barrier. There is associated ill-defined edema involving the cortex and subcortical white matter. Enhancement may occasionally be seen. Follow-up imaging after cessation of seizures demonstrates improvement or resolution. It is important to remember that the region of edema may be remote from the actual seizure focus.

■ Diagnosis

Focal cortical dysplasia

✓ Pearls

- FCD presents with abnormal cortical/subcortical signal intensity and blurring of the gray-white matter junction.
- Cortically based low-grade neoplasms may cause seizures; gliomas and gangliogliomas are most common.

- Encephalitis refers to focal parenchymal infection; meningeal enhancement, if present, is a helpful discriminator.

Suggested Readings

Lee BC, Schmidt RE, Hatfield GA, et al. MRI of focal cortical dysplasia. Neuroradiology 1998; 40: 675–683

O'Brien WT. Imaging of CNS infections in immunocompetent patients. J Am Osteopath Coll Radiol 2012; 1: 3–9

Venkatramana R, Vattipally MD, Bronen RA. MR imaging of epilepsy: strategies for successful interpretation. Radiol Clin North Am 2006; 44: 111–133

Case 24

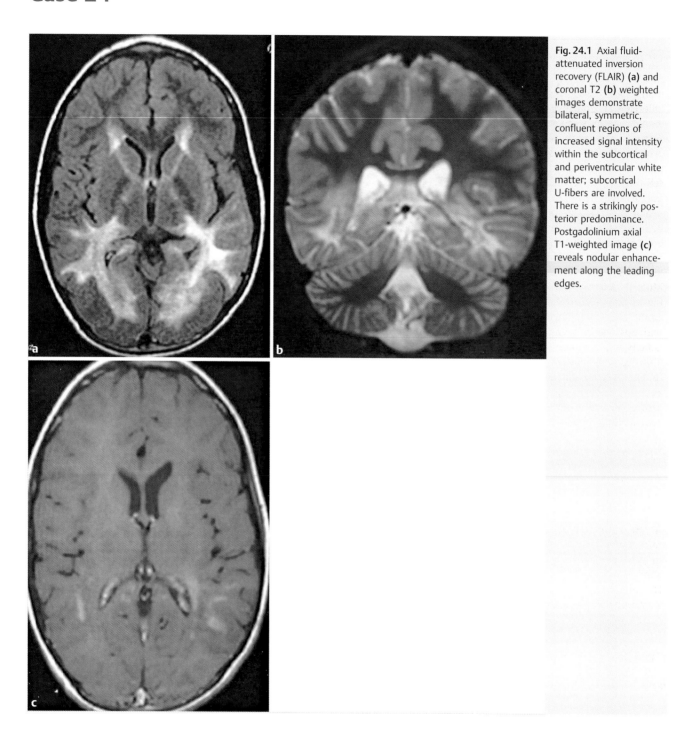

Fig. 24.1 Axial fluid-attenuated inversion recovery (FLAIR) **(a)** and coronal T2 **(b)** weighted images demonstrate bilateral, symmetric, confluent regions of increased signal intensity within the subcortical and periventricular white matter; subcortical U-fibers are involved. There is a strikingly posterior predominance. Postgadolinium axial T1-weighted image **(c)** reveals nodular enhancement along the leading edges.

■ **Clinical Presentation**

A 4-year-old boy with new onset developmental delay (▶ Fig. 24.1)

■ Key Imaging Finding

Confluent white matter lesions in a child

■ Top 3 Differential Diagnoses

- **Acute disseminating encephalomyelitis (ADEM).** ADEM is a monophasic demyelinating disease that occurs in children following an antecedent viral infection or vaccination. The demyelination is thought to be secondary to an autoimmune response against myelin due to cross-reaction with a viral protein. Patients present with neurological deficits that mimic multiple sclerosis (MS). Disease course varies from self-limiting to fulminant, hemorrhagic encephalitis. Computed tomography and magnetic resonance imaging (MRI) reveal large, usually bilateral, white matter lesions that are high signal on T2. Postcontrast images may demonstrate open-ring or nodular enhancement, corresponding to active regions of demyelination. Compared with MS, ADEM is more likely to be confluent and involve gray matter.

- **Multiple sclerosis (MS).** MS is the most common demyelinating disease. It occurs preferentially in young to middle-aged women, but also affects men and children. Patients present with optic neuritis, cranial neuropathies, and/or sensorimotor deficits, which typically resolve prior to subsequent episodes. Most patients have a relapsing and remitting course. MR findings include increased T2 signal intensity within the periventricular white matter, optic pathways, corpus callosum, cerebellum, cerebellar peduncles, and brain stem/cord. Periventricular lesions are ovoid and oriented perpendicular to the ventricles, resulting in characteristic lesions referred to as "Dawson fingers." Active regions of demyelination may enhance in a nodular or ring pattern with the open ring toward the overlying cortex. Compared with adults, children with MS tend to have fewer but larger lesions with less enhancement. The Marburg variant of MS is a fulminant, aggressive form that leads to rapid death. Schilder disease is a rare progressive form of MS that begins in childhood. Devic disease (neuromyelitis optica) affects the optic nerves and spinal cord with sparring of the brain parenchyma; Devic disease is now considered a separate entity from MS because it responds differently to therapy.

- **Dysmyelinating disease.** Leukodystrophies are a group of rare metabolic disorders characterized by dysmyelination secondary to accumulation of toxic metabolites as a result of enzyme deficiencies (lysosomal, peroxisomal, or mitochondrial disorders). Patients present most commonly at an early age with visual or behavioral disturbances. MRI demonstrates bilateral symmetric increased T2 signal intensity along white matter tracts. Metachromatic leukodystrophy has a predilection for the occipital lobes and splenium of the corpus callosum with sparing of subcortical U-fibers; adrenoleukodystrophy has a similar pattern, commonly affects males (x-linked), also affects the adrenal glands, and involves subcortical U-fibers in late stages of the disease; Alexander disease has frontal lobe predominance; and Canavan disease is associated with increased levels of N-acetyl aspartate on spectroscopy. Both Alexander and Canavan disease often result in macrocephaly in addition to the white matter manifestations.

■ Additional Differential Diagnoses

- **Atypical infection.** The human immunodeficiency virus (HIV) may primarily affect the central nervous system, resulting in confluent, symmetric regions of periventricular signal abnormality, along with disproportionate atrophy for age. No enhancement should be seen. Progressive multifocal leukoencephalopathy is an atypical viral (JC virus) infection that occurs in immunosuppressed patients, most commonly in the acquired immune deficiency syndrome population. The infection affects oligodendrocytes, resulting in confluent regions of increased T2 signal intensity within the periventricular and subcortical white matter. Enhancement is unusual. White matter involvement may be bilateral but is typically asymmetric.

■ Diagnosis

Dysmyelinating disease (adrenoleukodystrophy)

✓ Pearls

- ADEM is a monophasic demyelinating process that follows an antecedent viral infection or vaccination.
- MS is the most common demyelinating process; multiple forms exist with varying presentations.
- Leukodystrophies are rare metabolic disorders that result in diffuse dysmyelination.
- HIV may result in confluent, symmetric regions of signal abnormality, along with disproportionate atrophy for age.

Suggested Readings

Banwell B, Shroff M, Ness JM, Jeffery D, Schwid S, Weinstock-Guttman B International Pediatric MS Study Group. MRI features of pediatric multiple sclerosis. Neurology 2007; 68 Suppl 2: S46–S53

Cheon JE, Kim IO, Hwang YS et al. Leukodystrophy in children: a pictorial review of MR imaging features. Radiographics 2002; 22: 461–476

Case 25

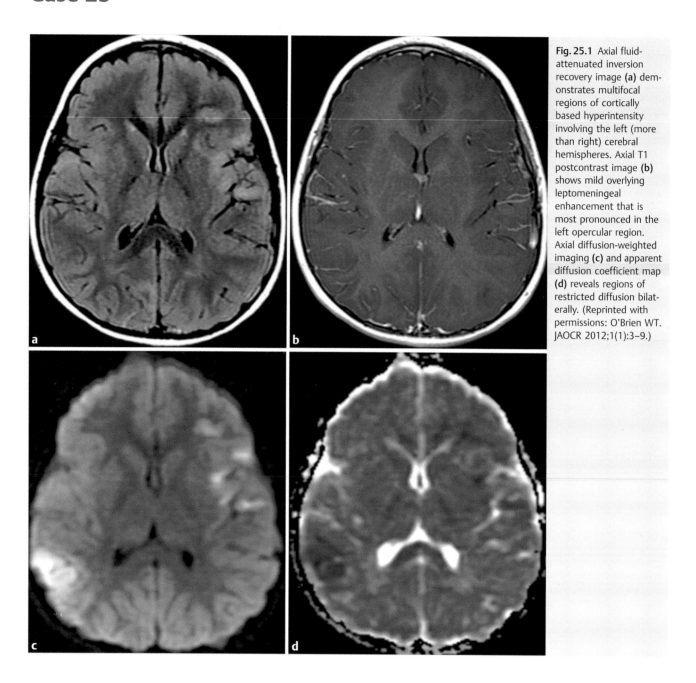

Fig. 25.1 Axial fluid-attenuated inversion recovery image (a) demonstrates multifocal regions of cortically based hyperintensity involving the left (more than right) cerebral hemispheres. Axial T1 postcontrast image (b) shows mild overlying leptomeningeal enhancement that is most pronounced in the left opercular region. Axial diffusion-weighted imaging (c) and apparent diffusion coefficient map (d) reveals regions of restricted diffusion bilaterally. (Reprinted with permissions: O'Brien WT. JAOCR 2012;1(1):3–9.)

■ Clinical Presentation

Adolescent with new onset headache and seizures (▶ Fig. 25.1)

■ Key Imaging Finding

Multifocal regions of cortical signal abnormality

■ Top 3 Differential Diagnoses

- **Cerebritis.** Cerebritis refers to focal infection of the brain parenchyma and may result from hematogenous spread, direct spread, or as a complication of meningitis. Direct spread tends to result in focal infection, whereas hematogenous spread and meningitis typically present with multifocal involvement. Patients present with fever, headache, seizures, or focal neurological deficits. On imaging, cerebritis presents as ill-defined cortical and subcortical hypoattenuation (computed tomography, CT) and increased T2/fluid-attenuated inversion recovery signal intensity (magnetic resonance imaging, MRI). Restricted diffusion may be seen, which may mimic an infarct acutely. Enhancement, if present, is ill-defined or thin and linear. Meningeal enhancement may also be seen.
- **Ischemia/infarcts.** Infarcts result from thromboembolic disease in older patients and vasculitis and arterial dissection in younger patients. They present as wedge-shaped regions of cortical and subcortical hypoattenuation on CT and T2 hyperintensity on MRI. Cytotoxic edema results in loss of gray-white matter differentiation and sulcal effacement. Acute infarcts demonstrate restricted diffusion. Gyral or patchy enhancement may be seen in the subacute phase. Perfusion imaging is useful in identifying the penumbra, which represents viable parenchyma at risk of infarct. CT angiography or MR angiography may show the region of vascular occlusion. Hemorrhagic transformation occurs in 15 to 20% of cases. Venous infarcts do not follow a vascular territory and are prone to hemorrhage.
- **Contusions.** Cerebral contusions result from traumatic injury as the brain parenchyma contacts the skull base or dural reflections. They occur most frequently along the inferior frontal lobes, anterior temporal lobes, and parasagittal locations. Contusions directly beneath the site of impact are referred to as coup injuries, whereas those on the opposite side of injury are referred to as contrecoup injuries. Acutely, there is cortical and subcortical edema and swelling. Foci of parenchymal or extraaxial hemorrhage are useful discriminators. Within the first 2 to 3 days, the contusions may expand with increase in amount of hemorrhage. In the chronic stage, regions of encephalomalacia are commonly seen.

■ Additional Differential Diagnoses

- **Vasculitis.** Vasculitides result in inflammation of arterial walls. Common etiologies include infectious, granulomatous (including primary angiitis of the central nervous system), collagen vascular diseases, radiation-induced, and drug-induced. Imaging findings range from normal to marked vascular and parenchymal abnormalities. Involved arteries demonstrate alternating regions of stenosis and dilatation. Parenchymal findings include regions of ischemia or infarct involving the superficial and deep gray and white matter. Restricted diffusion may be seen acutely. Lesions may enhance, especially in the subacute phase. Regions of microhemorrhage are seen as foci of hypointensity on gradient-echo and susceptibility-weighted imaging.
- **Cortical tubers.** Tuberous sclerosis is a neurocutaneous syndrome with a classic triad of facial angiofibromas, mental retardation, and seizures. Subependymal nodules and cortical tubers are present in the vast majority of cases. Tubers are composed of disorganized glial tissue and heterotopic neuronal elements. On imaging, they appear as wedge-shaped regions of cortical and subcortical signal abnormality with the tapered portion pointing medially. Prior to myelination, tubers may be hyperintense of T1; after myelination, they are typically T1 hypo- and T2 hyperintense. Tubers may occasionally enhance or calcify, which will alter the signal characteristics.
- **MELAS.** MELAS refers to mitochondrial encephalopathy with lactic acidosis and stroke-like episodes. It is an inherited mitochondrial disorder which is more common in boys and men. Patients present in adolescence or early adulthood with seizures and stroke-like episodes. Imaging reveals regions of attenuation and signal abnormality involving the cortex/subcortical white matter, as well as the basal ganglia and deep white matter. MR spectroscopy over the basal ganglia may reveal an elevated lactate peak, which is fairly characteristic of mitochondrial disorders.

■ Diagnosis

Cerebritis

✓ Pearls

- Cerebritis results from hematogenous or direct spread of infection or as a complication of meningitis.
- Thromboembolic disease, vasculitides, and arterial injury may result in cortical/subcortical ischemia or infarction.
- MELAS presents in adolescence or early adulthood with a seizures and stroke-like episodes.

Suggested Readings

O'Brien WT. Imaging of CNS infections in immunocompetent patients. J Am Osteopath Coll Radiol. 2012; 1: 3–9

Pomper MG, Miller TJ, Stone JH, Tidmore WC, Hellmann DB. CNS vasculitis in autoimmune disease: MR imaging findings and correlation with angiography. Am J Neuroradiol 1999; 20: 75–85

Case 26

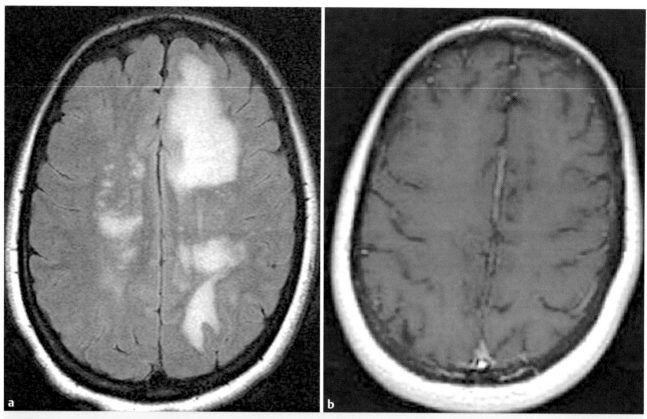

Fig. 26.1 Axial fluid-attenuated inversion recovery (FLAIR) **(a)** and T1 postgadolinium **(b)** MR images demonstrate extensive bilateral white matter FLAIR hyperintensity without significant mass effect and no enhancement. (Courtesy of Paul M. Sherman, MD.)

■ Clinical Presentation

A 45-year-old woman with seizures (▶ Fig. 26.1)

▨ Key Imaging Finding

Confluent white matter signal abnormality in an adult

■ Top 3 Differential Diagnoses

- **Demyelinating disease.** Multiple sclerosis (MS) demonstrates multiple perpendicular periventricular T2 hyperintensities with perivenular extension ("Dawson fingers"). The lesions are bilateral and asymmetric, often involving the optic pathways, corpus callosum, cerebellum, cerebellar peduncles (brachium pontis), and brain stem/cord. There is transient enhancement during active demyelination, which may be nodular or open ring-enhancing. Plaques may also be confluent or masslike (tumefactive). "Black holes" are hypointense on T1 and fluid-attenuated inversion recovery and represent chronic, burnt-out plaques. MS most commonly has a relapsing, remitting course, unlike acute disseminating encephalomyelitis, which is monophasic. Both processes may involve the spinal cord. Lyme disease is a tick-borne illness caused by the spirochete *Borrelia burgdorferi*. White matter lesions simulate MS, but there may be an associated viral-like illness or skin rash. Cranial nerve VII, leptomeningeal, and cauda equina involvement may be seen.
- **Neoplasm.** Gliomatosis cerebri is an infiltrating glial tumor that involves two or more lobes and may be bilateral. Although centered within the hemispheric white matter, the cortex may also be involved. There is relative preservation of the underlying brain morphology/architecture and no or minimal enhance-

ment. Anaplastic astrocytoma may be more discrete, with enhancement ranging from none to focal or patchy. Primary central nervous system (CNS) lymphoma characteristically involves the deep gray matter or periventricular white matter and classically involves the corpus callosum. There is often T2 hypointensity and computed tomography (CT) hyperdensity due to its high cellularity (small, round, blue cell tumor). Enhancement is typically homogeneous unless the patient is immunocompromised or steroids have been administered; then there may be ring enhancement.

- **Atypical infection.** The human immunodeficiency virus (HIV) may primarily affect the CNS, resulting in confluent, symmetric regions of periventricular signal abnormality, along with disproportionate atrophy for age. Progressive multifocal leukoencephalopathy is an atypical virus (JC virus) that affects oligodendrocytes. The vast majority of cases are seen in acquired immune deficiency syndrome patients. Magnetic resonance imaging (MRI) demonstrates confluent white matter T2 hyperintensities without mass effect and with characteristic involvement of the subcortical U-fibers. White matter involvement may be bilateral but is typically asymmetric. There is typically no enhancement; if present, it is faint and peripheral.

▨ Additional Differential Diagnoses

- **Microvascular ischemic disease.** Microvascular ischemic disease is common in the elderly population and can be advanced for age with comorbid conditions, such as hypertension, diabetes, and hyperlipidemia. Noncontrast CT reveals subcortical and periventricular white matter hypodensities; MRI demonstrates asymmetric white matter T2 hyperintense lesions without enhancement. White matter involvement may be confluent and extensive. Lacunar infarcts demonstrate signal intensity similar to cerebrospinal fluid with surrounding gliosis.

- **Autoimmune mediated vasculitis.** Vasculitis most commonly presents as multifocal gray and white matter lesions that are bilateral, usually cortical or subcortical, and often involve the basal ganglia and thalami. The lesions may mimic MS or infection if ring-enhancing. Gradient echo MR sequences may demonstrate foci of hemorrhage. Digital subtraction angiography (DSA) reveals alternating stenoses and dilatation involving the cerebral arterial vasculature.

■ Diagnosis

Progressive multifocal leukoencephalopathy (HIV patient)

✓ Pearls

- Demyelinating processes are a common cause of white matter lesions and may be confluent with extensive disease.
- Gliomatosis cerebri and lymphoma may present as infiltrating masses involving white matter tracts.

- Vasculitis presents as multifocal lesions with hemorrhage; DSA shows alternating stenoses and dilatations.
- Microvascular ischemic disease is common in elderly patients and can be advanced with comorbidities.

Suggested Readings

Bag AK, Curé JK, Chapman PR, Roberson GH, Shah R. JC virus infection of the brain. Am J Neuroradiol 2010; 31: 1564–1576

Filippi M, Rocca MA. MR imaging of multiple sclerosis. Radiology 2011; 259: 659–681

Case 27

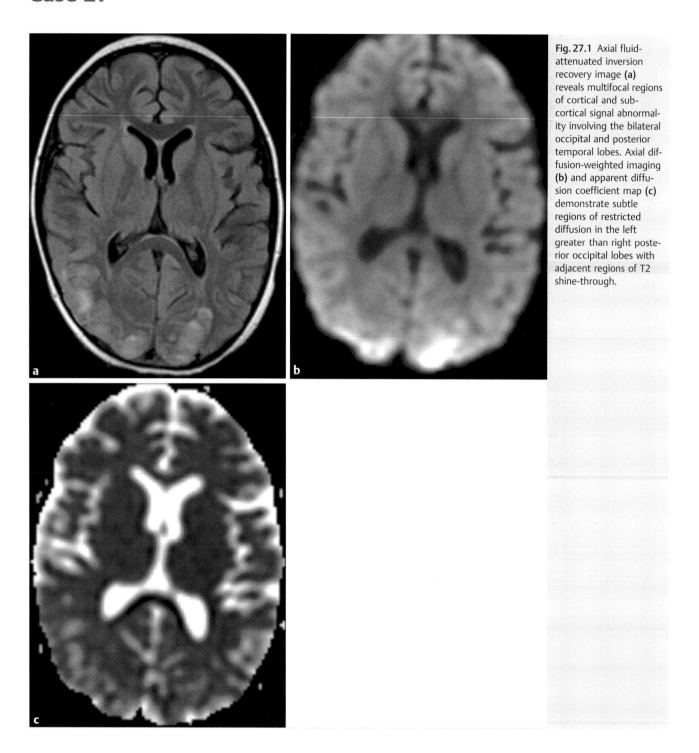

Fig. 27.1 Axial fluid-attenuated inversion recovery image (a) reveals multifocal regions of cortical and subcortical signal abnormality involving the bilateral occipital and posterior temporal lobes. Axial diffusion-weighted imaging (b) and apparent diffusion coefficient map (c) demonstrate subtle regions of restricted diffusion in the left greater than right posterior occipital lobes with adjacent regions of T2 shine-through.

■ **Clinical Presentation**

A young adult woman in acute renal failure with headache and visual changes (▶ Fig. 27.1)

▨ Key Imaging Finding

Posterior cortical/subcortical regions of signal abnormality

■ Top 3 Differential Diagnoses

- **Reversible hypertensive encephalopathy.** Reversible hypertensive encephalopathy (also referred to as posterior reversible encephalopathy syndrome, PRES) results in vasogenic edema secondary to failure of autoregulation during a hypertensive episode. The posterior circulation (occipital, parietal, and posterior temporal lobes) is most often involved due to relative decreased sympathetic innervation, limiting its ability to regulate intracerebral perfusion. Causative etiologies include preeclampsia/eclampsia, renal failure, and chemotherapeutic drug toxicities. Patients often present with headache and occasionally seizures. Increased perfusion pressures result in vasogenic edema with patchy regions of bilateral but usually asymmetric increased cortical and subcortical T2 signal intensity. The deep gray matter, brain stem, and cerebellum may also be involved. Restricted diffusion may be seen but is more worrisome for evolving infarct. There may be patchy enhancement. Magnetic resonance (MR) angiography may show regions of transient vasospasm in the posterior circulation. Regions of signal abnormality typically resolve after correction of the hypertensive episode, unless complicated by superimposed infarct.
- **Ischemia/infarct.** Bilateral posterior ischemic changes may result from arterial occlusion involving the vertebrobasilar system or generalized hypoperfusion affecting the posterior watershed distribution between the middle and posterior cerebral arteries. Arterial infarcts are often wedge-shaped with cytotoxic edema presenting as gyral swelling with sulcal effacement and loss of gray-white matter differentiation.

Restricted diffusion is seen in the acute setting; enhancement may be seen in the subacute phase. Bilateral ischemic changes may also be seen with venous infarcts, which typically occur in patients in a hypercoagulable state. Bilateral and often asymmetric regions of cytotoxic edema are seen. Venous infarcts are more likely to result in hemorrhage, especially when the thrombus extends into cortical veins. Computed tomography (CT) or MR venography is helpful in identifying the venous occlusion. The occlusion may also be seen as a region of increased T1 signal intensity or a region of central decreased enhancement (empty delta sign) on postcontrast CT and MR imaging (MRI).

- **Hypoglycemia.** Hypoglycemia may occur in neonates secondary to maternal diabetes or preeclampsia/eclampsia or in adults undergoing insulin therapy. The brain is especially susceptible to hypoglycemia because glucose is its main metabolite. Adult patients commonly present acutely with altered mental status and seizures. Pronounced hypoglycemia may result in coma. Neonates typically present with irritability, hypotonia, and seizures. Imaging demonstrates regions of cortical and subcortical hypoattenuation on CT and T2 hyperintensity with restricted diffusion (acutely) on MRI involving predominantly the occipital and parietal lobes. Temporal and frontal lobes are less often involved. The deep gray matter structures, to include the basal ganglia and thalami, may also be affected in more severe cases. The regions of restricted diffusion typically normalize with appropriate therapy; less often, they progress to frank infarcts.

■ Additional Differential Diagnoses

- **Seizure edema.** Seizures result in focal increased cerebral perfusion and disruption of the blood–brain barrier. There is associated edema involving the cortex and subcortical white matter with loss of gray-white matter differentiation and sulcal effacement. Enhancement may occasionally be seen. Follow-up imaging demonstrates improvement or resolution. It is important to remember that the region of edema may be remote from the actual seizure focus.

■ Diagnosis

Reversible hypertensive encephalopathy (PRES)

✓ Pearls

- PRES results in posterior (typically) edema secondary to failure of autoregulation during a hypertensive episode.
- Occlusion of the vertebrobasilar system, hypoperfusion, and venous infarcts may result in bilateral posterior ischemia.

- Hypoglycemia occurs in neonates and adults on insulin therapy; imaging findings mimic those of PRES.

Suggested Readings

Barkovich AJ, Ali FA, Rowley HA, Bass N. Imaging patterns of neonatal hypoglycemia. Am J Neuroradiol 1998; 19: 523–528

Lo L, Tan AC, Umapathi T, Lim CC. Diffusion-weighted MR imaging in early diagnosis and prognosis of hypoglycemia. Am J Neuroradiol 2006; 27: 1222–1224

McKinney AM, Short J, Truwit CL et al. Posterior reversible encephalopathy syndrome: incidence of atypical regions of involvement and imaging findings. Am J Roentgenol 2007; 189: 904–912

Case 28

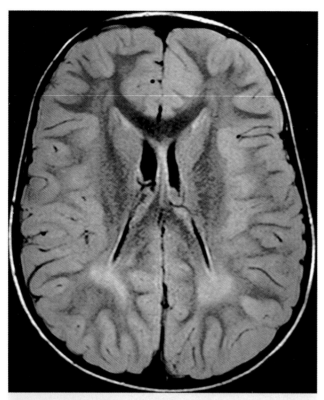

Fig. 28.1 Axial fluid-attenuated inversion recovery image demonstrates symmetric, hazy regions of increased signal intensity within the periatrial white matter.

■ Clinical Presentation

A 2-year-old boy with developmental delay (▶ Fig. 28.1)

▨ Key Imaging Finding

Periatrial signal abnormality in a young child

▨ Top 3 Differential Diagnoses

- **Delayed myelination.** Myelination occurs in a relatively predictable pattern with maturation progressing from central to peripheral, inferior to superior, and posterior to anterior. The pattern of myelination mirrors neurological development with early myelination of corticospinal and optic tracts, as well as the posterior brain stem. On magnetic resonance imaging (MRI), white matter approximates that of an adult brain on T1 sequences by 1 year of age and on T2 sequences by 2 years of age. The terminal zones of myelination include the periatrial white matter and subcortical white matter of the anterior frontal and temporal lobes. Patients with delayed myelination on imaging may be neurologically normal or demonstrate developmental delay.
- **Demyelinating disease.** Acute disseminated encephalomyelitis (ADEM) is the most common demyelinating disease in children. It is monophasic and occurs following an antecedent viral infection or vaccination. The disease course varies from self-limiting to fulminant, hemorrhagic encephalitis. MRI reveals regions of increased T2 signal abnormality within the white matter that may be confluent. Lesions are often bilateral but asymmetric. Involvement of the corpus callosum, optic pathways, cerebellar hemispheres, and brain stem is characteristic. Periventricular white matter lesions orient perpendicular to the ventricles, resulting in characteristic lesions referred to as "Dawson fin-

gers." Active lesions may demonstrate enhancement along the leading edge of demyelination in an "open ring" pattern. Multiple sclerosis (MS) occurs more frequently in adults and older children. As opposed to those with ADEM, patients with MS often have a relapsing and remitting rather than monophasic course. The imaging appearance may be identical to ADEM.
- **Metabolic disease.** Dysmyelinating diseases are rare metabolic disorders that occur secondary to accumulation of toxic metabolites as a result of enzyme deficiencies (lysosomal, peroxisomal, or mitochondrial disorders). Patients present at an early age with visual or behavioral disturbances. MRI demonstrates bilateral, symmetric regions of T2 hyperintensity along white matter tracts. Metachromatic leukodystrophy has a predilection for the occipital lobes and splenium of the corpus callosum with sparing of subcortical U-fibers; adrenoleukodystrophy has a similar pattern, commonly affects boys (x-linked), also affects the adrenal glands, and involves subcortical U-fibers; Alexander disease has frontal lobe predominance; and Canavan disease is associated with increased levels of N-acetyl aspartate on spectroscopy. Both Alexander and Canavan disease often result in macrocephaly. Canavan disease results in increased T2 signal within the thalami and globus pallidi. Krabbe disease characteristically results in hyperdensity of deep gray nuclei on computed tomography.

▨ Additional Differential Diagnoses

- **Neonatal hypoxic ischemic encephalopathy (HIE).** Parenchymal injury related to HIE is based upon the gestational age at the time of the insult, as well as the severity of the insult. Severe HIE affects the most metabolically active portions of the brain, including the deep gray and white matter. In preterm infants, mild to moderate HIE affects the periventricular white matter, resulting in signal abnormality and volume loss and often leading to periventricular leukomalacia. In full-term infants, mild to moderate HIE results in watershed ischemic changes, similar to the adult brain.

- **Atypical perivascular spaces.** Occasionally, regions of incidental, persistent, hazy periatrial signal abnormality may be associated with perivascular spaces. Perivascular spaces occur along a radial course from the periventricular region to the overlying cortex. Focal prominence is common in the basal ganglia, periatrial, and subcortical regions. Although they typically suppress on fluid-attenuated inversion recovery sequences, there may be atypical, hazy surrounding hyperintensity.

▨ Diagnosis

Hypo/delayed myelination

✓ Pearls

- Terminal zones of myelination include the periatrial and subcortical frontal and temporal lobe white matter.
- MS/ADEM result in asymmetric white matter lesions with characteristic morphology and distribution.

- Metabolic disorders result in bilateral, symmetric regions of confluent white matter signal abnormality.

Suggested Readings

Konishi Y, Kuriyama M, Hayakawa K et al. Periventricular hyperintensity detected by magnetic resonance imaging in infancy. Pediatr Neurol 1990; 6: 229–232

Nowell MA, Grossman RI, Hackney DB, Zimmerman RA, Goldberg HI, Bilaniuk LT. MR imaging of white matter disease in children. Am J Roentgenol 1988; 151: 359–365

Parazzini C, Baldoli C, Scotti G, Triulzi F. Terminal zones of myelination: MR evaluation of children aged 20–40 months. Am J Neuroradiol 2002; 23: 1669–1673

Case 29

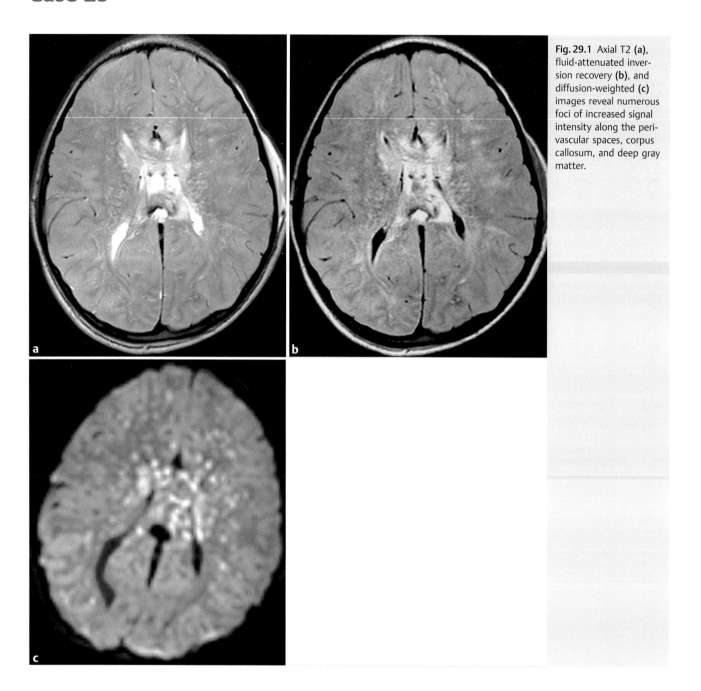

Fig. 29.1 Axial T2 **(a)**, fluid-attenuated inversion recovery **(b)**, and diffusion-weighted **(c)** images reveal numerous foci of increased signal intensity along the perivascular spaces, corpus callosum, and deep gray matter.

▓ Clinical Presentation

An 8-year-old boy with headache, fever, altered mental status, and diffuse petechial rash (▶ Fig. 29.1)

▓ Key Imaging Finding

Numerous foci of perivascular and deep gray/white matter signal abnormality

▓ Top 3 Differential Diagnoses

- **Cryptococcus.** Cryptococcus is a fungal infection that occurs in the setting of acquired immune deficiency syndrome (AIDS). It is the second most common opportunistic central nervous system (CNS) infection in AIDS after toxoplasmosis. It most often affects the CNS through hematogenous spread from a pulmonary infection. The most common imaging finding is multiple T2 hyperintense lesions involving the deep perivascular spaces, basal ganglia, and cerebral white matter. Four primary patterns of infection are recognized: granulomatous meningitis with nodular enhancement, dilated non-enhancing Virchow-Robin spaces representing cysts, "gelatinous pseudocysts" (which may or may not enhance) in the basal ganglia, and cryptococcomas with solid or ring-enhancing masses that often involve the choroid plexus. Hydrocephalus is commonly seen.
- **Lyme disease.** Lyme disease is a tick-borne illness caused by the spirochete *Borrelia burgdorferi*. It is endemic to northern climates and occurs during warm months. The infection is systemic with CNS involvement in more severe cases. The most common neurological imaging finding is abnormal cranial nerve (CN) enhancement, particularly of CN VII, which results in a Bell palsy. The infection may also spread to the meninges with associated clinical and imaging findings of meningitis, to include diffuse or focal leptomeningeal enhancement. Parenchymal involvement is relatively uncommon and results from small-vessel vasculitis. Magnetic resonance imaging (MRI) reveals multiple perivascular white matter lesions, which may simulate multiple sclerosis. Deep gray matter structures may also be involved. Parenchymal enhancement is variable. A key clinical distinction is the presence of a viral-like illness with a characteristic "bull's-eye" rash (erythema migrans) secondary to the tick bite.
- **Rocky Mountain spotted fever (RMSF).** RMSF is a tick-borne illness caused by the bacterium *Rickettsia rickettsii*. It typically occurs in wooded areas during late spring and early summer. The bacterium enters the bloodstream and results in a systemic small-vessel vasculitis. Patients most often present with fever, headache, and a rash that begins at the distal extremities and progresses proximally. The rash is maculopapular in its early stage and then becomes petechial with regions of necrosis. CNS manifestations vary from mild headache to a fulminant fatal meningoencephalitis. The small-vessel vasculitis preferentially involves the perivascular spaces, as well as the deep gray and white matter. MRI is more sensitive than computed tomography, better demonstrating involvement of perivascular spaces with surrounding gliosis. The perivascular involvement is somewhat similar to that of cryptococcus. Deep gray and white matter lesions are similar to that of other vasculitides, including Lyme disease. More extensive involvement of deep gray and white matter structures, to include the corpus callosum, is noted in severe cases. There may be restricted diffusion in the acute phase. If recognized early and treated appropriately, imaging findings may regress or resolve.

▓ Diagnosis

Rocky Mountain spotted fever

✓ Pearls

- Cryptococcus is a common fungal infection in the setting of AIDS; it preferentially involves perivascular spaces.
- Lyme disease is a tick-borne illness that is endemic to northern climates during warm months.
- CNS involvement with Lyme disease includes CN or meningeal enhancement and perivascular white matter lesions.
- RMSF causes small-vessel vasculitis that preferentially involves perivascular spaces and deep gray/white matter.

Suggested Readings

Baganz MD, Dross PE, Reinhardt JA. Rocky Mountain spotted fever encephalitis: MR findings. Am J Neuroradiol 1995; 16 Suppl: 919–922

Hildenbrand P, Craven DE, Jones R, Nemeskal P. Lyme neuroborreliosis: manifestations of a rapidly emerging zoonosis. Am J Neuroradiol 2009; 30: 1079–1087

Smith AB, Smirniotopoulos JG, Rushing EJ. From the archives of the AFIP: central nervous system infections associated with human immunodeficiency virus infection: radiologic-pathologic correlation. Radiographics 2008; 28: 2033–2058

Case 30

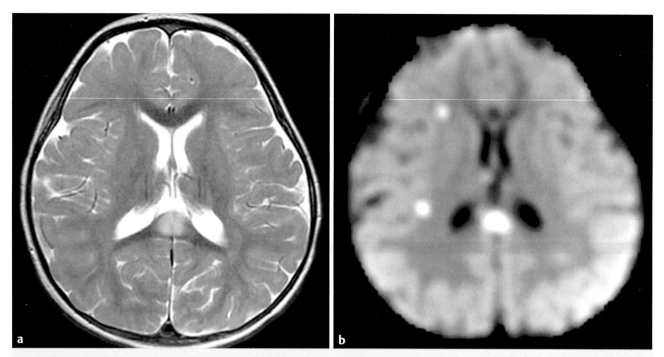

Fig. 30.1 Axial T2 image **(a)** demonstrates an ovoid region of increased signal intensity within the splenium of the corpus callosum. Diffusion-weighted image **(b)** reveals increased signal intensity, as well as additional lesions at the right insular gray-white matter junction and the medial right thalamus.

▨ Clinical Presentation

History withheld (▸ Fig. 30.1)

■ Key Imaging Finding

Corpus callosal signal abnormality

■ Top 3 Differential Diagnoses

- **Demyelinating disease.** Multiple sclerosis (MS) and acute disseminated encephalomyelitis (ADEM) are the most common demyelinating diseases. MS is more common in adults and ADEM primarily affects children. Characteristic imaging features include ovoid T2/fluid-attenuated inversion recovery hyperintense periventricular white matter lesions oriented perpendicular to the ventricles ("Dawson fingers"). High-specificity locations include the optic tracts, corpus callosum, cerebellum, brain stem, and cord. Transient enhancement (nodular or ring-enhancing) and restricted diffusion may be seen during periods of active demyelination. Tumefactive MS (large masslike enhancing lesions) is rare but may mimic neoplasm.
- **Diffuse axonal injury (DAI).** DAI results from white matter shear injury and presents as multifocal hemorrhagic or non-hemorrhagic lesions involving the gray-white matter junction (grade 1), corpus callosum (grade 2), deep gray matter, and dorsolateral brain stem (grade 3). Gradient-echo (T2*GRE) and susceptibility-weighted imaging sequences are sensitive for hemorrhagic shear injury due to susceptibility from blood products. Associated traumatic brain injury (contusions and extraaxial hemorrhage) is commonly seen.
- **Neoplasm (glioblastoma multiformes [GBM] and lymphoma).** GBM and lymphoma typically present as masses, as opposed to regions of signal abnormality. GBM is an aggressive World Health Organization grade IV astrocytoma and is the most common primary malignant brain tumor in adults. It extends across white matter tracts to involve the contralateral hemisphere, hence the term *butterfly glioma* of corpus callosum. It rapidly enlarges with central necrosis and neovascularity. There is marked mass effect; thick, irregular enhancement; and adjacent T2 hyperintensity that represents edema and tumor invasion. The tumor is primarily T2 hyperintense with necrosis and hemorrhage. Flow voids may be seen. Foci of restricted diffusion correspond to high cellularity or hemorrhage. GBM occurs at any age but is most common in middle-aged and elderly adults. Primary central nervous system lymphoma is almost exclusively of the non-Hodgkin variant. It occurs within the deep gray and white matter and commonly involves the corpus callosum and ependymal surfaces of the ventricles. Lymphoma may be solitary or multiple and circumscribed or infiltrative. Lesions are characteristically hyperdense on computed tomography, iso- to hypointense on T1 and T2 sequences, and demonstrate increased signal on diffusion sequences due to high cellularity. There is surrounding edema. Enhancement is homogenous in immunocompetent patients and peripheral or ring-enhancing in immunocompromised patients or after treatment. Unlike toxoplasmosis, lymphoma is hypermetabolic on thallium single-photon emission tomography and positron emission tomography imaging.

■ Additional Differential Diagnoses

- **Ischemia/edema.** In general, the corpus callosum is less prone to ischemic change due to the compact nature of white matter tracts; however, ischemic change and edema are increasingly more common. Ischemic change may occur anywhere within the corpus callosum, but is more common in the posterior body and splenium. Restricted diffusion may be seen acutely. Seizure-related edema has a propensity for the splenium, especially in children. The edema typically resolves after the seizure activity subsides, unless there are superimposed ischemic changes.
- **Toxic demyelination.** Chronic alcoholism (classically Italian red wine) and poor nutrition may result in focal demyelination, involving predominantly the splenium of the corpus callosum, termed *Marchiafava-Bignami*. Imaging findings of Wernicke encephalopathy are typically absent. Additional causes of toxic demyelination include medication toxicity secondary to chemotherapy, antiepileptic drugs, some antibiotics, and illicit drug abuse.

■ Diagnosis

Diffuse axonal injury (motor vehicle collision)

✓ Pearls

- Characteristic MS lesions include "Dawson fingers" and involvement of the corpus callosum and posterior fossa.
- DAI is due to shear injury and may involve the corpus callosum; GRE is most sensitive for hemorrhagic lesions.
- GBM and lymphoma are the most common neoplasms to involve and cross the corpus callosum.
- Ischemic changes and seizure-related edema may involve the corpus callosum.

Suggested Readings

McKinney AM, Kieffer SA, Paylor RT, SantaCruz KS, Kendi A, Lucato L. Acute toxic leukoencephalopathy: potential for reversibility clinically and on MRI with diffusion-weighted and FLAIR imaging. Am J Roentgenol 2009; 193: 192–206

Slone HW, Blake JJ, Shah R, Guttikonda S, Bourekas EC. CT and MRI findings of intracranial lymphoma. Am J Roentgenol 2005; 184: 1679–1685

Case 31

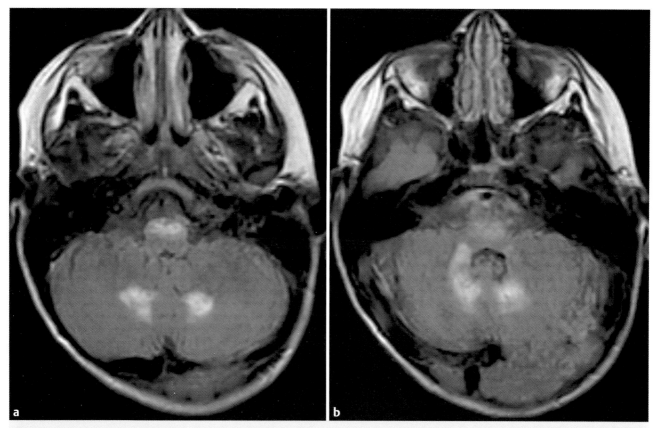

Fig. 31.1 Axial fluid-attenuated inversion recovery images reveal symmetric regions of signal abnormality involving the medial cerebellar hemispheres/nuclei, cerebellar peduncles, and brain stem [medulla **(a)** and pons **(b)**] without significant mass effect.

■ **Clinical Presentation**

A 5-year-old boy with developmental delay and altered mental status (▶ Fig. 31.1)

■ Key Imaging Finding

Diffuse cerebellar and brain stem signal abnormality in a child

■ Top 3 Differential Diagnoses

- **Rhombencephalitis.** Encephalitis refers to parenchyma infection due to hematogenous or direct spread of infectious and inflammatory cells. Causative organisms may be viral or bacterial. Bacterial infections are more common in immunosuppressed patients and are prone to abscess formation with delayed treatment. Viral meningitis favors the deep gray and white matter. Involvement of the hindbrain (cerebellum, pons, and medulla) is referred to as rhombencephalitis. On magnetic resonance imaging (MRI), viral encephalitis demonstrates regions of increased T2 signal intensity involving the deep gray and white matter structures, to include the cerebellum and brain stem. Enhancement is variable but typically patchy and ill-defined. Patients present with seizures or focal neurological deficits. Treatment is supportive with antibiotics for suspected bacterial infection. The infection may resolve or progress to abscess formation.

- **Demyelinating disease.** Acute disseminated encephalomyelitis (ADEM) is the most common demyelinating disease in children. It is monophasic and occurs following an antecedent viral infection or vaccination. MRI reveals increased T2 signal intensity within the white matter that may be confluent. Lesions are often bilateral but asymmetric. Involvement of the corpus callosum, cerebellar hemispheres, optic pathways, and brain stem is characteristic. Periventricular lesions are ovoid and perpendicular to the ventricles, resulting in characteristic "Dawson fingers." Active lesions may demonstrate solid or "open ring" enhancement. Multiple sclerosis (MS) occurs more frequently in adults and older children. Patients with MS typically have a relapsing and remitting rather than monophasic course. The imaging appearance may be identical to ADEM.

- **Infiltrating neoplasm.** Diffuse infiltrating pontine glioma (DIPG) is the most common brain stem neoplasm in children. It is a fibrillary World Health Organization grade II tumor; however, approximately half will develop anaplsia with progression to grade III (anaplastic) or IV (glioblastoma multiforme). The tumor is centered within the pons with spreading throughout the brain stem and into the cerebellum via the cerebellar peduncles. Exophytic components may engulf the basilar artery anteriorly or project into the fourth ventricle posteriorly. DIPG is hyperintense on T2/fluid-attenuated inversion recovery sequences. More aggressive components generally demonstrate increased enhancement, perfusion, and restricted diffusion. Prognosis is dismal with < 25% 10-year survival.

■ Additional Differential Diagnoses

- **Metabolic disease.** Maple syrup urine disease results from deficient metabolism of branched chain amino acids. Patients often present within the first 2 weeks of life with failure to thrive and an odor similar to maple syrup. Magnetic resonance imaging (MRI) reveals symmetric edema and restricted diffusion involving the brain stem, cerebellar white matter, thalami, globus pallidi, and perirolandic regions. Leigh syndrome is a mitochondrial disease that can affect infants and children. Patients present with failure to thrive, motor deficits, and seizures. MRI reveals symmetric increased T2 signal involving the deep gray matter, particularly the basal ganglia and thalami; dorsal brain stem; and, less frequently, the supra and infratentorial white matter. MR spectroscopy reveals an elevated lactate peak.

- **Neurofibromatosis type 1 (NF1) spots.** NF1 is the most common neurocutaneous syndrome. It is caused by a defect of chromosome 17 and results in increased incidence of neurofibromas and gliomas. Patients with NF1 have regions of myelin vacuolization that present as foci of increased T2 signal abnormality, most often involving the basal ganglia, thalami, dentate nuclei, cerebellar peduncles, brain stem, and optic radiations. These are commonly referred to as NF spots. Lesions wax and wane for the first decade of life and then regress.

■ Diagnosis

Metabolic disease (Leigh syndrome)

✓ Pearls

- Rhombencephalitis refers to infection of hindbrain structures, including the cerebellum, pons, and medulla.
- Demyelinating disease commonly involves the cerebellum and brain stem; ADEM is more common in children.
- Metabolic diseases are rare neurodegenerative processes with overlapping clinical and imaging manifestations.

Suggested Readings

Barkovich AJ, Good WV, Koch TK, Berg BO. Mitochondrial disorders: analysis of their clinical and imaging characteristics. Am J Neuroradiol 1993; 14: 1119–1137

Brismar J, Aqeel A, Brismar G, Coates R, Gascon G, Ozand P. Maple syrup urine disease: findings on CT and MR scans of the brain in 10 infants. Am J Neuroradiol 1990; 11: 1219–1228

Case 32

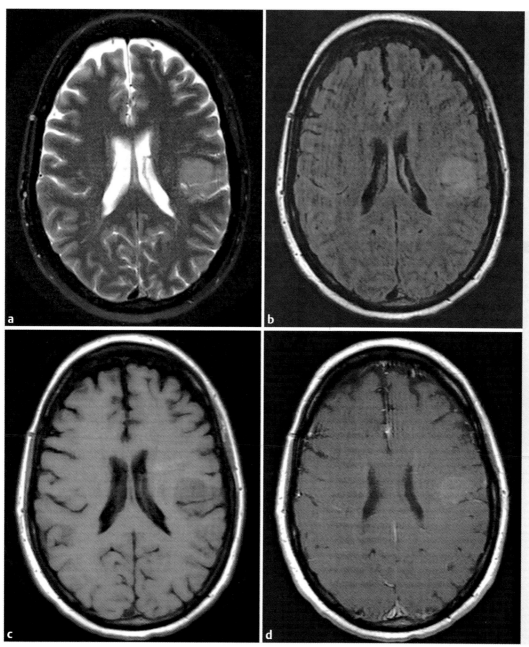

Fig. 32.1 Axial T2 (a) and fluid-attenuated inversion recovery (b) images of the brain demonstrate a relatively well-defined region of increased cortical and subcortical signal intensity within the left frontal lobe. The corresponding region is hypointense on T1 (c) and demonstrates mild enhancement after contrast administration (d).

▪ Clinical Presentation

A young adult woman with seizures (▶ Fig. 32.1)

■ Key Imaging Finding

Solitary region of cortical and subcortical signal abnormality in an adult

■ Top 3 Differential Diagnoses

- **Ischemia/infarct.** Cerebrovascular disease is common, especially in older patients, and most often results from thromboembolic arterial occlusion. In younger patients, vasculitis and dissection are prevalent. Patients present with focal neurological deficits, altered mental status, and/or aphasia. Arterial infarcts result in wedge-shaped regions of cortical and subcortical hypoattenuation (computed tomography, CT) and T2 hyperintensity (magnetic resonance imaging, MRI). Cytotoxic edema results in cortical swelling with effacement of adjacent sulci. Acute infarcts demonstrate restricted diffusion on MRI. Gyral or patchy enhancement may be seen in the subacute phase, beginning as early as 2 days and peaking around 10 to 14 days. CT angiography and MR angiography may show vascular occlusion. Perfusion imaging is useful in identifying the penumbra, which represents viable parenchyma that is at risk of infarct. Hemorrhagic transformation occurs in 15 to 20% of cases. Venous infarcts do not follow a vascular territory and are more prone to hemorrhage. CT venography or MR venography reveal the region of thrombosis.
- **Neoplasm.** Astrocytomas are the most common primary brain tumors in adults. Variants that present with cortical signal abnormality include fibrillary (World Health Organization [WHO] grade II) and anaplastic (WHO grade III). Fibrillary astrocytoma typically presents with indistinct or less commonly well-defined signal abnormality centered within the white matter with or without overlying cortical involvement. Enhancement, when present, is mild. Anaplastic astrocytoma is more aggressive with regions of increased perfusion, edema, and enhancement. MR spectroscopy reveals increased choline and decreased *N*-acetyl aspartate. Unlike infarcts, restricted diffusion is not typically seen, unless there is focal progression to a high-grade tumor. Oligodendrogliomas occur in middle-aged adults who present with seizures. They are centered within the subcortical white matter and commonly extend to the overlying cortex. The frontal lobe is the most common location. Lesions are well defined with little edema and mild enhancement. Regions of calcification are typically seen.
- **Cerebritis.** Cerebritis refers to focal infection of the brain parenchyma and may result from hematogenous spread, direct spread, or as a complication of meningitis. Patients present with fever, headache, seizures, or focal neurological deficits. On imaging, cerebritis presents as ill-defined cortical and subcortical hypoattenuation (CT) and increased T2/fluid-attenuated inversion recovery signal intensity (MRI). Restricted diffusion may be seen, which may mimic an infarct acutely. Enhancement, if present, is ill-defined or thin and linear. Meningeal enhancement is a useful discriminator.

■ Additional Differential Diagnoses

- **Contusion.** Cerebral contusions result from trauma as the brain parenchyma contacts the adjacent skull base or dural reflections. Common locations include the inferior frontal lobes, anterior temporal lobes, and parasagittal locations. Contusions directly beneath the site of impact are referred to as coup injuries, whereas those on the opposite side of injury are referred to as contrecoup injuries. Acutely, there is cortical and subcortical edema and swelling. Foci of parenchymal or extraaxial hemorrhage are hyperdense on CT and variable in signal on MRI depending upon the timing of imaging. MRI is more sensitive than CT and typically demonstrates additional foci of parenchymal injury, to include diffuse axonal injury, if present. Within the first 2 to 3 days, contusions may enlarge. Encephalomalacia is often seen chronically.
- **Seizure edema.** Seizure-related edema results in cortical and subcortical edema that is transient. It most often occurs in the setting of status epilepticus with continuous seizure activity that lasts for at least 30 minutes. Acutely, there is gyral swelling and sulcal effacement. Restricted diffusion and patchy enhancement may be seen. On follow-up imaging, the edema should decrease or resolve if the patient remains seizure-free. The regions of edema may or may not be in the same location as the underlying seizure focus.

■ Diagnosis

Low-grade (fibrillary) astrocytoma

✓ Pearls

- Infarcts typically result from thromboembolic disease; vasculitis and dissection are common in younger patients.
- Astrocytomas and oligodendrogliomas are the most common primary tumors with focal cortical signal abnormality.
- Contusions occur in characteristic locations with focal edema, swelling, and hemorrhage.

Suggested Readings

Koeller KK, Rushing EJ. From the archives of the AFIP: oligodendroglioma and its variants: radiologic-pathologic correlation. Radiographics 2005; 25: 1669–1688

O'Brien WT. Imaging of CNS infections in immunocompetent patients. JAOCR J Am Osteopath Coll Radiol. 2012; 1: 3–9

Case 33

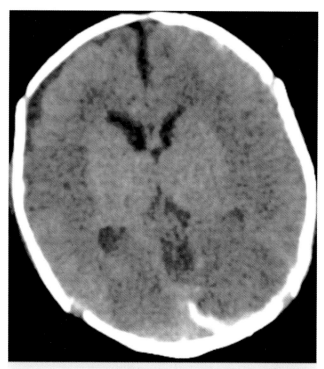

Fig. 33.1 Axial noncontrast CT image reveals diffuse cerebral edema with loss of gray-white matter differentiation and sulcal effacement bilaterally. Hyperdense subdural hemorrhage is noted along the posterior aspect of the falx and tentorium on the left.

■ Clinical Presentation

A 4-week-old boy with failure to thrive (▶ Fig. 33.1)

■ Key Imaging Finding

Diffuse cerebral edema in an infant

■ Top 3 Differential Diagnoses

- **Hypoxic-ischemic encephalopathy (HIE).** The neurological sequela of HIE depends upon a number of factors, including the severity of the insult, timing of the insult with respect to neuronal maturation, and duration of the insult. In the preterm infant, mild to moderate HIE results in injury to the periventricular white matter, resulting in periventricular leukomalacia. Early ultrasound imaging reveals hyperechoic periventricular white matter that may progress to cystic change with volume loss. Follow-up computed tomography (CT) or magnetic resonance imaging (MRI) will show abnormal signal and volume loss within the periatrial white matter with focal ventricular enlargement. The ventricles will have irregular margins. More severe HIE affects the deep gray matter structures (especially the thalami), brain stem, cerebellum, and cerebral cortex, particularly the perirolandic region. In full-term infants, mild to moderate HIE results in watershed ischemia, similar to adults. Abnormal hypoattenuation (CT) or signal (MRI) is seen in the cortex, subcortical white matter, and centrum semiovale of the watershed regions between the vascular distributions of the middle cerebral artery and the anterior and posterior cerebral arteries. More severe HIE is similar in the premature infant with less involvement of the cerebellum and increased involvement of the basal ganglia and cerebral cortex.
- **Trauma.** Trauma may be accidental or nonaccidental (NAT) with the main distinction being a history that is or is not compatible with the severity and pattern of injury. In direct blunt trauma (accidental or NAT), similar findings are seen as with adults, including skull fractures, extraaxial hemorrhage, and coup and contrecoup parenchymal injuries. It is important to describe the type, location, and pattern of injury, as well as to evaluate complications, such as herniation syndromes or ischemic changes. A subset of NAT includes "shaken baby" syndrome. With this type of injury, more specific findings are noted, including subdural hemorrhages with extension into the interhemispheric fissure and hypoxic-ischemic changes.

Rarely, retinal hemorrhages may be seen on imaging, although they are readily evident on physical examination. CT angiography or MR angiography may show regions of vascular injury or spasm. In the setting of NAT, it is important to remember that the density or signal of subdural hemorrhage is dependent upon numerous factors; therefore, pinpointing the precise age of an extraaxial collection is fraught with error. Additionally, the predictable pattern of hemorrhage evolution on MRI is derived from intraparenchymal hemorrhages and not extraaxial collections. If NAT is suspected, a skeletal survey should be performed and appropriate notifications must be made and documented.

- **Metabolic disease.** Numerous rare metabolic diseases may result in diffuse cerebral edema. Although the pattern of parenchymal involvement may suggest a particular process, a clinical workup is required to establish the diagnosis. Causes of diffuse cerebral edema in a neonate or infant include mitochondrial disorders, urea cycle disorders, and nonketotic hyperglycinemia. There are numerous variants of mitochondrial disorders that ultimately affect energy production due to enzyme deficiencies. Patients often present with encephalopathy or seizures. Imaging reveals abnormal attenuation (CT) and signal (MRI) involving the basal ganglia, cerebral white matter, cerebellum, and/or brain stem. Basal ganglia involvement is characteristic. In addition to parenchymal findings, Menkes disease (enlarged tortuous vasculature) and glutaric aciduria type 1 (widened Sylvian fissures with bilateral middle cranial fossa "cysts") may also present with subdural collections. Urea cycle disorders present acutely with diffuse cerebral swelling and abnormal hypoattenuation and signal involving the cortex, subcortical white matter, and deep gray nuclei. There is decreased swelling and parenchymal atrophy in the chronic phase. Nonketotic hyperglcinemia presents with abnormal attenuation and signal within the basal ganglia, corpus callosum, and cerebral cortex.

■ Diagnosis

Nonaccidental trauma

✓ Pearls

- Neurological sequela of HIE depends upon severity, duration, and timing of the insult with respect to brain maturation.
- HIE with cerebral edema may occur as a direct result or complication of trauma.

- Rare metabolic diseases may result in cerebral edema; an extensive workup is needed to establish the diagnosis.

Suggested Readings

Chao CP, Zaleski CG, Patton AC. Neonatal hypoxic-ischemic encephalopathy: multi-modality imaging findings. Radiographics 2006; 26 Suppl 1: S159–S172

Choi CG, Yoo HW. Localized proton MR spectroscopy in infants with urea cycle defect. Am J Neuroradiol 2001; 22: 834–837

Lonergan GJ, Baker AM, Morey MK, Boos SC. From the archives of the AFIP. Child abuse: radiologic-pathologic correlation. Radiographics 2003; 23: 811–845

Case 34

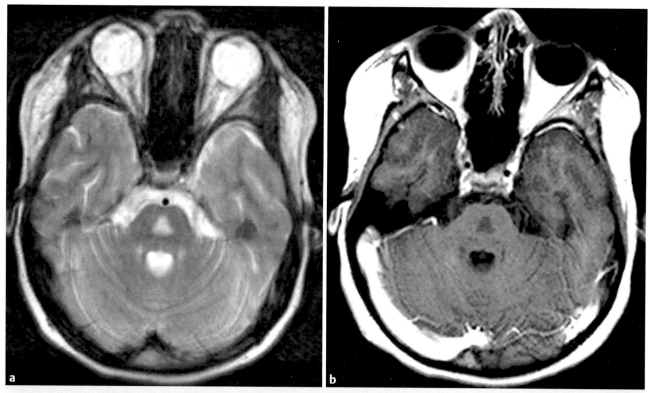

Fig. 34.1 Axial T2 **(a)** and T1 postcontrast **(b)** images reveal a triangular-shaped region of increased T2 and decreased T1 signal intensity within the central pons without enhancement.

■ Clinical Presentation

A young adult man with altered mental status (▶ Fig. 34.1)

■ Key Imaging Finding

Focal pontine signal abnormality

■ Top 3 Differential Diagnoses

- **Ischemia.** Microvascular ischemic disease (MVID) of the pons is relatively common in middle-aged and elderly patients, especially in the setting of hypertension, hyperlipidemia, and diabetes. As with other foci of MVID, lesions are hypodense on computed tomography and hyperintense on T2 sequences. Pontine infarcts typically result from occlusion of small perforators from the basilar artery. Infarcts from basilar artery occlusion are less common and may be catastrophic. Acutely, lesions demonstrate restricted diffusion; enhancement may be seen in the subacute phase. Lacunar infarcts follow cerebrospinal fluid signal intensity with a rim of gliosis.

- **Demyelinating disease.** Multiple sclerosis (MS) and acute disseminated encephalomyelitis (ADEM) are the most common demyelinating diseases. MS most commonly affects adults and has a relapsing and remitting course; ADEM is more common in children and is monophasic. Magnetic resonance imaging (MRI) reveals regions of increased T2 signal within the white matter that may be confluent. Lesions are often bilateral but asymmetric. Involvement of the corpus callosum, cerebellar hemispheres, optic pathways, and brain stem is characteristic. Periventricular lesions orient perpendicular to the ventricles, resulting in ovoid lesions referred to as "Dawson fingers." Active lesions may demonstrate solid or "open ring" enhancement, as well as restricted diffusion.

- **Osmotic demyelination.** Also known as central pontine myelinolysis, osmotic demyelination results from a rapid shift in osmolality, classically described with overzealous correction of hyponatremia. Approximately half of cases involve the central pons where lesions present as triangular or confluent T2 hyperintensities with sparing of corticospinal tracts. The remaining cases involve the deep gray and white matter, also referred to as extrapontine myelinolysis, with or without pontine involvement. Restricted diffusion may be seen acutely. Signal abnormality may regress over time.

■ Additional Differential Diagnoses

- **Vascular malformation (VM).** Cavernous malformations (CMs) and capillary telangiectases are the most common VMs to involve the brain stem. CMs are dilated vascular channels without intervening brain parenchyma. Lesions have a peripheral T2 hypointense hemosiderin rim and central regions of T1 and T2 hyper- and hypointensity, giving the characteristic "popcorn" appearance. Signal characteristics result from hemorrhages of different ages. Enhancement occurs in ~15% of cases. Surrounding edema may be seen with acute hemorrhage. Capillary telangiectases represent dilated capillaries with normal intervening brain parenchyma. They are asymptomatic, incidental lesions. Half will demonstrate subtle T2 hyperintensity; the remaining are occult on T2 sequences. Hypointensity is seen on gradient echo and susceptibility-weighted imaging. Lesions demonstrate faint brushlike enhancement.

- **Brain stem glioma.** Brain stem glioma represents approximately 10 to 20% of pediatric brain tumors and commonly presents in the first 2 decades of life. It typically presents as a diffuse, infiltrating pontine mass (World Health Organization grade II to III) that may have exophytic components. It is hyperintense on T2/fluid-attenuated inversion recovery sequences. More aggressive components demonstrate increased enhancement, perfusion, and restricted diffusion. Prognosis is dismal. The low-grade pilocytic variant is less common and presents as a cystic mass with enhancing nodule. It has an overall better prognosis.

- **Brain stem encephalitis.** Encephalitis refers to focal infection of the brain parenchyma. Viral etiologies more commonly affect the brain stem. Bacterial infections are more common in immunosuppressed patients. On MRI, encephalitis demonstrates regions of increased T2 signal intensity. Restricted diffusion may be seen. Enhancement is variable but typically patchy and ill-defined. The infection may resolve or progress to abscess formation.

■ Diagnosis

Osmotic demyelination (central pontine myelinolysis)

✓ Pearls

- MVID commonly involves the pons in older patients secondary to occlusion of perforating vessels.
- Osmotic demyelination results from rapid shift in osmolality; central pontine signal spares the corticospinal tracts.
- CMs have a characteristic "popcorn" appearance on MRI; capillary telangiectases have faint brushlike enhancement.

Suggested Readings

Smith AB. Vascular malformations of the brain: radiologic and pathologic correlation. J Am Osteopath Coll Radiol. 2012; 1: 10–22

Venkatanarasimha N, Mukonoweshuro W, Jones J. AJR teaching file: symmetric demyelination. Am J Roentgenol 2008; 191 Suppl: S34–S36

Case 35

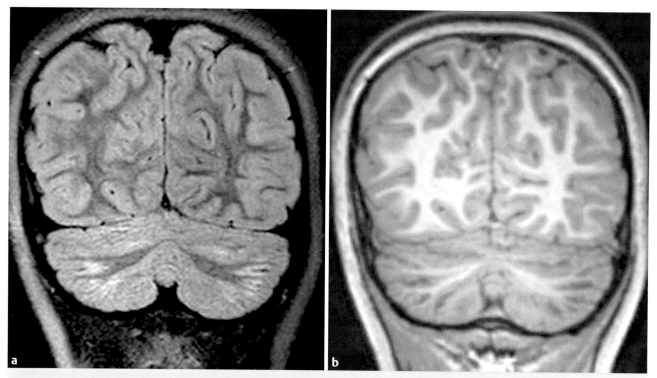

Fig. 35.1 Coronal fluid-attenuated inversion recovery (FLAIR) **(a)** and T1 **(b)** images demonstrate confluent regions of increased FLAIR and decreased T1 signal intensity involving predominantly the subcortical white matter of the cerebellar hemispheres. No enhancement was seen on postcontrast sequences (not shown).

■ Clinical Presentation

A 10-year-old boy with new onset ataxia (▶ Fig. 35.1)

■ Key Imaging Finding

Diffuse abnormal cerebellar signal

■ Top 3 Differential Diagnoses

- **Cerebellitis.** Cerebellitis most often involves children and young adults. Affected patients typically present with nausea, vomiting, and ataxia with or without systemic signs of infection. In some cases, the central nervous system manifestations occur weeks after an antecedent viral infection, similar to acute disseminated encephalomyelitis (ADEM). On imaging, cerebellitis often presents with patchy or confluent regions of hypoattenuation (computed tomography) or increased T2 and decreased T1 signal (magnetic resonance imaging, MRI) involving the cerebellar gray and white matter bilaterally. Patchy parenchymal or overlying meningeal enhancement may be seen. There is often T2 shine-through on diffusion-weighted imaging without restricted diffusion.
- **Demyelinating disease.** Multiple sclerosis (MS) and ADEM are the most common demyelinating diseases. ADEM is most common in children, is monophasic, and occurs following an antecedent viral infection or vaccination. Disease course varies from self-limiting to fulminant, hemorrhagic encephalitis. MRI reveals regions of increased T2 signal abnormality, some of which may be confluent, involving predominantly white matter. Gray matter involvement is more common with ADEM than MS. Lesions are often bilateral but asymmetric. Although isolated posterior fossa involvement may occur, supratentorial lesions are typically seen. Involvement of the corpus callosum, optic pathways, cerebellar hemispheres, and brain stem is characteristic of demyelinating disease. Periventricular demyelinating disease occurs along the perivenule spaces, resulting in ovoid white matter lesions oriented perpendicular to the ventricles, referred to as "Dawson fingers." Active lesions may demonstrate solid or "open ring" enhancement along the leading edge of demyelination; the open ring points toward the cortex. MS occurs more frequently in adults and older children. As opposed to those with ADEM, patients with MS typically have a relapsing and remitting rather than monophasic course. The imaging appearance may be identical to ADEM, although lesions are usually less confluent except in cases of advanced disease.
- **Infiltrating neoplasm.** The most common posterior fossa tumors in children include medulloblastoma, juvenile pilocytic astrocytoma, ependymoma, brain stem glioma, and atypical teratoid rhabdoid tumor. Aside from a diffuse infiltrating pontine glioma (DIPG), these tumors tend to be circumscribed and occur either midline (medulloblastoma and ependymoma) or within a cerebellar hemisphere. Isolated infiltrating cerebellar tumors without brain stem involvement are uncommon. Astrocytomas are most common with fibrillary (World Health Organization [WHO] grade II) or anaplastic (WHO grade III) variants. With higher-grade tumors, imaging demonstrates regions of enhancement and increased perfusion. Foci of restricted diffusion may also be seen. In adults, the most common cerebellar neoplasms include metastases (by far the most common) and hemangioblastoma. Infiltrating tumors in adults are exceedingly uncommon.

■ Diagnosis

Cerebellitis

✓ Pearls

- Cerebellitis presents as patchy or confluent regions of signal abnormality; meningeal enhancement may be seen.
- MS/ADEM may present as confluent cerebellar signal abnormality; supratentorial lesions are typically present.
- Isolated infiltrating cerebellar tumors are uncommon; DIPG may extend posteriorly to involve the cerebellum.

Suggested Readings

De Bruecker Y, Claus F, Demaerel P et al. MRI findings in acute cerebellitis. Eur Radiol 2004; 14: 1478–1483

Kornreich L, Schwarz M, Karmazyn B et al. Role of MRI in the management of children with diffuse pontine tumors: a study of 15 patients and review of the literature. Pediatr Radiol 2005; 35: 872–879

Case 36

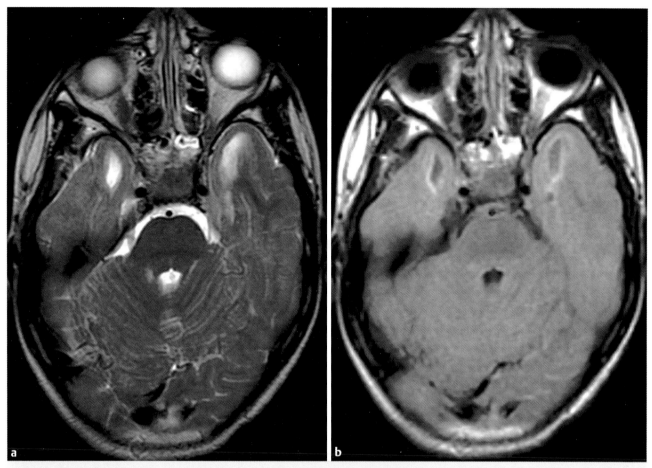

Fig. 36.1 Axial T2 **(a)** and fluid-attenuated inversion recovery **(b)** images demonstrate bilateral subcortical cysts within the anterior temporal lobes with surrounding gliosis **(b)**.

■ Clinical Presentation

Young girl with developmental delay (▶ Fig. 36.1)

■ Key Imaging Finding

Subcortical cysts in a child

■ Top 3 Differential Diagnoses

- **Cytomegalovirus (CMV).** CMV is the most common in utero TORCH infection. It may result from a primary infection during gestation or reactivation of a latent virus. Affected infants suffer from developmental delay and sensorineural hearing loss. As with other TORCH infections, the degree of insult is mostly dependent on the timing of infection in terms of development with more severe manifestations occurring earlier in gestation. The disease is often systemic with growth retardation, hepatosplenomegaly, jaundice, and a petechial rash. Central nervous system (CNS) manifestations include microcephaly, cortical malformations, ventriculomegaly, parenchymal calcifications with a periventricular distribution, and hypomyelination with increased T2 signal intensity predominantly within the deep white matter. Germinolytic cysts commonly form with a predilection for the subependymal region, periventricular white matter, and subcortical white matter of the anterior temporal lobes.
- **Megalencephalic leukeoencephalopathy with subcortical cysts (MLC).** Also known as van der Knaap disease, MLC is a leukodystrophy that results in diffuse white matter signal abnormality and regions of vacuolization. The white matter becomes edematous early in the disease process, resulting in macrocephaly. In this phase, the primary differentials include other leukodystrophies with macrocephaly, such as Canavan and Alexander disease. Enhancement is not typically seen. With time, the white matter edema dissipates, with persistence of diffuse signal abnormality, and vacuolating cysts appear. Subcortical cysts affecting the anterior temporal lobes are common and characteristic of MLC. Subcortical cysts may also be seen in the frontal and parietal lobes.
- **CADASIL.** Cerebral autosomal dominant arteriopathy with subcortical infarcts and leukoencephalopathy (CADASIL) is an inherited disorder that affects young to middle-aged adults. The arteriopathy primarily affects small vessels of the CNS. Patients present with a history of migraine-type headaches and transient ischemic attacks. Early in the disease process, imaging demonstrates multifocal regions of nonspecific hypoattenuation (computed tomography) or T2 hyperintensity (magnetic resonance imaging) within the subcortical and deep white matter. As the disease progresses, frank infarcts occur with associated restricted diffusion in the acute setting. Subcortical infarcts affecting the frontal lobes and anterior temporal lobes are fairly characteristic.

■ Diagnosis

Megalencephalic leukeoencephalopathy with subcortical cysts

✓ Pearls

- CMV infection results in numerous CNS abnormalities and malformations, including subcortical germinolytic cysts.
- MLC is a leukodystrophy that results in diffuse white matter signal abnormality and regions of vacuolization/cysts.
- CADASIL affects young to middle-aged adults with small-vessel ischemia and characteristic subcortical infarcts.

Suggested Readings

de Vries LS, Gunardi H, Barth PG, Bok LA, Verboon-Maciolek MA, Groenendaal F. The spectrum of cranial ultrasound and magnetic resonance imaging abnormalities in congenital cytomegalovirus infection. Neuropediatrics 2004; 35: 113–119

Tu YF, Chen CY, Huang CC, Lee CS. Vacuolating megalencephalic leukoencephalopathy with mild clinical course validated by diffusion tensor imaging and MR spectroscopy. Am J Neuroradiol 2004; 25: 1041–1045

van den Boom R, Lesnik Oberstein SAJ, Ferrari MD, Haan J, van Buchem MA. Cerebral autosomal dominant arteriopathy with subcortical infarcts and leukoencephalopathy: MR imaging findings at different ages—3rd-6th decades. Radiology 2003; 229: 683–690

Case 37

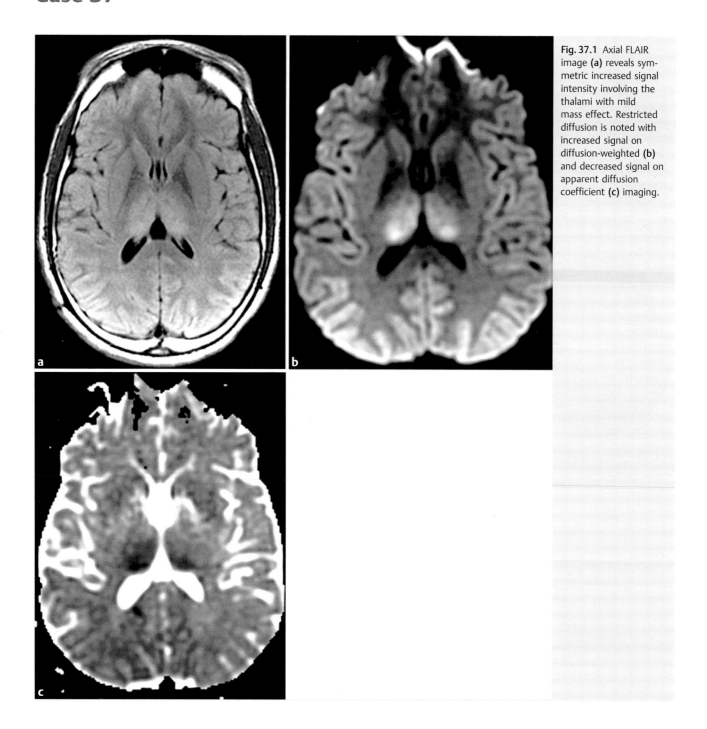

Fig. 37.1 Axial FLAIR image (a) reveals symmetric increased signal intensity involving the thalami with mild mass effect. Restricted diffusion is noted with increased signal on diffusion-weighted (b) and decreased signal on apparent diffusion coefficient (c) imaging.

■ Clinical Presentation

Young man found down (▶ Fig. 37.1)

■ Key Imaging Finding

Bilateral thalamic signal abnormality

■ Top 3 Differential Diagnoses

- **Ischemia/infarct.** Thalamic arterial supply arises from perforating branches of the posterior cerebral artery (PCA) and the posterior communicating artery (PComA). The PComA (when present) supplies the anterior thalami and the PCA supplies the medial and lateral thalami. An artery of Percheron (AOP) is an anatomic variant where a single perforator supplies the bilateral medial thalami and anterior midbrain. Occlusion of the AOP results in bilateral medial thalamic infarcts with or without midbrain involvement. Occlusion of the distal basilar artery is an additional cause of bilateral thalamic infarcts but is characterized by more extensive ischemic changes. Acutely, there is bilateral hypoattenuation (computed tomography, CT) and increased T2/fluid-attenuated inversion recovery (FLAIR)/diffusion-weighted imaging signal with edema. Deep venous infarcts are more common with hypercoagulable states and typically result from internal cerebral vein occlusion. Venous infarcts do not follow a vascular distribution. Thrombosed venous structures are often hyperdense on CT. Venous infarcts are more prone to hemorrhage.
- **Infiltrating neoplasm.** Thalamic gliomas may result as an extension of a brain stem glioma or as primary thalamic neoplasms. They occur more frequently in children and young adults. Most are fibrillary (World Health Organization [WHO] grade II) but commonly degenerate to high-grade tumors, such as anaplastic (WHO grade III). Imaging reveals thalamic expansion with hypoattenuation (CT) and increased T2/FLAIR signal (magnetic resonance imaging, MRI). Higher grade components demonstrate restricted diffusion, increased perfusion, and enhancement. Prognosis is poor. Central nervous system lymphoma can also involve the thalami but is characteristically hypointense on T2 sequences due to high cellularity and avidly enhances.
- **Viral encephalitis.** Mosquito-borne viral encephalitides such as West Nile, Eastern equine, and Japanese encephalitis are relatively common in endemic regions. Patients present with flu-like symptoms initially, followed by rapid progression to meningitis or encephalitis with seizures and focal neurological deficits. Imaging reveals hypoattenuation (CT) and increased T2/FLAIR signal (MRI) with edema involving the thalami, lentiform nuclei, caudate, mesial temporal lobes, and brain stem. Patchy or meningeal enhancement, hemorrhage, and restricted diffusion may be seen.

■ Additional Differential Diagnoses

- **Osmotic demyelination.** Osmotic demyelination results from rapid shifts in osmolality. It is classically due to rapid correction of hyponatremia, but may also be seen in malnourished and diabetic children. Fifty percent of cases involve the central pons, whereas the remaining are extrapontine with involvement of the basal ganglia, thalami, and cerebral white matter. Findings are typically bilateral and symmetric. Lesions are hypodense on CT and on T2/FLAIR hyperintense.
- **Wernicke encephalopathy.** Werncike encephalopathy is caused by thiamine deficiency. It is most common in alcoholic patients, but may also be seen with malabsorption or nutritional deficiencies. The classic clinical triad consists of altered mental status, ataxia, and ocular dysfunction. MRI features include symmetric increased T2 signal within the medial thalami, periaqueductal gray matter, tectal plate, and mamillary bodies. Enhancement may be seen.
- **Acute disseminated encephalomyelitis (ADEM).** ADEM is a monophasic demyelinating process that follows an antecedent viral infection or immunization. It occurs most often in children and young adults. White matter lesions may mimic those of multiple sclerosis (MS) with ovoid periventricular lesions and involvement of the corpus callosum, cerebellar hemispheres, and brain stem. Compared with MS, ADEM is more likely to be confluent and involve gray matter, including the thalami. Lesions are hyperintense on T2/FLAIR and may demonstrate enhancement and restricted diffusion with active demyelination. Presence of characteristic white matter lesions is a useful discriminator.

■ Diagnosis

Infarct (venous)

✓ Pearls

- Arterial and venous ischemia are important causes of abnormal bithalamic signal; restricted diffusion is seen acutely.
- Thalamic gliomas occur in children and young adults; they may be primary or an extension of a brain stem glioma.
- Infectious and parainfectious etiologies of thalamic signal abnormality include viral encephalitis and ADEM.

Suggested Readings

Hegde AN, Mohan S, Lath N, Lim CC. Differential diagnosis for bilateral abnormalities of the basal ganglia and thalamus. Radiographics 2011; 31: 5–30

Lazzaro NA, Wright B, Castillo M et al. Artery of percheron infarction: imaging patterns and clinical spectrum. Am J Neuroradiol 2010; 31: 1283–1289

Case 38

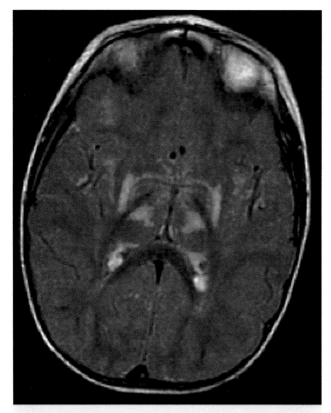

Fig. 38.1 Axial FLAIR image demonstrates symmetric hyperintense signal in the posterolateral putamina and ventral thalami, as well as within the bilateral insula.

▨ Clinical Presentation

An 8-year-old child; history otherwise withheld (▶ Fig. 38.1)

■ Key Imaging Finding

Increased T2 signal in basal ganglia/thalami in a child

■ Top 3 Differential Diagnoses

- **Hypoxic-ischemic or anoxic injury.** Severe hypoxic-ischemic injury predominantly affects the deep gray matter, which is particularly vulnerable to hypoxia. The posterior putamina and ventrolateral thalami are most commonly involved. There is also involvement of the gray-white matter junction, especially in watershed regions. Affected areas demonstrate T2/fluid-attenuated inversion recovery (FLAIR) hyperintensity; restricted diffusion is seen in the acute setting. Common etiologies in children include trauma, hypoperfusion, and anoxic events. Deep venous infarcts are an important cause of bilateral increased T2 signal within the thalami and are prone to hemorrhage. Thrombosed venous structures are often hyperdense on computed tomography (CT). Anoxic injury due to inhalation of carbon monoxide gas results in symmetric hypodensity (CT) and T2 hyperintensity (magnetic resonance imaging, MRI) of the globus pallidi. A hypointense hemosiderin rim may be seen. The caudate and putamina may also be affected. Confluent white matter hyperintensity reflects diffuse demyelination. Methanol poisoning preferentially involves the putamina with hemorrhagic putaminal necrosis. Optic nerves may also be involved.
- **Wilson disease.** Wilson disease (hepatolenticular degeneration) is an autosomal recessive disorder characterized by excessive copper accumulation in the liver and brain (particularly the basal ganglia), resulting in chronic ischemia. It results from deficiency of ceruloplasmin, which transports copper. There is increased T2/FLAIR signal in the lentiform nuclei, midbrain, thalami, and white matter tracts. The characteristic "face of the panda" sign on axial T2 images through the midbrain is due to hyperintense tegmentum and hypointense superior colliculi. Associated abnormalities include neuropsychiatric illnesses, Kayser-Fleischer corneal rings, and cirrhosis.
- **Metabolic disorder.** Mitochondrial disorders result from damage to energy-producing mitochondria. MELAS (mitochondrial myopathy, encephalopathy, lactic acidosis, and stroke-like episodes) is an uncommon but important cause of stroke in children. There are ischemic findings in nonvascular distributions. Chronic atrophy of the basal ganglia and cortex occurs with T2 hyperintensity in the deep gray and white matter. Leigh syndrome affects infants and children who present with failure to thrive, motor deficits, and seizures. MRI reveals symmetric increased T2 signal involving the deep gray matter, particularly the basal ganglia and thalami; dorsal brain stem; and less frequently, the supra- and infratentorial white matter. MR spectroscopy reveals an elevated lactate peak. Canavan disease is a leukodystrophy that results in diffuse abnormal signal within the white matter, thalami, and globus pallidus; macrocephaly; and increased N-acetyl aspartate on spectroscopy. Juvenile Huntington disease is associated with caudate atrophy.

■ Additional Differential Diagnoses

- **Kernicterus.** Kernicterus refers to encephalopathy from deposition of unconjugated bilirubin. Acutely (within the first 2 to 5 days of life), there is T1 and subtle T2 hyperintensity in the bilateral globus pallidi, hippocampi, and substantia nigra. Chronically, there is T2 hyperintensity in the posteromedial globus pallidi and dentate nuclei with normal T1 signal.
- **Osmotic demyelination.** Osmotic demyelination results from rapid shifts in osmolality. It is classically due to rapid correction of hyponatremia, but may also be seen in malnourished and diabetic children. Fifty percent of cases involve the central pons, whereas the remaining are extrapontine with involvement of the basal ganglia, thalami, and cerebral white matter. Findings are typically bilateral and symmetric. Lesions are hypodense on CT and on T2/FLAIR hyperintense.
- **Neurofibromatosis type 1 (NF1) spots.** NF1 is the most common neurocutaneous syndrome. It is caused by a defect of chromosome 17 that results in increased incidence of neurofibromas and gliomas. Patients with NF1 have regions of myelin vacuolization that are hyperintense on T2 sequences and involve the basal ganglia, thalami, dentate nuclei, cerebellar peduncles, brain stem, and optic radiations. Lesions wax and wane for the first decade and then regress.

■ Diagnosis

Hypoxic-ischemic insult (near drowning)

✓ Pearls

- Deep gray matter is vulnerable to hypoxic-ischemic and anoxic encephalopathy, particularly in at-risk children.
- Deposition disorders (Wilson disease and kernicterus) involve the deep gray matter, particularly the basal ganglia.
- Metabolic disorders affect deep gray matter structures; mitochondrial diseases demonstrate a lactate peak on MR spectroscopy.

Suggested Reading

Hegde AN, Mohan S, Lath N, Lim CC. Differential diagnosis for bilateral abnormalities of the basal ganglia and thalamus. Radiographics 2011; 31: 5–30

Case 39

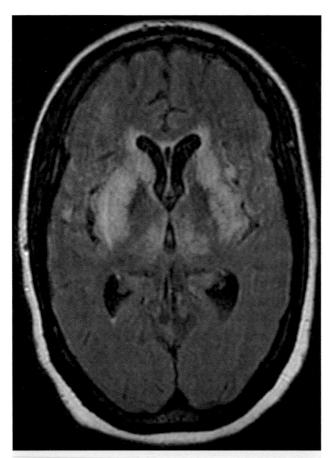

Fig. 39.1 Axial FLAIR image through the level of the deep gray matter structures reveals symmetric regions of increased signal intensity involving the bilateral thalami, lentiform nuclei, caudate, and subinsular white matter. Foci of increased signal are also seen within the insular cortex on the left and operculum on the right. (Reprinted with permission: O'Brien WT. J Am Osteopath Coll Radiol 2012;1[1]:3–9.)

■ Clinical Presentation

Adult man with altered mental status (▶ Fig. 39.1)

■ Key Imaging Finding

Symmetric increased T2 signal in basal ganglia/thalami in an adult

■ Top 3 Differential Diagnoses

- **Hypoxic-ischemic injury (HII).** HII may result from severe hypoperfusion, hypoxia, or anoxia. Common causes include near-drowning in young adults and cardiac arrest or vascular occlusion in older adults. Toxic exposures including carbon monoxide poisoning (globus pallidus involvement) and methanol toxicity (putaminal necrosis) are less common. Deep gray matter structures are most susceptible to severe HII due to their increased metabolic activity. The medial temporal lobes and cortical gray matter may also be involved, especially in watershed regions. Computed tomography (CT) reveals hypoattenuation and magnetic resonance imaging (MRI) demonstrates increased T2/fluid-attenuated inversion recovery (FLAIR) signal within the involved structures. Restricted diffusion is seen in the acute setting. Deep venous infarcts are an important cause of bilateral increased T2 signal within the thalami. Thrombosed venous structures are often hyperdense on CT. Venous infarcts are more prone to hemorrhage, which will result in heterogeneous signal on MRI based upon the age of hemorrhage.

- **Osmotic demyelination.** Osmotic demyelination is classically due to rapid correction of hyponatremia, but may also occur in alcoholic, diabetic, or malnourished patients. Approximately half of cases involve the central pons with sparing of descending corticospinal tracts, whereas the remaining are extrapontine with involvement of the basal ganglia, thalami, and cerebral white matter. Extrapontine involvement may occur with pontine involvement or in isolation. Findings are typically bilateral and symmetric. Lesions are hypodense on CT and on T2/FLAIR hyperintense.

- **Viral encephalitis.** Mosquito-borne viral encephalitides such as West Nile, Eastern equine, and Japanese encephalitis are relatively common in endemic regions. Patients present with flu-like symptoms initially, followed by rapid progression to meningitis or encephalitis with seizures and focal neurological deficits. Imaging reveals hypoattenuation (CT) and increased T2/FLAIR signal (MRI) with edema involving the thalami, lentiform nuclei, caudate, mesial temporal lobes, and brain stem. Patchy or meningeal enhancement, hemorrhage, and restricted diffusion may be seen.

■ Additional Differential Diagnoses

- **Wilson disease.** Wilson disease (hepatolenticular degeneration) is an autosomal recessive disorder characterized by excessive copper accumulation in the brain (particularly the basal ganglia) and liver, secondary to a deficiency of ceruloplasmin. Excessive copper deposition results in chronic ischemia. MRI reveals increased T2/FLAIR signal in the lentiform nuclei, midbrain, thalami, and white matter tracts. The characteristic "face of the panda" sign on axial T2 images through the midbrain is due to hyperintense tegmentum and hypointense superior colliculi. Associated abnormalities include neuropsychiatric illnesses, Kayser-Fleischer corneal rings, and cirrhosis.

- **Creutzfeldt-Jakob disease (CJD).** CJD is a rare spongiform encephalopathy caused by a prion. It may be acquired, sporadic, or inherited with sporadic being the most common. Acquired causes include consumption of contaminated foods (e.g., cases caused by contaminated beef in the United Kingdom) and medical procedures such as corneal transplant, blood transfusions, and electrode placement. The disease is fulminant and rapidly fatal. Patients present with confusion, dementia, gait abnormalities, personality changes, and myoclonic jerks. MRI demonstrates symmetric increased T2/FLAIR signal within the basal ganglia and thalami. Symmetric thalamic involvement of pulvinar and medial thalami results in the characteristic "hockey stick" sign. Increased signal may also be seen in the cortical gray matter. Increased diffusion-weighted imaging signal is commonly seen. Atrophy occurs in the chronic stage. Prognosis is dismal with death usually within months.

■ Diagnosis

Viral encephalitis

✓ Pearls

- Severe arterial ischemia, venous infarct, and toxic exposures may result in HII affecting deep gray matter structures.
- Osmotic demyelination results from rapid shifts in osmolality; correction of hyponatremia is the classic presentation.

- Viral encephalitides commonly affect deep gray matter structures; meningeal enhancement is a useful discriminator.
- CJD is a neurodegenerative disorder involving prions; medial thalamic and pulvinar involvement is characteristic.

Suggested Readings

Hegde AN, Mohan S, Lath N, Lim CC. Differential diagnosis for bilateral abnormalities of the basal ganglia and thalamus. Radiographics 2011; 31: 5–30

O'Brien WT. Imaging of CNS infections in immunocompetent patients. J Am Osteopath Coll Radiol 2012; 1: 3–9

Case 40

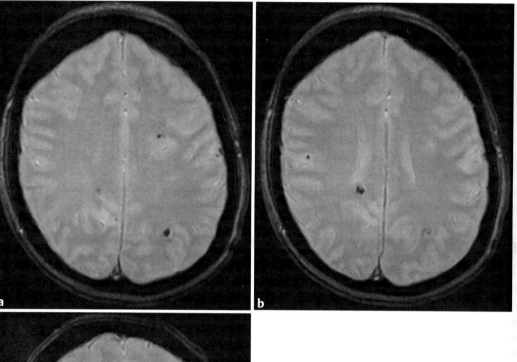
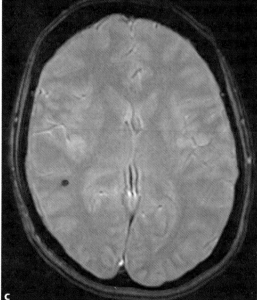

Fig. 40.1 Axial GRE images reveal numerous foci of susceptibility (hypointensity) with involvement of the gray-white matter junction (a–c) and along the superior aspect of the splenium of the corpus callosum on the right (b). Regions of increased signal are visualized posterior to the left frontal centrum semiovale lesion (a) and within the subinsular regions (c).

■ **Clinical Presentation**

Adult woman with headaches and neurological deficits (▶ Fig. 40.1)

▨ Key Imaging Finding

Multiple hypointense lesions on gradient echo (GRE) or suscep-tibility-weighted imaging (SWI)

■ Top 3 Differential Diagnoses

- **Hypertension.** Chronic, long-standing hypertension results in accelerated arteriosclerosis and fibrinoid necrosis of penetrating arteries. The increased perfusion pressures and weakening of the arterial wall result in true (Charcot-Bouchard) and false aneurysms of distal arterioles, which are prone to microhemorrhage. Microhemorrhages occur most commonly within the putamen, thalamus, pons, and cerebellar hemispheres. Involvement of the deep and lobar white matter may also be seen. Lesions are subtle on routine magnetic resonance imaging (MRI) sequences but readily evident on GRE or SWI.
- **Vasculitis.** Vasculitis results in inflammatory infiltration of arterial walls. Causative etiologies include autoimmune, infectious or granulomatous disease, radiation, and elicit drugs. MRI demonstrates bilateral regions of superficial and deep gray and white matter signal abnormality (increased T2/fluid-attenuated inversion recovery [FLAIR] signal intensity). GRE and SWI commonly reveal multifocal regions of microhemorrhage. Patchy enhancement may be seen. Angiography is often necessary to visualize alternating regions of stenosis and dilatation because MR angiography and computed tomography (CT) angiography are less sensitive in evaluating distal arterial branches. Biopsy is diagnostic.
- **Diffuse axonal injury.** DAI results from acceleration-deceleration injury with white matter shearing. The number and location of lesions correspond to the severity of injury. Grade 1 injury involves the gray-white matter junction. Grade 2 injury also involves the corpus callosum. Grade 3 injury is most severe with involvement of the deep gray matter and posterolateral brain stem. On CT, lesions may be imperceptible or demonstrate increased (hemorrhagic) or decreased (nonhemorrhagic) attenuation. On MRI, nonhemorrhagic lesions are T2 hyperintense, whereas hemorrhagic lesions are more variable in signal. GRE and SWI are sensitive for hemorrhagic lesions, detecting those not visible on routine sequences. Additional findings of traumatic brain injury (contusions and extraaxial hemorrhage) are often seen.

■ Additional Differential Diagnoses

- **Multiple cavernous malformations (CMs).** CMs consist of variable-sized blood-filled sinusoids and larger cavernous spaces without intervening brain parenchyma. The majority of lesions are solitary. Multiple lesions are inherited in an autosomal dominant pattern or acquired following radiation therapy, especially in children. Lesions have little or no edema or mass effect unless hemorrhage disrupts the capsule. CT may be normal or show regions of calcification or hemorrhage. Lesions have alternating foci of increased and decreased T1 and T2 signal centrally with a T2 dark capsule. Lesions are hypointense and conspicuous on GRE and SWI. Enhancement may be seen in ~15% of cases.
- **Cerebral amyloid angiopathy (CAA).** CAA occurs in elderly patients, typically older than 60 years of age. It is a common cause of lobar hemorrhage in this age group and is associated with an increased incidence of Alzheimer dementia. The amyloid deposition results in fibrinoid necrosis and microaneurysms of penetrating arteries. MRI often demonstrates moderate to marked microvascular ischemic disease, as well as multifocal regions of GRE and SWI hypointensity with a lobar, rather than deep, predominance.
- **Hematogenous spread of tumor or infection.** Hemorrhagic metastases present as multiple foci of decreased signal intensity on GRE and SWI. T1 and T2 signal intensity depends on the size of the lesions and age of hemorrhage. Lung, breast, melanoma, thyroid, renal cell, and choriocarcinoma are the most common primary hemorrhagic neoplasms. Aside from cortically based metastases, lesions will have surrounding vasogenic edema. Hematogenous septic emboli may calcify or have associated hemorrhage, resulting in hypointensity on GRE and SWI. Neurocysticercosis in its chronic stage demonstrates multiple calcified lesions without edema or enhancement. Tuberculosis and fungal infections may also produce calcified lesions; enhancement and edema are commonly seen.

▨ Diagnosis

Vasculitis

✓ Pearls

- Chronic hypertension results in microhemorrhages within the putamen, thalamus, pons, and cerebellar hemispheres.
- Vasculitis results in inflammatory infiltration of vascular walls; microhemorrhage and enhancement may be seen.
- DAI results from white matter shearing; the number and location of lesions correspond to severity of injury.
- CAA occurs in elderly patients, is a common cause of lobar hemorrhage, and is associated with Alzheimer dementia.

Suggested Reading

Thomas B, Somasundaram S, Thamburaj K et al. Clinical applications of susceptibility weighted MR imaging of the brain—a pictorial review. Neuroradiology 2008; 50: 105–116

Case 41

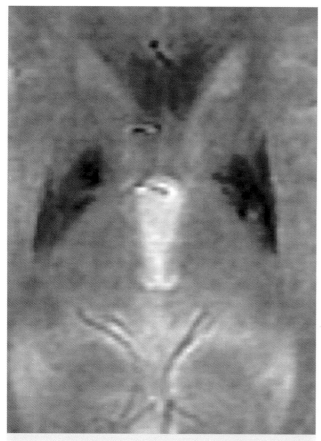

Fig. 41.1 Coned-down axial T2 image reveals symmetric hypointensity within the posterior lentiform nuclei.

▪ Clinical Presentation

A 50-year-old woman with gait abnormality (▶ Fig. 41.1)

▣ Key Imaging Finding

Decreased T2 signal in basal ganglia

▣ Top 3 Differential Diagnoses

- **Normal aging.** In middle-aged and older patients, decreased T2 signal may be seen within the basal ganglia, predominantly the globus pallidus, secondary to a combination of increased iron deposition and age-related senescent calcifications. Early onset of senescent calcification may occur in patients with Down syndrome. Associated findings of parenchymal atrophy and microvascular ischemic disease are commonly seen.
- **Basal ganglia calcification.** There are numerous causes of basal ganglia calcifications with senescent age-related calcifications being the most common. Additional causes of basal ganglia calcifications include metabolic disorders (mitochondrial disorders), endocrinopathies (abnormalities of calcium and phosphate or hypothyroidism), severe hypoxic-ischemic encephalopathy, postinfection (TORCH, congenital human immunodeficiency virus, tuberculosis, and neurocysticercosis), prior radiation and chemotherapy treatment, and Fahr disease. In general, nonsenescent calcifications have more extensive involvement of additional deep gray matter structures and occasionally the subcortical white matter. Calcifications are typically hypointense on T2 and variable in signal intensity on T1 sequences.

- **Neurodegenerative disorder.** Panthothenate kinase-associated neurodegeneration (PKAN), formerly known as Halloverden-Spatz disease, is an uncommon neurodegenerative disorder characterized by iron deposition in the globus pallidus and substantia nigra. Patients most often present in childhood with ataxia, dystonia, and visual abnormalities. Imaging reveals bilateral T2 hypointensity within the globus pallidus with central hyperintensity, referred to as the "eye of the tiger" sign. Hypointensity of additional deep gray matter structures and nuclei may be seen. Less common disorders of neurodegeneration with brain iron accumulation (NBIA) or neuroferrinopathies demonstrate decreased T2 signal in a similar distribution but without the eye of the tiger appearance. Parkinson, Alzheimer, and Huntington disease have been associated with increased iron deposition. Parkinson disease is a movement disorder that involves the pars compacta of the substantia nigra. It typically affects older adult patients who present with bradykinesia, resting tremor, "cogwheel" rigidity, and a shuffling gait. Huntington disease is an autosomal dominant disorder (chromosome 4) that results in progressive dementia and choreatic movement disorder. Imaging reveals caudate atrophy.

▣ Additional Differential Diagnoses

- **Demyelinating disease.** Demyelinating disease consists of multiple sclerosis (MS) and acute disseminated encephalomyelitis (ADEM). MS is most often relapsing and remitting, whereas ADEM is monophasic following an antecedent viral infection or immunization. Compared with MS, ADEM more often involves children, tends to be more confluent, and more commonly involves gray matter. Focal lesions within the deep gray matter are typically T2 hyperintense. With chronic disease, increased iron deposition results in decreased T2 signal intensity within the deep gray matter structures. Associated white matter lesions with characteristic morphology (ovoid,

perivenular) and distribution (periventricular, corpus callosum, cerebellum, and brain stem) are also seen.
- **Hemochromatosis.** Hemochromatosis is a disorder of iron overload and may be primary (inherited) or secondary (usually acquired from multiple transfusions). In the abdomen, primary hemochromatosis involves the liver and pancreas, whereas secondary hemochromatosis involves the liver and spleen. Central nervous system involvement is relatively uncommon and occurs late in the disease process. Imaging findings, when present, include decreased T2 signal within the basal ganglia; patients may demonstrate extrapyrimidal findings.

▣ Diagnosis

Neurodegenerative disorder (Parkinson disease)

✓ Pearls

- With aging, increased iron deposition and senescent calcifications result in decreased T2 signal in the globus pallidus.
- Iron deposition is common in neurodegenerative diseases, including PKAN, Alzheimer, Parkinson, and Huntington.

- Chronic MS plaques may have iron deposition; characteristic T2 hyperintense demyelinating lesions are often seen.

Suggested Readings

Hegde AN, Mohan S, Lath N, Lim CC. Differential diagnosis for bilateral abnormalities of the basal ganglia and thalamus. Radiographics 2011; 31: 5–30

Stankiewicz J, Panter SS, Neema M, Arora A, Batt CE, Bakshi R. Iron in chronic brain disorders: imaging and neurotherapeutic implications. Neurotherapeutics 2007; 4: 371–386

Case 42

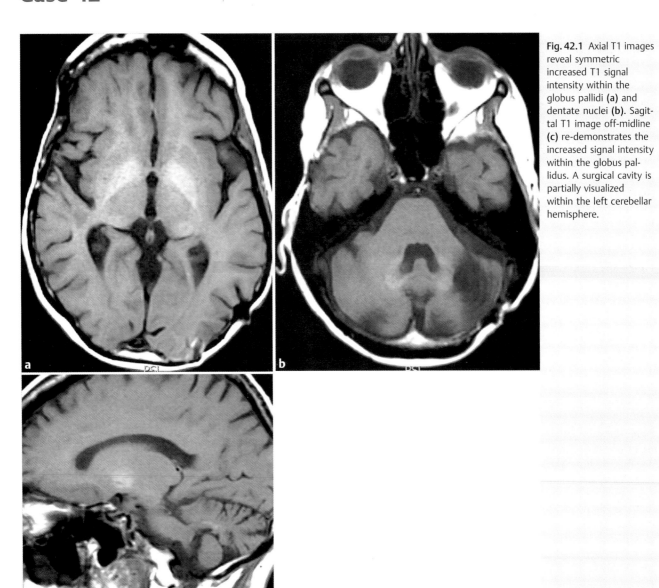

Fig. 42.1 Axial T1 images reveal symmetric increased T1 signal intensity within the globus pallidi (a) and dentate nuclei (b). Sagittal T1 image off-midline (c) re-demonstrates the increased signal intensity within the globus pallidus. A surgical cavity is partially visualized within the left cerebellar hemisphere.

■ Clinical Presentation

Adult patient with chronic neurological issues (▶ Fig. 42.1)

■ Key Imaging Finding

Symmetric increased T1 signal in basal ganglia

■ Top 3 Differential Diagnoses

• **Basal ganglia (BG) calcification or mineralization.** There are numerous causes of BG calcification with senescent age-related calcifications being the most common. Senescent calcifications occur in adults and preferentially involve the globus pallidi. Early onset of senescent calcification may occur in patients with Down syndrome. Additional causes of BG calcification or mineralization include metabolic disorders (mitochondrial disorders), endocrinopathies (abnormalities of calcium and phosphate or hypothyroidism), severe hypoxic-ischemic encephalopathy, postinfection, prior radiation and chemotherapy, and Fahr disease. Nonsenescent calcification or mineralization has more extensive involvement of deep gray matter structures and occasionally involves white matter.

• **Manganese deposition.** Excess manganese deposition results in increased T1 signal intensity within the basal ganglia secondary to paramagnetic effects. Common etiologies include hepatic encephalopathy secondary to chronic or occasionally acute hepatic failure, as well as patients receiving long-term parenteral feeding for chronic illnesses. The manganese deposition predominantly affects the globus pallidi and substantia nigra.

• **Hypoxic-ischemic or anoxic encephalopathy.** Severe hypoxic-ischemic and anoxic encephalopathy affects the most metabolically active portions of the brain, particularly the deep gray matter structures. Causes include hypoperfusion, near drowning, and toxic exposures, such as carbon monoxide poisoning. Computed tomography reveals hypoattenuation of the deep gray matter structures, as well as the perirolandic gray and white matter. On magnetic resonance imaging, regions of increased T1 and T2 signal may be seen. Restricted diffusion is noted with acute infarcts. Chronically, there is volume loss with calcifications.

■ Additional Differential Diagnoses

• **Neurodegenerative disorders.** Neurodegenerative disorders commonly involve the basal ganglia. Those that may result in hyperintense T1 signal include Wilson disease and pantothenate kinase-associated neurodegeneration (PKAN or Hallovorden-Spatz disease). Wilson disease results in excessive copper deposition within deep gray matter structures, particularly the BG, secondary to a deficiency in ceruloplasmin. The liver is also affected. In children, increased T1 signal intensity is seen in the BG. In adults, there is increased T2/fluid-attenuated inversion recovery signal in the lentiform nuclei, midbrain, thalami, and white matter tracts. The characteristic "face of the panda" sign on axial T2 images through the midbrain is due to hyperintense tegmentum and hypointense superior colliculi. PKAN results in excessive iron deposition within the globus pallidi. Imaging reveals central T2 hyperintensity with peripheral hypointensity, referred to as the "eye of the tiger" sign. T1 signal intensity is variable with regions that are hypo- and hyperintense.

• **Neurofibromatosis type 1 (NF1).** Central nervous system manifestations of NF1 include characteristic NF "spots," which are thought to represent regions of myelin vacuolization. They involve the BG, thalami, dentate nuclei, cerebellar peduncles, optic radiations, and brain stem. The lesions are hyperintense on T2 and typically mildly hyperintense on T1 images. There may be apparent but not true mass effect, especially with lesions located within the thalami, cerebellar peduncles, and brain stem. However, there should be no enhancement; the presence of enhancement suggests development of a low-grade glioma. Lesions wax and wane for the first decade of life and then regress.

• **Kernicterus.** Kernicterus refers to encephalopathy from deposition of unconjugated bilirubin. Acutely (within the first 2 to 5 days of life), there is T1 and subtle T2 hyperintensity in the globus pallidi, hippocampi, and substantia nigra. Chronically, there is T2 hyperintensity in the posteromedial globus pallidi and dentate nuclei with normal T1 signal.

■ Diagnosis

Basal ganglia mineralization (postradiation therapy)

✓ Pearls

• Calcification or mineralization are common causes of increased T1 signal intensity in the BG.
• Manganese deposition most often results from hepatic failure (typically chronic) or long-term parenteral nutrition.

• Neurodegenerative disorders (Wilson disease and PKAN) may occasionally result in increased BG T1 signal.
• NF1 spots are mildly hyperintense on T1 sequences; they wax and wane for the first decade of life and then regress.

Suggested Readings

Lai PH, Chen C, Liang HL, Pan HB. Hyperintense basal ganglia on T1-weighted MR imaging. Am J Roentgenol 1999; 172: 1109–1115

Rovira A, Alonso J, Córdoba J. MR imaging findings in hepatic encephalopathy. Am J Neuroradiol 2008; 29: 1612–1621

Case 43

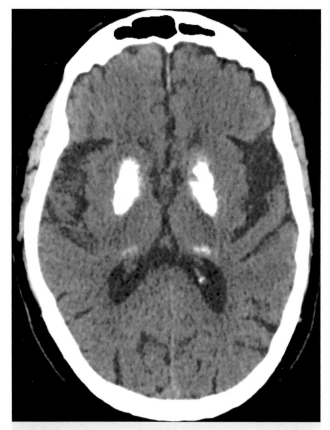

Fig. 43.1 Axial computed tomography image demonstrates bilateral symmetric calcifications involving the lentiform nuclei and posterior thalami.

■ Clinical Presentation

Adult man with muscle pains (▶ Fig. 43.1)

▣ Key Imaging Finding

Basal ganglia calcifications

▣ Top 3 Differential Diagnoses

- **Senescent calcifications.** Senescent calcifications involve the lentiform nuclei in adult patients. They are incidental, considered a normal part of the aging process, and may increase over time. The globus pallidi are involved to a greater degree than the putamina. Involvement of the caudate or thalami should suggest an underlying condition other than senescent calcifications. Patients with Down syndrome experience accelerated effects of aging within the central nervous system. These include early onset of senescent basal ganglia calcifications, parenchymal atrophy, and dementia.
- **Metabolic or Endocrine disease.** Abnormalities of calcium or phosphorus are common causes of parenchymal calcifications. The lentiform nuclei are most often involved. The caudate, thalami, dentate nuclei, and subcortical white matter may also be affected. Tertiary hyperparathyroidism may result in dural and scleral calcifications along with or in absence of parenchymal calcifications. Hypothyroidism is another cause of parenchymal calcification with a similar distribution. There are numerous variants of mitochondrial disorders that ultimately affect energy production due to enzyme deficiencies. Basal ganglia involvement is characteristic. Mitochondrial encephalopathy with lactic acidosis and stroke-like episodes (MELAS) and Leigh syndrome are the two most common to result in basal ganglia calcifications in the chronic setting. The putamina are involved to a greater extent than the caudate or globus pallidi. Associated basal ganglia and white matter signal abnormalities are commonly seen.
- **Ischemic or infectious injury.** Severe hypoxic-ischemic injury affects the most metabolically active portions of the brain, including the deep gray matter structures. There is edema acutely with hypoattenuation on computed tomography and increased T2 and diffusion-weighted imaging signal on magnetic resonance imaging. In the chronic stages, atrophy and calcification may be seen. Carbon monoxide poisoning may produce similar findings with a predilection for the globus pallidi. An appropriate history is the key to making the diagnosis. Numerous infectious agents may result in basal ganglia calcifications, although additional findings are commonly present to aid in identifying the organism. In utero cytomegalovirus (CMV) or toxoplasmosis infections result in parenchymal calcifications; CMV has a periventricular distribution, while toxoplasmosis is more random. Tuberculosis most often results in a basilar meningitis. Intraparenchymal tuberculomas occur in a minority of patients and present with intraparenchymal lesions that enhance and may calcify. Neurocysticercosis is the most common cause of acquired seizures worldwide and occurs in endemic locations. Imaging appearance depends on the stage of infection; the chronic, nodular stage results in calcified parenchymal lesions. Basal ganglia calcifications may also be seen in patients with human immunodeficiency virus, particularly children.

▣ Additional Differential Diagnoses

- **Treatment-related.** Radiation and chemotherapy treatment result in a mineralizing microangiopathy with associated parenchymal injury and calcifications. The mineralizing angiopathy generally occurs a few years after treatment and most often involves the deep gray matter structures and subcortical white matter. Atrophy occurs in chronic stages. Patients treated at a younger age are more prone to treatment-related parenchymal injury.
- **Fahr disease.** Fahr disease is a rare inherited neurodegenerative disorder that leads to symmetric intracranial calcifications involving predominantly the deep gray matter structures. Characteristic locations include the globus pallidi (most common), putamina, caudate, thalami, and dentate nuclei. Calcifications within the white matter are often seen. Fahr disease most often affects young and middle-aged adults with neurocognitive or neuromotor deficits.

▣ Diagnosis

Endocrine disease (hyperparathyroidism)

✓ Pearls

- Senescent calcifications are considered a normal part of aging and preferentially involve the globus pallidi.
- Endocrinopathies result in extensive deep gray matter calcifications and occasional white matter involvement.
- Radiation and chemotherapy may cause a mineralizing microangiopathy with resultant parenchymal calcifications.
- Fahr disease is an inherited disorder with extensive parenchymal calcifications and cognitive and motor deficits.

Suggested Readings

Hegde AN, Mohan S, Lath N, Lim CC. Differential diagnosis for bilateral abnormalities of the basal ganglia and thalamus. Radiographics 2011; 31: 5–30

Makariou E, Patsalides AD. Intracranial calcifications. Appl Radiol 2009; 38: 48–60

Case 44

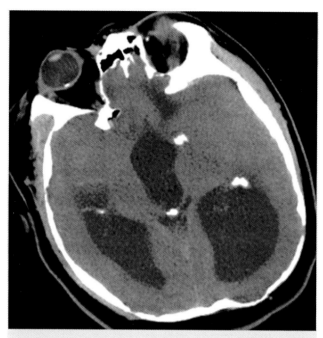

Fig. 44.1 Axial CT image demonstrates multiple periventricular calcifications in a subependymal distribution, as well as ventriculomegaly. An additional calcification is noted along the posterior aspect of the right globe.

■ Clinical Presentation

Young child with history of developmental delay and seizures (▶ Fig. 44.1)

■ Key Imaging Finding

Periventricular calcifications in an infant/child

■ Top 3 Differential Diagnoses

- **TORCH infection.** The TORCH infections consist of toxoplasmosis, syphilis, rubella, cytomegalovirus (CMV), herpes simplex virus, and human immunodeficiency virus (HIV). CMV and toxoplasmosis are both the most common in incidence, as well as the most common to result in parenchymal calcifications. The calcifications in CMV are characteristically periventricular in distribution, whereas those associated with toxoplasmosis are more random. Associated central nervous system (CNS) findings with TORCH infections include microcephaly, neuronal migration abnormalities, and cortical malformations, particularly with CMV. Clinically, patients often suffer from seizures, mental retardation, and varying degrees of hearing and visual loss.

- **Tuberous sclerosis (TS).** TS may occur sporadically or in an autosomal dominant fashion with variable penetrance. The classic clinical triad consists of facial angiofibromas, mental retardation, and seizures but is only seen in approximately 30% of cases. CNS manifestations include subependymal nodules, cortical tubers, white matter lesions, and retinal hamartomas. The majority of subependymal nodules calcify by end of the second decade and many demonstrate enhancement. Nodules have variable T1 and T2 signal, but demonstrate T2 gradient echo susceptibility when calcified. Subependymal giant cell astrocytomas (World Health Organization grade I) are seen in approximately 15% of cases. They are located at the foramen of Monro, enhance, and enlarge over time. Cortical tubers and white matter lesions occur in the vast majority of cases. Tubers are wedge-shaped and T1 hyperintense prior to myelination with variable T1 and hyperintense T2 signal intensity after myelination. White matter lesions are linear T2/fluid-attenuated inversion recovery hyperintensities along the radial migration lines from the ventricle to the overlying cortex.

- **Prior germinal matrix hemorrhage (GMH).** GMH occurs in premature infants with a low birth weight, typically within the first few days to the first week of life. The underdeveloped, highly vascular GM is prone to hemorrhage associated with the stresses of prematurity. The degree and distribution of hemorrhage is divided into four grades with grades 1 and 2 having a favorable prognosis and grades 3 and 4 having a worse prognosis. Grade 1 hemorrhage is limited to the caudothalamic groove. In grade 2, there is intraventricular extension of the hemorrhage without ventriculomegaly. With grade 3, there is intraventricular hemorrhage, which causes ventriculomegaly. Grade 4 presents with GMH, intraventricular hemorrhage, and parenchymal hemorrhage within the periventricular white matter, likely due to venous infarction. Head ultrasound (US) reveals regions of increased echogenicity within the regions of hemorrhage. The hemorrhage is hyperdense on computed tomography (CT). Magnetic resonance imaging (MRI) appearance is dependent upon the location and age of hemorrhage. Blooming hypointensity is noted on gradient echo and susceptibility-weighted sequences. With chronic hemorrhage and/or ischemia, dystrophic subependymal and periventricular calcifications may be seen. Overall, CT and MRI are more sensitive than US.

■ Diagnosis

Tuberous sclerosis (subependymal nodules and retinal hamartoma)

✓ Pearls

- CMV and toxoplasmosis are the most common TORCH infections to result in parenchymal calcifications.
- CMV calcifications are characteristically periventricular in distribution; toxoplasmosis calcifications are random.

- Classic triad of TS includes facial angiofibromas, mental retardation, and seizures; subependymal nodules calcify.
- Chronic GMH and associated ischemia may result in dystrophic subependymal and periventricular calcifications.

Suggested Readings

Blankenberg FG, Loh NN, Bracci P et al. Sonography, CT, and MR imaging: a prospective comparison of neonates with suspected intracranial ischemia and hemorrhage. Am J Neuroradiol 2000; 21: 213–218

Makariou E, Patsalides AD. Intracranial calcifications. Appl Radiol 2009; 38: 48–60

Case 45

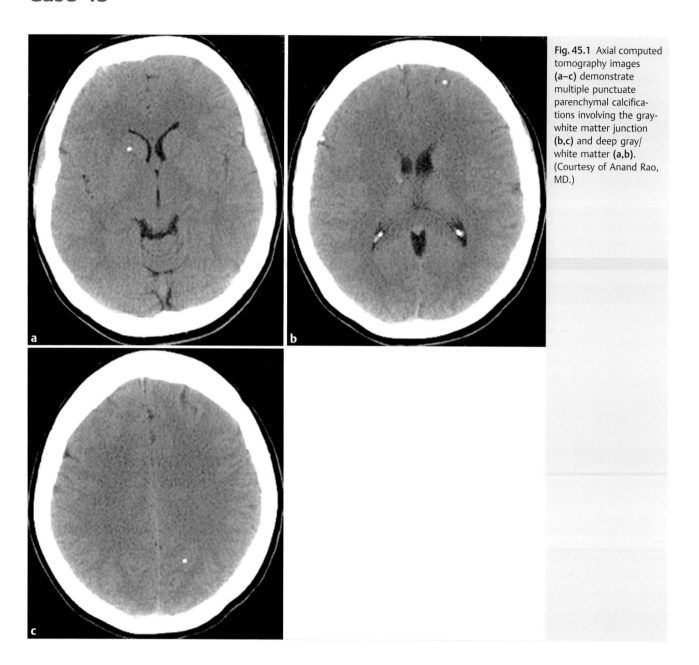

Fig. 45.1 Axial computed tomography images **(a–c)** demonstrate multiple punctuate parenchymal calcifications involving the gray-white matter junction **(b,c)** and deep gray/white matter **(a,b)**. (Courtesy of Anand Rao, MD.)

■ **Clinical Presentation**

Young adult woman with history of headaches and seizures (▶ Fig. 45.1)

■ Key Imaging Finding

Multiple parenchymal calcifications

■ Top 3 Differential Diagnoses

- **Disseminated infection.** Neurocysticercosis is a parasitic infection that occurs after ingestion of contaminated fruits and vegetables or undercooked pork. The causative organism is *Taenia solium*, a pork tapeworm. It is endemic in Central and South America and is the most common acquired cause of seizures worldwide. Imaging appearance depends on the stage of infection. In the early vesicular stage, there is a nonenhancing cyst with a mural nodule referred to as a scolex. The colloidal and granular stages are intermediate and occur after the cyst dies. Inflammatory vasogenic edema and ring enhancement is seen. The chronic, nodular stage presents with multiple calcified parenchymal lesions without enhancement or adjacent edema. In utero cytomegalovirus (CMV) or toxoplasmosis infections result in parenchymal calcifications; CMV has a periventricular distribution. Tuberculosis infection most often results in a basilar meningitis with avid meningeal enhancement and cranial neuropathies. Intraparenchymal tuberculomas occur in a minority of patients and present with intraparenchymal lesions, which enhance and may calcify.
- **Cavernous malformations (CMs).** CMs consist of variable-sized blood-filled sinusoids and larger cavernous spaces without intervening brain parenchyma. The majority of lesions are solitary. Multiple lesions may be inherited in an autosomal dominant pattern or acquired following radiation therapy, especially in children. Lesions have little or no edema or mass effect unless hemorrhage disrupts the capsule. Computed tomography may be normal or show regions of calcification or hemorrhage with increased attenuation. Lesions have alternating foci of increased and decreased T1 and T2 signal centrally with a T2 dark capsule on magnetic resonance imaging. Lesions are hypointense and more conspicuous on gradient echo and susceptibility-weighted imaging. Enhancement may be seen in ~15% of cases.
- **Metastases.** Calcified metastases are rare in the absence of treatment. Radiation therapy in particular may lead to multiple regions of parenchymal calcification. Primary tumors prone to calcification include mucinous adenocarcinomas, which typically arise within the gastrointestinal tract or from breast or lung primaries. Rarely, primary bone-forming tumors may result in calcified parenchymal metastases. Prominent surrounding edema and enhancement are seen.

■ Additional Differential Diagnoses

- **Treatment-related.** Radiation and chemotherapy treatment result in a mineralizing microangiopathy with associated parenchymal injury and calcifications. The mineralizing angiopathy generally occurs a few years after treatment and most often involves the deep gray matter structures and subcortical white matter. Atrophy occurs in chronic stages. Patients treated at a younger age are more prone to treatment-related parenchymal injury.
- **Endocrine disease.** Abnormalities of calcium or phosphorus are common causes of parenchymal calcifications. The lentiform nuclei are most often involved. The caudate, thalami, dentate nuclei, and subcortical white matter may also be affected. Hypothyroidism is another cause of parenchymal calcification with a similar distribution.
- **Tuberous sclerosis (TS).** TS may occur sporadically or in an autosomal dominant fashion. The classic clinical triad consists of facial angiofibromas, mental retardation, and seizures. CNS manifestations include subependymal nodules, cortical tubers, white matter lesions, and retinal hamartomas. The majority of subependymal nodules calcify by age 20. Cortical tubers may show regions of calcification, more often after the first decade of life.

■ Diagnosis

Disseminated infection (neuorcysticercosis)

✓ Pearls

- Neurocysticercosis is the most common acquired cause of seizures worldwide; lesions calcify in the nodular stage.
- Multiple cavernous malformations may be inherited or acquired after radiation therapy, especially in children.
- Metastases may calcify after treatment or result from mucinous adenocarcinoma or bone-forming primaries.
- Radiation and chemotherapy may cause a mineralizing microangiopathy with parenchymal calcifications.

Suggested Readings

Makariou E, Patsalides AD. Intracranial calcifications. Appl Radiol 2009; 38: 48–60

O'Brien WT. Imaging of CNS infections in immunocompetent patients. J Am Osteopath Coll Radiol. 2012; 1: 3–9

Smith AB. Vascular malformations of the brain: radiologic and pathologic correlation. J Am Osteopath Coll Radiol. 2012; 1: 10–22

Case 46

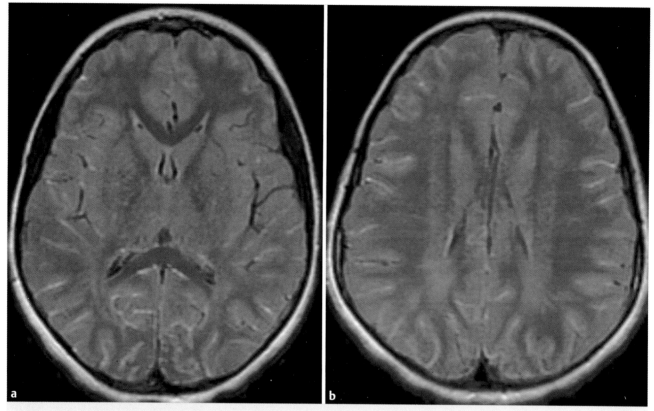

Fig. 46.1 Axial FLAIR images **(a,b)** reveal diffuse abnormal increased signal intensity throughout the subarachnoid spaces overlying the cerebral hemispheres. Hazy increased periatrial signal intensity corresponds to perivascular spaces (not optimally shown).

■ Clinical Presentation

Young girl with altered mental status and headache (▶ Fig. 46.1)

■ Key Imaging Finding

Increased subarachnoid fluid-attenuated inversion recovery (FLAIR) signal

■ Top 3 Differential Diagnoses

- **Subarachnoid hemorrhage (SAH)**. Computed tomography (CT) is the modality of choice in identifying acute SAH, followed by lumbar puncture. However, magnetic resonance imaging (MRI; specifically FLAIR sequences) may be as—if not more—sensitive than CT in evaluating for subtle SAH in regions where CT is limited (e.g., regions of beam-hardening artifact). MRI is still insufficient, however, to entirely exclude SAH if negative. Increased protein content and inflammatory cells result in FLAIR hyperintensity in the region of hemorrhage, which may be focal or diffuse depending on the etiology and amount of hemorrhage. Trauma and ruptured aneurysms are the most common etiologies of SAH.
- **Meningitis**. Similar to SAH, increased protein content and the presence of infectious and inflammatory cells result in FLAIR hyperintensity within the subarachnoid space in the setting of meningitis. There is associated inflammation of the meninges with leptomeningeal involvement being more common than pachymeningeal involvement. The regions of FLAIR signal abnormality may be localized or diffuse. Leptomeningeal enhancement is commonly seen in a similar distribution, and may also be noted in regions with no discernible FLAIR signal abnormality.
- **Leptomeningeal carcinomatosis**. Leptomeningeal malignancy results in increased cellular and protein content in the subarachnoid space, which is hyperintense on FLAIR sequences. It is most often due to hematogenous spread of a distant primary tumor versus less often direct spread from a primary central nervous system tumor or skull/dura-based metastases. The regions of involvement are often focal but may be diffuse with extensive, disseminated disease. Associated meningeal enhancement is typically seen. Additional parenchymal or calvarial metastatic foci are useful discriminators, if present. FLAIR and postcontrast T1 sequences are complementary in the metastatic workup.

■ Additional Differential Diagnoses

- **Hyperoxygenation**. Patients receiving supplemental oxygenation and those sedated with propofol often demonstrate diffuse increased FLAIR signal intensity throughout the subarachnoid spaces. The etiology is thought to be due to paramagnetic effects of oxygen when increased 4- to 5-fold from normal levels. The resultant signal abnormality within the cerebrospinal fluid (CSF) is diffuse, rather than focal. Excluding superimposed leptomeningeal pathology is difficult/limited.
- **Slow/collateral venous flow**. With acute large-vessel high-grade stenosis or occlusion, intravascular FLAIR hyperintensity may be seen within the subarachnoid space. This finding may precede signal abnormalities on other MRI sequences, including the presence of restricted diffusion. The cause of increased signal is thought to represent occlusion, slow flow, or collateral flow. Similar findings are noted in patients with moyamoya disease where numerous leptomeningeal collaterals develop secondary to a carotid terminus or proximal cerebral artery occlusion. In this setting, the appearance is termed the *"climbing ivy" sign*. Sturge-Weber is a neurocutaneous syndrome characterized by pial angiomatosis overlying a portion of a cerebral hemisphere. Increased FLAIR signal intensity is noted within the pial angiomatosis; there is also ipsilateral parenchymal atrophy and cortical calcifications in the chronic setting.
- **MR artifact**. Metallic artifact disrupts the local magnetic field, resulting in loss of the null signal associated with CSF on FLAIR sequences. Common causes include braces, surgical clips, and shunt catheter reservoirs. The susceptibility artifact is localized to the region adjacent to the metallic object and is fairly characteristic in imaging appearance.

■ Diagnosis

Slow/collateral venous flow (patient with moyamoya)

✓ Pearls

- Increased protein and cellular content results in FLAIR hyperintensity with SAH, meningitis, and carcinomatosis.
- Supplemental oxygen and propofol sedation may result in diffuse FLAIR hyperintensity in the subarachnoid spaces.
- Subarachnoid FLAIR hyperintensity may be seen with vessel occlusion, slow or collateral flow, or pial angiomatosis.
- Metallic artifact results in characteristic loss of the null signal associated with CSF on FLAIR sequences.

Suggested Reading

Stuckey SL, Goh TD, Heffernan T, Rowan D. Hyperintensity in the subarachnoid space on FLAIR MRI. Am J Roentgenol 2007; 189: 913–921

Case 47

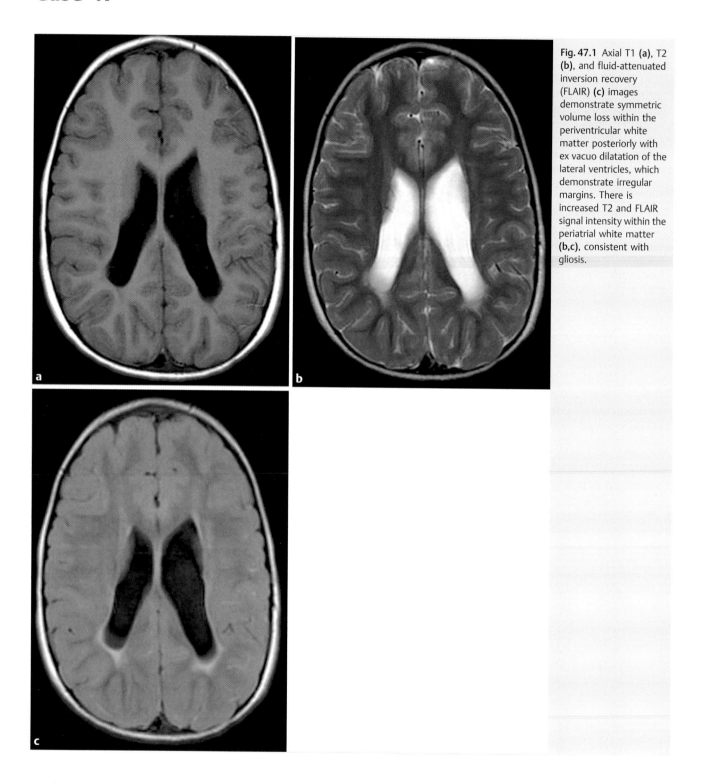

Fig. 47.1 Axial T1 (a), T2 (b), and fluid-attenuated inversion recovery (FLAIR) (c) images demonstrate symmetric volume loss within the periventricular white matter posteriorly with ex vacuo dilatation of the lateral ventricles, which demonstrate irregular margins. There is increased T2 and FLAIR signal intensity within the periatrial white matter (b,c), consistent with gliosis.

▨ Clinical Presentation

A 6-year-old girl with spastic quadriplegia (▶ Fig. 47.1)

Key Imaging Finding

Periventricular volume loss and ventriculomegaly with irregular margins

Diagnosis

Periventricular leukomalacia. In the setting of diffuse hypoxic-ischemic encephalopathy (HIE), the pattern and degree of insult depends upon the status of brain maturity, severity of the insult, and duration of the insult. In the setting of mild to moderate hypoxemia or ischemia, blood flow is preferentially diverted to regions of increased metabolic activity, including the deep gray matter structures, cerebellum, and brain stem. In full-term infants, children, and adults, the cortex and white matter of the centrum semiovale in the watershed regions between vascular territories are most susceptible to injury. With preterm infants, the penetrating vessels in the periventricular regions represent the most vulnerable watershed regions.

Imaging findings mirror the pathogenesis of HIE. Initial head ultrasound often demonstrates increased echotexture within the periventricular white matter, most pronounced posteriorly in the periatrial regions. Computed tomography is insensitive in this stage in the absence of hemorrhage due to the decreased attenuation associated with unmyelinated white matter. Magnetic resonance imaging demonstrates regions of increased signal in the periventricular white matter on T1, T2, and proton density sequences. Increased signal on diffusion-weighted imaging may be seen acutely.

As the injury progresses, volume loss and cystic change may occur, typically 2 to 6 weeks after the initial insult. There is resultant ex vacuo dilatation of the ventricles with irregular margins. The white matter volume loss also results in thinning of the corpus callosum. Gliosis is noted within the periventricular white matter, manifested by increased T2 signal intensity.

Clinically, patients typically experience seizures and/or apneic episodes in the acute setting. Chronically, patients suffer from spastic plegia or cerebral palsy.

✓ Pearls

- With HIE, the pattern of injury depends upon the status of brain maturity, severity of insult, and duration of insult.
- Clinically, patients suffer from spastic plegia or cerebral palsy.
- Imaging findings include periatrial white matter volume loss, gliosis, and ventriculomegaly with irregular margins.

Suggested Reading

Chao CP, Zaleski CG, Patton AC. Neonatal hypoxic-ischemic encephalopathy: multi-modality imaging findings. Radiographics 2006; 26 Suppl 1: S159–S172

Case 48

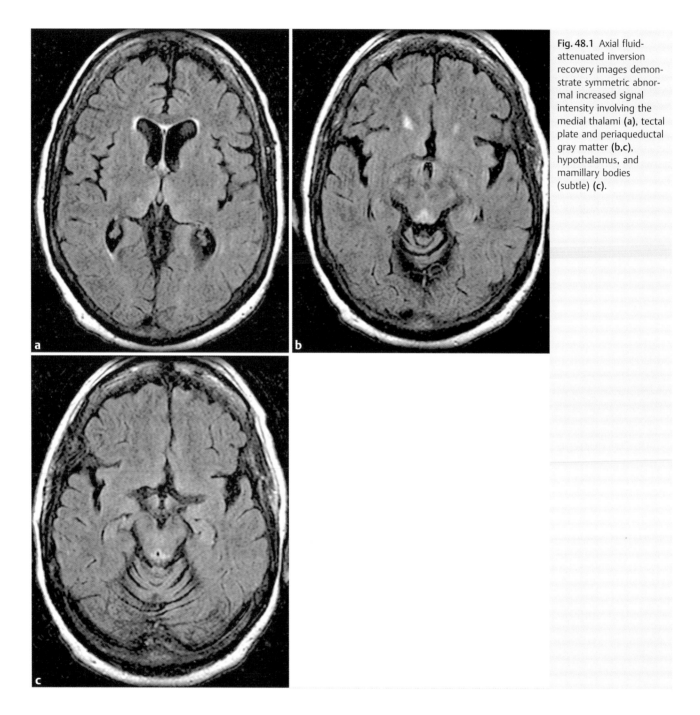

Fig. 48.1 Axial fluid-attenuated inversion recovery images demonstrate symmetric abnormal increased signal intensity involving the medial thalami **(a)**, tectal plate and periaqueductal gray matter **(b,c)**, hypothalamus, and mamillary bodies (subtle) **(c)**.

■ Clinical Presentation

A 59-year-old man with altered mental status (▶ Fig. 48.1)

■ Key Imaging Finding

Symmetric signal abnormality within the medial thalami, periaqueductal gray matter, and mamillary bodies

■ Diagnosis

Wernicke encephalopathy. Wernicke encephalopathy is a neurological disorder caused by thiamine deficiency. It most often occurs in alcoholic patients, but it may also be seen in nonalcoholic patients with malabsorption or nutritional deficiencies, including gastrointestinal neoplasms, prior gastric surgery, prolonged starvation, hyperemesis, and anorexia nervosa. Although the degree of clinical symptoms varies, the classic triad consists of altered consciousness, ataxia, and ocular dysfunction. Wernicke encephalopathy is a neurological emergency that requires prompt replenishment of thiamine.

Magnetic resonance imaging (MRI) features include symmetric increased T2/fluid-attenuated inversion recovery signal intensity within the medial thalami (most common), periaqueductal gray matter, tectal plate, and mamillary bodies. Mamillary body involvement is fairly specific and occurs in just over half of patients. Mass effect may be seen acutely. In alcoholic patients, there may be enhancement of the involved regions, particularly within the mamillary bodies; enhancement is less common in nonalcoholic patients for reasons that remain unknown. With appropriate treatment, clinical symptoms and imaging findings may regress or resolve.

✓ Pearls

- Wernicke encephalopathy is a neurological disorder caused by thiamine deficiency.
- Wernicke encephalopathy occurs in alcoholic patients or nonalcoholic patients with malabsorption or nutritional deficiencies.

- MRI reveals symmetric increased signal in the medial thalami, periaqueductal gray matter, and mamillary bodies.

Suggested Reading

Zuccoli G, Gallucci M, Capellades J et al. Wernicke encephalopathy: MR findings at clinical presentation in twenty-six alcoholic and nonalcoholic patients. Am J Neuroradiol 2007; 28: 1328–1331

Case 49

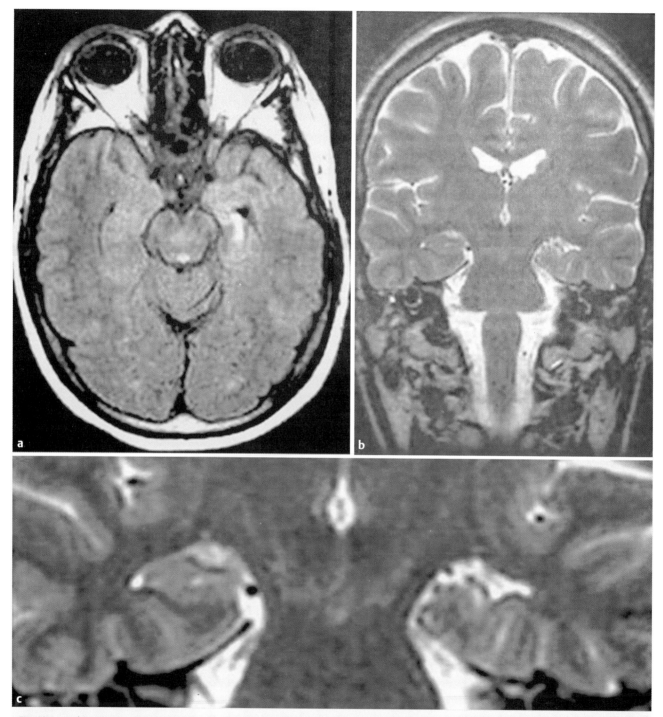

Fig. 49.1 Axial FLAIR image **(a)** demonstrates increased signal intensity and volume loss within the left mesial temporal lobe. The atrophy of the left mesial temporal lobe/hippocampus is better depicted on routine **(b)** and magnified **(c)** coronal T2 images.

■ Clinical Presentation

A 14-year-old boy with complex partial seizures (► Fig. 49.1)

▥ Key Imaging Finding

Atrophy and increased T2/fluid-attenuated inversion recovery (FLAIR) signal intensity within the mesial temporal lobe

▥ Diagnosis

Mesial temporal sclerosis (MTS). Temporal lobe epilepsy is relatively common in adolescents and young adults and typically manifests as complex partial seizures. Within this patient population, MTS is thought to represent the most common identifiable cause of temporal lobe seizures. Debate exists as to whether MTS is acquired or a developmental abnormality. Some studies show an increased incidence in patients with a history of infant febrile seizures.

Magnetic resonance imaging is the mainstay in the workup of seizure disorders because computed tomography is often normal. Seizure protocols for children and young adults typically include high-resolution coronal sequences through the mesial temporal lobes/hippocampal formations. Imaging findings of MTS include hippocampal atrophy with associated dilatation of the ipsilateral temporal horn of the lateral ventricle. Increased T2/FLAIR signal intensity is also commonly seen and increases the specificity in terms of suggesting the diagnosis. MR spectroscopy shows decreased *N*-acetyl aspartate in the affected temporal lobe and may be helpful in localizing certain cases. Interictal FDG-PET (18F-fluorodeoxyglucose positron emission tomography) imaging demonstrates hypometabolism with decreased uptake within the affected mesial temporal lobe.

Medical treatment is successful in approximately 25% of cases of MTS. Anterior temporal lobe resection is often necessary for persistent seizure activity.

✓ Pearls

- Temporal lobe epilepsy is common in adolescents and young adults; it typically manifests as complex partial seizures.
- MTS is characterized by atrophy and increased T2/FLAIR signal intensity within the involved hippocampus.
- Interictal FDG-PET shows hypometabolism with decreased uptake within the affected mesial temporal lobe.

Suggested Readings

Bocti C, Robitaille Y, Diadori P et al. The pathological basis of temporal lobe epilepsy in childhood. Neurology 2003; 60: 191–195

Castillo M, Smith JK, Kwock L. Proton MR spectroscopy in patients with acute temporal lobe seizures. Am J Neuroradiol 2001; 22: 152–157

Case 50

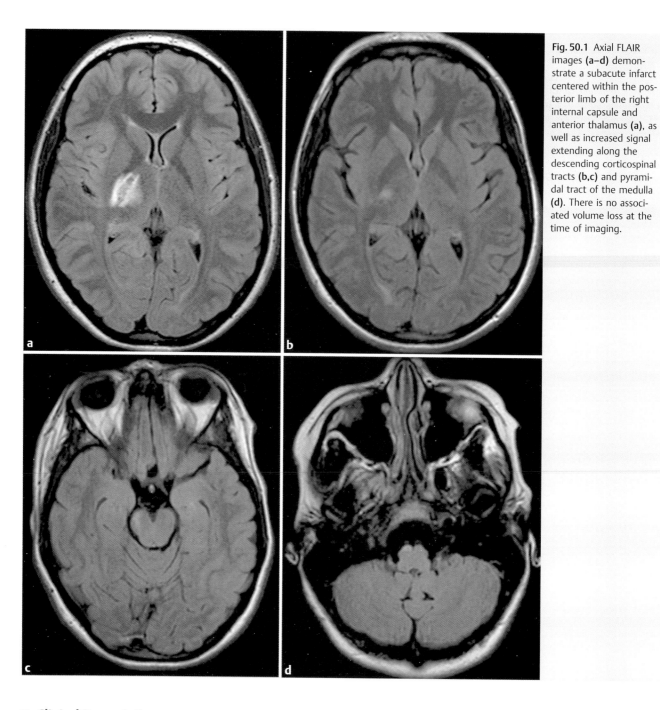

Fig. 50.1 Axial FLAIR images (**a–d**) demonstrate a subacute infarct centered within the posterior limb of the right internal capsule and anterior thalamus (**a**), as well as increased signal extending along the descending corticospinal tracts (**b,c**) and pyramidal tract of the medulla (**d**). There is no associated volume loss at the time of imaging.

▧ Clinical Presentation

A young adult man with known subacute infarct (▶ Fig. 50.1)

■ Key Imaging Finding

Increased signal intensity along descending tracts with corresponding parenchymal abnormality

■ Diagnosis

Wallerian degeneration (WD). WD refers to ipsilateral degeneration of descending axons/white matter tracts secondary to a more proximal neuronal or axonal injury. Infarcts are the most common cause of WD, followed by hemorrhage and tumors. Corticospinal tracts (CSTs) are most commonly involved; corpus callosal, cerebellar peduncle, and optic radiation involvement may occasionally be seen. The extent of WD often correlates with the degree of clinical impairment.

Acutely, contiguous increased T2/fluid-attenuated inversion recovery (FLAIR) signal is noted extending through the internal capsule and brain stem along the CSTs, often referred to as Wallerian edema at this stage. Increased signal may also be seen on diffusion-weighted imaging, which may precede abnormal signal on conventional sequences. Diffusion tensor imaging may show reduced fractional anisotropy within the descending CSTs. In the chronic stage, atrophy is noted with volume loss that is most conspicuous within the cerebral peduncle.

✓ Pearls

- WD refers to degeneration of descending white matter tracts secondary to proximal neuronal or axonal injury.
- Infarcts are the most common cause of WD, followed by hemorrhage and tumors; CSTs are most commonly affected.

- Magnetic resonance imaging findings include increased T2/FLAIR signal along descending tracts; atrophy is seen in the chronic stage.

Suggested Readings

Uchino A, Sawada A, Takase Y, Egashira R, Kudo S. Transient detection of early wallerian degeneration on diffusion-weighted MRI after an acute cerebrovascular accident. Neuroradiology 2004; 46: 183–188

Uchino A, Takase Y, Nomiyama K, Egashira R, Kudo S. Brainstem and cerebellar changes after cerebrovascular accidents: magnetic resonance imaging. Eur Radiol 2006; 16: 592–597

Case 51

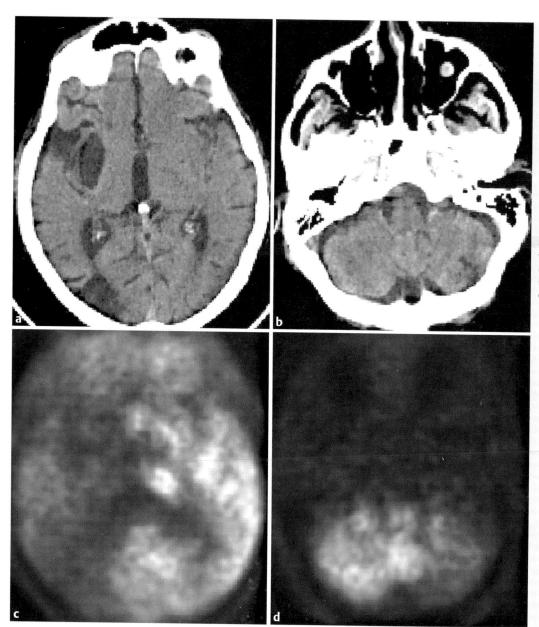

Fig. 51.1 Axial computed tomography (CT) image (a) demonstrates a remote infarct with encephalomalacia involving the right cerebral cortex, lentiform nuclei, and deep white matter. Axial CT image through the posterior fossa (b) reveals very subtle volume loss and a small infarct within the left cerebellar hemisphere. Corresponding PET images (c,d) show decreased metabolism within the right cerebral (c) and left cerebellar (d) hemispheres. (Courtesy of Kamal Singh, MD.)

■ Clinical Presentation

A 65-year-old man with prior stroke (▶ Fig. 51.1)

■ Key Imaging Finding

Cerebral insult with ipsilateral cerebral and contralateral cerebellar volume loss and decreased metabolism

■ Diagnosis

Crossed cerebellar diaschisis. Cross cerebellar diaschisis refers to volume loss of one cerebellar hemisphere secondary to an insult involving the contralateral cerebral hemisphere. Common etiologies include cerebral infarcts, hemorrhage, postoperative changes, large vascular malformations, and tumors. Patients with chronic seizures originating from one cerebral hemisphere may also demonstrate volume loss in the contralateral cerebellum.

After injury, neurons undergo secondary degeneration. Two types of secondary degeneration are recognized: Wallerian and transneuronal. Wallerian degeneration occurs along descending tracts ipsilateral to the insult, extending through the cerebral peduncle and into the brain stem. Most of the afferent tracts originate from the frontal and parietal cortices. Transneuronal degeneration results from interference and disruption of tracts that synapse within the brain stem and cross midline to the contralateral cerebellar hemisphere. In crossed cerebellar diaschisis, transneuronal degeneration affects the pontocerebellar tract, which synapses in the superior aspect of the pons.

Crossed cerebellar diaschisis is a late finding, typically occurring at least one year after the initial insult. Positron emission tomography (PET) imaging studies reveal hypometabolism within the involved cerebral hemisphere and contralateral cerebellar hemisphere. Cross-sectional imaging reveals unilateral cerebellar volume loss, which is often subtle. The affected cerebellar hemisphere may show normal or slightly increased T2 signal intensity. A hemosiderin rim (hypointense on T2) may also be seen. The degree of cerebellar volume loss is relatively proportional to the supratentorial volume loss. Clinical symptoms are related to the degree of supratentorial injury; the degree of cerebellar atrophy poorly correlates with clinical outcomes.

✓ Pearls

- Cross cerebellar diaschisis refers to cerebellar volume loss due to an insult involving the contralateral cerebrum.
- PET imaging reveals hypometabolism in the involved cerebral hemisphere and contralateral cerebellum.
- Magnetic resonance imaging shows cerebral and contralateral cerebellar volume loss; there may be subtle increased T2 cerebellar signal.

Suggested Readings

Tien RD, Ashdown BC. Crossed cerebellar diaschisis and crossed cerebellar atrophy: correlation of MR findings, clinical symptoms, and supratentorial diseases in 26 patients. Am J Roentgenol 1992; 158: 1155–1159

Uchino A, Takase Y, Nomiyama K, Egashira R, Kudo S. Brainstem and cerebellar changes after cerebrovascular accidents: magnetic resonance imaging. Eur Radiol 2006; 16: 592–597

Case 52

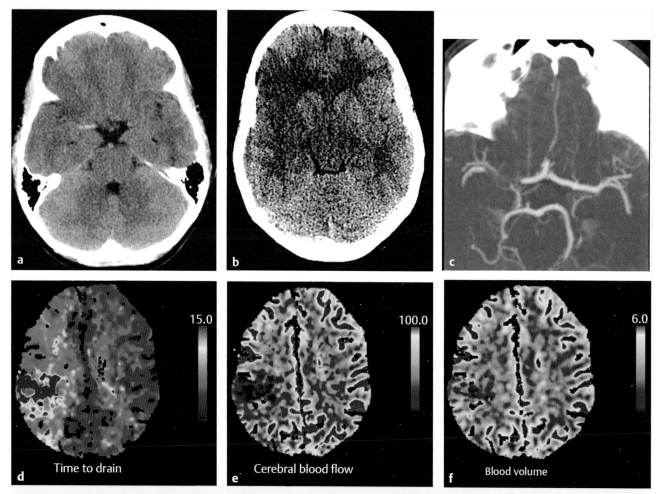

Fig. 52.1 Axial CT image **(a)** demonstrates a hyperdense right MCA; normal attenuation is noted within the contralateral MCA and basilar artery. Axial image more superiorly in stroke/ischemia windows **(b)** shows loss of gray-white matter differentiation involving the right insular ribbon and operculum with mild sulcal effacement. Maximum intensity projection from a CT angiogram **(c)** reveals occlusion of the proximal-mid right MCA. Axial time to drain **(d)**, cerebral blood flow **(e)**, and blood volume **(f)** images from a CTP scan in a different patient with similar clinical presentation reveal a central region of significantly decreased cerebral blood flow and increased time to drain with a smaller region of moderately decreased blood volume involving the posterior right MCA vascular territory. This is surrounded by regions of moderately decreased blood flow and increased time to drain with minimal decrease in blood volume. (Images d–f courtesy of Rocky Saenz, DO.)

■ **Clinical Presentation**

Adult men with acute onset left-sided neurological deficits (▶ Fig. 52.1)

■ Key Imaging Finding

Perfusion imaging with an ischemic penumbra surrounding a central infarct

■ Diagnosis

Stroke. Stoke is a leading cause of morbidity and mortality, especially in adults. Early recognition and treatment are key to optimizing patient outcomes. Computed tomography (CT) and magnetic resonance imaging (MRI) provide useful diagnostic information, evaluate for potential complications, and aid in directing therapy. Angiography is primarily utilized in cases where intraarterial thrombolysis is a consideration.

The imaging workup of stroke begins with a noncontrast head CT. CT is useful in identifying early signs of ischemia and evaluating for contraindications to thrombolytic therapy, including a large middle cerebral artery (MCA) infarct or the presence of intracranial hemorrhage. Early CT findings of stroke include a hyperdense MCA due to intraluminal clot; loss of gray-white matter differentiation involving the deep gray matter, insular ribbon, and cerebral cortex; and sulcal effacement. Loss of gray-white matter differentiation and sulcal effacement result from cytotoxic edema and neuronal swelling. In hyperacute stroke, CT may initially be normal with follow-up imaging hours later better depicting the regions of ischemia. By 24 hours, nearly all strokes are detectable on CT.

MRI is more sensitive than CT, especially within the first few hours of symptom onset. Diffusion sequences may show restricted diffusion within minutes, manifesting as hyperintensity on diffusion-weighted imaging (DWI) and hypointensity on corresponding apparent diffusion coefficient maps. Development of cytotoxic edema over the next few hours results in increased T2/fluid-attenuated inversion recovery signal in the involved vascular distribution with loss of gray-white matter differentiation and sulcal effacement. In the setting of vessel occlusion, there is loss of the normal T2 flow void in the affected arterial segment. The thrombus typically demonstrates blooming artifact on gradient echo and may appear hyperintense on unenhanced T1 sequences.

An important aspect of the imaging workup includes vessel analysis and evaluation for a penumbra, which refers to salvageable brain parenchyma at risk for infract. Typically, strokes have a central region of infarct and a peripheral penumbra. Both CT angiography (CTA) and MR angiography (MRA) are useful to evaluate for vessel patency. CTA is quicker and more readily available; however, MRA does not require the use of contrast. On CTA, occlusion presents as an intraluminal filling defect, most commonly in the proximal MCA. On MRA, time-of-flight imaging is most often utilized; regions of diminished or occluded flow present with loss of flow signal intensity in the affected segment. Increased enhancement or flow signal within collateral vessels may be seen.

Perfusion imaging is designed to evaluate for the presence of a penumbra, which may affect management. In general, the window for intravenous (IV) thrombolytics is 3 hours from the onset of symptoms; however, thrombolytic therapy may be considered beyond this point in certain patients with a penumbra. CT perfusion (CTP) is relatively quick and more readily available than MR perfusion (MRP); however, both may be utilized in the workup of stroke. On CTP, the region of infarct demonstrates significantly decreased blood flow and blood volume and increased mean transit time/time to drain (time between arterial inflow and venous outflow); the penumbra, on the other hand, typically shows moderately decreased blood flow, increased mean transit time, and normal or mildly decreased blood volume. MRP may be done with IV contrast (most common) or arterial spin labeling. Parenchyma that shows both restricted diffusion and decreased perfusion corresponds to an infarct; regions of decreased perfusion and normal DWI signal represent the penumbra.

The advent of intraarterial thrombolysis has greatly improved stroke outcomes. Patients with acute large vessel occlusion (often the proximal MCA) < 5 to 6 hours from symptom onset are potential candidates. Numerous systems are currently available with most combining pharmaceutical and mechanical thrombolytic techniques. Treatment of basilar occlusions may be performed as late as 24 hours after symptom onset in some cases. Potential complications include distal emboli, vessel injury, and parenchymal hemorrhage.

✓ Pearls

- CT is useful in identifying early signs of ischemia and evaluating for contraindications to thrombolytic therapy.
- MRI is more sensitive than CT, especially within the first few hours; restricted diffusion is the first abnormality.

- Assessment of vessel patency and the presence of a penumbra are important in directing therapeutic options.

Suggested Reading

Srinivasan A, Goyal M, Al Azri F, Lum C. State-of-the-art imaging of acute stroke. Radiographics 2006; 26 Suppl 1: S75–S95

Case 53

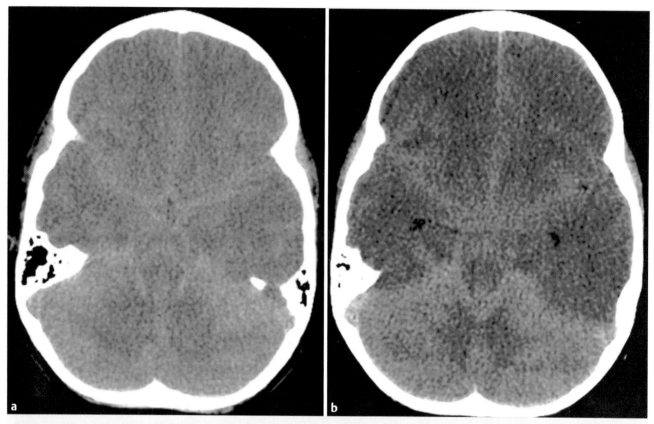

Fig. 53.1 Axial computed tomography images **(a,b)** demonstrate diffuse cerebral edema with hypodensity throughout the brain parenchyma. There is effacement of extraaxial CSF spaces with relative increased density of the basal cisterns.

▨ Clinical Presentation

A young boy with acute onset altered mental status and loss of consciousness (▶ Fig. 53.1)

▣ Key Imaging Finding

Diffuse cerebral edema with hyperdense basal cisterns

▣ Diagnosis

Pseudosubarachnoid hemorrhage. Pseudosubarachnoid hemorrhage (pseudo-SAH) refers to the hyperdense appearance of the basal cisterns in the setting of diffuse cerebral edema; less commonly, it has been described in association with intracranial hypotension. Pseudo-SAH is believed to result from a variety of factors affecting both the extraaxial cerebrospinal fluid (CSF) spaces and the underlying brain parenchyma. In the setting of diffuse cerebral edema, there is increased intracranial pressure, which results in engorgement of the blood-filled pial veins, as well as effacement of the hypodense extraaxial CSF. This combined with underlying cortical hypodensity secondary to cytotoxic edema, results in relative increased attenuation within the basal cisterns, simulating SAH. The Hounsfield unit (HU) measurement of pseudo-SAH (approximately 30 HU) is considerably less than that expected with SAH in a patient with a normal hematocrit (~55 to 70 HU), which helps distinguish between the two entities.

✓ Pearls

- Pseudo-SAH refers to the hyperdense appearance of the basal cisterns in the setting of diffuse cerebral edema.
- With cerebral edema, increased density in the basal cisterns and decreased density of the parenchyma simulates SAH.

- The HU of pseudo-SAH is considerably less than that expected with SAH in a patient with a normal hematocrit.

Suggested Reading

Given CA, II, Burdette JH, Elster AD, Williams DW, III. Pseudo-subarachnoid hemorrhage: a potential imaging pitfall associated with diffuse cerebral edema. Am J Neuroradiol 2003; 24: 254–256

Case 54

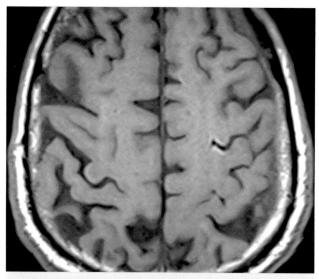

Fig. 54.1 Axial unenhanced T1 magnetic resonance image demonstrates bandlike regions of cortical hyperintensity in the left precentral gyrus.

■ Clinical Presentation

Adult man with long-standing history of hypertension, diabetes, and microvascular ischemic disease (▶ Fig. 54.1)

▦ Key Imaging Finding

Bandlike increased T1 cortical signal intensity

▦ Diagnosis

Cortical laminar necrosis. Hypoxic-ischemic encephalopathy (HIE) may result from a variety of causes, to include cardiac arrest (most common), pulmonary disease, trauma, near-drowning, status epilepticus, drug overdose, toxins, and so forth. The pattern of brain injury and prognosis varies based upon patient age and the duration and severity of the underlying condition. In general, gray matter is more prone to injury than white matter due to its increased metabolic activity; it is even more susceptible when located in watershed regions between two different vascular territories.

The normal cortex consists of six layers, each with differing degrees of susceptibility to hypoxic-ischemic insults. Layer three is most susceptible, followed by layers five and six. Cortical laminar necrosis refers to regions of nonhemorrhagic

necrosis isolated to a particular cortical band, typically the third layer. On magnetic resonance imaging, cortical laminar necrosis characteristically presents as bandlike regions of increased signal intensity on unenhanced T1 sequences. They typically first appear in the late subacute phase at approximately 2 weeks, peak at around 2 months, and then become less conspicuous. There may be bandlike cortical enhancement on postcontrast sequences during the early subacute phase, preceding the signal abnormality on unenhanced T1 sequences, although this finding is not specific to cortical laminar necrosis. A corresponding region of hyperdensity may be seen on computed tomography. Adjacent white matter injury is common and often demonstrates chronic volume loss with encephalomalacia.

✓ Pearls

- The pattern of HIE depends upon patient age and the duration and severity of the underlying condition.
- Cortical laminar necrosis refers to bandlike nonhemorrhagic necrosis usually involving the third cortical layer.

- Cortical laminar necrosis characteristically presents as bandlike regions of increased T1 signal intensity.

Suggested Readings

Komiyama M, Nakajima H, Nishikawa M, Yasui T. Serial MR observation of cortical laminar necrosis caused by brain infarction. Neuroradiology 1998; 40: 771–777

Takahashi S, Higano S, Ishii K et al. Hypoxic brain damage: cortical laminar necrosis and delayed changes in white matter at sequential MR imaging. Radiology 1993; 189: 449–456

Case 55

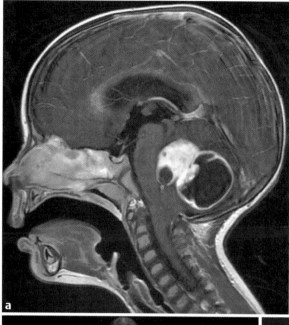

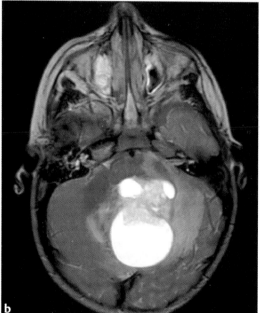

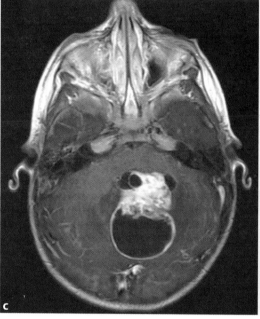

Fig. 55.1 Sagittal contrast-enhanced T1 image (a) demonstrates a large posterior fossa mass with cystic and enhancing solid components. There is obstruction of the fourth ventricle with hydrocephalus and inferior displacement of the cerebellar tonsils. On axial T2 (b) and T1 post-contrast (c) images, the mass is slightly eccentric to the left. There is solid enhancement, as well as enhancement along the walls of the cystic components (c). The fourth ventricle is effaced and there is surrounding edema in the cerebellar hemispheres (b).

■ **Clinical Presentation**

An 8-year-old boy with headaches, vomiting, and ataxia (▶ Fig. 55.1)

■ Key Imaging Finding

Posterior fossa mass in child

■ Top 3 Differential Diagnoses

• **Medulloblastoma.** Medulloblastoma is an aggressive (World Health Organization [WHO] grade IV) primitive neuroectodermal tumor (PNET) and is the most common posterior fossa tumor in children. The peak incidence is within the first decade of life. As with all posterior fossa tumors, patients often present with headache or symptoms related to obstructive hydrocephalus. The tumor typically arises from the superior medullary velum or roof of the fourth ventricle. Although characteristically midline, lateral (cerebellar hemisphere) origin may be seen in older children and young adults. Medulloblastomas are hyperdense on computed tomography (CT) (~90%) and demonstrate regions of restricted diffusion on magnetic resonance imaging due to high cellular content. They are T1 hypointense, T2 iso- to hyperintense, and fluid-attenuated inversion recovery (FLAIR) hyperintense. Cystic changes occur in approximately half of cases; calcification occurs in ~20%. Enhancement is heterogeneous but avid. Subarachnoid seeding is present in up to one-third of cases at presentation; therefore, evaluation of the entire neuroaxis is required prior to surgical intervention for any posterior fossa tumor.

• **Juvenile pilocytic astrocytoma (JPA).** JPA (WHO grade I astrocytoma) is the second most common primary posterior fossa tumor in children with an incidence slightly below that for medulloblastoma. They may occur sporadically or in association with neurofibromatosis type 1. Peak incidence is 5 to 15 years of age. The tumor arises from the cerebellar hemisphere; therefore, it is typically off-midline. The most common presentation is a cystic mass with an enhancing mural nodule. The cystic component is T1 iso- to hypointense and T2/FLAIR hyperintense. The solid component is T2 and FLAIR hyperintense and enhances avidly. Enhancement of the cyst wall suggests the presence of tumor cells. A less common imaging appearance includes a solid mass with a cystic/necrotic center.

• **Ependymoma.** Ependymoma is a slow-growing, midline posterior fossa tumor of ependymal cells that originates along the floor of the fourth ventricle. It characteristically squeezes through the fourth ventricle foramina into the foramen magnum, cerebellopontine angle, or cisterna magna. Mean age of presentation is 6 years. On CT, calcification is seen in ≈50% of cases; cystic change and foci of hemorrhage occur in ≈20%. Two-thirds arise from the fourth ventricle and approximately one-third are supratentorial and centered within the brain parenchyma. The tumor is heterogeneous and iso- to hypointense on T1 and hyperintense on T2 sequences. Tumor cysts are often hyperintense to cerebrospinal fluid (CSF) on T1 and FLAIR images. There is mild to moderate heterogeneous enhancement of the solid components. CSF dissemination is less common than with medulloblastoma.

■ Additional Differential Diagnoses

• **Brain stem glioma.** Brain stem glioma represents ≈10 to 20% of pediatric brain tumors and commonly presents within the first and second decades of life. It typically presents as a diffuse, infiltrating pontine mass (WHO grade II to III) with exophytic components that may engulf the basilar artery or project into the fourth ventricle. It is typically hypointense on T1 and hyperintense on T2 sequences with variable enhancement. Higher-grade regions demonstrate restricted diffusion, increased enhancement, and increased perfusion. Prognosis is poor.

• **Atypical teratoid rhabdoid tumor (ATRT).** ATRT is a rare, aggressive embryonal tumor composed of rhabdoid cells and PNET components. It typically presents within the first few years of life with the majority located within the posterior fossa and the remainder occurring supratentorially. Its appearance on gross examination and imaging is nearly identical to medulloblastoma, including hyperdensity on CT and regions of restricted diffusion. The key distinction is the age of presentation. Subarachnoid seeding is common at presentation. Prognosis is dismal; mean survival is < 6 months if the patient is < 3 years of age at time of presentation.

■ Diagnosis

Juvenile pilocytic astrocytoma

✓ Pearls

• Medulloblastoma is the most common posterior fossa mass in a child, is midline, and often seeds the CSF.

• JPA most commonly presents as an off-midline cystic mass with enhancing mural nodule.

• Ependymoma is a midline tumor that extends through the ventricular foramina.

Suggested Readings

O'Brien WT. Imaging of posterior fossa brain tumors in children. J Am Osteopath Coll Radiol. 2013; 2: 2–12

Poretti A, Meoded A, Huisman TAGM. Neuroimaging of pediatric posterior fossa tumors including review of the literature. J Magn Reson Imaging 2012; 35: 32–47

Case 56

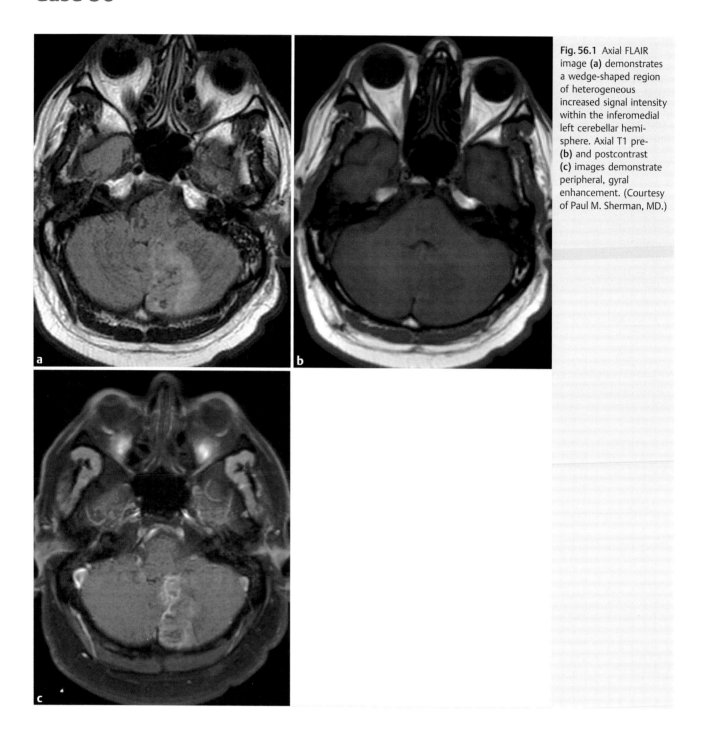

Fig. 56.1 Axial FLAIR image **(a)** demonstrates a wedge-shaped region of heterogeneous increased signal intensity within the inferomedial left cerebellar hemisphere. Axial T1 pre- **(b)** and postcontrast **(c)** images demonstrate peripheral, gyral enhancement. (Courtesy of Paul M. Sherman, MD.)

■ Clinical Presentation

A 52-year-old man with headache and new onset gait disturbances for one week (▶ Fig. 56.1)

Key Imaging Finding

Posterior fossa mass in adult

Top 3 Differential Diagnoses

- **Infarction.** Ischemic changes commonly affect the posterior fossa and may have a masslike appearance. The morphology of an infarct is often wedge-shaped and corresponds to the vascular territory of the involved vessel (posterior inferior, anterior inferior, and superior cerebellar arteries). Other differentiating features include restricted diffusion in the acute and early subacute stages and occasionally vascular occlusion demonstrated on computed tomography (CT) angiography or magnetic resonance (MR) angiography. Edema, mass effect, hemorrhagic transformation, and subacute enhancement may mimic a mass.

- **Metastatic disease.** Metastatic disease represents the most common posterior fossa parenchymal neoplasm in middle-aged and older adults. Lung, breast, and gastrointestinal (GI) malignancies are among the most common primary neoplasms. Metastases are more often multiple, although solitary lesions are not uncommon. Tumors are typically solid; cystic change and calcification occasionally occur with mucinous adenocarcinomas (breast, lung, and GI). Hemorrhagic metastases, which may occur with breast, lung, renal cell, thyroid, melanoma, and choriocarcinoma primaries, tend to have strong enhancement and an incomplete hemosiderin rim. Renal cell carcinoma metastases may mimic hemangioblastoma, as they are very vascular.

- **Hemangioblastoma.** Hemangioblastomas are low-grade (World Health Organization grade I) meningeal neoplasms and are the most common primary posterior fossa neoplasms in adults. Ninety to ninety-five percent occur within the posterior fossa, typically within the cerebellar hemispheres, whereas 5 to 10% are supratentorial. Supratentorial lesions commonly occur in the setting of von Hippel-Lindau (VHL) disease (autosomal dominant, chromosome 3). Larger lesions present as cystic masses with enhancing mural nodules (similar to juvenile pilocytic astrocytoma) that abut the pial surface; smaller lesions commonly present as solid enhancing masses. Cystic components may be slightly hyperintense to cerebrospinal fluid on T1 and fluid-attenuated inversion recovery (FLAIR) sequences. The cyst and nodule are hyperintense on T2/FLAIR images. The solid components avidly enhance, abut the pial surface, and may demonstrate flow voids. When identified, the entire neuroaxis should be imaged to look for additional lesions, especially within the spinal cord. Approximately one-quarter to one-half of patients with posterior fossa hemangioblastomas will have VHL. Patients with VHL may also have retinal hemangioblastomas, endolymphatic sac tumors, renal cell carcinoma, pheochromocytoma, islet cell tumors, and visceral cysts.

Additional Differential Diagnoses

- **Vascular malformation.** Arteriovenous malformations consist of a nidus of abnormal connections between arteries and veins without intervening capillaries. CT may demonstrate regions of increased attenuation or calcification. MR imaging (MRI) reveals a tangle of enlarged vessels; perinidal aneurysms are a common source of hemorrhage. Cavernous malformations consist of blood-filled sinusoids and cavernous spaces without intervening parenchyma. CT may be normal or show subtle regions of calcification or hemorrhage. Lesions have foci of increased and decreased T1 and T2 signal centrally with a T2 dark (hemosiderin) capsule on MRI.

- **Hypertensive hemorrhage.** Hypertensive hemorrhage commonly involves the posterior fossa, including the pons and cerebellar hemispheres. Hemorrhagic foci are typically round or oval. Acute hemorrhage is hyperdense on CT with mass effect and surrounding edema. MRI appearance varies based upon the age of blood products and composition of the hemoglobin moiety. Gradient echo and susceptibility-weighted imaging often identify additional foci of microhemorrhage associated with hypertension in the lentiform nuclei and thalami.

Diagnosis

Subacute posterior inferior cerebellar artery territory infarct

✓ Pearls

- Ischemia commonly affects the posterior fossa, follows a vascular distribution, and has restricted diffusion.
- Metastases are the most common posterior fossa parenchymal tumors in adults and may be multiple.

- Hemangioblastomas present as cystic masses with mural nodules; they may be sporadic or inherited (VHL).
- Hypertensive hemorrhages commonly involve the lentiform nuclei, thalami, and posterior fossa.

Suggested Readings

Cormier PJ, Long ER, Russell EJ. MR imaging of posterior fossa infarctions: vascular territories and clinical correlates. Radiographics 1992; 12: 1079–1096

Poretti A, Meoded A, Huisman TAGM. Neuroimaging of pediatric posterior fossa tumors including review of the literature. J Magn Reson Imaging 2012; 35: 32–47

Case 57

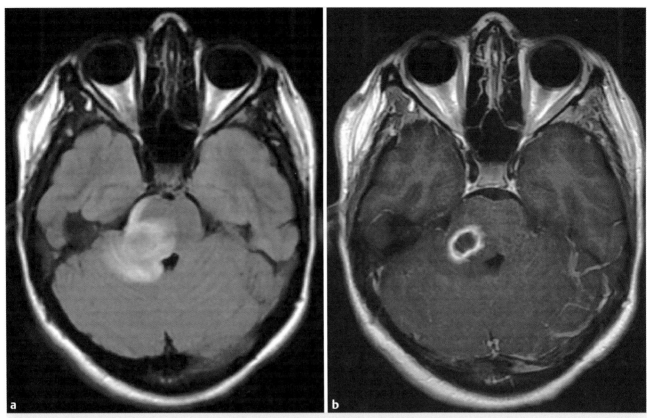

Fig. 57.1 1 Axial fluid-attenuated inversion recovery image **(a)** demonstrates diffuse abnormal increased signal within the pons on the right with extension into the middle cerebellar peduncle and right cerebellar hemisphere. Axial T1 postcontrast image **(b)** reveals ring enhancement centrally with surrounding hypointensity.

■ Clinical Presentation

A teenage girl with ataxia and headaches (▶ Fig. 57.1)

▨ Key Imaging Finding

Enhancing pontine mass in a child

▨ Top 3 Differential Diagnoses

- **Brain stem glioma.** Brain stem glioma represents approximately 10 to 20% of pediatric brain tumors. Patients most often present in the first or second decades of life with cranial neuropathies, motor deficits, ataxia, headache, and/or nausea/vomiting. The most common variant is the diffuse infiltrating pontine glioma (DIPG), which is a World Health Organization [WHO] grade II tumor (fibrillary) but often has regions that are higher grade (anaplastic). The tumor results in brain stem enlargement with diffuse increased T2/fluid-attenuated inversion recovery signal abnormality. Abnormal signal may extend posteriorly into the cerebellar peduncles or superiorly through the cerebral peduncles and into the deep gray and white matter. Exophytic components may extend anteriorly and engulf the basilar artery or extend posteriorly into the fourth ventricle. Regions of enhancement, restricted diffusion, and increased perfusion are often noted within the tumor, correspond to regions of higher grade, and are the preferred sites for biopsy, if necessary. Prognosis is dismal with the majority of cases progressing to higher-grade tumors. A less common variant is the juvenile pilocytic astrocytoma, which is a low-grade (WHO grade I) tumor that presents as a cystic brain stem mass with an enhancing nodule, as is commonly seen in the cerebellum.

- **Demyelinating disease.** Acute disseminated encephalomyelitis (ADEM) is the most common demyelinating disease in children. It is monophasic and occurs following an antecedent viral infection or vaccination. The disease course varies from self-limiting to fulminant, hemorrhagic encephalitis. Magnetic resonance imaging (MRI) reveals regions of ovoid increased T2 signal abnormality within the white matter that may be confluent. Lesions are often bilateral but asymmetric. Involvement of the corpus callosum, cerebellar hemispheres, optic pathways, and brain stem is characteristic of demyelinating disease. Compared with multiple sclerosis (MS), ADEM lesions tend to be more confluent and are more likely to involve gray matter. Active lesions may demonstrate enhancement along the leading edge of demyelination in an "open ring" pattern. MS occurs more frequently in adults and older children. As opposed to those with ADEM, patients with MS characteristically have a relapsing and remitting rather than monophasic course. The imaging appearance may be identical to ADEM.

- **Rhombencephalitis.** Encephalitis refers to focal infection of the brain parenchyma due to spread of infectious and inflammatory cells hematogenously or directly. Involvement of the hindbrain (cerebellum, pons, and medulla) is referred to as rhombencephalitis. Causative organisms may be viral or bacterial. Bacterial infections are more common in immunosuppressed patients. Viral meningitis tends to favor the deep gray and white matter. On MRI, viral encephalitis demonstrates regions of increased T2 signal intensity involving the deep gray and white matter structures, including the cerebellum and brain stem. Enhancement is variable but typically patchy and ill-defined. Overlying leptomeningeal enhancement occasionally may be seen in some infections. Patients with brain stem involvement often present with relatively acute onset ataxia, headaches, and cranial nerve deficits. Cortical involvement results in seizures and focal neurological deficits. Treatment includes supportive care along with intravenous antibiotics for suspected bacterial infection. Symptoms may resolve or the infection may progress to abscess formation, in which case rim enhancement of the abscess capsule is seen.

▨ Diagnosis

Rhombencephalitis (with abscess)

✓ Pearls

- DIPG is the most common variant of brain stem glioma; prognosis is dismal.
- High-grade regions within DIPG show restricted diffusion, increased perfusion, and increased enhancement.
- ADEM results in ovoid or confluent regions of signal abnormality; "open ring" enhancement may be seen.
- Rhombencephalitis refers to infection of the hindbrain, including the cerebellum, pons, and medulla.

Suggested Readings

Mialin R, Koob M, de Seze J, Dietemann JL, Kremer S. Case 173: acute disseminated encephalomyelitis confined to the brainstem. Radiology 2011; 260: 911–914

O'Brien WT. Imaging of posterior fossa brain tumors in children. J Am Osteopath Coll Radiol. 2013; 2: 2–12

Poretti A, Meoded A, Huisman TAGM. Neuroimaging of pediatric posterior fossa tumors including review of the literature. J Magn Reson Imaging 2012; 35: 32–47

Case 58

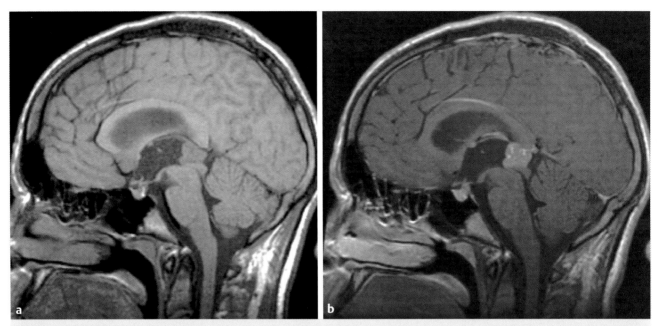

Fig. 58.1 Sagittal T1 pre- **(a)** and postcontrast **(b)** images demonstrate a lobulated, enhancing pineal region mass that causes mass effect on the tectal plate and obstruction of the cerebral aqueduct with associated hydrocephalus. There is also a small, nodular enhancing focus within the superior third ventricle.

▓ Clinical Presentation

A 15-year-old boy with headaches and vomiting (▶ Fig. 58.1)

▦ Key Imaging Finding

Pineal region mass

▦ Top 3 Differential Diagnoses

- **Pineal cyst.** Pineal cysts are common and usually incidental. Rarely, large cysts (> 15 mm) may produce symptoms secondary to local mass effect resulting in headache or visual disturbances. Simple cysts follow fluid signal intensity on magnetic resonance imaging (MRI) and lack central, solid enhancement; surrounding enhancement involving the cyst wall and within the pineal substance is commonly seen. The cysts may demonstrate increased signal intensity on T1 sequences due to proteinaceous content or occasionally hemorrhage with trauma. Cysts > 10 mm are often followed with serial imaging to ensure stability, if atypical features are identified.
- **Germ cell tumor (GCT).** GCTs are the most common malignant neoplasms of the pineal gland with germinomas representing more than 60% of cases. Most cases occur in adolescent and young adult males. Presenting symptoms are usually secondary to mass effect resulting in obstructive hydrocephalus, Parinaud syndrome (paralysis of upward gaze), or endocrine dysfunction. Germinomas are hyperdense on computed tomography (CT) due to the high nuclear-to-cytoplasmic ratio and may contain calcifications centrally. On MRI, germinomas are typically intermediate in signal intensity on T1 and T2 sequences with avid enhancement. On occasion, germinomas may appear cystic. As cerebrospinal fluid (CSF) dissemination is common, the entire spine must be imaged to evaluate for drop metastases. Other GCTs include teratomas, yolk sac tumors, and choriocarci-nomas. Teratomas will typically have macroscopic fat and calcification. Yolk sac tumors may be cystic and associated with elevated levels of alpha-fetoprotein. Choriocarcinomas have a propensity to bleed and are associated with elevated levels of human chorionic gonadotropin.
- **Pineal cell tumor.** Pineal cell origin tumors consist of pineoblastomas, pineocytomas, and pineal parenchymal tumors of intermediate differentiation (PPTID). Pineoblastomas are more malignant with a peak incidence in the first decade of life. Seeding of the CSF is common. Pineocytomas (World Health Organization [WHO] grade I) have a peak incidence in the third and fourth decades of life and are less aggressive. PPTID are intermediate tumors (WHO grade II or III) that occur most commonly in young adults. Presenting symptoms are usually due to mass effect resulting in obstructive hydrocephalus, Parinaud syndrome, or endocrine dysfunction. On imaging, the tumors may closely resemble one another. On average, pineoblastomas are larger at the time of presentation. All may be hyperdense on CT due to the high cellularity. When calcifications occur with pineal cell tumors, they are typically along the periphery in an "exploded" pattern. On MRI, pineal cell tumors are of intermediate signal intensity on T1 and intermediate to hyperintense on T2 sequences with avid enhancement. As with GCTs, the spine must be imaged to evaluate for drop metastases.

▦ Additional Differential Diagnoses

- **Tectal plate glioma.** Tectal gliomas are slow growing, low-grade astrocytomas that occur primarily in children. Patients present with symptoms related to increased intracranial pressure. Imaging reveals bulbous enlargement of the tectal plate with narrowing or obstruction of the cerebral aqueduct. There is increased T2 signal intensity and typically no or minimal enhancement. Treatment is geared toward CSF diversion.
- **Meningioma.** Meningiomas are the most common extraaxial intracranial tumors. They may occur along the margin of the tentorium, mimicking a pineal gland mass. The pineal gland and internal cerebral veins are often displaced superiorly. On noncontrast CT, meningiomas may be hyperdense; calcification is common. The enhancement pattern is typically avid and homogenous with a dural tail.

▦ Diagnosis

Pineal germinoma (with CSF dissemination)

✓ Pearls

- Pineal cysts are often asymptomatic and incidentally found; no internal enhancement should be seen.
- GCTs are the most common pineal neoplasms and commonly result in CSF dissemination.
- Pineal origin tumors are the second most common pineal neoplasms and may also result in CSF dissemination.
- Tectal plate gliomas are low-grade T2 hyperintense astrocytomas that obstruct the cerebral aqueduct.

Suggested Reading

Smith AB, Rushing EJ, Smirniotopoulos JG. From the archives of the AFIP: lesions of the pineal region: radiologic-pathologic correlation. Radiographics 2010; 30: 2001–2020

Case 59

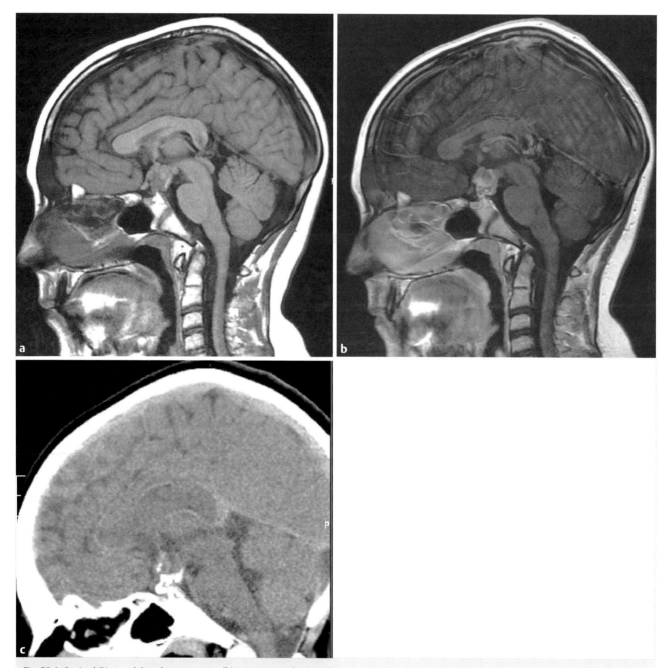

Fig. 59.1 Sagittal T1 pre- **(a)** and postcontrast **(b)** images reveal a mixed cystic and solid iso- to hypointense suprasellar mass with regions of enhancement. There is mass effect on the hypothalamus and optic chiasm. Sagittal reformatted CT image **(c)** shows regions of calcification within the mass.

■ Clinical Presentation

An 11-year-old boy with headache and visual changes (▹ Fig. 59.1)

▦ Key Imaging Finding

Suprasellar mass in child

▦ Top 3 Differential Diagnoses

- **Craniopharyngioma.** Craniopharyngiomas represent the most common suprasellar masses in children. They are benign tumors that arise from Rathke pouch epithelium. There are two subtypes, each with varying age peaks and imaging features: adamantinomatous (peak age 5 to 15 years) and papillary (peak age > 50 years). Pediatric adamantinomatous craniopharyngiomas present as multicystic suprasellar masses that may extend into the sella, anterior and middle cranial fossae, and retroclival regions. Computed tomography (CT) demonstrates amorphous calcifications in more than 90% of cases. There is often sellar expansion and clival remodeling or erosion. Both CT and magnetic resonance imaging (MRI) reveal a mixed cystic and solid suprasellar mass with enhancement of the solid components and cyst walls. The cystic content may be hyperdense on CT, hyperintense on T1, and variable on T2 sequences due to increased protein content, which is described as "crank case oil" on gross pathologic examination. In contrast, the adult variant (papillary) most commonly presents as a solid enhancing suprasellar mass without calcifications.
- **Germ cell tumor (GCT).** GCTs are most common in the pediatric population. They occur most frequently in the pineal region, followed by the suprasellar region and are often midline. Germinomas are the most common subtype and present as infiltrating sellar and/or suprasellar masses that typically follow gray matter signal and homogeneously enhance. With sellar involvement, there is often absence of the posterior pituitary bright spot on precontrast T1 images. Teratomas are more heterogeneous and usually have regions of macroscopic fat and calcification, which are useful discriminators. Dermoid cysts may follow cerebrospinal fluid (CSF) signal on T2-weighted sequences but are often slightly hyperintense to CSF on T1 and may have wall calcification. When present, fat-fluid levels are characteristic. GCTs may seed the CSF due to direct extension (germinomas) or rupture (dermoid cysts).
- **Rathke cleft cyst.** Rathke cleft cysts are non-neoplastic lesions that arise from remnants of Rathke cleft. The lesions are intrasellar; however, many will have suprasellar extension. Approximately 10 to 15% of the cysts will have curvilinear wall calcification. On MRI, the cystic fluid may have variable signal intensity based upon mucinous content. Lesions with high mucin content will be hyperintense on T1 sequences. An intracystic nodule is commonly seen, which is a useful discriminator. There is no internal enhancement, but a rim of enhancing pituitary gland is typically seen.

▦ Additional Differential Diagnoses

- **Optic nerve/hypothalamic glioma.** Optic nerve gliomas are low-grade neoplasms that most often occur between 5 and 15 years of age. They may occur sporadically or be associated with neurofibromatosis type 1 (NF1); bilateral optic nerve involvement is pathognomonic for NF1. Tumors cause enlargement, elongation and "buckling" of the optic nerve. Enhancement is variable. The tumor may extend along the optic pathway. Non-NF1 cases tend to involve the optic chiasm/hypothalamus, are typically larger and more masslike, commonly have cystic degeneration, and often extend beyond the optic pathways. Hypothalamic gliomas are similar in imaging appearance but are centered within the hypothalamus. Mild enhancement is often seen.
- **Hypothalamic hamartoma.** Hypothalamic hamartomas are rare, benign masses that occur in children who present with gelastic seizures or precocious puberty. The hamartomas are isointense to gray matter on T1 and iso- to hyperintense on T2 sequences. No enhancement should be seen; the presence of enhancement suggests a hypothalamic glioma rather than hamartoma. Characteristic clinical features combined with imaging findings are key to making the diagnosis.

▦ Diagnosis

Craniopharyngioma

✓ Pearls

- Pediatric craniopharyngiomas present as mixed cystic and solid suprasellar masses with regions of calcification.
- Germ cell tumors occur in the midline and may seed the CSF; germinoma is the most common subtype.
- Optic nerve and hypothalamic gliomas may occur sporadically or be associated with NF1.
- Patients with hypothalamic hamartomas often present with precocious puberty or gelastic seizures.

Suggested Reading

Hershey BL. Suprasellar masses: diagnosis and differential diagnosis. Semin Ultrasound CT MR 1993; 14: 215–231

Case 60

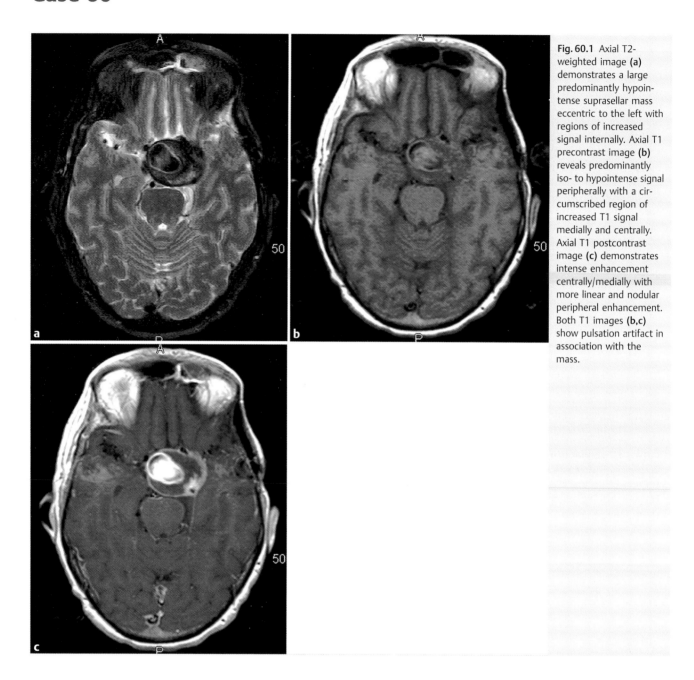

Fig. 60.1 Axial T2-weighted image **(a)** demonstrates a large predominantly hypointense suprasellar mass eccentric to the left with regions of increased signal internally. Axial T1 precontrast image **(b)** reveals predominantly iso- to hypointense signal peripherally with a circumscribed region of increased T1 signal medially and centrally. Axial T1 postcontrast image **(c)** demonstrates intense enhancement centrally/medially with more linear and nodular peripheral enhancement. Both T1 images **(b,c)** show pulsation artifact in association with the mass.

▨ Clinical Presentation

A 57-year-old woman with headache and blurred vision (▶ Fig. 60.1)

■ Key Imaging Finding

Suprasellar mass in adult

■ Top 3 Differential Diagnoses

- **Pituitary macroadenoma.** Upward extension of a pituitary macroadenoma (> 10 mm) from the sella is the most common suprasellar mass in adults. The best diagnostic clue is a sellar mass without a separate identifiable pituitary gland. The classic appearance is a "snowman" configuration due to impression on the mass by the diaphragma sella at its "waist." The tumor is most commonly isodense on computed tomography (CT), isointense on T1, and iso- to hyperintense on T2 sequences compared with gray matter. The imaging appearance is more heterogeneous in cases of hemorrhage (10%), calcification (1 to 2%), or cystic/necrotic change. Nearly all macroadenomas demonstrate some degree of enhancement, which is usually heterogeneous. There may be lateral displacement of the ipsilateral internal carotid artery. With cavernous sinus invasion, there is carotid artery encasement (> two-thirds is typically considered a sign of cavernous sinus invasion), typically without narrowing of the vessel lumen. Malignant transformation is exceedingly rare, but macroadenomas can appear locally aggressive with skull base/clival invasion. The peak age of onset is 20 to 40 years of age. Patients often present with visual field defects or cranial nerve palsy due to local mass effect. Treatment of choice is resection.

- **Craniopharyngioma.** Craniopharyngiomas are more common in children than adults. The classic pediatric case will present as a mixed cystic and solid suprasellar mass with calcifications. In adults > 50 years of age, craniopharyngiomas are of the papillary subtype and present as a solid, round suprasellar masses without calcification.

- **Aneurysm.** Aneurysm of the parasellar internal carotid artery should always be considered when a suprasellar mass is identified. Aneurysms tend to be eccentric and not directly suprasellar in location. The presence of flow voids and pulsation artifact on magnetic resonance imaging (MRI) are useful discriminators. Calcification is more common than with pituitary adenomas and is typically peripheral along the arterial wall. The patent lumen of the aneurysm will often avidly enhance, whereas thrombosed portions will be more heterogeneous in signal and enhancement. The pituitary gland will be seen separate from an aneurysm. CT angiography, MR angiography, or digital subtraction angiography can be used to characterize the aneurysm.

■ Additional Differential Diagnoses

- **Meningioma.** Meningiomas arising from the diaphragma sella can appear similar to a pituitary neoplasm; however, the pituitary gland often will be identified separate from the mass. Look for the low MR signal line of the diagphragma sella between the mass (above) and the pituitary gland (below). Dural thickening associated with meningioma is more extensive than with a pituitary macroadenoma. With cavernous sinus invasion, meningiomas often result in narrowing of the internal carotid artery with encasement, a finding that is not typically seen with pituitary macroadenomas. Classically, there is avid, homogenous enhancement with a dural tail, which is a useful supportive finding for meningioma. On unenhanced CT, meningiomas are typically iso- to hyperdense. Calcification and adjacent bony remodeling or hyperostosis may be seen.

■ Diagnosis

Aneurysm (with mural thrombus)

✓ Pearls

- Macroadenomas are the most common suprasellar masses in adults; a "snowman" configuration is classic.
- Craniopharyngiomas are solid in adults without calcification; in children, cysts and calcification are seen.
- Aneurysms must be a consideration with a suprasellar mass; look for flow voids and pulsation artifact.
- Meningiomas are commonly hyperdense and avidly enhance; calcification and hyperostosis may be seen.

Suggested Reading

Hershey BL. Suprasellar masses: diagnosis and differential diagnosis. Semin Ultrasound CT MR 1993; 14: 215–231

Case 61

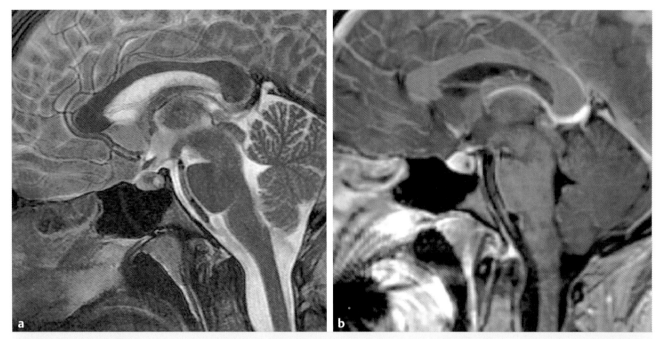

Fig. 61.1 Sagittal T2 image **(a)** reveals a circumscribed hyperintense cystic lesion within the posterior aspect of the pituitary gland with a tiny hypointense nodule along its posteroinferior margin. Sagittal T1 postcontrast image **(b)** shows a lack of enhancement within the cystic portion of the lesion.

▓ Clinical Presentation

A 16-year-old girl with chronic headaches (▶ Fig. 61.1)

▩ Key Imaging Finding

Intrasellar cystic lesion

▩ Top 3 Differential Diagnoses

- **Pars intermedia cyst.** The pars intermedia serves as the boundary between the adenohypophysis (anterior pituitary) and neurohypophysis (posterior pituitary). Cysts in this region are typically small, asymptomatic, and incidental. On magnetic resonance imaging (MRI), pars intermedia cysts are hypointense on T1 and hyperintense on T2 sequences (fluid signal) without enhancement or an intracystic nodule.
- **Rathke cleft cyst.** Rathke cleft cysts are benign, non-neoplastic cysts that arise from persistent remnants of the embryological Rathke cleft. Smaller lesions are purely intrasellar, whereas larger lesions may extend into the suprasellar region. The vast majority are asymptomatic and discovered incidentally. Large lesions may result in pituitary dysfunction or headaches. Acute hemorrhage into an underlying cyst occasionally results in pituitary apoplexy. The imaging appearance of Rathke cleft cysts varies. Computed tomography may be normal or demonstrate a noncalcified sellar lesion that is hypo- (most common), iso-, or hyperdense (least common). The most common appearance on MRI is a nonenhancing T2 hyperintense sellar lesion with a hypointense intracystic nodule. Approximately one-third of lesions will be iso- to hypointense on T2 sequences. The T1 signal within the cyst is variable with approximately half of cases hypo- and the remaining hyperintense. The intracystic nodule is typically hyperintense on T1. When purely intrasellar, the cysts are surrounded by enhancing pituitary tissue.
- **Cystic pituitary microadenoma.** Pituitary adenomas are benign, low-grade tumors and are most often discovered incidentally if nonsecreting. Microadenomas measure < 10 mm, and macroadenomas are > 10 mm. In general, microadenomas are prone to hormone secretion and thus will present earlier when symptomatic. Prolactin-secreting adenomas are the most common, followed by those that secrete growth hormone. Macroadenomas tend to be nonsecreting and present later with symptoms related to mass effect on sellar and suprasellar structures. MRI is the modality of choice to evaluate for a suspected microadenoma. They are best seen as regions of relative decreased enhancement within the pituitary substance on dynamic contrast-enhanced images. Lesions are typically less conspicuous on delayed images as contrast continues to perfuse into the lesions and approximates the signal intensity of the surrounding glandular tissue. Occasionally, adenomas undergo cystic degeneration in which case they appear as nonenhancing intrasellar cysts.

▩ Additional Differential Diagnoses

- **Intrasellar craniopharyngioma.** There are two variants of craniopharyngioma: adamantinomatous, which occurs in children and presents as a cystic and solid enhancing mass with calcifications, and papillary, which occurs in middle-aged adults and presents as a solid enhancing mass without calcifications. The vast majority of craniopharyngiomas are suprasellar with or without extension into the sella. A purely intrasellar craniopharyngioma is rare. Mixed cystic and solid components with calcification are distinguishing features.
- **Dermoid/epidermoid cyst.** Dermoids and epidermoids represent inclusion cysts, which are congenital in the sellar region. Both are lined by squamous epithelium; dermoid cysts also contain dermal elements, such as sebaceous glands and hair follicles. On imaging, epidermoids follow cerebrospinal fluid signal on nearly all pulse sequences but also demonstrate increased signal on diffusion-weighted imaging (DWI). Dermoid cysts may contain macroscopic fat or fat-fluid levels. Purely intrasellar dermoid or epidermoid cysts are rare. From a practical standpoint, these lesions should be included in the differential of an intrasellar cystic lesion if hyperintense DWI or fat signal intensity is visualized.

▩ Diagnosis

Rathke cleft cyst (presumed)

✓ Pearls

- Pars intermedia is the boundary between the anterior and posterior pituitary; incidental cysts are common.
- Rathke cleft cysts most often present as T2 hyperintense sellar lesions with a hypointense intracystic nodule.
- Microadenomas present as regions of decreased enhancement; cystic degeneration may occasionally occur.

Suggested Readings

Byun WM, Kim OL, Kim D. MR imaging findings of Rathke's cleft cysts: significance of intracystic nodules. Am J Neuroradiol 2000; 21: 485–488

Schroeder JW, Vezina LG. Pediatric sellar and suprasellar lesions. Pediatr Radiol 2011; 41: 287–298, quiz 404–405

Case 62

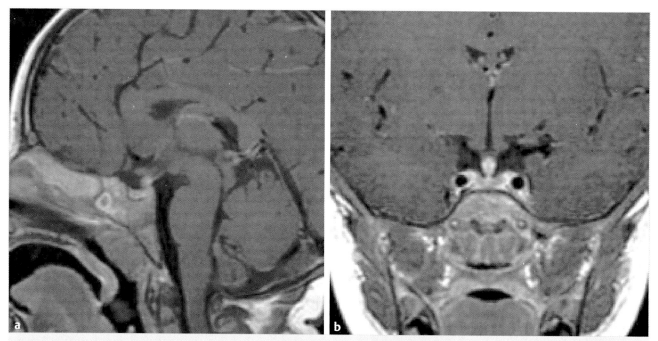

Fig. 62.1 Sagittal **(a)** and coronal **(b)** postcontrast T1 images demonstrate abnormal enlargement and enhancement of the pituitary infundibulum.

■ Clinical Presentation

A 9-year-old girl with stunted growth (▶ Fig. 62.1)

■ Key Imaging Finding

Enlarged, enhancing pituitary infundibulum in a child

■ Top 3 Differential Diagnoses

- **Germinoma.** Germinoma is the most common central nervous system germ cell tumor and commonly involves the suprasellar and pineal regions. Patients often present in the second decade of life with symptoms localized to the region of involvement. Hypothalamic-infundibular involvement typically manifests as diabetes insipidus (DI), pituitary dysfunction, or visual deficits associated with compression of the optic chiasm. Pineal region masses often result in Parinaud syndrome (paralysis of upward gaze) due to mass effect on the tectal plate or obstructive hydrocephalus. Cerebrospinal fluid (CSF) dissemination is common. Magnetic resonance imaging (MRI) of suprasellar involvement may show absence of the normal posterior pituitary bright spot on precontrast T1 sequences. The mass itself involves the pituitary stalk and/or hypothalamus, often with extension into the sella. It is typically iso- to hyperintense compared with brain parenchyma on T2 and isointense on T1 sequences with avid enhancement. In the setting of DI, follow-up imaging should be performed if initial imaging studies are normal because clinical manifestations may precede MRI visualization of the mass.
- **Langerhans cell histiocytosis (LCH).** The most common neuroimaging manifestations of LCH include a lytic skull lesion with beveled edges, a destructive temporal bone lesion, and infiltration of the hypothalamic-pituitary axis centered on the infundibulum. Hypothalamic-pituitary involvement typically presents clinically with DI early in childhood. MRI demonstrates abnormal enlargement and enhancement of the pituitary stalk or hypothalamus with or without extension into the sella; absence of the normal posterior pituitary bright spot on precontrast T1 sequences is also a common finding. The degree and pattern of hypothalamic or infundibular enlargement varies widely from a focal mass to more ill-defined infiltration.
- **Lymphoma/leukemia.** Leptomeningeal involvement of lymphoma and leukemia results from secondary, hematogenous spread. Sellar or suprasellar involvement occurs as an extension of the leptomeningeal disease. Imaging features vary from diffuse or nodular regions of meningeal enhancement to focal extraaxial masses. Calvarial lesions may also be seen. MRI of the sella demonstrates abnormal enlargement and enhancement of involved sellar and suprasellar structures, including the infundibulum; in general, lymphomatous or leukemic infiltration tends to result in more diffuse rather than focal enlargement. Additional regions of meningeal or extraaxial enhancement are typically seen. A focal myeloid cell tumor associated with leukemia is referred to as a chloroma.

■ Additional Differential Diagnoses

- **Leptomeningitis.** Leptomeningitis results from hematogenous spread of a distant infection or from direct spread of paranasal or mastoid infections. Infectious/inflammatory infiltration results in regions of abnormal meningeal enhancement with a leptomeningeal pattern being more common than pachymeningeal. Sellar/suprasellar involvement results from extension of leptomeningeal disease. MRI demonstrates regions of smooth or nodular enhancement along the infundibulum, sella, and pial surfaces of the hypothalamus. Additional regions of leptomeningeal disease are commonly seen.

■ Diagnosis

Langerhans cell histiocytosis

✓ Pearls

- Germinomas most often involve the sellar/suprasellar and pineal regions; CSF dissemination is common.
- LCH occurs in children and may involve the calvarium, temporal bone, or hypothalamic-pituitary axis.
- Sellar/suprasellar involvement of lymphoma and leukemia occurs as an extension of leptomeningeal disease.
- Leptomeningitis results in smooth or nodular enhancement along the infundibulum, sella, and hypothalamus.

Suggested Reading

Demaerel P, Van Gool S. Paediatric neuroradiological aspects of Langerhans cell histiocytosis. Neuroradiology 2008; 50: 85–92

Case 63

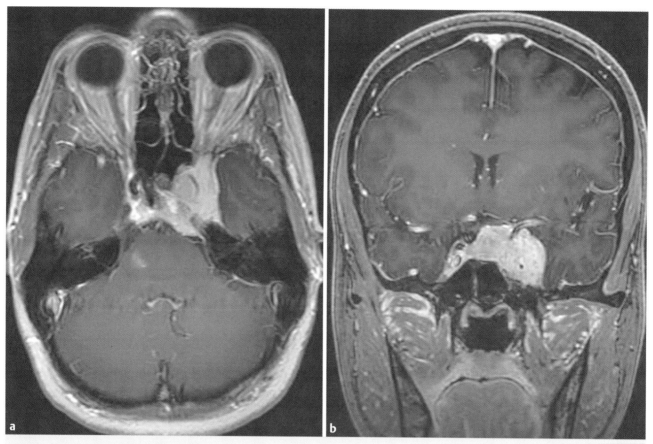

Fig. 63.1 Axial (**a**) and coronal (**b**) T1 postcontrast images demonstrate an avidly enhancing left cavernous sinus mass with encasement and marked narrowing of the cavernous segment of the left ICA. There is extension into the prepontine cistern on the left. Hyperintense signal intensity overlying the pons on the right (**a**) was artifactual.

■ **Clinical Presentation**

A 31-year-old post-partum woman complaining of facial numbness (► Fig. 63.1)

■ Key Imaging Finding

Cavernous sinus mass/enhancement

■ Top 3 Differential Diagnoses

- **Meningioma.** Meningiomas are benign dural-based masses and represent the most common extraaxial masses. When located in the cavernous sinus, patients often present with oculomotor symptoms related to mass effect on the cranial nerves (CNs). They may also characteristically encase and narrow the internal carotid artery (ICA). Most meningiomas are hyperdense on computed tomography (CT) with or without calcification; the remainder are isodense to brain parenchyma. Overlying bony hyperostosis may be seen. Meningiomas are typically iso- to hypointense on T1 and variable but generally hyperintense on T2 sequences. There is avid enhancement with a dural tail.
- **Schwannoma.** Schwannomas are nerve sheath tumors and represent the second most common extraaxial masses. Cavernous sinus schwannomas most often involve the trigeminal nerve. On CT, schwannomas are typically isodense compared with brain parenchyma with heterogeneous enhancement.

Unlike meningiomas, calcification is rare. When located near the skull base or exiting foramina, smooth bony remodeling and foraminal enlargement is commonly seen. On magnetic resonance imaging (MRI), schwannomas are iso- to hypointense on T1, variably hyperintense on T2, and demonstrate heterogeneous but avid enhancement.

- **Pituitary macroadenoma.** Pituitary macroadenoma (> 10 mm) is the most common suprasellar mass in adults. The best diagnostic clue is a sellar mass without a separate identifiable pituitary gland. The tumor is most commonly isodense on CT, isointense on T1, and iso- to hyperintense on T2 sequences compared with gray matter. Enhancement is usually heterogeneous. With cavernous sinus invasion, there may be carotid artery encasement (> two-thirds is typically considered a sign of cavernous sinus invasion) without narrowing. Patients often present with visual field defects or CN palsy due to local mass effect.

■ Additional Differential Diagnoses

- **Tolosa-Hunt syndrome.** Tolosa-Hunt syndrome is an idiopathic, inflammatory process of the cavernous sinus that is pathologically related to orbital pseudotumor. The syndrome is characterized by recurrent, painful ophthalmoplegia with involvement of the oculomotor nerve from the superior orbital fissure to the cavernous sinus. MRI features are similar to inflammatory orbital pseudotumor, demonstrating iso- to hypointense signal intensity on both T1 and T2 sequences. Enhancement may be ill-defined or masslike.
- **Carotid-cavernous fistula (CCF).** A CCF is an abnormal communication between the carotid artery and the venous spaces of the cavernous sinus. They are most often direct fistulas involving the ICA from trauma; aneurysm rupture and indirect fistulas involving dural arterial branches are less common. Patients present with headaches, exophthalmos,

ophthalmoplegia, and bruit. Angiographically, a CCF will demonstrate early venous filling of the cavernous sinus, superior ophthalmic vein, and/or inferior petrosal sinus. On CT or MRI, there is prominent enlargement and enhancement of the cavernous sinus; flow voids may be seen on T2 MRI sequences. Endovascular treatment options are favored and include glue or coil embolization.

- **Perineural spread of tumor or infection.** Infiltrating sinonasal or head and neck carcinomas or invasive infections (e.g., fungal) may extend into the cavernous sinus via entry through the skull base foramina. Postcontrast fat saturated MRI is most helpful in demonstrating intracranial extension, especially when asymmetric or unilateral. Oftentimes, the primary origin may be identified if not already known clinically.

■ Diagnosis

Meningioma

✓ Pearls

- Cavernous sinus meningiomas avidly enhance with a dural tail; they may encase and narrow the ICA.
- Cavernous sinus schwannomas most commonly involve CN V; skull base foraminal remodeling may be seen.

- Pituitary macroadenomas present as sellar/suprasellar masses without a separate identifiable pituitary gland.
- Tolosa-Hunt is an inflammatory process of the cavernous sinus that is related to orbital pseudotumor.

Suggested Reading

Lee JH, Lee HK, Park JK, Choi CG, Suh DC. Cavernous sinus syndrome: clinical features and differential diagnosis with MR imaging. Am J Roentgenol 2003; 181: 583–590

Case 64

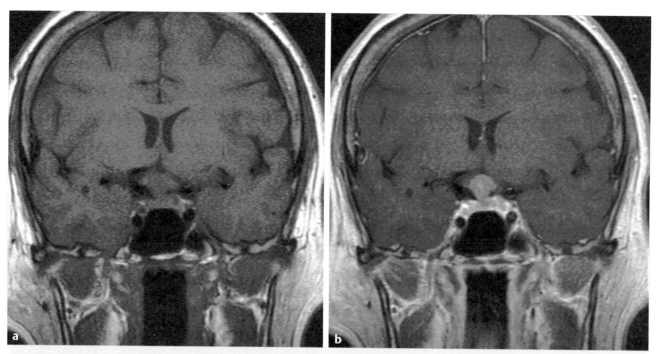

Fig. 64.1 Coronal T1 pre- **(a)** and postcontrast **(b)** images demonstrate abnormal thickening and enhancement of the pituitary infundibulum, most pronounced superiorly. (Courtesy of Paul M. Sherman, MD.)

■ Clinical Presentation

An adult man with headache and visual disturbances (▶ Fig. 64.1)

■ Key Imaging Finding

Enlarged, enhancing pituitary infundibulum in an adult

■ Top 3 Differential Diagnoses

- **Neurosarcoidosis.** Sarcoidosis is a systemic inflammatory disease characterized by noncaseating granulomas. It primarily affects adults with an onset typically in the third and fourth decades. Neurosarcoidosis is relatively uncommon, with symptomatic central nervous system (CNS) involvement in approximately 5% of cases. CNS manifestations include smooth or nodular (more common) dural and/or leptomeningeal enhancement, most pronounced along the basal cisterns. There is often involvement of the optic chiasm, hypothalamus, infundibulum, internal auditory canals, and cranial nerves at the skull base. Brain parenchymal involvement includes multiple focal or perivascular lesions, some of which may enhance, and changes associated with vasculitis. Hydrocephalus is a potential complication with leptomeningeal disease. If not already obtained, look for lymphadenopathy with or without interstitial lung disease on chest X-ray.
- **Lymphocytic hypophysitis.** Lymphocytic hypophysitis results from inflammation of the pituitary stalk and anterior pituitary gland. Its exact etiology remains unclear. It most often affects pregnant or recently postpartum patients who present with headache and endocrinopathies. Imaging demonstrates a thickened and enhancing stalk with absence of normal tapering as it descends from the hypothalamus. There may also be sellar extension with enlargement of the anterior pituitary. Loss of the normal posterior pituitary bright spot on precontrast T1 sequences is commonly seen. Treatment consists of steroids and hormone replacement.
- **Metastases/lymphoma.** Leptomeningeal carcinomatosis typically results from hematogenous spread of a remote primary, with breast and lung cancer being the most common; secondary spread of lymphoma also commonly results in meningeal involvement. Sellar or suprasellar metastatic disease is fairly uncommon; when seen, additional regions of metastases are often visualized, including meningeal, parenchymal, and/or calvarial involvement. Metastases or lymphoma result in infundibular enlargement, abnormal enhancement, and lack of normal tapering. In general, lymphomatous infiltration tends to result in more diffuse enlargement, whereas metastases tend to result in more focal enlargement.

■ Additional Differential Diagnoses

- **Pituicytoma.** A pituicytoma is a rare tumor that originates from pituicytes along the pituitary stalk and neurohypophysis (posterior pituitary). It typically occurs in middle-aged to older adults and has a slight male predominance. Patients often present with headache and pituitary dysfunction.

Magnetic resonance imaging demonstrates an enhancing mass within the infundibulum with or without extension into the neurohypophysis. The mass is typically isointense to hypointense compared with brain parenchyma on both T2 and precontrast T1 sequences.

■ Diagnosis

Metastases

✓ Pearls

- Dural enhancement along the basilar cisterns is the most common CNS manifestation of neurosarcoidosis.
- Lymphocytic hypophysitis typically affects pregnant or postpartum patients with headache and endocrinopathy.
- Metastases and lymphoma may affect the leptomeninges with extension into the sella and suprasellar region.
- Pituicytoma is a rare tumor that originates from pituicytes along the pituitary stalk and neurohypophysis.

Suggested Readings

Gibbs WN, Monuki ES, Linskey ME, Hasso AN. Pituicytoma: diagnostic features on selective carotid angiography and MR imaging. Am J Neuroradiol 2006; 27: 1639–1642

Sato N, Sze G, Endo K. Hypophysitis: endocrinologic and dynamic MR findings. Am J Neuroradiol 1998; 19: 439–444

Smith JK, Matheus MG, Castillo M. Imaging manifestations of neurosarcoidosis. Am J Roentgenol 2004; 182: 289–295

Case 65

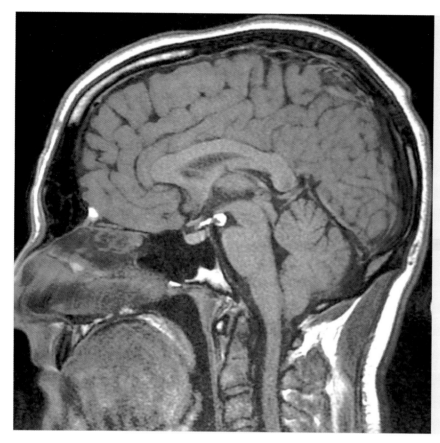

Fig. 65.1 Sagittal T1 image demonstrates a lobulated hyperintense mass within the interpeduncular cistern and extending into the posterior aspect of the suprasellar cistern.

■ Clinical Presentation

A 14-year-old boy with migraine headaches (► Fig. 65.1)

▤ Key Imaging Finding

Midline suprasellar T1 hyperintense mass

▤ Top 3 Differential Diagnoses

- **Lipoma.** Intracranial lipomas result from persistence of the meninx primitiva, which usually involutes early in gestation. They may occur throughout the central nervous system cisterns, but the vast majority are midline. The most common midline locations include pericallosal, quadrigeminal plate cistern, and suprasellar cistern. Clinical symptoms are variable, ranging from asymptomatic and incidental to seizures and developmental delay in association with multiple developmental anomalies. Lipomas are hypodense on computed tomography (CT) and follow fat signal intensity on all magnetic resonance imaging (MRI) sequences; fat-suppression is the key to diagnosis.
- **Germ cell tumor.** Sellar/suprasellar GCTs are most common in the pediatric population. Germinomas are the most common subtype and present as infiltrating masses that typically follow gray matter signal and homogeneously enhance. With sellar involvement, there is often absence of the posterior pituitary bright spot on precontrast T1 images. Teratomas are more heterogeneous and usually have regions of macroscopic fat, which are hyperintense on T1 and T2, which is a useful discriminator. Dermoid cysts may follow cerebrospinal fluid (CSF) signal on T2 sequences but are often slightly hyperintense to CSF on T1 and may have wall calcification. Fat-fluid levels may be seen. GCTs may seed the CSF due to direct extension (germinomas) or rupture (dermoid cysts).
- **Craniopharyngioma.** Craniopharyngiomas are the most common suprasellar masses in children and arise from Rathke pouch epithelium. There are two subtypes: adamantinomatous (peak age 5 to 15 years) and papillary (peak age > 50 years). Pediatric variants present as multicystic suprasellar masses that may extend into the sella, anterior and middle cranial fossae, and retroclival regions. CT demonstrates amorphous calcifications in more than 90% of cases. There is often sellar expansion and clival remodeling or erosion. Both CT and MRI reveal a mixed cystic and solid suprasellar mass with enhancement of the solid components and cyst walls. The cystic content may be hyperdense on CT, hyperintense on T1, and variable on T2 sequences due to increased protein content, which is described as "crank case oil" on gross pathologic examination, or hemorrhage.

▤ Additional Differential Diagnoses

- **Ectopic posterior pituitary.** An ectopic posterior pituitary refers to failure of the decent of the neurohypophysis. On MRI, it is seen as a focal "bright spot" on T1 sequences along the inferior aspect of the hypothalamus. The increased T1 signal is thought to be secondary to the presence of vasopressin. In isolation, an ectopic posterior pituitary may be incidental and asymptomatic. When associated with transection or absence of the pituitary stalk, however, patients often experience pituitary dysfunction affecting hormones of the anterior pituitary/adenohypophysis. Growth hormone deficiency and diabetes insipidus are the most common clinical manifestations. An ectopic pituitary may also be seen in association with septo-optic dysplasia and holoprosencephaly.
- **Blood products.** Intra- and extracellular methemoglobin is hyperintense on T1 sequences. Common causes of blood products within the sellar/suprasellar region include subarachnoid hemorrhage (SAH), pituitary apoplexy, traumatic or nonapoplexy hemorrhage into an underlying mass (macroadenoma, Rathke cleft cyst), and a partially thrombosed aneurysm of the parasellar internal carotid artery. Fluid-fluid levels may be seen in the setting of hemorrhage into an underlying lesion. The presence of pulsation artifact is a helpful discriminator in the setting of aneurysm.

▤ Diagnosis

Lipoma

✓ Pearls

- Causes of increased T1 signal include lesions with fat, protein, hemorrhage, and an ectopic posterior pituitary.
- Common sellar/suprasellar masses with T1 hyperintensity include lipomas, craniopharyngiomas, and GCTs.
- Ectopic posterior pituitary may be incidental or associated with hypopituitarism or additional malformations.
- Blood products may be due to SAH, hemorrhage into an underlying mass, or aneurysm thrombosis.

Suggested Reading

Bonneville F, Cattin F, Marsot-Dupuch K, Dormont D, Bonneville JF, Chiras J. T1 signal hyperintensity in the sellar region: spectrum of findings. Radiographics 2006; 26: 93–113

Case 66

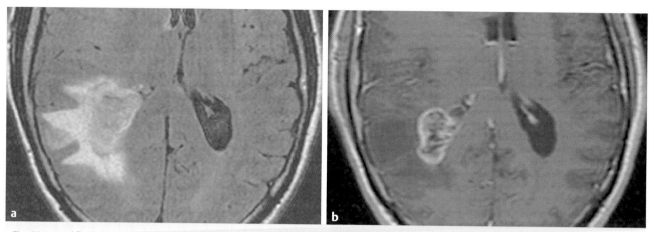

Fig. 66.1 Axial fluid-attenuated inversion recovery image **(a)** shows an intermediate to hypointense mass along the periatrial region of the right lateral ventricle with surrounding vasogenic edema. Axial T1 postcontrast image **(b)** demonstrates enhancement, which is more prominent along the periphery.

▓ Clinical Presentation

A 43-year-old woman with headaches (▶ Fig. 66.1)

▣ Key Imaging Finding

Periventricular mass/enhancement with edema

▣ Top 3 Differential Diagnoses

- **Primary central nervous system (CNS) lymphoma.** Primary CNS lymphoma is almost exclusively of the non-Hodgkin variant. It typically occurs within the periventricular white matter and basal ganglia and commonly involves the corpus callosum and ependymal surfaces of the ventricles. Leptomeningeal and dural involvement occurs more often with secondary lymphoma. Lymphoma may present as a solitary mass or multiple lesions and can be circumscribed or infiltrative. There is typically mild surrounding edema. The lesions are characteristically hyperdense on computed tomography (CT) and iso- to hypointense on both T1 and T2 sequences due to high cellularity. Increased signal on diffusion sequences may also be seen. Hemorrhage and necrosis are uncommon. Enhancement is intense and homogenous in immunocompetent patients and may be peripheral or ring-enhancing in immunocompromised patients. Unlike toxoplasmosis, lymphoma is hypermetabolic on Thallium single-photon emission CT (SPECT) and positron emission tomography imaging and demonstrates increased perfusion.

- **Glial neoplasm.** Aggressive glial tumors commonly involve the deep gray and white matter and may extend into the ventricles along the ependymal surface. Glioblastoma multiforme (World Health Organization grade IV astrocytoma) is the most common subtype and results in thick, irregular enhancement and central necrosis. The tumor is heterogeneous but primarily T2 hyperintense and T1 iso- to hypointense with associated cysts, hemorrhage, and fluid debris. There is prominent surrounding edema; viable tumor cells extend beyond the margin of signal abnormality on pathological evaluation. Regions of diffusion restriction and increased perfusion are noted within solid components. Prominent flow voids may be seen and are associated with neovascularity. As with primary CNS lymphoma, the corpus callosum is commonly involved and expanded. Prognosis is poor.

- **Ventriculitis/Ependymitis.** Ventricular or ependymal spread of infection may occur from hematogenous spread to the choroid plexus or direct extension from a parenchymal infection, such as intraventricular rupture of a periventricular abscess. Immunocompromised patients and those with intraventricular drainage catheters are more prone to intraventricular infections. Cytomegalovirus, toxoplasmosis, and tuberculosis are common causative agents in immunosuppressed patients. Magnetic resonance imaging (MRI) demonstrates increased T2/fluid-attenuated inversion recovery signal along the ventricular margin and avid, thin ependymal enhancement. There is often layering of dependent debris, which may demonstrate restricted diffusion in the setting of pyogenic infection. Short- and long-term complications include hydrocephalus, which is most often communicating. Periventricular extension may result in toxic or ischemic parenchymal injury.

▣ Diagnosis

Primary CNS lymphoma

✓ Pearls

- CNS lymphoma and aggressive glial tumors often involve the periventricular region and corpus callosum.
- Regions of tumor with high cellularity are often hyperdense on CT and hypointense on T2 MRI sequences.

- GBM is an aggressive tumor with thick, irregular enhancement; central necrosis and flow voids are common.
- Ventriculitis is more common in immunosuppressed patients; there is enhancement and layering of debris.

Suggested Reading

Smirniotopoulos JG, Murphy FM, Rushing EJ, Rees JH, Schroeder JW. Patterns of contrast enhancement in the brain and meninges. Radiographics 2007; 27: 525–551

Case 67

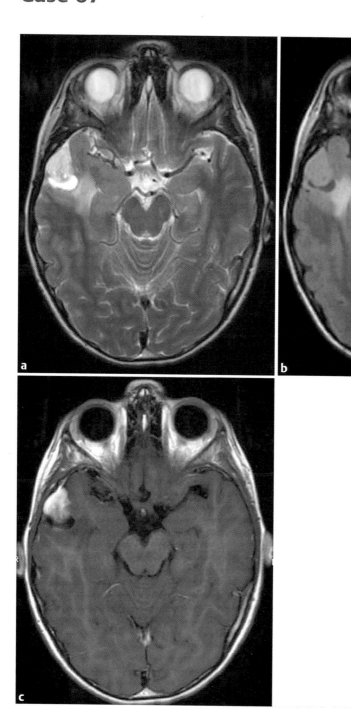

Fig. 67.1 Axial T2 (a) and fluid-attenuated inversion recovery (b) images reveal a cystic and solid cortically based mass in the right temporal lobe with surrounding vasogenic edema. Axial enhanced T1 image demonstrates enhancement of the solid components, as well as mild overlying meningeal enhancement.

■ Clinical Presentation

A 14-year-old boy with headache and seizures (▶ Fig. 67.1)

■ Key Imaging Finding

Cortically based cystic temporal lobe mass in a patient with seizures

■ Top 3 Differential Diagnoses

- **Ganglioglioma.** Ganglioglioma is a low-grade (typically World Health Organization grade I), cortically based neuroepithelial tumor, which is composed of neoplastic ganglion and glial cells. It most often occurs in the temporal lobes and is the most common neoplastic cause of temporal lobe seizures in adolescents and young adults. Additional symptoms include headache and focal neurological deficits. Although its imaging appearance varies, the most common presentation is a superficial mixed cystic and solid mass; the solid components often present as a mural nodule and are hyperintense on T2 sequences. Because the lesion is cortically based, cortical expansion and overlying bony remodeling is often seen. Calcifications and enhancement of solid components are noted in approximately half of cases. Meningeal enhancement and surrounding edema are mild, when present.
- **Dysembryoplastic neuroepithelial tumor (DNET).** DNET is a benign tumor that is composed of both glial and neuronal elements. A unique feature is its association with adjacent regions of cortical dysplasia. It typically occurs in adolescents and young adults; the most common presentation is seizures. Surgical resection must include the foci of cortical dysplasia to ensure resolution of seizures. DNET most often occurs in the temporal lobes. On magnetic resonance imaging (MRI), DNET presents as a circumscribed, wedge-shaped, cortically based mass. It is hyperintense on T2 sequences with a characteristic "bubbly" or multicystic appearance. Calcification and enhancement are relatively uncommon, occurring in approximately one-fifth to one-third of cases. There is typically no significant edema. Because the mass is cortically based, expansion of the cortex and remodeling of the overlying calvarium are commonly seen.
- **Pleomorphic xanthoastrocytoma (PXA).** PXA is a low-grade, cortically based astrocytoma that most often occurs during childhood and early adulthood. Patients commonly present with seizures, headache, and occasionally focal neurological deficits. The majority of cases involve the temporal lobe, resulting in temporal lobe epilepsy. On MRI, PXA presents as a T2 hyperintense cortically based cystic and solid mass with a solid mural nodule. The solid nodular component extends along the pial surface. Prominent enhancement and surrounding vasogenic edema is typically seen. The majority of cases demonstrate overlying meningeal enhancement, which is a useful discriminator. Computed tomography may show calcification, as well as bony remodeling.

■ Additional Differential Diagnoses

- **Balloon cell (Taylor) cortical dysplasia.** Focal cortical dysplasia (FCD) is a neuronal migrational disorder characterized by abnormal cortical development secondary to some form of insult. There are two distinct subtypes: type 1 in which there is abnormal cortical development without abnormal neurons, and type 2 in which there are both abnormal cortical development and dysmorphic neurons. Taylor dysplasia is a specific subset of type 2 that contains characteristic balloon cells on pathological examination. On MRI, cortical dysplasia presents with focal abnormal increased T2/fluid-attenuated inversion recovery signal intensity involving the cortex and subcortical white matter with blurring of the gray-white matter junction. The signal abnormality is commonly wedge-shaped with tapered signal pointing toward the ventricles. The overlying cortex may be thickened. Regions of increased cortical signal intensity on heavily T1-weighted sequences are fairly characteristic and helpful in distinguishing from neoplasms. There is no enhancement or surrounding edema. Patients often present with seizures or focal neurological deficits.

■ Diagnosis

Pleomorphic xanthoastrocytoma

✓ Pearls

- Gangliogioma is a common cause of temporal lobe epilepsy in young adults; it is mixed cystic and solid.
- DNET presents as a nonenhancing, "bubbly," multicystic mass with adjacent regions of cortical dysplasia.
- PXA presents as a cystic mass with enhancing mural nodule; meningeal enhancement is often seen.
- Taylor dysplasia presents as wedge-shaped cortical/subcortical signal abnormality tapering toward ventricles.

Suggested Readings

Colombo N, Tassi L, Galli C et al. Focal cortical dysplasias: MR imaging, histopathologic, and clinical correlations in surgically treated patients with epilepsy. Am J Neuroradiol 2003; 24: 724–733

Koeller KK, Henry JM Armed Forces Institute of Pathology. From the archives of the AFIP: superficial gliomas: radiologic-pathologic correlation. Radiographics 2001; 21: 1533–1556

Case 68

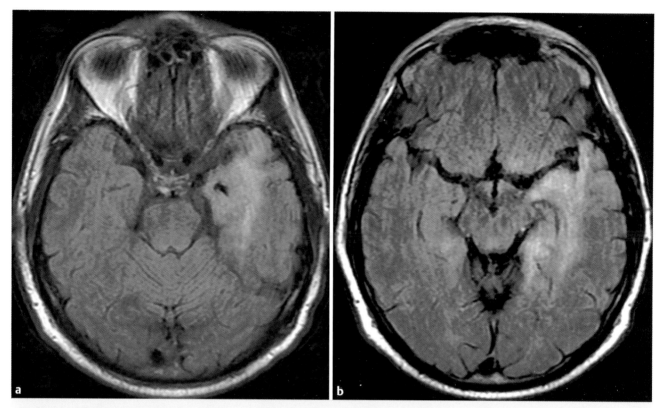

Fig. 68.1 Axial fluid-attenuated inversion recovery images **(a,b)** demonstrate confluent regions of cortical and subcortical signal abnormality with mild mass effect throughout the left temporal lobe. There is also subtle signal abnormality involving the inferior left frontal and medial right temporal lobes **(b)**.

▩ Clinical Presentation
....

A 64-year-old man with new onset seizures (▶ Fig. 68.1)

▧ Key Imaging Finding

Diffuse, infiltrating temporal lobe mass/edema

▧ Top 3 Differential Diagnoses

- **Herpes encephalitis.** Brain parenchymal infection secondary to Herpes simplex virus type 1 in adults characteristically involves the limbic system, including the temporal lobes, insula, inferior frontal lobes, and cingulate gryi. Patients present with acute onset of fever, headaches, seizures, and/or focal neurological deficits. Imaging reveals bilateral, asymmetric involvement of the cortex and subcortical white matter with sparing of the basal ganglia. There is edema with loss of gray-white differentiation and local mass effect, typically in a nonvascular distribution. Foci of hemorrhage and restricted diffusion are commonly seen. Mild, patchy enhancement may be seen acutely, developing into gyriform enhancement usually within one week. Mortality is 50 to 70% if not recognized and treated promptly.
- **Ischemia/infarction.** Infarcts result from arterial or venous occlusion. Patients present acutely with focal neurological deficits, altered mental status, and/or aphasia. Arterial etiologies include thromboembolic disease (most common), dissection, vasculitis, and hypoperfusion. Imaging reveals cytotoxic edema with loss of gray-white matter differentiation and sulcal effacement in a vascular distribution. Occlusion of the proximal middle cerebral artery (MCA) may show a characteristic "dense MCA" sign on computed tomography (CT) with hypoattenuation involving the basal ganglia and insula. Both

CT angiography and magnetic resonance angiography may demonstrate the site of vascular occlusion. Acute infarcts show restricted diffusion. Gyral or patchy enhancement may be seen in the subacute stage. Perfusion imaging evaluates the ischemic penumbra, or potentially viable parenchyma. Hemorrhagic transformation occurs in 15 to 20% of cases. Venous infarcts occur in patients with one of many hypercoagulable states. Temporal lobe involvement is common and may result from occlusion of the vein of Labbe. Imaging reveals cytotoxic edema in a nonvascular distribution. Hemorrhage is common, especially when thrombus extends into the cortical veins.
- **Gliomatosis cerebri.** Gliomatosis cerebri is a World Health Organization grade III infiltrating astrocytoma with a peak incidence in the fifth and sixth decades of life. Patients often present with headaches, seizures, or focal neurological deficits. Imaging reveals diffuse, confluent regions of T2/fluid-attenuated inversion recovery hyperintensity with mass effect, often centered within the centrum semiovale. There is characteristic involvement of two or more lobes, and there may be extension across white matter tracts to involve the contralateral hemisphere. There is typically no or minimal patchy enhancement. Involvement of the cortex, deep gray matter, cerebellum, brain stem, and spinal cord may be seen.

▧ Additional Differential Diagnoses

- **Limbic encephalitis.** Limbic encephalitis is a paraneoplastic syndrome associated with a primary malignancy, typically lung or breast cancer. Imaging findings may be indistinguishable from Herpes encephalitis with unilateral or bilateral regions of signal abnormality with a predilection for the limbic system; however, hemorrhage does not occur. Clinically, the onset of symptoms is usually more insidious (weeks to months) rather than acute. Treatment of the primary malignancy may result in stabilization or improvement of symptoms.
- **Status epilepticus.** Seizures result in focal increased cerebral perfusion and disruption of the blood–brain barrier. There is associated ill-defined edema involving the cortex and subcortical white matter; the temporal lobe is commonly involved. Enhancement may occasionally be seen. Follow-up imaging after cessation of seizures demonstrates improvement or resolution. It is important to remember that the region of edema may be remote from the actual seizure focus.

▧ Diagnosis

Herpes encephalitis

✓ Pearls

- Herpes encephalitis is a life-threatening infection that preferentially involves the limbic system.
- Ischemia results in cortical edema, sulcal effacement, and restricted diffusion in a vascular distribution.
- Gliomatosis cerebri is an infiltrating neoplasm involving two or more lobes.
- Limbic encephalitis is a paraneoplastic syndrome with insidious rather than acute onset of symptoms.

Suggested Reading

PeerAully T, Landolfi JC. Herpes encephalitis masquerading as tumor. ISRN Neurol 2011; 2011: 474672

Case 69

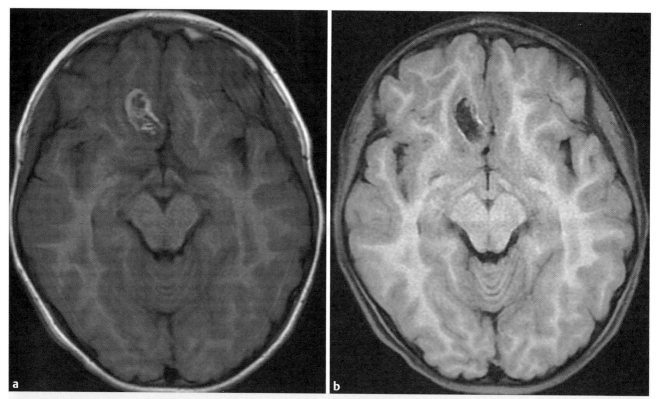

Fig. 69.1 Axial T1 image **(a)** demonstrates an ovoid mass within the right frontal lobe that contains linear striations of increased signal intensity. The majority of the increased signal is hypointense on the T1 fat-suppressed image **(b)**.

■ Clinical Presentation

An adolescent boy with headaches (▶ Fig. 69.1)

▧ Key Imaging Finding

T1 hyperintense parenchymal mass

▧ Top 3 Differential Diagnoses

- **Hemorrhage.** Intraparenchymal hemorrhage results from a variety of conditions, including hypertension, trauma, arterial or venous infarction, underlying vascular malformation or malignancy, illicit drug use, and amyloid angiopathy. Parenchymal hematomas undergo a predictable pattern of evolution with T1 and T2 signal intensity varying based upon alterations in the hemoglobin moiety. In the hyperacute stage, oxyhemoglobin results in isointense T1 and hyperintense T2 signal. As the oxyhemoglobin converts to deoxyhemoglobin in the acute stage, the T1 signal remains isointense, whereas the T2 signal becomes hypointense. In the early (intracellular methemoglobin) and late (extracellular methemoglobin) subacute stages, the T1 signal is hyperintense and the T2 signal is hypointense and hyperintense, respectively. In the chronic stage, hemosiderin forms, which is hypointense on T1 and T2 sequences. Gradient echo or susceptibility-weighted imaging sequences will show hypointense blooming. Diffusion-weighted imaging, patterns of enhancement, and follow-up imaging are important in identifying (and treating) the cause of hemorrhage.
- **Fat.** Macroscopic fat is hyperintense on T1 and non-fat-suppressed T2 sequences and hypodense on computed tomography. Chemical shift artifact is often seen and presents as a band of hyperintensity along one margin and a band of hypo-intensity along the opposite margin. Intracranial lesions that may contain macroscopic fat include lipomas, dermoids, and teratomas. Rarely, primary and metastatic tumors may contain fatty elements. Congenital lipomas are typically midline in location and most often found along the corpus callosum, tectal plate, or suprasellar cistern. Linear lipomas are often incidental; the tubulonodular variant is more commonly associated with additional anomalies. Lipomas may also be seen in the cerebellopontine angle and internal auditory canal. Dermoids and teratomas most often occur in the suprasellar region or off-midline where they may be intra- or extraaxial. Ruptured dermoids may result in diffuse subarachnoid spread with a chemical meningitis. Teratomas often have regions of soft tissue, cysts, and calcification in addition to macroscopic fat.
- **Melanin.** Melanin results in hyperintense T1 signal. Metastatic melanoma is the most common cause of intracranial melanin. It may present as solitary or multiple parenchymal lesions. Surrounding edema is seen, but may be subtle with cortical lesions. The increased T1 signal is typically due to a combination of melanin and hemorrhage. Most lesions enhance. Neurocutaneous melanosis is a rare phakomatosis that results in parenchymal and meningeal T1 hyperintense lesions. Diffuse meningeal enhancement is commonly seen.

▧ Additional Differential Diagnoses

- **Protein.** Fluid signal is hypointense on T1 and hyperintense on T2 sequences. As the protein content increases, the T1 signal increases and the T2 signal decreases. When the proteinaceous content increases significantly, the signal will be low on all pulse sequences. Aside from some forms of adenocarcinoma (particularly mucinous), most protein-containing lesions are extraaxial, including craniopharyngiomas and dermoid cysts.
- **Calcification/ossification.** Calcification or ossification may result in increased T1 signal. This most often occurs along the falx and inner margins of the calvarium. Occasionally, calcifications within a mass, such as arteriovenous malformation, tuberculoma, and benign and malignant neoplasms, may have increased T1 signal.
- **Enhancement.** Regions of enhancement are hyperintense on T1 sequences and are best evaluated by directly comparing pre- and postcontrast sequences. Delayed and continuous enhancement may be seen in patients with recent enhanced magnetic resonance imaging (MRI) and in cases of renal failure.

▧ Diagnosis

Fat (dermoid)

✓ Pearls

- MRI signal intensity of intraparenchymal hematomas varies based upon alterations in the hemoglobin moiety.
- Fat-containing intracranial masses include lipoma, dermoid, teratoma, and, rarely, primary or metastatic tumors.
- Metastatic melanoma is hyperintense on T1 sequences secondary to both melanin content and hemorrhage.

Suggested Reading

Cakirer S, Karaarslan E, Arslan A. Spontaneously T1-hyperintense lesions of the brain on MRI: a pictorial review. Curr Probl Diagn Radiol 2003; 32: 194–217

Case 70

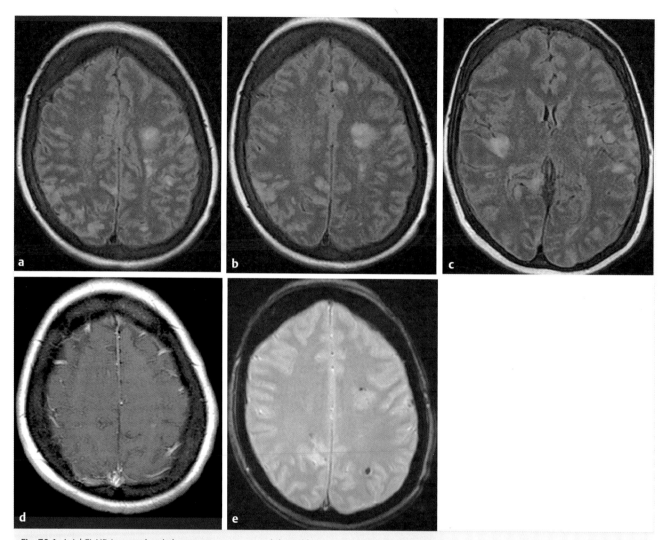

Fig. 70.1 Axial FLAIR images **(a–c)** demonstrate numerous bilateral hyperintense lesions centered at the gray-white matter junction with regions of overlying cortical signal abnormality. Axial T1 postcontrast image **(d)** demonstrates nodular enhancement of a lesion within the left parietal lobe along the central sulcus. Several of the lesions reveal GRE susceptibility **(e)**. The corpus callosum, posterior fossa, and brain stem were not involved (not shown).

■ Clinical Presentation

A 62-year-old woman with altered mental status and focal neurological deficits (▶ Fig. 70.1)

■ Key Imaging Finding

Multiple lesions at gray-white matter junction

■ Top 3 Differential Diagnoses

- **Ischemic emboli.** Ischemic emboli most often occur in older patients with carotid artery atherosclerosis. Soft plaques are prone to rupture with resultant distal emboli that lodge in end arterioles at the gray-white matter junction and within deep penetrating vessels. Unilateral disease is typically seen due to the carotid vascular distribution; the middle cerebral artery (MCA) territory is involved to a greater extent than the anterior cerebral artery territory. Cardiac emboli are an additional source of ischemic emboli. Patients with cardiac arrhythmias and collagen vascular diseases are most susceptible. As opposed to atherosclerotic disease, lesions tend to be bilateral due to the central etiology of the emboli. Atherosclerotic and cardiac emboli present as multifocal regions of cortical and subcortical T2/fluid-attenuated inversion recovery (FLAIR) hyperintensity, many of which will have a wedge-shaped configuration. Restricted diffusion is seen in the acute setting; enhancement may be seen in the subacute phase.
- **Metastases.** Hematogenous spread of metastases may result in solitary or multiple parenchymal lesions with approximately equal incidence. They are typically small (< 2 cm) and located at the gray-white matter junction or in the region of end arterioles of deep penetrating vessels. Less often, metastases may spread along venous channels that preferentially involve the posterior fossa. The majority of metastases are supratentorial and in the MCA distribution because that is the largest blood supply to the brain. Computed tomography (CT) and magnetic resonance imaging (MRI) demonstrate cortical or subcortical enhancing lesions with surrounding edema. The edema is more pronounced with subcortical lesions; isolated cortical metastases may have little surrounding edema. As metastatic foci enlarge, enhancement may become heterogeneous and cystic change may occur. Primary tumors prone to hemorrhage include breast, lung, melanoma, renal cell carcinoma, thyroid carcinoma, and choriocarcinoma.
- **Septic emboli.** Septic emboli spread hematogenously to the brain parenchyma and are centered at the gray-white matter junction and end arterioles of deep penetrating vessels. As with other hematogenous processes, the majority of lesions are located within the MCA vascular distribution. Lesions initially present as cerebritis with ill-defined regions of hypoattenuation on CT and increased T2/FLAIR signal intensity on MRI. There may be regions of restricted diffusion and ill-defined enhancement. Hematogenous septic emboli may calcify or have associated hemorrhage, resulting in hypointensity on gradient echo (GRE) and susceptibility-weighted imaging. If the infectious process progresses, it may become more organized with formation of an abscess capsule, which is typically smooth and thinner toward the ventricles, as well as characteristically hypointense on T2 sequences. With abscess formation, there is pronounced vasogenic edema. Pyogenic abscesses demonstrate central restricted diffusion.

■ Additional Differential Diagnoses

- **Vasculitis.** Vasculitis results in inflammatory infiltration of arterial walls. Causative etiologies include autoimmune, infection or granulomatous disease, radiation, and drugs. MRI demonstrates bilateral regions of superficial and deep gray and white matter signal abnormality. GRE imaging may reveal hemorrhage, which is common in vasculitis. Patchy enhancement may be seen. Angiography is often necessary to visualize alternating regions of stenosis and dilatation because MR angiography and CT angiography are less sensitive. Biopsy is diagnostic.

■ Diagnosis

Vasculitis

✓ Pearls

- Atherosclerotic ischemic emboli produce ipsilateral parenchymal lesions; cardiac emboli are typically bilateral.
- Hematogenous spread involves the gray-white matter junction and end arterioles of penetrating vessels.
- Septic emboli present initially as regions of cerebritis that may progress to abscess formation.
- Vasculitis presents with multifocal regions of gray/white matter signal abnormality; hemorrhage is common.

Suggested Reading

Smirniotopoulos JG, Murphy FM, Rushing EJ, Rees JH, Schroeder JW. Patterns of contrast enhancement in the brain and meninges. Radiographics 2007; 27: 525–551

Case 71

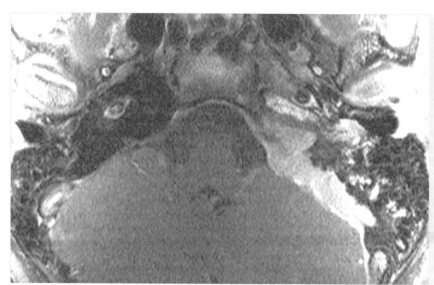

Fig. 71.1 Axial T1 postcontrast image through the posterior fossa demonstrates an avidly enhancing dural-based mass along the inner margin of the mastoid and petrous portions of the left temporal bone. An enhancing dural tail is seen both anteriorly and posteriorly.

■ Clinical Presentation

A young adult with headaches (▶ Fig. 71.1)

▨ Key Imaging Finding

Dural-based mass

▨ Top 3 Differential Diagnoses

- **Meningioma.** Meningiomas are benign dural-based masses and represent the most common extraaxial masses. Common locations include parasagittal, convexities, middle cranial fossa, and planum sphenoidale. Less common locations include the sellar/suprasellar region and cerebellopontine angle. They occur most frequently in adult women and are typically solitary. Multiple meningiomas occur sporadically, in patients with neurofibromatosis type 2 (NF2), or as a complication of radiation therapy. Lesions have a broad, dural base and may be circumscribed or plaque-like. The majority are hyperdense on computed tomography (CT); the remainder are isodense to brain parenchyma. Calcification is noted in about one-quarter of cases. Overlying bony remodeling or hyperostosis is common. There is often mass effect on the underlying parenchyma; edema is not uncommon with larger lesions. On CT and magnetic resonance imaging (MRI), there is avid enhancement with a dural tail. MRI shows the extra-axial location with a cerebrospinal fluid cleft separating the lesion from the underlying parenchyma. Meningiomas are typically iso- to hypointense on T1, variable in signal on T2, and hyperintense on fluid-attenuated inversion recovery (FLAIR). Calcification is typically hypointense on all sequences. As with CT, vasogenic edema may be seen.
- **Metastases/Lymphoma.** Metastatic disease may involve the dura primarily or represent extension from calvarial metastases. The most common primaries with dural-based metastases include breast, lung, non-Hodgkin lymphoma, leukemia, prostate, and neuroblastoma. Skull-based metastases with dural extension are most often seen with lung, breast, prostate, and renal cell carcinoma. Lesions present as enhancing dural-based masses that may mimic meningiomas, especially lymphoma, which may also be hyperdense on CT. Lymphoma is also typically hypointense on T2 sequences due to its high cellularity. Calvarial destruction is a useful discriminator, as is the presence of additional lesions, especially parenchymal masses.
- **Hemangiopericytoma.** Hemangiopericytoma is a dural-based mesenchymal tumor of pericytes. It occurs in middle-aged adults and is histologically more aggressive (World Health Organization grade II or III) than meningioma. It presents as a heterogeneous dural-based mass that is iso- to hyperdense to parenchyma on CT without calcification. Cystic change is common, as is underlying mass effect and vasogenic edema. Calvarial erosion is common without hyperostosis. On MRI, hemangiopericytomas demonstrate heterogeneous signal and enhancement; prominent flow voids are commonly seen. There may be a dural tail; however, it is a less characteristic feature.

▨ Additional Differential Diagnoses

- **Granulomatous disease.** Tuberculosis and sarcoidosis are granulomatous processes that involve the dura. Most often, these present as regions of dural thickening and enhancement with a propensity for the basal cisterns, resulting in cranial neuropathies. A less common presentation is a focal or plaque-like dural-based mass that may mimic a meningioma. Regions of nodular leptomeningeal enhancement are a useful discriminator.
- **Extramedullary hematopoiesis.** Extramedullary hematopoiesis occurs in patients with severe anemia secondary to chronic disease or marrow infiltrative processes. Imaging findings include calvarial thickening with well-defined, smooth extra-dural masses. Multiple lesions are more common than a solitary lesion. On CT, foci of hematopoiesis are iso- to hyperdense, mimicking hematomas, meningiomas, or lymphoma. Lesions are typically T1 isointense, T2 hypointense, and FLAIR hyperintense with avid, homogeneous enhancement.
- **Rosai-Dorfman.** Rosai-Dorfman disease is a non-Langerhans cell histiocytosis that most often occurs in children and young adults. The most common imaging feature is cervical lymphadenopathy, which is often massive. Less common presentations include dural-based and orbital masses. Dural-based lesions are typically multiple, isointense on T1, hyperintense on T2, and diffusely enhance.

▨ Diagnosis

Meningioma (plaque-like in a patient with NF2)

✓ Pearls

- Meningiomas are the most common extraaxial masses; they are benign and occur most often in adult women.
- Metastases and lymphoma may involve the meninges primarily or result from extension of calvarial metastases.
- Hemangiopericytomas are more aggressive than meningiomas and lack calcification or bony hyperostosis.

Suggested Reading

Johnson MD, Powell SZ, Boyer PJ, Weil RJ, Moots PL. Dural lesions mimicking meningiomas. Hum Pathol 2002; 33: 1211–1226

Case 72

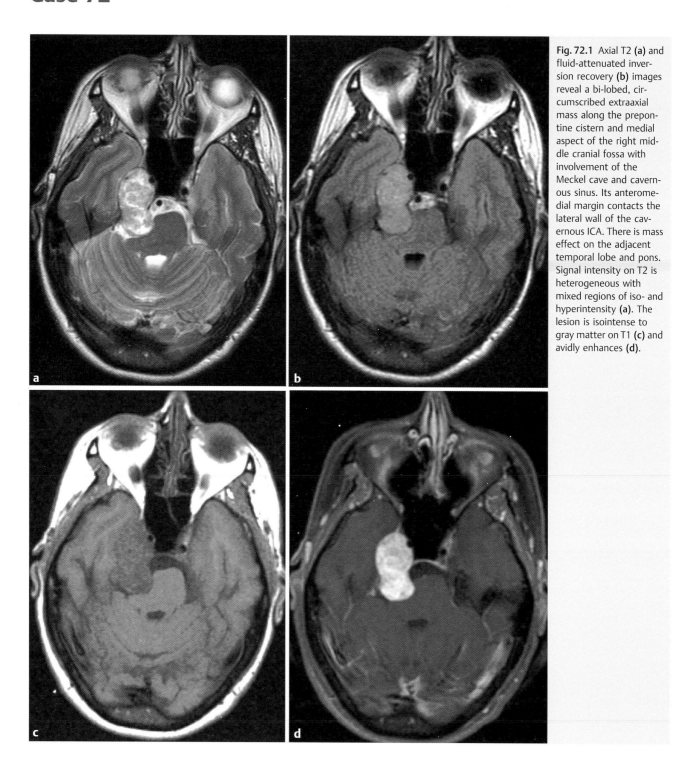

Fig. 72.1 Axial T2 (a) and fluid-attenuated inversion recovery (b) images reveal a bi-lobed, circumscribed extraaxial mass along the prepontine cistern and medial aspect of the right middle cranial fossa with involvement of the Meckel cave and cavernous sinus. Its anteromedial margin contacts the lateral wall of the cavernous ICA. There is mass effect on the adjacent temporal lobe and pons. Signal intensity on T2 is heterogeneous with mixed regions of iso- and hyperintensity (a). The lesion is isointense to gray matter on T1 (c) and avidly enhances (d).

Clinical Presentation

A 53-year-old woman with migraine headaches (▶ Fig. 72.1)

▣ Key Imaging Finding

Circumscribed extraaxial mass at the skull base

▣ Top 3 Differential Diagnoses

- **Meningioma.** Meningiomas are benign dural-based masses and represent the most common extraaxial masses. Common locations include parasagittal, convexities, middle cranial fossa, and planum sphenoidale. Less common locations include the sellar/suprasellar region and cerebellopontine angle. They occur most frequently in adult women and are typically solitary. Multiple meningiomas occur sporadically, in patients with neurofibromatosis type 2 (NF2), or as a complication of radiation therapy. Lesions have a broad, dural base and may be circumscribed or plaque-like. The majority are hyperdense on computed tomography (CT); the remainder are isodense to brain parenchyma. Calcification is noted in about one-quarter of cases. Overlying bony remodeling or hyperostosis is common. There is often mass effect on the underlying parenchyma; edema is not uncommon with larger lesions. On CT and magnetic resonance imaging (MRI), there is avid enhancement with a dural tail. MRI shows the extra-axial location with a cerebrospinal fluid cleft separating the lesion from the underlying parenchyma. Meningiomas are typically iso- to hypointense on T1, variable in signal on T2, and hyperintense on fluid-attenuated inversion recovery. Calcification is typically hypointense on all sequences. As with CT, vasogenic edema may be seen.
- **Schwannoma.** Schwannomas are nerve sheath tumors that arise from perineural Schwann cells. They are the second most common extraaxial masses after meningiomas. Common locations include the cerebellopontine angle (CPA); the skull base, basal cisterns, and exiting foramina along the course of the cranial nerves; and within the cavernous sinus.

After vestibular schwannoma, trigeminal schwannomas are the next most common. Schwannomas are composed of two tissue types: Antoni A and B. Antoni A tissue is densely packed, whereas Antoni B tissue is loosely packed. On CT, schwannomas are typically isodense compared with brain parenchyma with heterogeneous enhancement. There is often mass effect on adjacent parenchyma without edema. Unlike meningiomas, calcification is rare. When located near the skull base or exiting foramina, smooth bony remodeling and enlargement of foramina is commonly seen. On MRI, schwannomas are iso- to hypointense on T1 sequences with heterogeneous but avid enhancement. The T2 signal intensity varies based upon tissue composition. Antoni A components are iso- to hyperintense, whereas Antoni B components are prominently hyperintense. The vast majority of lesions are solitary; multiple lesions may be seen in the setting of NF2.

- **Hemangiopericytoma.** Hemangiopericytoma is a dural-based mesenchymal tumor of pericytes. It occurs in middle-aged adults and is histologically more aggressive (World Health Organization grade II or III) than meningioma. It presents as a heterogeneous dural-based mass that is iso- to hyperdense to parenchyma on CT without calcification. Cystic change is common, as is underlying mass effect and vasogenic edema. Calvarial erosion is common without hyperostosis. On MRI, hemangiopericytomas demonstrate heterogeneous signal and enhancement; prominent flow voids are commonly seen. There may be a dural tail; however, it is a less characteristic feature.

▣ Additional Differential Diagnoses

- **Lymphoma.** Dural-based or extraaxial lymphoma typically results from hematogenous spread of non-Hodgkin lymphoma. Lesions commonly present as dural-based masses (well-defined) or (plaque-like) that may mimic meningiomas. They are often hyperdense on CT and iso- to hypointense on T2 MRI sequences due to high cellularity.

▣ Diagnosis

Schwannoma (trigeminal)

✓ Pearls

- Meningiomas are the most common extraaxial masses; calcification and a dural tail are characteristic features.
- Schwannomas are the second most common extraaxial masses; they occur along the course of cranial nerves.
- Hemangiopericytoma is a relatively rare vascular tumor that mimics an aggressive meningioma on imaging.
- Dural-based or extraaxial lymphoma typically results from hematogenous spread of non-Hodgkin lymphoma.

Suggested Reading

Yuh WTC, Wright DC, Barloon TJ, Schultz DH, Sato Y, Cervantes CA. MR imaging of primary tumors of trigeminal nerve and Meckel's cave. Am J Roentgenol 1988; 151: 577–582

Case 73

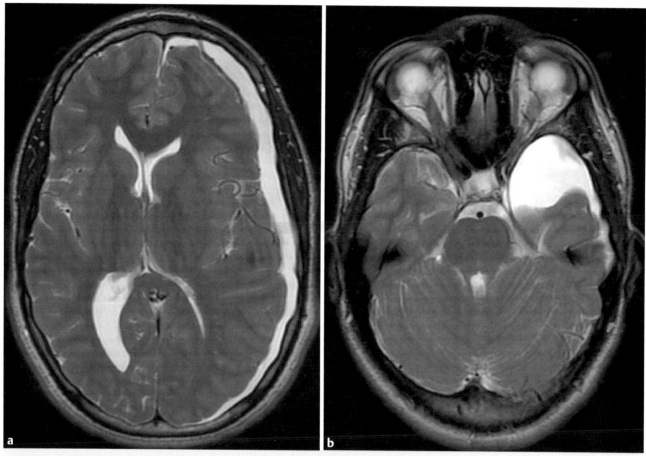

Fig. 73.1 Axial T2 images **(a,b)** demonstrate a subdural collection over the left convexity **(a)** with inward mass effect on the underlying parenchyma and left lateral ventricle, as well as midline shift to the right. The collection is isointense to CSF. Axial T2 image through the middle cranial fossa **(b)** reveals an arachnoid cyst on the left that is contiguous with the subdural collection.

■ Clinical Presentation

A 17-year-old boy with headache; history otherwise withheld (▶ Fig. 73.1)

▓ Key Imaging Finding

Subdural fluid collection

■ Top 3 Differential Diagnoses

- **Subdural hematoma.** Subdural hematomas (SDHs) result from tearing of bridging cortical veins as they pass between the arachnoid and dura. They are most often seen in the setting of trauma, both accidental and nonaccidental. Patients undergoing anticoagulation or those with enlarged extraaxial cerebrospinal fluid (CSF) spaces are more prone to developing SDH with relatively minor trauma. The subdural space is bound by midline dural attachments. Because of these attachments, SDH appears as a crescent-shaped collection overlying a cerebral convexity. It may cross sutures and extend along the interhemispheric fissure and falx, but it may not cross midline. The appearance of a SDH depends upon the timing of imaging, presence of re-bleeding, hemoglobin/coagulation state, and presence or absence of inter-mixed CSF within the subdural collection. In general, acute SDH is hyperdense on computed tomography (CT). As time progresses, the hemorrhage evolves through stages during which it becomes isodense (late subacute) and then finally hypodense (chronic stage) compared with brain parenchyma. Timing of SDH on magnetic resonance imaging (MRI) is fraught with error, as the predictable pattern of hemorrhage evolution applies to intraparenchymal hemorrhages. Although the general sequence of evolution is similar, the timing may vary significantly due to intermixture of CSF and differences in oxygen tension within the extraaxial spaces. Gradient echo and susceptibility weighted imaging sequences are sensitive for SDH. Mild meningeal enhancement may be seen. Mass effect, herniation, and secondary ischemia increase morbidity and mortality.

- **Subdural hygroma.** Subdural hygromas represent CSF collections within the subdural space. They most often occur in the setting of trauma with resultant arachnoid tearing. The term has also been used to describe chronic subdural hematomas that follow CSF signal on all pulse sequences. Rarely, they may result from rupture of an arachnoid cyst into the subdural space. Subdural hygromas are differentiated from prominence of the subarachnoid space by inward displacement of the venous structures that traverse the subarachnoid space. Subdural hygromas may cross sutures and extend along the interhemispheric fissure, but do not cross midline. When large, there may be mass effect on the underlying brain parenchyma.

- **Subdural empyema.** Subdural empyemas most often result as a complication of meningitis or from direct spread of adjacent parenchymal, sinonasal, or otomastoid infections. Post-traumatic or postoperative subdural empyemas are less common. As with other subdural collections, subdural empyemas are crescent-shaped, may cross sutures and extend along the interhemispheric fissure, and do not cross midline. On CT, subdural empyemas are hypodense and typically have enhancement of the overlying dura and underlying leptomeninges. On MRI, the collections are hypointense on T1 and hyperintense on T2 sequences. Restricted diffusion is often seen with pyogenic infections. Adjacent meningeal enhancement is better seen on MRI compared with CT.

■ Additional Differential Diagnoses

- **Subdural effusion.** Subdural effusions are sterile collections that occur in the setting of meningitis. They are most often seen in children with *Haemophilus influenza* meningitis. On CT, subdural effusions are hypodense without discernible enhancement. On MRI, effusions follow CSF signal on all sequences, do not show restricted diffusion, and typically have no or minimal meningeal enhancement.

■ Diagnosis

Subdural hygroma (due to ruptured arachnoid cyst)

✓ Pearls

- SDHs result from traumatic tearing of bridging cortical veins as they pass between the arachnoid and dura.
- Subdural hygromas are CSF collections that are most often post-traumatic with resultant arachnoid tearing.

- Subdural empyemas are infectious collections that often have adjacent meningeal enhancement.
- Subdural effusions are sterile collections that occur in the setting of *H. influenza* meningitis.

Suggested Readings

O'Brien WT. Imaging of CNS infections in immunocompetent hosts. J Am Osteopath Coll Radiol. 2012; 1: 3–9

Vezina G. Assessment of the nature and age of subdural collections in nonaccidental head injury with CT and MRI. Pediatr Radiol 2009; 39: 586–590

Case 74

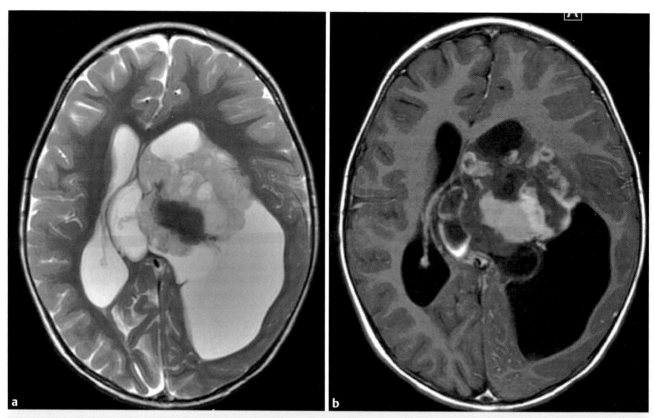

Fig. 74.1 Axial T2 image **(a)** demonstrates a large cystic and solid mass centered within the deep gray/white matter on the left with mass effect on the body of the left lateral ventricle and entrapment of the atria. There is midline shift to the right with mass effect on and enlargement of the right lateral ventricle as well. Solid components are heterogeneous with regions that are hyper- and hypointense. Axial T1 postcontrast image **(b)** reveals enhancement of the solid components and along the walls of some of the cystic components.

▨ Clinical Presentation

A 2 ½-year-old boy with chronic headache, vomiting, and developmental delay (▶ Fig. 74.1)

Key Imaging Finding

Large supratentorial mass in an infant or young child

Top 3 Differential Diagnoses

- **Astrocytoma.** Astrocytomas are glial tumors that may present as superficial or deep parenchymal masses. Juvenile pilocytic astrocytomas (JPA) and pleomorphic xanthoastrocytomas (PXA) are low-grade variants that present as cystic masses with solid mural nodules. Glioblastoma multiforme is the most aggressive variant (World Health Organization grade IV) and is relatively uncommon in children. Fibrillary (grade II) and anaplastic (grade III) are additional variants. Aside from JPA and PXA, as lesions become more aggressive, there is increased enhancement, edema, and perfusion. Magnetic resonance spectroscopy shows a tumor spectra with increased choline and decreased N-acetyl aspartate. High-grade lesions have an elevated lipid-lactate peak; low-grade astrocytomas will have increased myoinositol.
- **Teratoma.** Teratomas are germ cell tumors with components from all three germinal layers. They may present in newborns, infants, children, or young adults, depending upon the size and location of the lesion. It is a leading differential in a newborn with a parenchymal mass. Teratomas are often midline and may be associated with developmental anomalies. They may contain regions of fat, calcification, and soft tissue with or without cystic components. Identifying the presence of macroscopic fat is key to suggesting the diagnosis.
- **Supratentorial PNET.** Primitive neuroectodermal tumors (PNET) are highly aggressive, cellular masses with an overall poor prognosis. They are most common in the posterior fossa. When supratentorial, they present as large, heterogeneous parenchymal masses with vasogenic edema. Solid components heterogeneously but avidly enhance. Regions of calcification, hemorrhage, and cystic necrosis are common. Due to the high cellularity, there is often restricted diffusion, which is a useful discriminator. Lesions are prone to meningeal spread.

Additional Differential Diagnoses

- **Desmoplastic infantile ganglioglioma** (DIG). DIG is a rare tumor that most often occurs in infancy but may also be seen in early childhood. Classic teaching is that it is a benign entity composed of neoplastic astrocytes on a background of desmoplastic tissue; however, malignant cases have been described. In infancy, patients present with macrocephaly and occasionally seizures. The most common imaging appearance is a large, peripheral, supratentorial cystic and solid mass that abuts the pial surface. Solid components are heterogeneous in signal and demonstrate enhancement. Overlying meningeal enhancement is characteristic. Calcifications typically do not occur. A less common presentation is a cystic and solid mass centered within the deep gray and white matter with otherwise similar imaging characteristics.
- **Atypical teratoid rhabdoid tumor** (ATRT). ATRT is a rare, aggressive embryonal tumor composed of rhabdoid and PNET cells. It typically occurs in children < 3 years of age and has a dismal prognosis. There is an equal incidence of supratentorial and infratentorial involvement. Imaging appearance is often indistinguishable from medulloblastoma, demonstrating a large mass with avidly enhancing solid components and surrounding edema. Solid components are often hyperdense (computed tomography) with restricted diffusion (magnetic resonance imaging). Cysts, calcification, and hemorrhage may be seen. Subarachnoid seeding is common at presentation.
- **Choroid plexus tumors.** Choroid plexus papillomas occur most commonly in children within the atria of the lateral ventricles and less commonly in adults within the fourth ventricle. Infants and toddlers present with enlarging head size and symptoms related to hydrocephalus that results from overproduction and likely impaired resorption of cerebrospinal fluid. They are circumscribed with frondlike projections and a vascular pedicle. Calcification is seen in 25% of cases. Lesions intensely and homogeneously enhance. Heterogeneous enhancement and brain parenchymal invasion suggests choroid plexus carcinoma.

Diagnosis

Desmoplastic infantile ganglioglioma

✓ Pearls

- Astrocytomas are glial tumors; more aggressive variants have increased enhancement, edema, and perfusion.
- Teratomas are germ cell tumors with components from all three germinal layers; they are common in newborns/infants.
- Supratentorial PNET and ATRT are highly aggressive tumors that may occur in infants and young children.

Suggested Reading

Buetow PC, Smirniotopoulos JG, Done S. Congenital brain tumors: a review of 45 cases. Am J Roentgenol 1990; 155: 587–593

Case 75

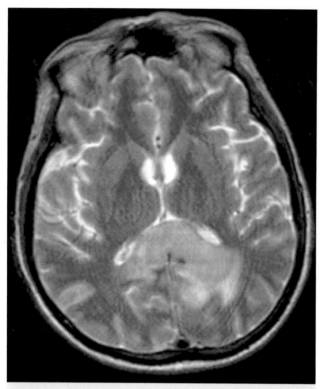

Fig. 75.1 Axial T2 image through the brain demonstrates a large intermediate to hyperintense mass involving and expanding the splenium of the corpus callosum. (Image courtesy of Paul M. Sherman, MD)

■ Clinical Presentation

A 53-year-old man with altered mental status (▶ Fig. 75.1)

■ Key Imaging Finding

Expansile corpus callosal mass

■ Top 3 Differential Diagnoses

- **Glioblastoma multiforme (GBM).** GBM is a highly aggressive, World Health Organization grade IV astrocytoma and is the most common primary intracranial neoplasm in adults. Although it may occur at any age, the peak incidence is between 45 and 70 years of age. GBM crosses white matter tracts to involve the contralateral hemisphere, hence the term *butterfly glioma* of corpus callosum. It is a rapidly enlarging tumor with central necrosis and neovascularity. There is marked mass effect; thick, irregular enhancement of solid components; and adjacent T2/fluid-attenuated inversion recovery (FLAIR) hyperintensity that represents vasogenic edema and tumor invasion. Viable tumor cells extend beyond the margin of abnormal signal on magnetic resonance imaging (MRI). The tumor is heterogeneous but primarily T2 hyperintense and T1 iso- to hypointense with associated cysts, hemorrhage, and fluid debris. Regions of diffusion restriction and increased perfusion are noted within solid components. Prominent flow voids may be seen due to neovascularity. MR spectroscopy shows significantly elevated choline, decreased *N*-acetyl aspartate, and a lipid-lactate peak. Prognosis is poor.
- **Lymphoma.** Primary central nervous system (CNS) lymphoma is almost exclusively of the non-Hodgkin variant. It typically occurs within the periventricular white matter and basal ganglia and commonly involves the corpus callosum and ependymal surfaces of the ventricles. Leptomeningeal and dural involvement occurs more often with secondary lymphoma. Lymphoma may present as a solitary mass or multiple lesions and can be circumscribed or infiltrative. There is typically mild surrounding edema. The lesions are characteristically hyperdense on computed tomography (CT) and iso- to hypointense on both T1 and T2 sequences due to increased nuclear-to-cytoplasmic ratio. Restricted diffusion may be seen and is also associated with high cellularity. Hemorrhage and necrosis are uncommon. Enhancement is intense and homogenous in immunocompetent patients and may be peripheral or ring-enhancing in immunocompromised patients. Unlike toxoplasmosis, lymphoma is hypermetabolic on thallium single-photon emission computed tomography and positron emission tomography imaging and demonstrates increased perfusion.
- **Demyelinating disease.** Multiple sclerosis is the most common primary demyelinating disease, is more common in women, and typically presents between 20 and 40 years of age. Disease course is most often relapsing and remitting. Acute disseminated encephalomyelitis is a monophasic demyelinating process that is more common in children and young adults. Characteristic imaging features include ovoid T2/fluid-attenuated inversion recovery hyperintense white matter lesions in a periventricular location and oriented perpendicular to the ventricles ("Dawson fingers"). High-specificity locations include the corpus callosum, cerebellum, brain stem/brachium pontis, and cord. Transient enhancement and occasionally restricted diffusion may be seen during periods of active demyelination. The enhancement pattern may be nodular or "open ring" with the enhancement along the leading edge of demyelination and open portion of the ring facing the cortex. Tumefactive demyelination presents as a large mass with variable enhancement, simulating a neoplasm.

■ Diagnosis

CNS lymphoma

✓ Pearls

- GBM is highly aggressive with central necrosis and neovascularity; it often involves the corpus callosum.
- Lymphoma is hyperdense on CT and low in T2 signal on MRI due to high cellularity.
- Lymphoma commonly involves the deep gray/white matter; enhancement pattern depends upon immune status.
- Classic demyelinating lesions include "Dawson fingers" and involvement of the corpus callosum and brain stem.

Suggested Reading

Bourekas EC, Varakis K, Bruns D et al. Lesions of the corpus callosum: MR imaging and differential considerations in adults and children. Am J Roentgenol 2002; 179: 251–257

Case 76

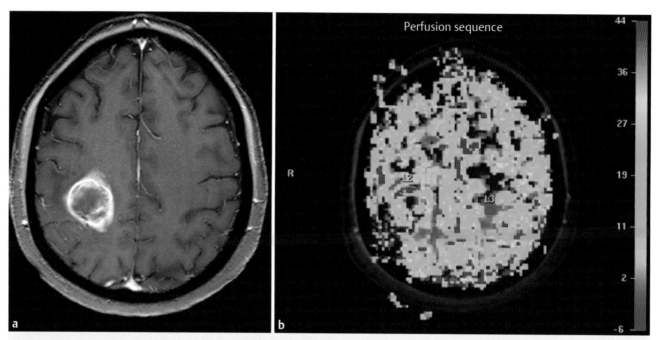

Fig. 76.1 Axial T1 postcontrast image with fat suppression **(a)** demonstrates a ring-enhancing mass within the right centrum semiovale. The margins are relatively thick and irregular. Adjacent vasogenic edema is subtly seen. Corresponding axial perfusion image **(b)** shows increased perfusion along the peripheral margins of the mass (focal areas of red and green) compared with the adjacent and contralateral white matter (blue).

■ Clinical Presentation

A 28-year-old woman with headaches and left-sided weakness (▶ Fig. 76.1)

■ Key Imaging Finding

Ring-enhancing mass

■ Top 3 Differential Diagnoses

- **Neoplasm.** High-grade gliomas, lymphoma, and metastases represent the majority of ring-enhancing tumors. Glioblastoma multiforme is the most common primary brain tumor in adults and is highly aggressive (World Health Organization grade IV). There is rapid growth with neovascularity. Lesions are typically solitary with marked mass effect, surrounding vasogenic edema, thick irregular peripheral enhancement, and central necrosis. Although heterogeneous, the tumor is predominantly T2 hyperintense. Regions of hemorrhage and restricted diffusion (due to high cellularity) are common. Involvement of the corpus callosum is often seen. Primary central nervous system lymphoma characteristically involves the deep gray and white matter. Involvement of the corpus callosum and ependymal surface of the ventricles is common. Lesions may show characteristic hypointensity on T2 images due to high cellularity. There is solid enhancement in immunocompetent patients; ring enhancement may be seen following treatment or in immunosuppressed patients. Positron emission tomography or thallium imaging demonstrates increased metabolic activity, which distinguishes lymphoma from toxoplasmosis. As with other tumors, there is increased perfusion. Metastatic lesions may be solitary (~45%) or multiple. They often involve the gray-white matter junction, deep gray/white matter, and posterior fossa. There is often pronounced edema, except for cortically based metastases that show little edema. Ring enhancement occurs with cystic metastases or central necrosis.

- **Abscess.** Abscesses result from hematogenous spread; direct spread from sinonasal or otomastoid infections, trauma, or surgery; or as a complication of meningitis. They may be solitary or multiple. Well-formed abscesses have smooth rim enhancement with surrounding vasogenic edema. On magnetic resonance imaging (MRI), they have a characteristic T2 hypointense capsule that is thinner toward the ventricles and thus prone to intraventricular rupture. Pyogenic abscesses demonstrate central restricted diffusion. Toxoplasmosis, a common ring-enhancing parasitic infection in immunosuppressed patients, does not typically show restricted diffusion. As opposed to tumors, abscesses have decreased perfusion. MR spectroscopy shows an elevated lipid-lactate doublet.

- **Subacute infarct.** Cortically based infarcts are typically located in a vascular distribution; deep infarcts may be more difficult to characterize. The presence of edema, mass effect, hemorrhagic transformation, and subacute enhancement may mimic a mass lesion, especially if rim-enhancing. Infarcts show restricted diffusion acutely that may persist into the subacute phase. This is helpful but nonspecific, as abscesses and cellular neoplasms may also demonstrate restricted diffusion. Enhancement begins as early as 2 days and peaks at 2 weeks.

■ Additional Differential Diagnoses

- **Demyelinating disease.** Multiple sclerosis is the most common primary demyelinating disease; acute disseminating encephalomyelitis is monophasic and more common in children. Characteristic features include ovoid T2/fluid-attenuated inversion recovery hyperintense lesions oriented perpendicular to the ventricles ("Dawson fingers"). High-specificity locations include the corpus callosum, optic pathways, and posterior fossa. Enhancement suggests active demyelination. The enhancement pattern may be nodular or "open ring" with the open portion facing the cortex. Tumefactive lesions mimic neoplasms.

- **Resolving contusion.** A history of trauma is important in differentiating a contusion from other ring-enhancing lesions. Blood products are present in varying stages, depending upon the age of the hematoma. Rim enhancement occurs within a few days in a vascularized capsule. Acute blood products are isointense on T1 and hypointense on T2. Subacute blood products (intra- or extracellular methemoglobin (MetHb)) are T1 hyperintense. Intracellular MetHb is T2 hypointense; extracellular MetHb is T2 hyperintense.

■ Diagnosis

Neoplasm (high-grade glioma)

✓ Pearls

- Glioblastoma multiforme, lymphoma, and metastases are the most common tumors to present as ring-enhancing lesions.
- Abscesses characteristically have a T2 hypointense capsule with smooth enhancement and restricted diffusion.

- Enhancement pattern of demyelinating plaques may be "open ring" with the open portion facing the cortex.

Suggested Reading

Smirniotopoulos JG, Murphy FM, Rushing EJ, Rees JH, Schroeder JW. Patterns of contrast enhancement in the brain and meninges. Radiographics 2007; 27: 525–551

Case 77

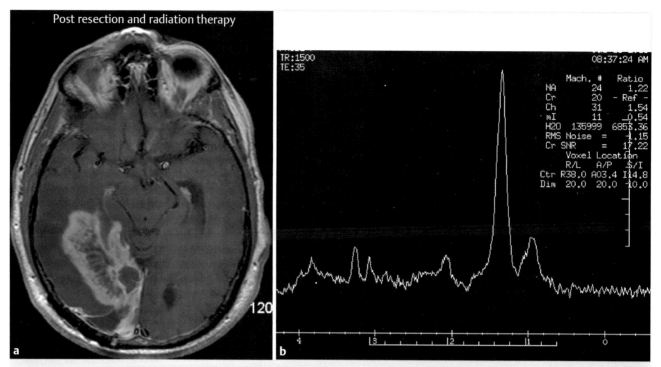

Fig. 77.1 Axial T1 postcontrast MR image **(a)** demonstrates masslike enhancement within a surgical cavity located in the right occipitotemporal region with surrounding hypointense vasogenic edema. Short echo MR spectroscopy **(b)** performed over the region of enhancement reveals suppression of metabolites with a prominent lipid (0.9 ppm) and lipid-lactate (1.3 to 1.33 ppm) peaks. (Courtesy of Aaron Betts, MD and Mary Gaskill-Shipley, MD.)

■ Clinical Presentation

A 70-year-old man with high-grade glioma postexcision and radiation therapy (► Fig. 77.1)

■ Key Imaging Finding

Enhancement in surgical bed

■ Top 3 Differential Diagnoses

- **Recurrent or residual tumor.** Glioblastoma multiforme is the most common primary brain tumor in adults; it may also occasionally be seen in children. It is highly aggressive (World Health Organization grade IV) and presents as an infiltrating mass with vasogenic edema, thick peripheral enhancement, and central necrosis. Involvement of the corpus callosum is common. Treatment consists of resection with radiation therapy to the surgical/tumor bed. Tumor cells often extend beyond the regions of T2/fluid-attenuated inversion recovery signal abnormality; therefore, complete resection is difficult. Adjuvant therapies include steroids, chemotherapy, and antiangiogenic agents. Recurrent tumor most often occurs within the surgical bed. It presents as increased mass effect, edema, and enhancement. Patients often suffer from new or progressive neurological deficits. Imaging appearance of recurrent tumor, treatment changes, and radiation necrosis overlaps on conventional magnetic resonance imaging (MRI) sequences. Perfusion imaging in the setting of recurrence reveals increased cerebral blood flow (CBF) and volume (CBV) compared with adjacent white matter. On MR spectroscopy, high-grade tumors demonstrate elevated choline, decreased *N*-acetyl aspartate (NAA), and elevated lipid-lactate peak.

- **Post-treatment changes.** Treatment of high-grade tumors often involves surgical resection with radiation therapy within the surgical/tumor bed. Adjuvant chemotherapy and antiangiogenic therapies are becoming commonplace in clinical practice. Steroid therapy results in decreased edema, decreased enhancement, and improvement in neurological symptoms. Expected postoperative changes include regions of hemorrhage and enhancement within and overlying the surgical bed. Postoperative enhancement is often linear; nodular foci may be seen due to the presence of granulation tissue. These regions can be followed to ensure stability or resolution. Newer therapies have resulted in findings that present a challenge in determining response to therapy. Pseudoprogression is seen most often in patients treated with radiation and chemotherapy. It presents as increased enhancement in the surgical bed 2 to 6 months after therapy. It stabilizes or decreases on follow-up imaging. Interestingly, pseudoprogression is associated with better treatment outcomes. Also, these patients are typically asymptomatic. Perfusion imaging demonstrates similar perfusion characteristics compared with white matter, whereas recurrent tumor shows increased perfusion. Pseudoresponse is another post-treatment change that typically results from a combination of chemotherapy and antiangiogenic agents. These therapies result in significant decrease in enhancement within the surgical/tumor bed without decrease in tumor volume. Although patients who demonstrate pseudoresponse have short-term survival benefits, long-term outcomes are variable.

- **Radiation necrosis.** High-grade tumors are typically treated with fractionated radiotherapy over several weeks. Radiation necrosis is a severe complication that results in tissue necrosis due to radiation toxicity. It most often occurs 3 to 12 months after therapy, but delayed occurrences may be seen years and even decades later. The incidence of radiation necrosis is between 5 and 25% and is proportional to the radiation dose. On MRI, radiation necrosis presents as regions of prominent enhancement with foci of central necrosis, often referred to as a "soap bubble" or "Swiss cheese" appearance. There is mass effect and surrounding vasogenic edema. It occurs in the region of highest radiation dose, which is typically within the postoperative bed. On conventional sequences, it is difficult if not impossible to distinguish from recurrent tumor. New regions of enhancement within the radiation bed but in regions remote from prior tumor are more likely to represent radiation necrosis. On perfusion imaging, radiation necrosis has similar CBF and CBV compared with normal white matter, whereas high-grade tumors have increased CBF and CBV that is similar to gray matter. On MR spectroscopy, radiation necrosis demonstrates decreased choline, NAA, and creatine with an elevated lipid-lactate doublet. This pattern reflects the absence of tumor and presence of necrotic parenchyma.

■ Diagnosis

Radiation necrosis

✓ Pearls

- Recurrent tumor typically occurs in the surgical bed; there is increased perfusion and a tumor spectra on MR spectroscopy.
- Treatment choices affect imaging findings; knowledge of these is critical in determining treatment response.

- Radiation necrosis mimics recurrent tumor on conventional sequences; perfusion imaging and MR spectroscopy are helpful.

Suggested Reading

Fatterpekar GM, Galheigo D, Narayana A, Johnson G, Knopp E. Treatment-related change versus tumor recurrence in high-grade gliomas: a diagnostic conundrum —use of dynamic susceptibility contrast-enhanced (DSC) perfusion MRI. Am J Roentgenol 2012; 198: 19–26

Case 78

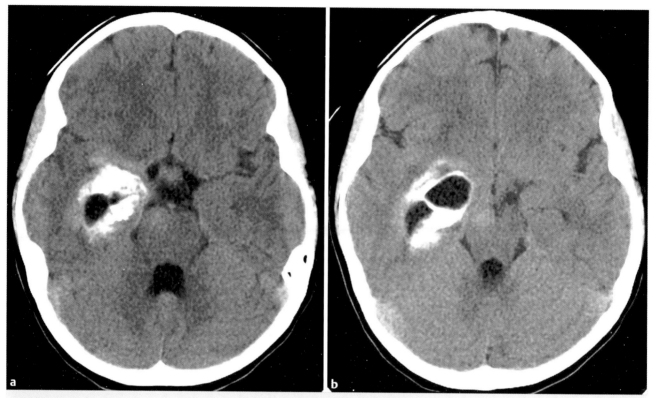

Fig. 78.1 Axial CT images **(a,b)** demonstrate a cystic and solid right temporal lobe mass with prominent calcifications extending into the deep white matter.

▓ Clinical Presentation

A young adult with new-onset seizures (▶ Fig. 78.1)

▨ Key Imaging Finding

Calcified supratentorial parenchymal mass

■ Top 3 Differential Diagnoses

- **Astrocytoma.** There are numerous variants of astrocytoma that range from low to high grade. They may present as superficial or deep parenchymal masses. The diffuse fibrillary variant (World Health Organization grade II) is the most common to calcify, although calcifications are only seen in ~20% of cases. The calcification pattern varies from punctate to diffuse and is nonspecific. Although astrocytomas have a lower frequency of calcification compared with oligodendrogliomas, they are more common in incidence.
- **Oligodendroglioma.** Oligodendroglioma is a glial tumor that most often occurs in adults. It typically involves the subcortical white matter and overlying cortex. Clinically, patients often present with seizures, headaches, or focal neurological deficits. Although they may occur anywhere, frontal lobe involvement is most common. On imaging, oligodendroglioma presents as a well-circumscribed (more common) or ill-defined mass with a high incidence of calcification (up to 90%). Calcifications may be punctate, ribbon-like, or diffuse.

There is typically no or mild surrounding vasogenic edema. Enhancement, if present, is subtle and ill-defined.
- **Vascular malformation.** Arteriovenous malformations (AVMs) consist of a nidus of abnormal connections between arteries and veins without an intervening capillary network. Patients often present in young adulthood with headaches, hemorrhage, seizures, or focal neurological deficits. Computed tomography (CT) may be normal or demonstrate regions of increased attenuation or calcification. Magnetic resonance imaging (MRI) reveals a tangle of enlarged vessels, corresponding to the nidus. Perinidal aneurysms are a common source of hemorrhage. Cavernous malformations (CMs) consist of variable-sized blood-filled sinusoids and larger cavernous spaces without intervening brain parenchyma. The majority of lesions are solitary. CT may be normal or show subtle regions of calcification or hemorrhage. Lesions have foci of increased and decreased T1 and T2 signal centrally with a T2 dark (hemosiderin) capsule on MRI.

■ Additional Differential Diagnoses

- **Ependymoma.** The majority of ependymomas present as fourth ventricular masses in children. However, they may also occur in the supratentorial compartment as a parenchymal mass centered in the white matter with surrounding edema. As with posterior fossa ependymomas, cystic components and calcification (≈50%) are relatively common. Solid components heterogeneously enhance. Ependymomas occur predominantly in children and young adults.
- **Infection.** Infectious processes prone to parenchymal calcifications include neurocysticercosis, tuberculosis (TB), cryptococcus, and human immunodeficiency virus in children. Of these, tuberculoma is the most common to present as a calcified mass. Cysticercosis most often presents as multiple parenchymal calcifications with or without additional cystic

or rim-enhancing lesions. Tuberculomas result from hematogenous spread; concurrent meningeal involvement may be seen, preferentially involving the basal cisterns. Imaging appearance varies widely from focal cerebritis to frank abscesses with rim enhancement. Calcifications occur in the minority of cases.
- **Metastases.** Metastatic mucinous adenocarcinoma may occasionally present as a calcified parenchymal mass. Common primaries include breast, lung, colon, and ovarian carcinoma. Bone-forming tumors such as osteosarcoma may also present with calcified or ossified lesions. Metastases may be solitary or multiple and typically have pronounced vasogenic edema, with the exception of cortically based metastases that may have little edema.

■ Diagnosis

Oligodendroglioma

✓ Pearls

- Tumors with calcification include astrocytoma, oligodendroglioma, ependymoma, and, rarely, metastases.
- AVMs and CMs may have regions of calcification; AVMs have a vascular nidus and are prone to hemorrhage.

- TB, fungal, and neurocysticercosis are the most common infections to result in calcified parenchymal lesions.

Suggested Readings

Koeller KK, Rushing EJ. From the archives of the AFIP: oligodendroglioma and its variants: radiologic-pathologic correlation. Radiographics 2005; 25: 1669–1688

Makariou E, Patsalides AD. Intracranial calcifications. Appl Radiol 2009; 38: 48–60

Smith AB. Vascular malformations of the brain: radiologic and pathologic correlation. J Am Osteopath Coll Radiol. 2012; 1: 10–22

Case 79

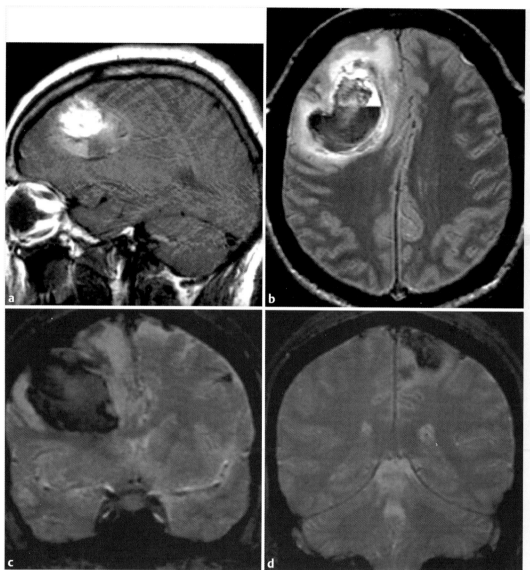

Fig. 79.1 Sagittal T1 (**a**) and axial T2 (**b**) images demonstrate a right frontal parenchymal hematoma with blood-fluid levels (blood products of different ages) and surrounding edema (T2 hyperintensity). The intraparenchymal hemorrhage is predominantly hyperintense on T1 and hypointense on T2 sequences, corresponding to an early subacute hemorrhage. Coronal T2* GRE images (**c,d**) demonstrate blooming artifact bilaterally, as well as within the superior sagittal sinus and superficial cortical veins, consistent with thrombus. MR venography (not shown) revealed absence of the normal flow signal within the superior sagittal sinus. (Courtesy of Paul M. Sherman, MD.)

▓ Clinical Presentation

A 46-year-old woman with new onset headache (▶ Fig. 79.1)

■ Key Imaging Finding

Intraparenchymal hemorrhage

■ Top 3 Differential Diagnoses

- **Hemorrhagic infarct.** Hypertensive infarcts occur in adults or in younger patients with malignant hypertension or illicit drug use. They most commonly involve the basal ganglia/external capsule, thalamus, and posterior fossa. Hemorrhage is typically round or elliptical with surrounding edema. There may be extension into the ventricles. There is typically no enhancement. Hemorrhagic transformation of an arterial infarct usually occurs in the subacute phase when gyral enhancement is seen or more acutely if thrombolytics are administered. Arterial infarcts are characteristically wedge-shaped and follow a vascular distribution. Restricted diffusion is seen in the acute setting. Hemorrhagic venous infarcts occur in patients with hypercoagulable states and associated dural venous sinus or cortical vein (more commonly associated with parenchymal hemorrhage) thrombosis. Clot is hyperdense on unenhanced computed tomography (CT; "cord sign" for cortical veins); the "empty delta" sign on contrast studies corresponds to enhancement of the sinus surrounding the nonenhancing thrombus. CT venography or magnetic resonance (MR) venography demonstrate the region of venous thrombosis. Gradient echo (GRE) and susceptibility-weighted imaging (SWI) sequences are sensitive for hemorrhage.

- **Vascular malformation.** Arteriovenous malformations (AVMs) are abnormal networks of arteries and veins with no intervening capillary bed. The vast majority are solitary and supratentorial. Unenhanced CT demonstrates iso- to hyperdense serpentine vessels; calcifications are common. MR imaging (MRI) reveals flow voids in a "bag of worms" pattern with avid contrast enhancement. Associated aneurysms (arterial, venous, or intranidal) are often seen and are a primary source of hemorrhage. AVMs are classified based upon size, location (eloquent or noneloquent brain), and venous drainage (superficial or deep). They may be treated endovascularly or surgically. Cavernous malformations consist of variable-sized blood-filled sinusoids and larger cavernous spaces without intervening brain parenchyma. The majority of lesions are solitary. CT may be normal or show subtle regions of calcification or hemorrhage. A "popcorn" appearance is noted on MRI secondary to mixed hyper- and hypointense blood products on T1 and T2 sequences. There is blooming on GRE and SWI sequences.

- **Hemorrhagic neoplasm.** Glioblastoma multiforme (GBM) is the most common primary brain neoplasm in adults. It is highly aggressive (World Health Organization grade IV) with vasogenic edema and regions of central necrosis, tumoral enhancement, and neovascularity, which makes it prone to hemorrhage. Hemorrhagic metastases may be solitary or multiple. Primary neoplasms prone to hemorrhage include lung, breast, renal cell carcinoma, thyroid, and melanoma. Metastases may involve the gray-white matter junction or end arterioles within the deep brain parenchyma.

■ Additional Differential Diagnoses

- **Contusion.** Contusions present as patchy, superficial parenchymal hemorrhages with surrounding edema. They involve characteristic locations where parenchyma contacts the adjacent calvarium, to include the anterior temporal, inferior frontal, and parasagittal parenchyma. Within the first few days following trauma, contusions may expand and then subsequently regress. Calvarial fractures and foci of extraaxial hemorrhage are associated findings. GRE and SWI (more sensitive) demonstrate blooming associated with hemorrhage.

- **Cerebral amyloid disease.** Amyloid angiopathy typically presents as spontaneous, lobar parenchymal hemorrhages in elderly patients. There is an association with underlying white matter disease and dementia. The parietal and occipital lobes are most common, although any lobe may be involved. Approximately one-third of patients who present with acute intracranial hemorrhage will have MRI findings of old lobar or petechial hemorrhages, best seen on GRE and SWI sequences.

■ Diagnosis

Hemorrhagic venous infarct

✓ Pearls

- AVMs are most commonly solitary and supratentorial, have flow voids, and avidly enhance.
- Hemorrhagic infarcts include hypertensive hemorrhages, hemorrhagic conversion, and venous infarcts.
- GBM and hypervascular metastases may present as hemorrhagic intraparenchymal masses.
- Contusions occur where brain abuts the calvarium—temporal, inferior frontal, and parasagittal regions.

Suggested Reading

Linn J, Brückmann H. Differential diagnosis of nontraumatic intracerebral hemorrhage. Klin Neuroradiol 2009; 19: 45–61

Case 80

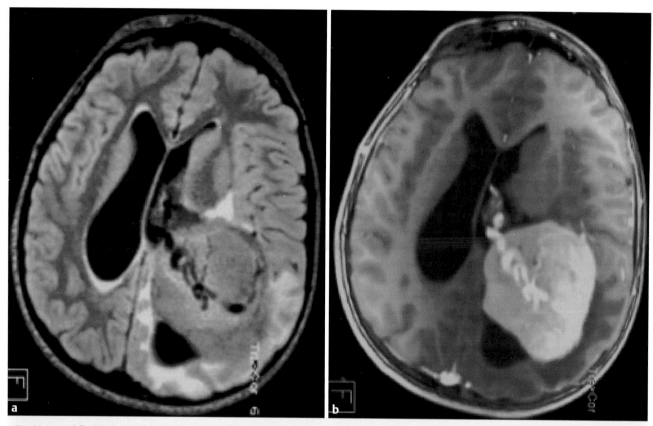

Fig. 80.1 Axial fluid-attenuated inversion recovery image **(a)** reveals a circumscribed iso- to hypointense mass within the atria of the left lateral ventricle with a prominent serpentine hypointense flow void. There is enlargement of the lateral ventricles with a rind of transependymal flow of CSF and edema within the left posterior temporal and occipital lobes. Axial T1 postcontrast image **(b)** demonstrates avid homogeneous enhancement of the mass, as well as enhancement of the prominent serpentine vasculature.

■ **Clinical Presentation**

Adolescent boy with increasing headaches (► Fig. 80.1)

Key Imaging Finding

Lateral ventricle mass

Top 3 Differential Diagnoses

- **Meningioma.** Meningiomas are the most common primary adult intracranial tumor and occur more frequently in women. Although intraventricular meningiomas are relatively uncommon, they still represent the most common atrial masses in adults. They may also be seen in children, especially in the setting of neurofibromatosis type 2. Meningiomas arise from arachnoid cap cells within the choroid plexus or velum interpositum. On computed tomography (CT), they are circumscribed and typically hyperdense compared with brain parenchyma; calcification is frequently seen. On magnetic resonance imaging (MRI), meningiomas are iso- to hypointense on T1 and variable but typically hyperintense on T2 sequences, although regions of calcification may be T2 hypointense. Mass effect may result in ventricular dilatation and parenchymal edema. Lesions intensely enhance.
- **Choroid plexus tumor.** Choroid plexus tumors consist of benign choroid plexus papilloma (CPP) and malignant choroid plexus carcinoma (CPC). They occur most commonly in children within the atria of the lateral ventricles and less commonly in adults within the fourth ventricle. Infants and toddlers present with enlarging head size, vomiting, and ataxia secondary to hydrocephalus due to overproduction of cerebrospinal fluid (CSF). They are well-circumscribed with frondlike projections and a vascular pedicle. Calcifications are seen in 25% of cases. The lesions are hypointense on T1 and hyperintense on T2 sequences. CPP intensely and homogeneously enhances. Heterogeneous enhancement and brain parenchymal invasion suggests a CPC rather than benign CPP.
- **Central neurocytoma.** Central neurocytomas are histologically distinct but similar to oligodendrogliomas. They arise from and have a broad attachment to the septum pellucidum or ventricular wall. Nearly half of cases occur near the foramina of Monro. Peak incidence is between 20 and 40 years of age. Patients may present with ventricular obstruction, visual disturbances, or hormonal changes. Lesions appear as circumscribed, lobulated masses with numerous cysts, often with a "soap bubble" appearance. Solid components are iso- to hyperdense on CT, variable on T1, and heterogeneously hyperintense on T2. There is moderate enhancement. Calcifications are visualized in ~50% of cases. Surrounding periventricular edema may be seen, especially with larger lesions.

Additional Differential Diagnoses

- **Ependymoma/Subependymoma.** Although ependymomas are common posterior fossa tumors in children, they may also be supratentorial, either within the ventricles or within the brain parenchyma (more common). Ependymomas are isointense on T1 and hyperintense on T2 with heterogeneous enhancement. Signal intensity varies in the setting of cystic change, calcification, and hemorrhage. Subependymomas occur more frequently in adults within the fourth and lateral ventricles. When located in the lateral ventricles, they may mimic central neurocytomas with a "bubbly" appearance. On MRI, lesions are iso- to hypointense on T1 and hyperintense on T2. Enhancement is variable but typically faint. They commonly calcify, especially in the fourth ventricle.
- **Metastases.** Metastases result from hematogenous spread to the choroid plexus, direct extension from parenchymal or infiltrative tumors (germ cell tumor, lymphoma), or as a result of CSF dissemination. Lateral ventricles are most often involved. The most common adult primary tumors include renal cell and lung carcinomas; melanoma, gastrointestinal tumors, and lymphoma are less common. In children, neuroblastoma, Wilms tumor, and retinoblastoma are most common. Metastatic lesions may be solitary or multiple. They are typically hypointense on T1 and hyperintense on T2 sequences with heterogeneous enhancement, especially with hemorrhage.

Diagnosis

Meningioma

✓ Pearls

- Meningiomas are the most common primary intracranial and intraventricular/atrial tumors in adults.
- Choroid plexus tumors most often occur in the atria of the lateral ventricles (children) and fourth ventricle (adults).
- Central neurocytoma occurs along the septum pellucidum or ventricular wall with a "soap bubble" appearance.
- Subependymomas occur in adults within the fourth and lateral ventricles; they may mimic central neurocytomas.

Suggested Reading

Koeller KK, Sandberg GD Armed Forces Institute of Pathology. From the archives of the AFIP. Cerebral intraventricular neoplasms: radiologic-pathologic correlation. Radiographics 2002; 22: 1473–1505

Case 81

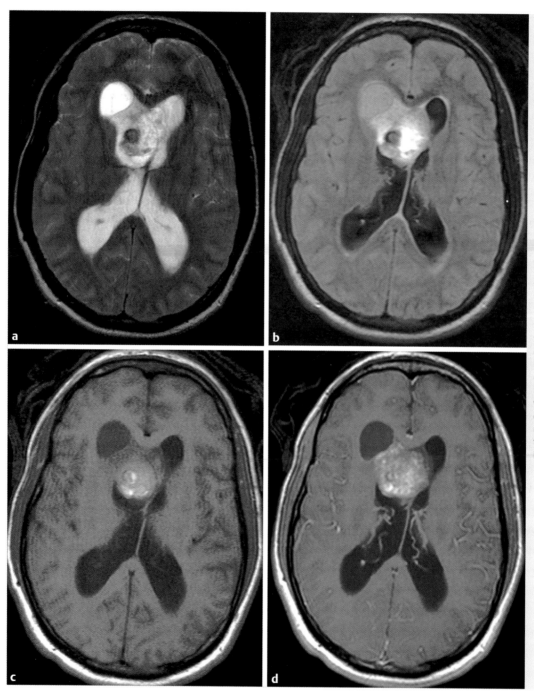

Fig. 81.1 Axial T2 **(a)** and fluid-attenuated inversion recovery (FLAIR) **(b)** images demonstrate a mixed cystic and solid mass centered along the anterior aspect of the septum pellucidum and frontal horn of the right lateral ventricle. The solid component is predominantly hyperintense with focal regions of hypointensity. The dominant cystic component in the frontal horn of the right lateral ventricle is hyperintense compared with CSF. Axial T1 image **(c)** reveals portions of the solid component to be intrinsically hyperintense, including the T2 hypointense foci, consistent with calcification. Solid enhancement is noted **(d)**. The dominant cystic component is slightly hyperintense compared with CSF. Lateral ventricles are enlarged with mild transependymal flow of CSF on the FLAIR image **(b)**.

■ **Clinical Presentation**

A young adult man with increasing headaches and intermittent nausea/vomiting (▶ Fig. 81.1)

■ Key Imaging Finding

Septum pellucidum/foramina of Monro mass

■ Top 3 Differential Diagnoses

- **Astrocytoma.** Primary gliomas of the septum pellucidum are typically low grade. Pilocytic variants present as cystic lesions with focal solid enhancement; they may occur sporadically or be associated with neurofibromatosis type 1. Subependymal giant cell astrocytomas (SEGAs) are mixed glioneuronal tumors that occur at the foramina of Monro in ~15% of tuberous sclerosis (TS) patients. Most lesions occur in the first and second decades of life. Lesions are identified based upon interval growth of a subependymal nodule in the characteristic location; enhancement pattern is not a distinguishing feature. Lesions may result in hydrocephalus. Primary treatment options include cerebrospinal fluid (CSF) diversion or tumor resection; newer medical therapies may be promising. On computed tomography (CT), SEGAs are iso- to hypodense and may have calcification. On magnetic resonance imaging (MRI), lesions are hypointense on T1 and heterogeneously hyperintense on T2 sequences; calcifications are typically T2 hypointense. The enhancement pattern is variable.

- **Oligodendroglioma.** Oligodendrogliomas are glial tumors involving oligodendrocytes. The vast majority occur superficially within the cerebral hemispheres. Intraventricular origin is relatively uncommon and most often involves the anterior aspect of the lateral ventricles and region of the foramina of Monro. Patients may present with symptoms related to obstructive hydrocephalus. CT reveals a circumscribed mass that is typically iso- to mildly hyperdense. Regions of cystic change and calcification are commonly seen. On MRI, lesions are variable but typically iso- to hypointense on T1 and hyperintense on T2 with heterogeneous enhancement. Signal characteristic are more heterogeneous in the presence of calcification or hemorrhage. Ventricular enlargement is a common finding. Parenchymal edema may be seen with large or more aggressive lesions.

- **Central neurocytoma.** Central neurocytomas are histologically distinct but similar to oligodendrogliomas. They arise from and have a broad attachment to the septum pellucidum or ventricular wall. Nearly half of cases occur near the foramina of Monro. Peak incidence is between 20 and 40 years of age. Patients may present with ventricular obstruction, visual disturbances, or hormonal changes. Lesions appear as circumscribed, lobulated masses with numerous cysts, often with a "soap bubble" appearance. Solid components are iso- to hyperdense on CT, variable on T1, and heterogeneously hyperintense on T2. There is moderate enhancement. Calcifications are visualized in ≈50% of cases. Surrounding periventricular edema may be seen, especially with larger lesions.

■ Additional Differential Diagnoses

- **Ependymoma/subependymoma.** Although ependymomas are common posterior fossa tumors in children, they may also be supratentorial, either within the ventricles or within the brain parenchyma (more common). Ependymomas are isointense on T1 and hyperintense on T2 with heterogeneous enhancement. Signal intensity varies in the setting of cystic change, calcification, and hemorrhage. Subependymomas occur more frequently in adults within the fourth and lateral ventricles. When located in the lateral ventricles, they may mimic central neurocytomas with a "bubbly" appearance. On MRI, lesions are iso- to hypointense on T1 and hyperintense on T2. Enhancement is variable but typically faint. They commonly calcify, especially in the fourth ventricle.

- **Metastases.** Metastases result from hematogenous spread to the choroid plexus, direct extension from parenchymal or infiltrative tumors (germ cell tumor, lymphoma), or as a result of CSF dissemination. Lateral ventricles are most often involved. The most common adult primary tumors include renal cell and lung carcinomas; melanoma, gastrointestinal tumors, and lymphoma are less common. In children, neuroblastoma, Wilms tumor, and retinoblastoma are most common. Metastatic lesions may be solitary or multiple. They are typically hypointense on T1 and hyperintense on T2 sequences with heterogeneous enhancement, especially with hemorrhage.

■ Diagnosis

Oligodendroglioma

✓ Pearls

- Gliomas of the septum pellucidum are often low grade; SEGAs occur at the foramina of Monro in patients with TS.
- Oligodendrogliomas occur along the septum pellucidum; cystic change and calcification are commonly seen.

- Central neurocytomas have a broad attachment to the septum and a characteristic "bubbly" appearance.

Suggested Reading

Koeller KK, Sandberg GD Armed Forces Institute of Pathology. From the archives of the AFIP. Cerebral intraventricular neoplasms: radiologic-pathologic correlation. Radiographics 2002; 22: 1473–1505

Case 82

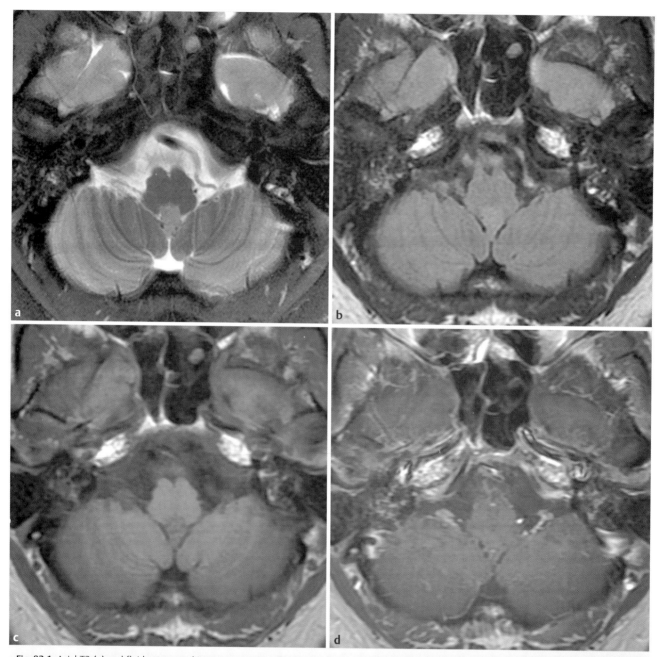

Fig. 82.1 Axial T2 (a) and fluid-attenuated inversion recovery (b) images reveal a lobulated hyperintense mass centered within the inferior aspect of the fourth ventricle. The mass is iso- to hypointense on T1 (c) and does not enhance (d).

▪ Clinical Presentation

A 56-year-old man with chronic headaches (▶ Fig. 82.1)

■ Key Imaging Finding

Fourth ventricle mass in an adult

■ Top 3 Differential Diagnoses

- **Subependymoma.** Subependymomas are relatively uncommon tumors that arise from the subependymal glial layer surrounding the ventricles. The vast majority occur within the fourth and lateral ventricles. Most are small and found incidentally in asymptomatic patients. When large, they may obstruct the fourth ventricle, leading to hydrocephalus. On computed tomography (CT), subependymomas are lobulated and typically iso- to hypodense. Calcification is seen in one-third of cases and cystic change is noted in ~20% of cases. Intratumoral hemorrhage may be seen but is uncommon. Most lesions demonstrate mild, focal enhancement. On magnetic resonance imaging (MRI), lesions are hypointense on T1 and heterogeneously hyperintense on T2 sequences. Enhancement, when present, is mild. Unlike ependymomas, subependymomas typically do not extend through the ventricular outlet foramina.

- **Choroid plexus tumor.** The choroid plexus consists of neuroepithelial tissue and is responsible for cerebrospinal fluid (CSF) production. It can be found within portions of the lateral (majority in the atria), third, and fourth ventricles. Tumors are classified as low-grade choroid plexus papillomas or higher-grade choroid plexus carcinomas. Lateral ventricle tumors occur predominantly in young children; tumors within the fourth ventricle occur more often in adults. Tumors are typically lobular or frondlike in morphology and have a vascular pedicle that attaches to the medullary velum in the fourth ventricle. Lesions are iso- to hyperdense on CT with avid enhancement. Calcification is seen in ≈10% of cases. Extension through outlet foramina into the cerebellopontine angle may be seen. On MRI, lesions are hypointense on T1 and heterogeneously hyperintense on T2 sequences with avid enhancement.

- **Ependymoma.** Ependymoma is a slow-growing, midline posterior fossa tumor of ependymal cells that originates most often along the floor of the fourth ventricle. It characteristically squeezes through the fourth ventricle foramina into the foramen magnum, cerebellopontine angle, or cisterna magna. It is far more common in children, but may also occur in adults. Calcification is seen in ≈50% of cases; cystic change and foci of hemorrhage occur in ≈20%. Two-thirds arise from the fourth ventricle and approximately one-third are supratentorial and may be within the brain parenchyma. The tumor is heterogeneous and iso- to hypointense on T1 and hyperintense on T2 sequences. There is mild to moderate heterogeneous enhancement of the solid components. The entire neuroaxis should be evaluated for CSF dissemination, which occurs in ~5 to 15% of cases.

■ Additional Differential Diagnoses

- **Metastases.** Hematogenous metastases to the choroid plexus are rare. When present, the lateral ventricle is by far the most common site, followed by the third ventricle, and lastly the fourth ventricle. Common primary tumors in adults include lung and renal cell carcinoma; melanoma, lymphoma, and gastrointestinal primaries are less common. In children, neuroblastoma, Wilms tumor, and retinoblastoma represent the most common primaries. Metastatic foci are typically hypodense on CT, hypointense on T1 MRI sequences (except melanoma), hyperintense on T2 sequences, and avidly enhance. The presence of additional parenchymal, extraaxial, or calvarial lesions is a useful discriminator.

- **Meningioma.** Meningiomas represent one of the most common intraventricular tumors in adults; the vast majority occur in the atria of the lateral ventricles. Fourth ventricular involvement, however, is rare. On CT, meningiomas present as circumscribed iso- to hyperdense masses with avid enhancement; calcification is common. Edema may be seen within the adjacent brain parenchyma. When large, there may be obstruction of the fourth ventricle. On MRI, lesions are hypointense on T1 and hyperintense on T2 with avid enhancement.

■ Diagnosis

Subependymoma

✓ Pearls

- Subependymomas occur most often in the fourth ventricle; the majority are asymptomatic and found incidentally.
- In adults, choroid plexus tumors occur in the fourth ventricle; they are lobular in morphology and avidly enhance.
- Ependymomas are more common in children than adults; extension through outlet foramina is characteristic.

Suggested Reading

Koeller KK, Sandberg GD Armed Forces Institute of Pathology. From the archives of the AFIP. Cerebral intraventricular neoplasms: radiologic-pathologic correlation. Radiographics 2002; 22: 1473–1505

Case 83

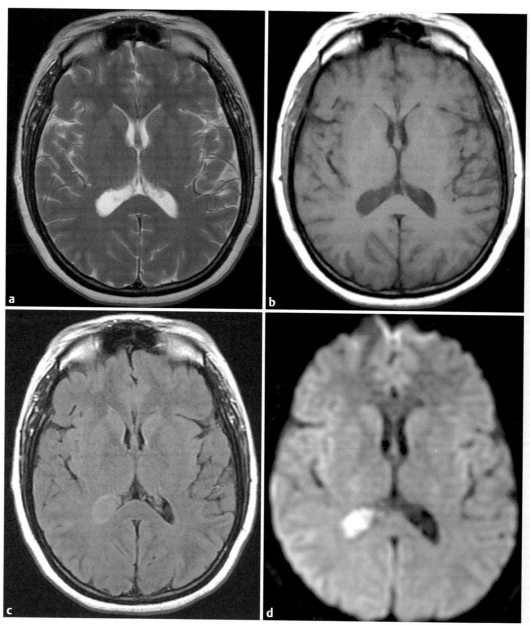

Fig. 83.1 Axial T2 (**a**) and T1 (**b**) images demonstrate a subtle cystic lesion in the atria of the right lateral ventricle. The lesion is isointense to CSF on T2 and iso- to slightly hyperintense on T1. Axial FLAIR (**c**) and DWI (**d**) images show increased signal. A similar lesion (not shown) was noted on the contralateral side.

▪ Clinical Presentation

A 47-year-old woman with headaches (▸ Fig. 83.1)

▨ Key Imaging Finding

Ventricular cyst

▨ Top 3 Differential Diagnoses

- **Choroid plexus cyst.** Choroid plexus cysts represent the most common neuroepithelial cysts. They most often occur within the body of the choroid plexus in the atria of the lateral ventricles. They may be unilocular or multilocular. The vast majority are unilateral, less than 1 cm in size, and asymptomatic. Rarely, there is an increased incidence on prenatal screening in patients with chromosomal abnormalities, particularly trisomy 18, especially when large and bilateral. On computed tomography (CT), choroid plexus cysts are iso- to slightly hyperdense compared with cerebrospinal fluid (CSF). On magnetic resonance imaging (MRI), lesions are iso- to slightly hyperintense on T1 and T2 sequences and isointense (suppress) compared with CSF on fluid-attenuated inversion recovery (FLAIR). Approximately two-thirds of cases show increased signal on diffusion-weighted imaging (DWI). Enhancement of the surrounding choroid plexus is noted, portions of which may appear nodular.

- **Ependymal cyst.** Ependymal cysts are uncommon neuroepithelial cysts that occur along margins of the lateral ventricles. They are thin-walled and contain fluid that is secreted from ependymal cells located within the cyst walls. Lesions vary in size from a few millimeters to several centimeters. The vast majority are asymptomatic and incidental; larger lesions may rarely be symptomatic. On CT and MRI, ependymal cysts are isodense and isointense to CSF, respectively. There is no enhancement.

- **Arachnoid cyst.** Arachnoid cysts are benign CSF collections contained within arachnoid. The vast majority are developmental due to embryonic failure of meningeal fusion; acquired cases have been described in the setting of trauma, infection, or in association with neoplasms. The most common locations include the middle cranial fossa, followed by the posterior fossa. Intraventricular arachnoid cysts are relatively uncommon. The cysts are typically isodense on CT and isointense on MRI compared with CSF. Slight increased signal may be seen on T2 sequences due to lack of normal CSF pulsations. There is no restricted diffusion. The presence of hemorrhage or protein within the cyst will alter the signal characteristics on MRI. Large intraventricular arachnoid cysts may result in obstruction of CSF flow.

▨ Additional Differential Diagnoses

- **Choroid plexus xanthogranuloma (CPX).** CPXs are benign lesions composed of chronic inflammatory debris, as well as cholesterol and lipid-laden macrophages. They are asymptomatic and typically seen bilaterally within the body of the choroid plexus in the atria of the lateral ventricles. Rare cases of CPX within the third ventricle may obstruct CSF flow. On CT, xanthogranulomas are ovoid and iso- to hyperdense compared with CSF. On MRI, lesions are iso- to hyperintense on T1 and T2 sequences and hyperintense on both FLAIR and DWI. Enhancement of surrounding choroid plexus is noted.

▨ Diagnosis

Choroid plexus xanthogranuloma

✓ Pearls

- Choroid plexus cysts are the most common neuroepithelial cysts; the vast majority are incidental.
- Ependymal cysts are relatively uncommon and typically follow CSF signal intensity on MRI sequences.

- Arachnoid cysts most often result from embryonic failure of meningeal fusion; acquired cases are less common.
- Xanthogranulomas are composed of inflammatory debris, as well as cholesterol and lipid-laden macrophages.

Suggested Readings

Naeini RM, Yoo JH, Hunter JV. Spectrum of choroid plexus lesions in children. Am J Roentgenol 2009; 192: 32–40

Osborn AG, Preece MT. Intracranial cysts: radiologic-pathologic correlation and imaging approach. Radiology 2006; 239: 650–664

Case 84

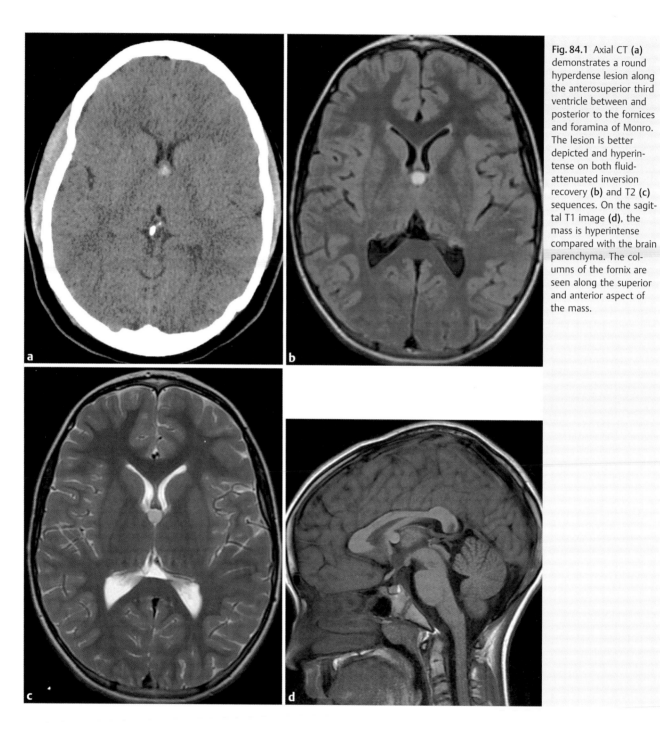

Fig. 84.1 Axial CT (**a**) demonstrates a round hyperdense lesion along the anterosuperior third ventricle between and posterior to the fornices and foramina of Monro. The lesion is better depicted and hyperintense on both fluid-attenuated inversion recovery (**b**) and T2 (**c**) sequences. On the sagittal T1 image (**d**), the mass is hyperintense compared with the brain parenchyma. The columns of the fornix are seen along the superior and anterior aspect of the mass.

■ **Clinical Presentation**

An adolescent girl with episodic headaches (▶ Fig. 84.1)

▩ Key Imaging Finding

Hyperdense/hyperintense, circumscribed mass along the anterosuperior third ventricle

▩ Diagnosis

Colloid cyst. Colloid cysts are benign lesions that originate along the anterosuperior aspect of the third ventricle. Most are incidental; however, they may cause headaches and intermittent acute hydrocephalus as a result of obstruction of the foramina of Monro. Therefore, they are typically treated with surgical resection, aspiration, or cerebrospinal fluid diversion.

The location and imaging appearance are fairly characteristic. Colloid cysts occur between and posterior to the forniceal columns as they pass along the formina of Monro. The internal contents have varying amounts of proteinaceous fluid and viscosity, which account for its imaging appearance. On computed tomography (CT), the lesions are most often hyperdense due to a high protein content and increased viscosity; however, lesions with relatively low protein content will be isodense and may be overlooked. On magnetic resonance imaging, colloid cysts are typically iso- to hyperintense on T1 sequences. The T2 signal is more variable. In general, as the protein content and viscosity increase, the T2 signal decreases. Subtle peripheral enhancement may be seen; however, the lesions themselves should not enhance.

✓ Pearls

- Colloid cysts are benign and originate along the anterosuperior aspect of the third ventricle.
- Colloid cysts may cause intermittent acute hydrocephalus as a result of obstruction of the foramina of Monro.
- Imaging appearance of colloid cysts depends upon the protein content and viscosity of the fluid.
- Colloid cysts are usually hyperdense on CT, iso- to hyperintense on T1, and variable in signal on T2 sequences.

Suggested Reading

Armao D, Castillo M, Chen H, Kwock L. Colloid cyst of the third ventricle: imaging-pathologic correlation. Am J Neuroradiol 2000; 21: 1470–1477

Case 85

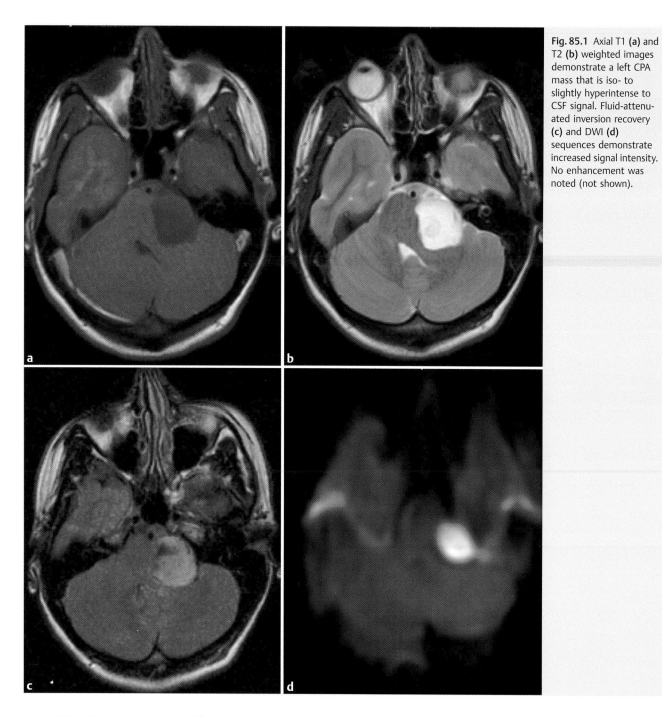

Fig. 85.1 Axial T1 (**a**) and T2 (**b**) weighted images demonstrate a left CPA mass that is iso- to slightly hyperintense to CSF signal. Fluid-attenuated inversion recovery (**c**) and DWI (**d**) sequences demonstrate increased signal intensity. No enhancement was noted (not shown).

▧ Clinical Presentation

A 23-year-old woman with headaches (▶ Fig. 85.1)

■ Key Imaging Finding

Extraaxial mass with signal characteristics similar to cerebrospinal fluid (CSF) and increased signal on diffusion-weighted imaging (DWI)

▨ Diagnosis

Epidermoid. Epidermoids represent congenital ectodermal inclusion cysts lined by stratified squamous epithelium. They are typically incidental and asymptomatic, although symptoms related to mass effect may occasionally be seen. The majority occur in the posterior fossa with the cerebellopontine angle (CPA) and prepontine cistern representing the most common locations, followed by the fourth ventricle. The parasellar region is the most common supratentorial location. Calvarial epidermoids occur in ~10% of cases and most often involve the lateral orbital rim.

On imaging, intracranial epidermoids typically present as well-defined, lobulated masses that insinuate throughout extraaxial CSF spaces and encase rather than displace vascular structures. They follow CSF attenuation on computed tomography and are similar to CSF signal on magnetic resonance imaging with slightly hyperintense fluid-attenuated inversion recovery and T1 signal intensity. There is increased signal intensity on DWI, which is a characteristic imaging feature. Epidermoids do not enhance, although mild peripheral enhancement may occasionally be seen.

✓ Pearls

- Epidermoids are ectodermal inclusion cysts; the CPA and prepontine cistern are the most common locations.
- Epidermoids present as well-defined, lobulated masses that insinuate throughout extraaxial CSF spaces.

- Epidermoids are similar in attenuation and signal to CSF; increased signal on DWI sequences is characteristic.

Suggested Reading

Osborn AG, Preece MT. Intracranial cysts: radiologic-pathologic correlation and imaging approach. Radiology 2006; 239: 650–664

Case 86

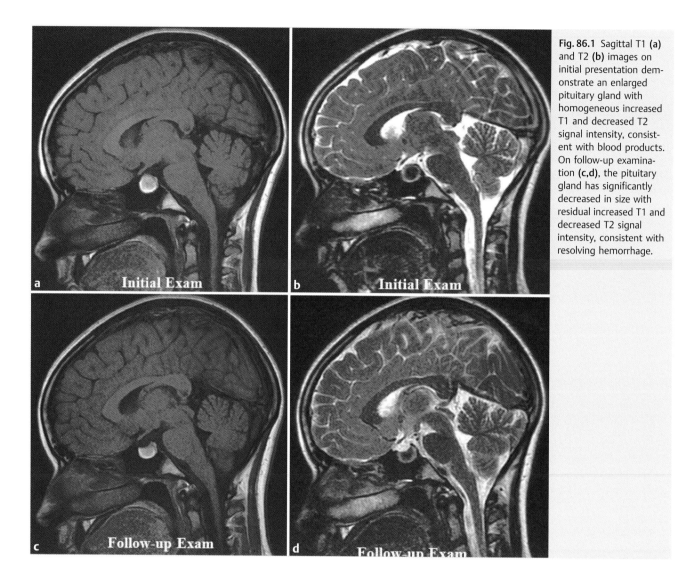

Fig. 86.1 Sagittal T1 **(a)** and T2 **(b)** images on initial presentation demonstrate an enlarged pituitary gland with homogeneous increased T1 and decreased T2 signal intensity, consistent with blood products. On follow-up examination **(c,d)**, the pituitary gland has significantly decreased in size with residual increased T1 and decreased T2 signal intensity, consistent with resolving hemorrhage.

■ Clinical Presentation

A young adult woman with acute onset headache, nausea, and visual disturbances (▶ Fig. 86.1)

■ Key Imaging Finding

Hemorrhage within an enlarged pituitary gland

■ Diagnosis

Pituitary apoplexy. Pituitary apoplexy refers to a clinical syndrome caused by pituitary infarction or hemorrhage, typically within an underlying lesion. Risk factors include pregnancy, trauma, systemic or intracranial hypertension, anticoagulation, and treatment with bromocriptine. Common presenting symptoms include headache (most common); nausea and vomiting; visual disturbances secondary to mass effect of the optic chiasm, nerves, and tracts; altered mental status; and pituitary dysfunction. Noncontrast head computed tomography should be performed acutely to evaluate for intracranial hemorrhage; hyperdensity may be seen within an enlarged pituitary gland in the setting of hemorrhagic apoplexy. Magnetic resonance imaging (MRI) is the modality of choice for detailed evaluation of the sella.

MRI findings in the setting of infarction typically show either an enlarged or normal-sized gland with peripheral enhancement and central necrosis. The central portion varies in signal intensity based upon the protein content of the fluid, as well as the presence or absence of hemorrhage. Pituitary infarct causing apoplexy in a postpartum woman is referred to as Sheehan syndrome and is considered a neurological emergency.

In hemorrhagic pituitary apoplexy, the gland is nearly always enlarged. An underlying lesion is usually present but is difficult to evaluate with superimposed hemorrhage. Common lesions include macroadenomas and Rathke cleft cysts. Although the signal characteristics may vary based upon the age of hemorrhage, the lesions are typically hyperintense on T1 and hypointense on T2 sequences. T2 shading or fluid-fluid levels within the gland are highly characteristic.

The classic teaching regarding treatment in the setting of hemorrhagic apoplexy is that urgent surgical intervention is required to decrease morbidity and mortality. More recently, patients with relatively mild clinical symptoms are being treated conservatively in the acute setting and followed with serial imaging to document hemorrhage resolution.

✓ Pearls

- Pituitary apoplexy refers to a clinical syndrome cause by pituitary infarction or hemorrhage.
- Infarcts present as an enlarged or normal-sized gland with peripheral enhancement and central necrosis.

- With pituitary hemorrhage, the gland is typically enlarged with increased T1 and decreased T2 signal.

Suggested Readings

Kyle CA, Laster RA, Burton EM, Sanford RA. Subacute pituitary apoplexy: MR and CT appearance. J Comput Assist Tomogr 1990; 14: 40–44

Mohr G, Hardy J. Hemorrhage, necrosis, and apoplexy in pituitary adenomas. Surg Neurol 1982; 18: 181–189

Tosaka M, Sato N, Hirato J et al. Assessment of hemorrhage in pituitary macroadenoma by T2*-weighted gradient-echo MR imaging. Am J Neuroradiol 2007; 28: 2023–2029

Case 87

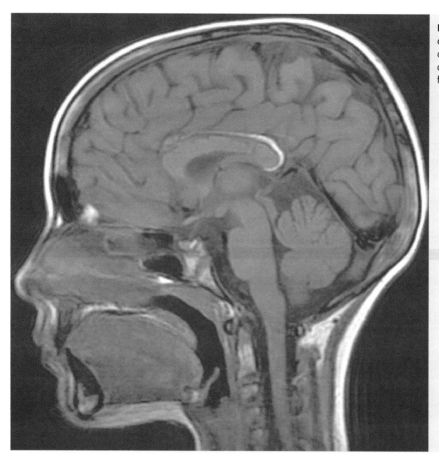

Fig. 87.1 Sagittal T1 midline image reveals a curvilinear hyperintensity along the outer margin of the splenium and posterior body of the corpus callosum. The corpus callosum appears normally formed.

▧ Clinical Presentation

An 8-year-old girl with chronic headaches (▶ Fig. 87.1)

■ Key Imaging Finding

Midline fat signal intensity along the margin of the corpus callosum

■ Diagnosis

Pericallosal lipoma. Intracranial lipomas result from persistence of the meninx primitiva that usually involutes early in gestation. They may occur throughout the central nervous system cisterns, but the vast majority are midline with the pericallosal region being most common. Clinical symptoms are variable, ranging from asymptomatic and incidental to seizures and developmental delay in association with multiple developmental anomalies. The morphology of the lipoma correlates well with patient presentation and associated findings.

Pericallosal lipomas occur in two distinct forms: tubulonodular and curvilinear. The tubulonodular variant is larger (typically > 2 cm) and has a rounded or lobular masslike configuration. It occurs more commonly along the anterior portion of the corpus callosum and has a higher incidence of associated callosal, parenchymal, and craniofacial anomalies. There may be extension into the lateral ventricles and choroid plexus, which is fairly characteristic. The curvilinear form is thin (< 1 cm), typically occurs along the posterior body and splenium of the corpus callosum, and is often incidental. The underlying corpus callosum may be mildly hypoplastic.

On computed tomography, lipomas are characteristically hypodense. Calcifications may be seen, especially with the tubulonodular variant. Lipomas may engulf vessels, so careful evaluation of the adjacent vasculature is important. On magnetic resonance imaging, lipomas follow fat signal with hyperintensity seen on both T1 and T2 sequences. There may be chemical shift artifact along its margins secondary to differences in the resonance frequencies of fat and water in the frequency encoding direction. This results in a band of hyperintensity on one margin and a band of hypointensity along the opposite margin. There should be no enhancement. Calcifications are best seen on gradient echo or susceptibility-weighted sequences. Vascular flow voids may be seen within the lipomas. Fat-suppressed sequences confirm the diagnosis. Interestingly, lipomas may occasionally enlarge secondary to lipomatous hypertrophy, especially during periods of somatic growth.

✓ Pearls

- Intracranial lipomas result from persistence of the meninx primitiva; the vast majority are midline.
- Pericallosal lipomas may be tubulonodular (more often associated with additional anomalies) or curvilinear.

- Lipomas follow fat signal or attenuation; calcifications may be seen, especially with the tubulonodular variant.

Suggested Readings

Ickowitz V, Eurin D, Rypens F et al. Prenatal diagnosis and postnatal follow-up of pericallosal lipoma: report of seven new cases. Am J Neuroradiol 2001; 22: 767–772

Tart RP, Quisling RG. Curvilinear and tubulonodular varieties of lipoma of the corpus callosum: an MR and CT study. J Comput Assist Tomogr 1991; 15: 805–810

Case 88

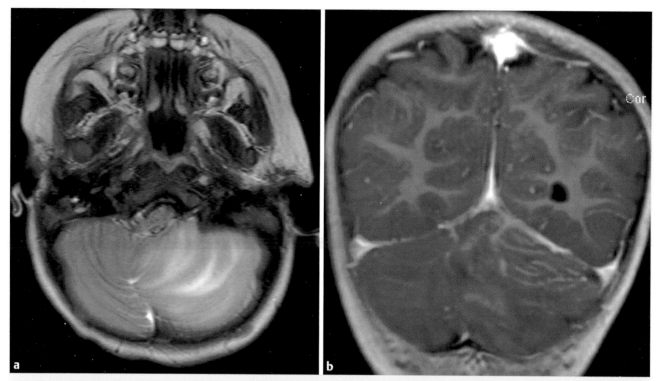

Fig. 88.1 Axial T2 image **(a)** demonstrates thickening of the left cerebellar cortex with regions of increased signal intensity within the underlying white matter, resulting in a striated or "corduroy" appearance. Coronal T1 postcontrast image **(b)** shows a similar striated appearance of the left cerebellar hemisphere secondary to decreased parenchymal signal intensity and enhancement of the overlying leptomeningeal venous structures.

■ **Clinical Presentation**

A young girl with chronic ataxia and gastrointestinal lesions (▶ Fig. 88.1)

▥ Key Imaging Finding

Cerebellar "mass" with a striated or "corduroy" appearance

▥ Diagnosis

Lhermitte-Duclos disease. Lhermitte-Duclos disease (LDD) refers to a dysplastic cerebellar gangliocytoma of uncertain etiology. Controversy exists over classification of this lesion because it may have pathological characteristics of both a hamartoma and a benign neoplasm. It is associated with Cowden syndrome, which is an autosomal dominant syndrome characterized by mucocutaneous lesions and increased incidence of neoplasms involving the gastrointestinal tract, genitourinary tract, breast, and thyroid.

LDD presents most often in young to middle-aged adults. It is also infrequently seen in children. Patients may be asymptomatic or present with ataxia, cranial nerve deficits, or symptoms related to mass effect, including obstructive hydrocephalus. Symptoms are usually insidious in onset.

On computed tomography, LDD presents as a relatively ill-defined region of enlargement and hypoattenuation within the cerebellar hemisphere(s) with mass effect. Calcifications may be seen. Findings on magnetic resonance imaging are more characteristic, demonstrating thickening of the cerebellar folia/cortex and increased T2 signal intensity within the underlying white matter, resulting in a striated or "corduroy" appearance. A similar striated appearance is seen on T1 postcontrast sequences with parenchymal hypoattenuation and enhancement of the overlying leptomeningeal veins. The lesion itself should not enhance. If symptomatic, surgery is the treatment of choice; recurrences have been described.

✓ Pearls

- LDD is a dysplastic cerebellar gangliocytoma; it often has characteristics of both a hamartoma and a neoplasm.
- LDD results in thickening of the cerebellar folia/cortex and underlying increased T2 and decreased T1 signal.

- Signal characteristics result in a "corduroy" appearance on T2 and postcontrast T1 sequences.
- LDD is associated with Cowden syndrome (mucocutaneous lesions and increased incidence of neoplasms).

Suggested Readings

Klisch J, Juengling F, Spreer J et al. Lhermitte-Duclos disease: assessment with MR imaging, positron emission tomography, single-photon emission CT, and MR spectroscopy. Am J Neuroradiol 2001; 22: 824–830

Shinagare AB, Patil NK, Sorte SZ. Case 144: dysplastic cerebellar gangliocytoma (Lhermitte-Duclos disease). Radiology 2009; 251: 298–303

Case 89

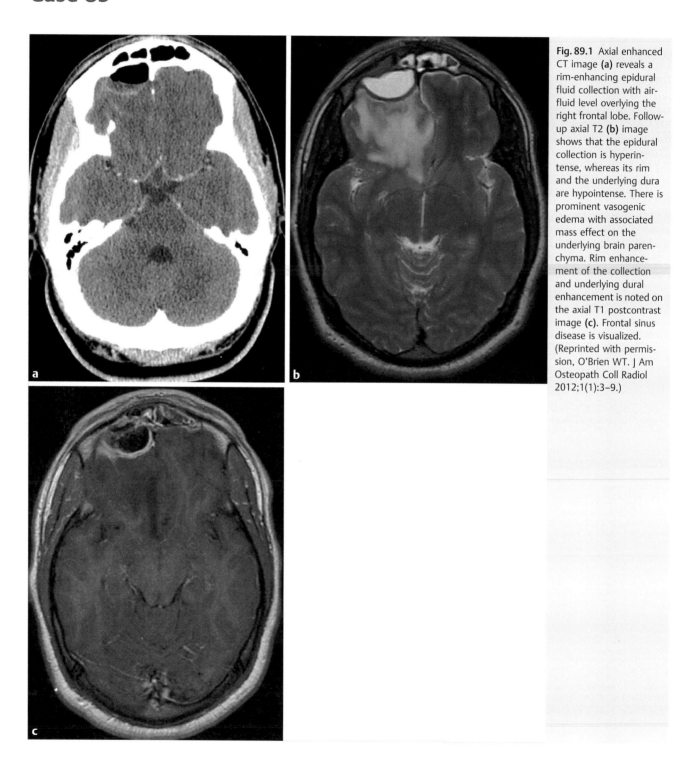

Fig. 89.1 Axial enhanced CT image **(a)** reveals a rim-enhancing epidural fluid collection with air-fluid level overlying the right frontal lobe. Follow-up axial T2 **(b)** image shows that the epidural collection is hyperintense, whereas its rim and the underlying dura are hypointense. There is prominent vasogenic edema with associated mass effect on the underlying brain parenchyma. Rim enhancement of the collection and underlying dural enhancement is noted on the axial T1 postcontrast image **(c)**. Frontal sinus disease is visualized. (Reprinted with permission, O'Brien WT. J Am Osteopath Coll Radiol 2012;1(1):3–9.)

▧ Clinical Presentation

Persistent headaches after upper respiratory infection (▶ Fig. 89.1)

■ **Key Imaging Finding**

Rim-enhancing epidural fluid collection with dural enhancement

■ **Diagnosis**

Epidural abscess. Epidural abscesses most often result from direct spread of paranasal sinus or otomastoid infections or as a result of post-traumatic or postoperative complications. They may also extend from adjacent calvarial processes, such as osteomyelitis. As with other epidural collections, epidural abscesses are biconvex or lenticular in shape, confined by sutures, and may cross midline.

On computed tomography (CT), epidural abscesses are hypodense and may have air-fluid levels. The abscess cavity demonstrates rim enhancement, often thick; enhancement of the underlying dura may also be seen. Similar findings are noted on magnetic resonance imaging (MRI) where the epidural collections are hypointense on T1 and hyperintense on T2 sequences with rim and dural enhancement. The rim of the abscess cavity and of the underlying dura are hypointense on T2 sequences. Foci of air are hypointense on all pulse sequences. The presence of restricted diffusion is variable but typically seen. When adjacent to dural venous sinuses, it is important to look for evidence of sinus thrombosis.

Treatment of epidural abscesses includes a combination of antibiotic therapy and surgical drainage. If left untreated, epidural abscesses may extend through the dura to involve the subdural space, leptomeninges, or brain parenchyma.

✓ **Pearls**

- Epidural abscesses often result from paranasal sinus/mastoid infections or from postoperative complications.
- On CT, epidural abscesses are hypodense, rim-enhancing, and may have air-fluid levels.

- On MRI, epidural abscesses are T2 hyperintense with rim and dural enhancement; restricted diffusion is common.

Suggested Reading

O'Brien WT. Imaging of CNS infections in immunocompetent hosts. J Am Osteopath Coll Radiol. 2012; 1: 3–9

Case 90

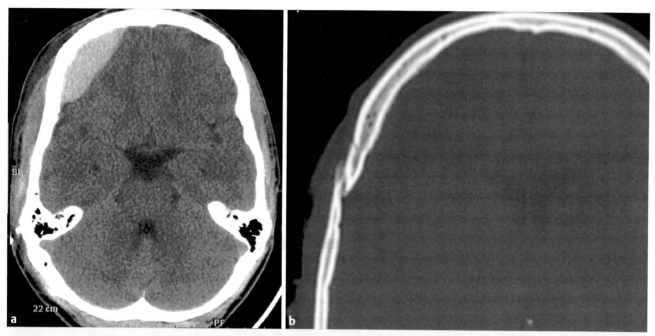

Fig. 90.1 Axial CT image (**a**) reveals a lenticular, biconvex hyperdense extraaxial hemorrhage with mass effect on the underlying right frontal lobe, as well as a superficial scalp hematoma with soft-tissue swelling. The hemorrhage is confined by the coronal suture. Coned-down axial CT image in bone window (**b**) reveals a nondisplaced fracture of the frontal bone (just anterior to the coronal suture) with mild sutural diastasis. An overlying scalp skin laceration with soft-tissue swelling is noted.

■ **Clinical Presentation**

Young adult patient in a motor vehicle crash (▶ Fig. 90.1)

Key Imaging Finding

Biconvex extraaxial hemorrhage confined by sutures

Diagnosis

Epidural hematoma. Epidural hematomas occur in the setting of trauma and appear as biconvex or lenticular regions of extraaxial hemorrhage. The vast majority are supratentorial and unilateral. The most common cause is tearing of the middle meningeal artery (MMA) (~90%) secondary to an adjacent skull fracture. Occasionally, meningeal arterial injury may occur in the absence of calvarial fracture, particularly in children. Because of dural attachments, epidural hematomas may cross midline but are confined by sutures. Rarely, sutural diastasis may allow an epidural process to extend beyond a sutural margin. Venous epidural hematomas are less common (≈10%) and occur more frequently in children or in cases of direct injury to a dural venous sinus. Unlike arterial epidural hematomas, venous epidurals may cross the sagittal suture and the tentorium.

Computed tomography (CT) demonstrates a hyperdense, biconvex or lenticular, epidural collection with mass effect and inward displacement of the underlying brain parenchyma. Midline shift is common. The parietal and temporal lobes are most commonly involved because the MMA courses superficial to these regions. Venous hematomas may be seen near the vertex or within the posterior fossa. Although nonspecific, heterogeneous attenuation within the epidural hematoma is suggestive of active bleeding, especially with a swirling pattern. It is important to evaluate for additional regions of hemorrhage, to include subarachnoid, parenchymal, and contrecoup subdural.

The imaging appearance of epidural hematomas on magnetic resonance imaging (MRI) is variable and dependent upon the stage of hemorrhage. The evolution pattern of hemorrhage

Table 90.1 Evolution of MR signal for intracranial hematomas.

	Hemoglobin State	T1 Signal	T2 Signal
Hyperacute	Oxyhemoglobin	Isointense	Hyperintense
Acute	Deoxyhemoglobin	Isointense	Hypointense
Early Subacute	Methemoglobin (intracellular)	Hyperintense	Hypointense
Late Subacute	Methemoglobin (extracellular)	Hyperintense	Hyperintense
Chronic	Hemosiderin	Hypointense	Hypointense

signal on T1 and T2 sequences for intraparenchymal hematomas is listed in ▶ Table 90.1. Unlike parenchymal hemorrhages, however, the timing of extraaxial hemorrhage stages is not reliable because external factors alter the breakdown of the hemoglobin moiety. Gradient echo and susceptibility-weighted sequences are sensitive for hemorrhage; regions of restricted diffusion may be seen within blood products.

Clinically, patients may experience a lucid interval where they appear neurologically intact despite the presence of an epidural hemorrhage. After the lucid interval, however, some may experience abrupt neurological decline that may be fatal. Larger hemorrhages with neurological deficits or significant mass effect require surgical intervention and evacuation. Smaller regions may be followed both clinically and with imaging.

✓ Pearls

- Epidural hematomas most often result from traumatic tearing of the MMA and are biconvex in shape.
- Venous epidural hematomas are more frequent in children or in cases of direct injury to a dural venous sinus.

- On CT, heterogeneous attenuation suggests active bleeding; MRI appearance is variable.

Suggested Readings

Al-Nakshabandi NA. The swirl sign. Radiology 2001; 218: 433

Provenzale J. CT and MR imaging of acute cranial trauma. Emerg Radiol 2007; 14: 1–12

Case 91

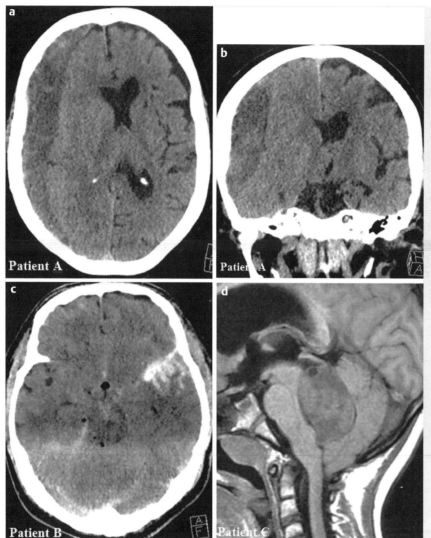

Fig. 91.1 Axial **(a)** and reformatted coronal **(b)** computed tomography (CT) images in Patient A demonstrate a mixed attenuation subdural hemorrhage overlying the right cerebral hemisphere with midline shift to the left and subfalcine herniation. There is compression of the right lateral ventricle and partial entrapment of the left lateral ventricle. Axial CT image in Patient B **(c)** reveals intraparenchymal, subarachnoid (SAH), and subdural (SDH) hemorrhage within and overlying the left temporal lobe; SAH within the interpeduncular fossa and overlying the right frontal lobe; SDH along the falx and interhemispheric fissure; pneumocephalus; diffuse cerebral edema; and bilateral uncal herniation with cisternal effacement and compression of the midbrain. Sagittal T1 magnetic resonance image in patient C, who is a child, **(d)** demonstrates a midline posterior fossa mass with mass effect on the brain stem, inferior displacement of the cerebellar tonsils through the foramen magnum, and obstructive hydrocephalus.

■ Clinical Presentation

Patients A and B are post-trauma; Patient C is a child with headaches and vomiting (▶ Fig. 91.1)

■ Key Imaging Finding

Intracranial mass effect with associated herniations

■ Diagnosis

Brain herniations. Brain herniations occur secondary to mass effect from underlying processes such as neoplasms, hemorrhage, infection, and infarctions. They are most severe in young to middle-aged adults due to the relative increased volume of brain parenchyma and limited potential for accommodation within the intracranial compartment. The presence of open sutures in young children and parenchymal atrophy in elderly adults allows for some degree of accommodation for increases in intracranial pressure. When these factors are overridden, however, brain herniation ensues with parenchyma extending beyond compartmental barriers. There are four basic types of brain herniation: subfalcine, uncal, transtentorial, and tonsillar.

Subfalcine herniation is the most common type and refers to brain parenchyma (typically the cingulate gyrus) extending beneath the rigid, midline falx cerebri. As the degree of herniation increases, there in increased mass effect on the ipsilateral lateral ventricle, which may become compressed or entrapped, and the branches of the anterior cerebral artery (ACA) that course along the interhemispheric fissure. Potential complications of subfalcine herniation include vascular injury or occlusion with ischemic changes in the ACA distributions. Herniations more posteriorly may compress or obstruct deep draining veins.

Uncal herniation refers to inferomedial displacement of the uncus over the tentorium cerebelli and most often results from mass effect within the inferior cerebral hemisphere, particularly the temporal lobe. The herniated uncus becomes situated between the tentorium and the midbrain with effacement of the suprasellar cistern and compression of the ipsilateral cerebral peduncle and oculomotor nerve. Third cranial nerve dysfunction results in a "blown" or dilated pupil; cerebral peduncle compression results in contralateral hemiparesis. Continued mass effect results in compression of the brain stem against the contralateral tentorium, referred to as the Kernohan notch, which may result in hemiparesis on the ipsilateral side of the uncal herniation, complicating clinical localization.

Complications of uncal herniation include compression of the posterior cerebral, superior cerebellar, and anterior choroidal arteries.

The tentorial notch is a confined space that includes the brain stem and surrounding cisterns. Transtentorial herniation refers to superior (ascending) or inferior (descending) displacement of brain parenchyma through the tentorial notch. Descending herniation most often occurs with masses located within the inferior aspect of the cerebral hemisphere. The mass effect causes inferior displacement of the parahippocampal gyrus through the tentorial notch with inferior displacement and compression of the diencephalon and midbrain. Effacement of basilar cisterns is common. As with uncal herniation, there may be compression of the oculomotor nerve, and posterior cerebral, superior cerebellar, and anterior choroidal arteries. Focal regions of pontine hemorrhage due to vascular injury are referred to as Duret hemorrhages. Ascending herniation results from mass effect in the posterior fossa. There is superior displacement of the superior cerebellum and central lobule through the tentorial notch with effacement of the superior vermian cistern; the fourth ventricle is often compressed. With increased herniation, there may be complete effacement of the basilar cisterns of compression of the cerebral aqueduct, resulting in obstructing hydrocephalus. Occlusion of deep venous structures may also occur.

Tonsillar herniation refers to inferior displacement of the cerebellar tonsils through the foramen magnum. It may occur in the setting of Chiari malformations or with posterior fossa mass effect. The tonsillar displacement may result in effacement of cerebrospinal fluid and fourth ventricular outflow obstruction. Severe herniation may cause vascular injury to the posterior inferior cerebellar arteries. It is important to look for the presence of coexistent ascending transtentorial herniation. In the setting of significant tonsillar herniation, lumbar puncture is contraindicated.

✓ Pearls

- Subfalcine herniation is most common and refers to parenchyma extending beneath the rigid, midline falx.
- Uncal herniation refers to inferomedial displacement of the uncus over the tentorium cerebelli.

- Transtentorial herniation refers to superior or inferior displacement of parenchyma through the tentorial notch.
- Tonsillar herniation refers to inferior displacement of the cerebellar tonsils through the foramen magnum.

Suggested Reading

Coburn MW, Rodriguez FJ. Cerebral herniations. Appl Radiol 1998; 27: 10–16

Case 92

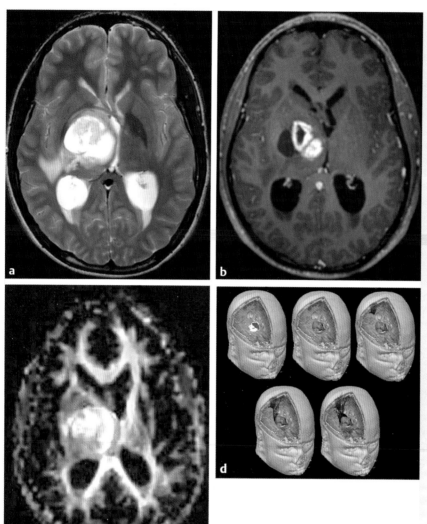

Fig. 92.1 Axial T2 image **(a)** demonstrates a mixed cystic and solid mass centered within the right thalamus, deep white matter, and medial lentiform nuclei with surrounding vasogenic edema. There is mass effect on the right lateral and third ventricles, midline shift to the left, and entrapment of the bilateral atria and occipital horns of the lateral ventricles. T1 postcontrast image with fat suppression **(b)** reveals solid and ring enhancement. Axial color-coded DTI **(c)** shows infiltration and displacement of various deep white matter tracts. Sequential reformatted three-dimensional functional images **(d)** identify the mass with respect to motor tracts for preoperative planning. (Courtesy of James L. Leach, MD.)

■ Clinical Presentation

An adolescent boy with high-grade glioma referred for preoperative planning (▶ Fig. 92.1)

■ Key Imaging Finding

High-grade tumor centered in deep gray and white matter with diffusion tensor imaging and functional imaging

■ Diagnosis

Preoperative tractography. Tractography refers to functional mapping of tracts, fibers, and interconnections within the brain. It has a multitude of applications in various clinical settings, including neurodegenerative, demyelinating, developmental, psychiatric, and neoplastic processes. DTI is the basis for tractography and consists of diffusion-weighted imaging (DWI) with directionality.

DWI is sensitive to the movement of water molecules within a particular voxel. Under normal circumstances, water molecule diffusion within gray matter is isotropic, meaning that water moves equally in all directions. In white matter, however, water molecule motion is anisotropic with movement of water molecules occurring predominantly along the orientation of the white matter tract. The presence of an intact myelin sheath is thought to be the greatest contributor to anisotropy in white matter tracts.

To obtain DTI maps, a certain minimum number of DWI sequences must be obtained: a $b0$ image and DW images with a b value between 700 and 1200 with at least 6 varying motion-probing gradients. In clinical use, 12 or more motion-probing gradients are typically obtained to improve reliability and image quality. Scan times must be short because patient motion will register as increased diffusivity. Tractography connects fiber orientation within adjacent voxels and infers the overall configuration of white matter. The direction of anisotropy, and thus the white matter tract orientation, is often color-coded to best identify specific white matter tracts on postprocessed images. Current and potential uses for tractography are vast, ranging from mapping of normal anatomic tracts for preoperative planning to evaluating focal or widespread white matter disease.

Preoperative tractography is useful in both neoplasm and epilepsy treatment planning. With tumors, tractography may be used to evaluate for white matter infiltration or displacement, as well as to map critical white matter pathways with regards to the tumor location to plan the best surgical approach. Similar benefits are noted in epileptic patients with mapping of critical functional centers and tracts in relation to the seizure focus. Additionally, tractography combined with functional imaging helps identify the locations of language, visual, and motor centers prior to surgical intervention.

✓ Pearls

- Tractography refers to functional mapping of white matter tracts, fibers, and interconnections within the brain.
- Water molecule motion in white matter is anisotropic, occurring along the orientation of the white matter tract.
- Preoperative tractography may help distinguish between tumor infiltration and displacement of white matter.
- Tractography combined with functional imaging helps identify language, visual, and motor centers.

Suggested Reading

Nucifora PGP, Verma R, Lee SK, Melhem ER. Diffusion-tensor MR imaging and tractography: exploring brain microstructure and connectivity. Radiology 2007; 245: 367–384

Case 93

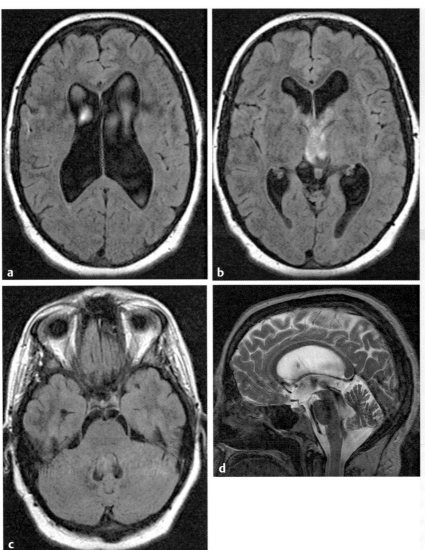

Fig. 93.1 Axial fluid-attenuated inversion recovery images demonstrate enlargement of the lateral **(a)**, third **(b)**, and fourth **(c)** ventricles with hyperdynamic CSF flow signal intensity. Sagittal T2 MR image **(d)** reveals ventriculomegaly with CSF flow voids within the third and fourth ventricles, as well as through the cerebral aqueduct and fourth ventricular outlet foramina. A ventricular drainage catheter is partially visualized within the lateral ventricle.

■ Clinical Presentation

Adult woman with cognitive impairment and ataxia (▶ Fig. 93.1)

■ Key Imaging Finding

Ventriculomegaly in an adult

■ Top 3 Differential Diagnoses

• **Central atrophy.** Atrophy refers to parenchymal volume loss secondary to a variety of conditions, including age-related changes, ischemic disease, infectious or inflammatory processes, trauma, demyelinating disease, and treatment-related changes (radiation and/or chemotherapy). When parenchymal volume loss occurs, the cerebrospinal fluid (CSF) spaces expand to fill the intracranial space. Depending upon the etiology and location, the volume loss may be diffuse or focal and characterized as central and/or cortical. Central atrophy is more pronounced with injury to the periventricular white matter and deep gray matter, as is commonly seen with microvascular ischemic disease. With most diffuse processes, there is typically proportional cortical atrophy as well. Focal injury with encephalomalacia results in regional expansion of the adjacent ventricle and overlying extraaxial CSF spaces.

• **Hydrocephalus.** Hydrocephalus is characterized as communicating or noncommunicating. Patients often present with headache, nausea, and vomiting. Communicating (extraventricular obstructive) hydrocephalus results from impaired CSF resorption, typically due to prior hemorrhage, infection, or neoplasm. On computed tomography (CT) and magnetic resonance imaging (MRI), the lateral, third, and fourth ventricles are proportionally enlarged. In adults, basilar cisterns may be normal or effaced. In infants and young children, there may be enlargement of the extraaxial CSF and macrocephaly. Noncommunicating (intraventricular obstructive) hydrocephalus refers to obstruction proximal to the fourth ventricular outlet foramina. There is enlargement of the ventricles proximal to the level of obstruction; distally, the ventricles may be normal

or relatively small in size. Common locations of obstruction include the foramina of Monro, cerebral aqueduct, and posterior fossa. Acute, uncompensated hydrocephalus results in transependymal flow of CSF, which manifests as a rind of signal abnormality along the ventricular margins.

• **Normal pressure hydrocephalus (NPH).** NPH is characterized by disproportionate enlargement of the ventricles compared with the sulci and overlying extraaxial CSF spaces. It affects elderly patients who present with varying degrees of dementia, ataxia, and/or incontinence. Approximately half of cases are idiopathic; the remainder occur in patients who typically have a history of intracranial hemorrhage or infection. Although the exact pathophysiology of NPH remains unclear, it is thought to result from impaired CSF resorption. On CT, NPH presents as ventriculomegaly that is disproportionate to the extraaxial CSF spaces. In some cases, there may be mild transependymal flow of CSF. MRI demonstrates similar findings, as well hyperdynamic CSF flow that manifests as a prominent flow void through an enlarged cerebral aqueduct, best visualized on sagittal T2 and cine sequences. Age-related microvascular ischemic disease is commonly seen. An indium CSF study may be useful, as the findings are characteristic. After 24 to 48 hours, patients with NPH demonstrate reflux of radiopharmaceutical into the ventricles and absence of activity over the cerebral convexities. Treatment consists of a therapeutic lumbar puncture or placement of a lumbar drain. Approximately one-third of patients will show clinical improvement, especially in cases treated early and when ataxia is the prominent clinical finding.

■ Additional Differential Diagnoses

• **Dementia complex.** Common dementia complexes include Alzheimer disease (AD), frontotemporal dementia (FTD), and multi-infarct dementia (MID). All result in parenchymal volume loss; occasionally, characteristic patterns of atrophy suggest the correct diagnosis. AD is the most common dementia complex and presents with disproportionate cortical atrophy of the parietal and temporal lobes, as well as hippocampal

atrophy. FTD results in disproportionate atrophy of the frontal and temporal lobes with somewhat characteristic tapered or knife-like gyri. MID presents with relatively diffuse volume loss and multiple prior lacunar and cortical infarcts. Positron emission tomography imaging demonstrates decreased metabolism that corresponds to the regions of preferential atrophy.

■ Diagnosis

Normal pressure hydrocephalus

✓ Pearls

• Hydrocephalus may be communicating (decreased CSF resorption) or noncommunicating (obstructive).
• NPH presents in the elderly with dementia, ataxia, and incontinence, as well as disproportionate ventriculomegaly.

• Dementia complexes are associated with parenchymal atrophy; the pattern of atrophy may suggest the etiology.

Suggested Reading

Kiefer M, Unterberg A. The differential diagnosis and treatment of normal-pressure hydrocephalus. Dtsch Arztebl Int 2012; 109: 15–25, quiz 26

Case 94

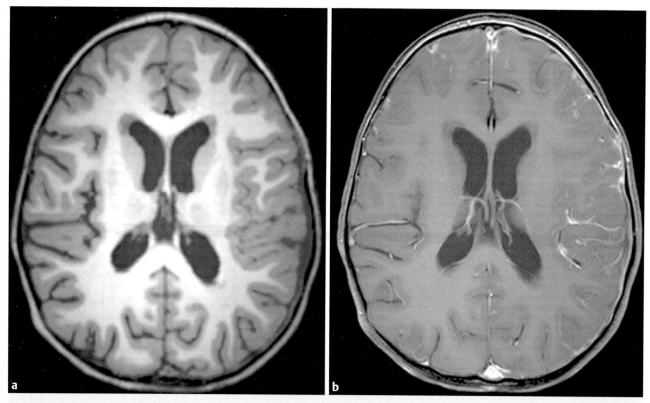

Fig. 94.1 Axial T1 pre- **(a)** and postcontrast **(b)** images reveal nodular leptomeningeal enhancement involving the left more than than right frontal and left temporal lobes. There is a small, left temporal subdural collection. Hypointensity adjacent to the frontal horns of the lateral ventricles corresponds to regions of gliosis. (Reprinted with permission, O'Brien WT. J Am Osteopath Coll Radiol 2012;1[1]:3–9.)

Clinical Presentation

A young girl with headache, altered mental status, and neck/back pain (▶ Fig. 94.1)

▓ Key Imaging Finding

Leptomeningeal enhancement

▓ Top 3 Differential Diagnoses

- **Meningitis.** Meningitis is an inflammatory infiltration of the pia, arachnoid, and cerebrospinal fluid most often due to hematogenous dissemination of a distant infection. Lumbar puncture is the most sensitive test, revealing increased white blood cells and protein with decreased glucose. The exact values vary based upon the etiology of infection (most often viral or bacterial). Magnetic resonance imaging (MRI) may show hyperintense fluid-attenuated inversion recovery (FLAIR) signal and enhancement of the subarachnoid space from the exudative inflammatory process. Potential complications include hydrocephalus, ventriculitis, cerebral abscesses, empyema, infarction, and venous thrombosis.
- **Leptomeningeal carcinomatosis.** Leptomeningeal carcinomatosis may be caused by hematogenous spread of malignancy (most commonly lung and breast), CSF dissemination of a central nervous system (CNS) primary tumor, secondary lymphoma, or direct extension by a CNS primary tumor. MRI is the most sensitive imaging modality; lumbar puncture demonstrates tumor cells on cytological examination. Overall sensitivity is increased when both procedures are performed. Postcontrast MRI sequences show smooth or nodular leptomeningeal enhancement, which may be focal or diffuse. The ependymal surfaces of the ventricles and cranial nerves may be coated. Hyperintense FLAIR signal within the subarachnoid space may be seen. Communicating hydrocephalous is a potential complication from interference with CSF resorption. CT is relatively insensitive for detection of leptomeningeal disease, but will show hydrocephalus as an early sign. The presence of additional parenchymal or calvarial metastatic foci is a useful discriminator.

- **Neurosarcoidosis.** Sarcoidosis is a systemic inflammatory granulomatous (noncaseating) disease with a peak onset in the third and fourth decades of life. Symptomatic CNS involvement is relatively uncommon (~5 of cases) and most often presents with smooth or nodular dural and/or leptomeningeal enhancement, especially along the basal cisterns. There is often involvement of the optic chiasm, hypothalamus, infundibulum, internal auditory canals, and cranial nerves at the skull base. Perivascular and ependymal enhancement may be seen. Brain parenchyma can also be involved in one-third of patients with the hypothalamus most often involved, followed by the brain stem and cerebral or cerebellar hemispheres. Hydrocephalus is a potential complication. If not already obtained, look for lymphadenopathy with or without interstitial lung disease on chest X-ray or CT.

▓ Additional Differential Diagnoses

- **Collateral vascular flow.** The leptomeningeal vasculature is an important source of collateral flow in the setting of proximal arterial stenosis or occlusion. Given the relatively slow flow seen in collateral vessels, leptomeningeal enhancement is noted on postcontrast imaging. Common etiologies of proximal stenoses include atherosclerosis, primary or secondary moyamoya, and vasculitis. On imaging, the appearance of leptomeningeal vascular enhancement has been referred to as the "climbing ivy" sign.

- **Subacute infarction.** Contrast-enhanced CT or MRI of a subacute infarction can show gyriform parenchymal enhancement and swelling of the cerebral or cerebellar cortex within a vascular distribution. In addition, there is often overlying leptomeningeal enhancement, representing collateral flow. Remember the "2–2–2" rule: gyriform enhancement begins as early as 2 days, peaks at 2 weeks, and typically resolves by 2 months.

▓ Diagnosis

Meningitis

✓ Pearls

- Meningitis results from hematogenous spread of infection; leptomeningeal enhancement is commonly seen.
- Leptomeningeal carcinomatosis may be due to distant metastases, direct extension, or CSF dissemination.

- Neurosarcoidosis presents with leptomeningeal enhancement, most often along the basal cisterns.
- Leptomeningeal collateral flow due to a proximal stenosis or occlusion is described as the "climbing ivy" sign.

Suggested Readings

Phillips ME, Ryals TJ, Kambhu SA, Yuh WT. Neoplastic vs inflammatory meningeal enhancement with Gd-DTPA. J Comput Assist Tomogr 1990; 14: 536–541

Smirniotopoulos JG, Murphy FM, Rushing EJ, Rees JH, Schroeder JW. Patterns of contrast enhancement in the brain and meninges. Radiographics 2007; 27: 525–551

Case 95

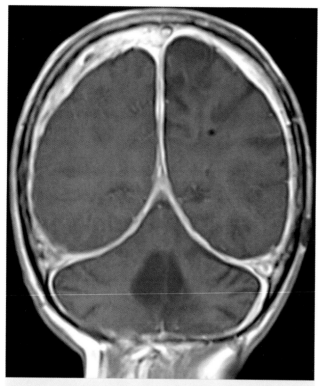

Fig. 95.1 Coronal T1 postcontrast image reveals abnormal, diffuse dural thickening and enhancement. Enlargement of the fourth ventricle is partially seen.

▓ Clinical Presentation

A young patient with headaches (▶ Fig. 95.1)

■ Key Imaging Finding

Pachymeningeal/dural enhancement

■ Top 3 Differential Diagnoses

- **Intracranial hypotension.** Intracranial hypotension results from decreased intracranial pressure due to a cerebrospinal fluid leak (CSF). Common etiologies include trauma, iatrogenia (lumbar puncture or postoperative), and idiopathic or spontaneous CSF leaks. Patients present clinically with orthostatic headaches. Classic imaging findings include diffuse pachymeningeal (dural) enhancement and caudal displacement of the cerebellar tonsils ("sagging brain" appearance). The presence of dural thickening, subdural fluid collections, venous engorgement/distention, and pituitary hyperemia may also be seen. If the site of the CSF leak is unknown, computed tomography (CT), magnetic resonance imaging (MRI), or radionuclide cisternography may be useful in determining the origin of the leak. Conservative therapies (bed rest, hydration, and caffeine) and epidural blood patches are the most common first-line treatments.
- **Metastases.** Metastatic disease commonly affects the pachymeninges/dura either from hematogenous spread or direct extension from calvarial lesions. Breast, lung, and prostate carcinoma are the most common primary neoplasms; hematologic malignancies, such as lymphoma and leukemia, may also demonstrate abnormal dural enhancement. The regions of abnormal enhancement may be smooth or nodular and focal or diffuse. Although dural lesions are often asymptomatic (depending on location), cranial neuropathies are common with skull-base involvement.
- **Pachymeningitis.** Meningeal infection may be due to bacterial, viral, or fungal etiology. The diagnosis is made clinically with CSF sampling; imaging is useful to evaluate for suspected complications. Meningeal enhancement is only evident in ~50% of patients with meningitis and commonly involves both the leptomeninges and pachymeninges. *Mycobacterium tuberculosis* (TB) classically results in meningeal disease involving the skull base, cerebritis, and intracranial abscess formation (tuberculoma); isolated TB pachymeningitis with associated enhancement has been described in immunocompromised patients.

■ Additional Differential Diagnoses

- **Sarcoidosis.** Approximately 5% of sarcoid patients develop symptomatic central nervous system involvement. Neurosarcoidosis most often presents with smooth or nodular dural and/or leptomeningeal enhancement, especially along the basal cisterns. There is often involvement of the optic chiasm, hypothalamus, infundibulum, internal auditory canals, and cranial nerves at the skull base. Brain parenchyma can also be involved in one-third of patients.
- **Subdural hemorrhage.** Subdural hemorrhage typically results from tearing of bridging veins and is most often due to trauma. In contrast to epidural hemorrhage, subdural collections may cross sutures but cannot cross midline. The blood products within the hemorrhage vary in attenuation (CT) and signal intensity (MRI) based upon the age of hemorrhage, as well as additional factors. Hyperdense or T1 hyperintense blood products may mimic dural enhancement. Also, blood products are a source of meningeal irritation, which may manifest as true meningeal enhancement on CT or MRI. Patients often have an antecedent history of trauma.

■ Diagnosis

Pachymeningeal carcinomatosis

✓ Pearls

- Intracranial hypotension results from a CSF leak; findings include dural enhancement and tonsillar ectopia.
- Dural-based metastases may result from hematogenous spread or direct spread from calvarial lesions.
- Common imaging findings of meningitis include leptomeningeal and/or pachymeningeal (dural) enhancement.
- Neurosarcoidosis often results in nodular meningeal enhancement; cranial neuropathies are common.

Suggested Readings

Castillo M. Imaging of meningitis. Semin Roentgenol 2004; 39: 458–464

Goyal M, Sharma A, Mishra NK, Gaikwad SB, Sharma MC. Imaging appearance of pachymeningeal tuberculosis. Am J Roentgenol 1997; 169: 1421–1424

Schievink WI, Maya MM, Louy C, Moser FG, Tourje J. Diagnostic criteria for spontaneous spinal CSF leaks and intracranial hypotension. Am J Neuroradiol 2008; 29: 853–856

Smirniotopoulos JG, Murphy FM, Rushing EJ, Rees JH, Schroeder JW. Patterns of contrast enhancement in the brain and meninges. Radiographics 2007; 27: 525–551

Case 96

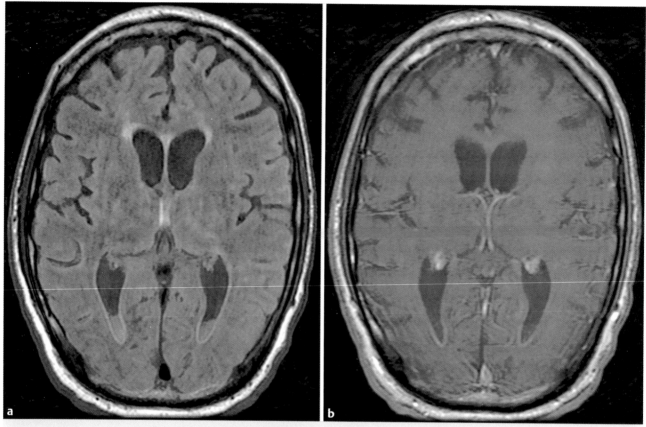

Fig. 96.1 Axial FLAIR MR image (**a**) demonstrates hyperintense signal layering in the dependent portions of the occipital horns of the lateral ventricles, along the ependymal surfaces bilaterally, and within the bilateral deep gray and white matter. Axial T1 postcontrast image (**b**) shows symmetric, abnormal ependymal enhancement posteriorly. There is disproportionate parenchymal volume loss for age.

Clinical Presentation

A 42-year-old immunocompromised man with headache, nausea, and vomiting (▶ Fig. 96.1)

■ Key Imaging Finding

Layering intraventricular debris

■ Top 3 Differential Diagnoses

- **Ventriculitis/Ependymitis.** Ventricular or ependymal spread of infection may occur from hematogenous spread to the choroid plexus or direct extension from a parenchymal infection, such as intraventricular rupture of a periventricular abscess. Immunocompromised patients and those with intraventricular drainage catheters are more prone to intraventricular infections. Cytomegalovirus, toxoplasmosis, and tuberculosis are common causative agents in immunosuppressed patients. Magnetic resonance imaging (MRI) demonstrates increased T2/fluid-attenuated inversion recovery (FLAIR) signal along the ventricular margin and avid, thin ependymal enhancement. There is often layering-dependent debris, which may demonstrate restricted diffusion in the setting of pyogenic infection. Short- and long-term complications include hydrocephalus, which is most often communicating. Periventricular extension may result in toxic or ischemic parenchymal injury.

- **Hemorrhage.** Intraventricular hemorrhage in adults most often results from reflux of subarachnoid hemorrhage (SAH) into the ventricular system (ruptured aneurysm or trauma) or intraventricular extension of a parenchymal hemorrhage. Parenchymal hemorrhages prone to intraventricular extension include hypertensive hemorrhages (most often in the basal ganglia or thalami), post-traumatic hemorrhage, rupture of a vascular malformation, or hemorrhage associated with a deep parenchymal neoplasm. Hemorrhage from a primary intraventricular neoplasm is less common. In premature infants, intraventricular hemorrhage may be seen in association with germinal matrix hemorrhage. Acute hemorrhage is hyperdense on computed tomography (CT). In the subacute phase, hemorrhage becomes isodense compared with brain parenchyma. Chronic hemorrhage is hypodense. The MRI signal intensity depends upon the stage of hemorrhage and evolution of blood products; the MRI appearance and evolution of intraventricular hemorrhage is less predictable compared with intraparenchymal hemorrhage. FLAIR and gradient echo or susceptibility-weighted sequences are the most sensitive for identifying blood products. In hospitalized patients, hemorrhagic blood products will layer within the dependent portions of the ventricles, particularly the occipital horns of the lateral ventricles. Communicating hydrocephalus may occur secondary to interference with cerebrospinal fluid (CSF) resorption.

- **Carcinomatosis.** Intraventricular carcinomatosis may result from intraventricular extension of a parenchymal tumor, CSF seeding, or hematogenous spread of a distant neoplasm to the choroid plexus. Primary central nervous system lymphoma and high-grade gliomas have a propensity for deep parenchymal involvement and intraventricular extension. Common tumors to result in CSF seeding include medulloblastoma, ependymoma, germ cell tumors, pineal cell tumors, and choroid plexus tumors. CSF seeding may be present at the time of initial diagnosis or present as a recurrence following therapy. Lung and breast carcinomas are the most common primary tumors in adults that may spread to the choroid plexus; the presence of additional parenchymal or calvarial lesions is often seen and is a useful discriminator. Intraventricular carcinomatosis most often presents as regions of irregular or nodular enhancement. In the setting of a periventricular tumor, there is often continuity with the primary neoplasm. Tumor cells may interfere with resorption of CSF, resulting in a communicating hydrocephalus.

■ Diagnosis

Ventriculitis

✓ Pearls

- Ventriculitis is more common in immunosuppressed patients; there is enhancement and layering debris.
- Intraventricular hemorrhage most often results from reflux of SAH or extension of parenchymal hemorrhage.
- In hospitalized patients, infectious debris and blood products layer in the dependent portions of the ventricles.
- Intraventricular carcinomatosis most often presents as regions of irregular or nodular enhancement.

Suggested Reading

Smirniotopoulos JG, Murphy FM, Rushing EJ, Rees JH, Schroeder JW. Patterns of contrast enhancement in the brain and meninges. Radiographics 2007; 27: 525–551

Case 97

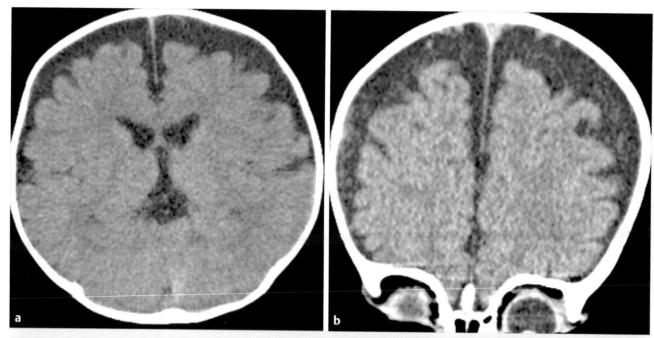

Fig. 97.1 Axial CT image **(a)** demonstrates symmetric extraaxial CSF-attenuation fluid collections overlying the frontal lobes. Reformatted coronal CT image **(b)** reveals the bifrontal extraaxial collection with vessels traversing through the fluid, indicating enlargement of the subarachnoid space rather than subdural collections.

■ Clinical Presentation

An 8-month-old boy with enlarged head circumference (▶ Fig. 97.1)

■ Key Imaging Finding

Enlarged extraaxial cerebrospinal fluid (CSF) spaces in an infant

■ Top 3 Differential Diagnoses

- **Benign macrocrania.** Benign macrocrania is characterized by idiopathic enlargement of the subarachnoid spaces in an infant with an enlarged head and normal neurological development. Patients typically present within the first year of life after macrocrania is noted on a well-baby visit. Oftentimes, there is a family history of macrocrania. The condition is self-limited and typically resolves by 24 months of age. The enlarged spaces may predispose the patient to subdural hemorrhage from trauma due to stretching of cortical bridging veins; however, this remains controversial. Computed tomography (CT) or magnetic resonance imaging (MRI) demonstrates enlargement of the subarachnoid spaces, most prominent over the frontal lobes. Ventricles are typically normal to slightly enlarged. The presence of bridging cortical veins within the extraaxial CSF confirms subarachnoid (and not subdural) location. Patients are followed clinically; follow-up imaging is not required in the setting of normal neurological development.

- **Communicating hydrocephalus.** Hydrocephalus is characterized as communicating or noncommunicating. Communicating hydrocephalus (extraventricular obstructive hydrocephalus) results from impaired CSF resorption, typically due to prior

hemorrhage, infection, or neoplasm. Patients often present with symptoms related to increased intracranial pressure, including nausea and vomiting. On CT and MRI, the lateral, third, and fourth ventricles are proportionally enlarged. In infants and young children, there may be enlargement of the extraaxial CSF and macrocephaly. Acute, uncompensated hydrocephalus results in transependymal flow of CSF, which manifests as a rind of signal abnormality along the margins of the ventricles.

- **Parenchymal injury/atrophy.** Parenchymal atrophy results from some form of insult. Common etiologies include ischemia, infectious or inflammatory insult, and hemorrhage. Parenchymal atrophy results in diffuse or focal enlargement of the extraaxial CSF spaces depending upon the nature and extent of the inciting event. Because parenchymal development affects calvarial development, patients often have a normal or decreased head circumference, which is a discriminating feature. Also, patients often suffer from neurological impairment or developmental delay. CT and MRI reveal decreased parenchymal volume with compensatory enlargement of the subarachnoid spaces. Regions of encephalomalacia and delayed or dysmyelination are commonly seen.

■ Additional Differential Diagnoses

- **Subdural collections.** Subdural collections may cross sutures but not extend beyond midline unless located within the posterior fossa. On CT, it may be difficult to differentiate enlarged subarachnoid spaces from subdural collections; MRI readily distinguishes between the two. The key imaging distinction is the presence or absence of cortical bridging veins within the fluid collection. With enlarged subarachnoid spaces, the bridging veins extend through the CSF; with subdural collec-

tions, the subarachnoid space (and bridging veins) is displaced inward against the brain parenchyma. Common etiologies of subdural collections include subdural hemorrhage (accidental or nonaccidental trauma), empyemas (infectious subdural collection), hygromas (CSF collections in the subdural space), and effusions (typically seen in children with *Haemophilus influenza* meningitis).

■ Diagnosis

Benign macrocrania

✓ Pearls

- Benign macrocrania is a self-limiting condition in infants with normal neurological development.
- Communicating hydrocephalus results in increased intracranial pressure and developmental delay.

- Parenchymal atrophy results in a normal or decreased head circumference, often with developmental delay.
- Subdural collections displace the subarachnoid space (and bridging veins) inward against brain parenchyma.

Suggested Readings

Wilms G, Vanderschueren G, Demaerel PH et al. CT and MR in infants with pericerebral collections and macrocephaly: benign enlargement of the subarachnoid spaces versus subdural collections. Am J Neuroradiol 1993; 14: 855–860

Zahl SM, Egge A, Helseth E, Wester K. Benign external hydrocephalus: a review, with emphasis on management. Neurosurg Rev 2011; 34: 417–432

Case 98

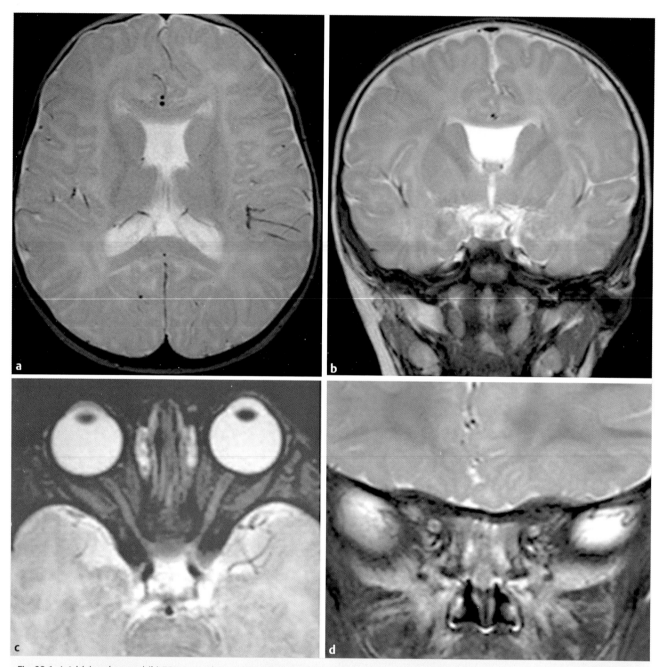

Fig. 98.1 Axial **(a)** and coronal **(b)** T2 images demonstrate absence of the septum pellucidum with characteristic flattening of the roof of the frontal horns of the lateral ventricles on the coronal image. Coned-down axial **(c)** and coronal **(d)** T2 images reveal bilateral optic nerve hypoplasia.

■ **Clinical Presentation**

Young girl with pituitary insufficiency (▶ Fig. 98.1)

■ Key Imaging Finding

Absent septum pellucidum

■ Top 3 Differential Diagnoses

- **Septo-optic dysplasia (SOD).** SOD, also known as de Morsier syndrome, is characterized by absence or hypoplasia of the septum pellucidum, hypoplastic optic nerves and chiasm, and hypothalamic-pituitary dysfunction with hypoplasia of the pituitary gland and occasionally an ectopic posterior pituitary. Some authors consider SOD as a mild form of holoprosencephaly; unlike classic forms of holoprosencephaly, however, the falx is intact. On magnetic resonance imaging, there is absence of the septum pellucidum with characteristic squaring of the frontal horns of the lateral ventricles on coronal sequences. The optic nerves and chiasm are hypoplastic; optic nerve involvement may be unilateral or asymmetric. The pituitary gland may be small. An ectopic posterior pituitary presents as a T1 hyperintensity (bright spot) at the base of the hypothalamus or along the infundibulum. Approximately 50% of cases of SOD will have associated schizencephaly, which is a cerebrospinal fluid–lined cleft that communicates with the ventricles and is lined by dysplastic gray matter.
- **Holoprosencephaly.** Holoprosencephaly is a spectrum of congenital forebrain malformations characterized as alobar, semilobar, and lobar variants. The lobar form is the least severe and is typically characterized by incomplete formation of the falx, absence of the septum pellucidum, partially fused thalami, and near-complete separation of the lateral ventricles. The cerebral hemispheres are essential normal. The alobar form is the most severe form and is characterized by absence of the single midline structures, to include the corpus callosum, anterior falx, and interhemispheric fissure; absent Sylvian fissures; fusion/failure of separation of the anterior cerebral hemispheres; fused thalami; and a large dorsal monoventricle/interhemispheric cyst. The semilobar form is the most variable form with abnormalities somewhere between lobar and alobar variants. It is typically characterized by absence of the septum pellucidum, partial formation of the falx and interhemispheric fissure, absence of the anterior portion of the corpus callosum (a relatively specific finding), and fused thalami and basal ganglia. An azygous anterior cerebral artery is commonly seen. Craniofacial abnormalities associated with alobar and severe semilobar variants include hypotelorism, fused metopic suture, and cleft palate.
- **Septal injury.** Absence of the septum pellucidum may occasionally result from septal injury. The most common etiologies are iatrogenic after instrumentation through the septum pellucidum or in the setting of pressure erosion. Pressure erosion may be seen with long-standing hydrocephalus or, less commonly, secondary to adjacent masses. Appropriate history and visualization of postoperative changes are helpful, as is absence of secondary findings commonly seen with SOD and holoprosencephaly.

■ Diagnosis

Septo-optic dysplasia

✓ Pearls

- SOD is characterized by absence of the septum pellucidum, hypoplastic optic nerves, and pituitary dysfunction.
- Approximately 50% of cases of SOD will have associated schizencephaly.
- Holoprosencephaly is a spectrum of forebrain malformations characterized as alobar, semilobar, and lobar.
- Absence of the septum pellucidum may occasionally result from septal injury, in hydrocephalus or postoperative.

Suggested Reading

Barkovich AJ, Norman D. Absence of the septum pellucidum: a useful sign in the diagnosis of congenital brain malformations. Am J Roentgenol 1989; 152: 353–360

Case 99

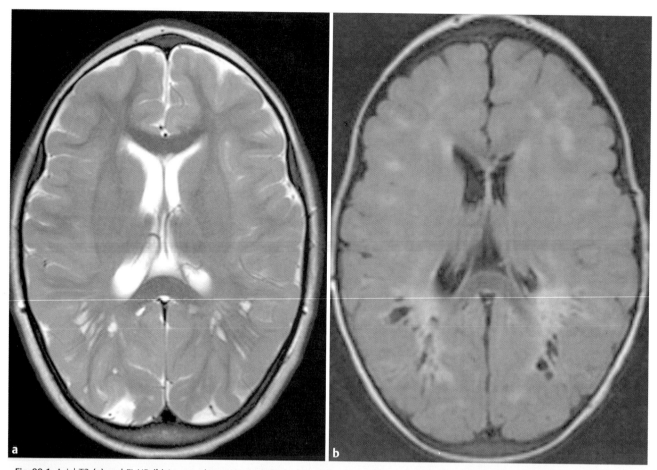

Fig. 99.1 Axial T2 **(a)** and FLAIR **(b)** images demonstrate multiple, bilateral enlarged perivascular spaces in the periatrial white matter. There is surrounding increased FLAIR signal intensity, as well as additional foci of subcortical FLAIR signal abnormality involving the cerebral hemispheres.

■ Clinical Presentation

An early adolescent girl with developmental and motor delay (▶ Fig. 99.1)

Key Imaging Finding

Enlarged perivascular spaces

Top 3 Differential Diagnoses

- **Virchow-Robin (VR) spaces.** VR spaces are pial-lined perivascular (PV) spaces that surround perforating arteries as they extend from the subarachnoid space into the brain parenchyma. They occur in characteristic locations, including the deep gray and white matter (inferior one-third of the basal ganglia and anterior perforated substance); along the course of the medullary veins, most pronounced in the periatrial regions; and within the midbrain. VR spaces are typically 2 to 5 mm in size; giant VR spaces are > 1.5 cm. They follow cerebrospinal fluid (CSF) signal on all magnetic resonance imaging sequences; atypical PV spaces have minimal surrounding fluid-attenuated inversion recovery (FLAIR) signal.
- **Ischemia.** Lacunar infarcts are small areas of encephalomalacia that result from occlusion of perforating vessels. Characteristic locations include the basal ganglia (upper two-thirds), thalami, internal and external capsules, periventricular white matter, and pons. Acutely, lacunar infarcts are hyperintense on T2/FLAIR and demonstrate restricted diffusion. In the subacute phase, enhancement may be seen. Chronic lacunes follow CSF signal intensity with variable surrounding FLAIR hyperintensity/gliosis. Lacunar infarcts are most commonly seen in elderly patients with associated small-vessel ischemic changes within the periventricular and subcortical white matter. In neonates, prenatal or perinatal hypoxemia/ischemia results in periventricular leukomalacia (PVL), which is characterized by abnormal, increased T2 signal intensity and volume loss within the periatrial white matter. Regions of necrosis result in cystic PVL with surrounding gliosis.
- **Infection.** Cryptococcus is an opportunistic fungal infection that affects immunosuppressed patients, especially those with acquired immune deficiency syndrome. The infection affects the meninges and spreads through the subarachnoid and perivascular spaces, which become distended. The most common finding is multiple T2 hyperintense lesions in the basal ganglia with surrounding gliosis. Restricted diffusion and enhancement may be seen. Larger lesions are referred to as "gelatinous pseudocysts" and most often occur in the basal ganglia. Cryptococcomas are solid or ring-enhancing masses that most often involve the deep gray matter. Neurocysticercosis is a parasitic infection caused by the pork tapeworm (*Taenia solium*). It is the most common cause of epilepsy in endemic regions. In the initial vesicular stage, the cystic lesions are isointense to CSF, mimicking VR spaces. A hyperintense eccentric scolex may be seen (hyperdense by computed tomography). In the colloidal and granular stages, there is ring and nodular enhancement with surrounding edema. Calcification occurs in the nodular stage. Lesions may involve the gray-white junction (most common), subarachnoid space, and ventricles.

Additional Differential Diagnoses

- **Mucopolysaccharidoses (MPS).** MPS are inherited disorders characterized by enzyme deficiencies that result in accumulation of glycosaminoglycan (GAG). Clinically, patients suffer from mental and motor retardation. Imaging reveals macrocephaly and dilated perivascular spaces due to accumulation of GAG. The dilated PV spaces are similar to CSF signal intensity; however, the surrounding white matter demonstrates confluent regions of increased T2/FLAIR signal abnormality, likely representing gliosis or de/dysmyelination.
- **Neuroepithelial cyst.** Neuroepithelial cysts are nonenhancing parenchymal cysts with minimal or no surrounding signal abnormality, similar to VR spaces. They most often occur within the cerebral hemispheres, thalami, brain stem, and choroidal fissures. They are smooth, round, and unilocular, and they follow CSF signal intensity on all sequences. There is no communication with the ventricles.
- **Cystic neoplasm.** Cystic tumors may occur within the deep gray and white matter. Unlike VR spaces, neoplasms have solid components and often demonstrate enhancement and surrounding vasogenic edema.

Diagnosis

Mucopolysaccharidoses (Hurler syndrome)

✓ Pearls

- VR spaces are perivascular spaces that occur in characteristic locations and follow CSF signal.
- Lacunar infarcts and infection (cryptococcus) mimic VR spaces but have surrounding signal abnormality.
- MPS result in mental and motor retardation; dilated PV spaces have adjacent, confluent signal abnormality.

Suggested Reading

Kwee RM, Kwee TC. Virchow-Robin spaces at MR imaging. Radiographics 2007; 27: 1071–1086

Case 100

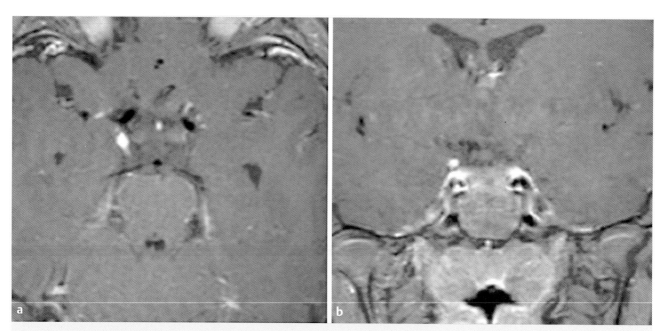

Fig. 100.1 Axial **(a)** and coronal **(b)** T1 postcontrast images with fat suppression demonstrate focal enlargement and enhancement involving the cisternal segment of the right oculomotor nerve (CN III).

▓ Clinical Presentation

Young girl with headaches and transient diplopia (▶ Fig. 100.1)

Key Imaging Finding

Oculomotor nerve enhancement

Top 3 Differential Diagnoses

- **Schwannoma.** Schwannomas are nerve sheath tumors that arise from perineural Schwann cells. They are the second most common extraaxial masses, following meningiomas. Common locations include the internal auditory canals, skull base and basal cisterns, and within the cavernous sinus. On magnetic resonance imaging (MRI), schwannomas are iso- to hypointense on T1, variably hyperintense on T2, and demonstrate heterogeneous but avid enhancement. The vast majority of lesions are solitary; multiple lesions may be seen in the setting of neurofibromatosis type 2 (NF2).
- **Meningitis.** Meningitis is an inflammatory infiltration of the pia, arachnoid, and cerebrospinal fluid (CSF) most often due to hematogenous dissemination of a distant infection. Atypical infections may be seen in immunocompromised patients. Lumbar puncture is the most sensitive test, revealing increased white blood cells and protein with decreased glucose. The exact values vary based upon the etiology of infection (bacterial or viral). MRI may be normal or show hyperintense fluid-attenuated inversion recovery (FLAIR) signal and/or smooth or nodular leptomeningeal enhancement. Complications include hydrocephalus, ventriculitis, abscesses, empyema, infarction, and venous thrombosis.
- **Leptomeningeal carcinomatosis.** Leptomeningeal carcinomatosis may be due to distant metastases, direct extension, or CSF dissemination. MRI is the most sensitive imaging modality, demonstrating hyperintense FLAIR CSF signal intensity and smooth or nodular leptomeningeal enhancement, which may be focal or diffuse. The ependymal surfaces of the ventricles and cranial nerves (CNs) may be coated. Communicating hydrocephalus is a potential complication from interference with CSF absorption. Additional parenchymal or calvarial metastatic foci are useful discriminators.

Additional Differential Diagnoses

- **Neurosarcoidosis.** Sarcoidosis is a systemic inflammatory granulomatous (noncaseating) disease with a peak onset in the third and fourth decades of life. Central nervous system involvement is relatively uncommon (~5 of cases) and most often presents with smooth or nodular dural and/or leptomeningeal enhancement, especially along the basal cisterns. There is often involvement of the optic chiasm, hypothalamus, infundibulum, internal auditory canals, and CNs at the skull base. Perivascular and ependymal enhancement may be seen. Regions of abnormal enhancement are typically multiple or confluent. Brain parenchyma can also be involved in one-third of patients. Look for lymphadenopathy with or without interstitial lung disease on chest X-ray or computed tomography (CT).
- **Ophthalmoplegic migraine.** Ophthalmoplegic migraine is a misnomer because it represents a form of cranial neuralgia rather than a variant of migraine headaches. It is a rare, self-limiting syndrome of unknown etiology that occurs in children and young adults and is characterized by headaches and oculomotor nerve dysfunction. Enhanced CT or MRI demonstrate transient, focal enlargement and enhancement of the cisternal segment of the oculomotor nerve (CN III), most commonly near the root entry zone. In a young patient with characteristic imaging and clinical findings, a presumptive diagnosis of ophthalmoplegic migraine may be made with close clinical and imaging follow-up; both imaging and clinical findings typically resolve within a few weeks.
- **Miller-Fisher syndrome.** Miller-Fisher syndrome is thought to represent a variant of Gullain-Barré syndrome (GBS) and is characterized by the clinical triad of ophthalmoplegia, ataxia, and areflexia. MRI demonstrates abnormal CN enhancement. Evaluation of the spine may demonstrate enhancement of the cauda equina as well. Prognosis is generally good with complete resolution of clinical and imaging findings.

Diagnosis

Ophthalmoplegic migraine

✓ Pearls

- Infectious, neoplastic, and granulomatous causes of CN enhancement are often multiple or confluent.
- The vast majority of schwannomas are solitary; multiple lesions may be seen in the setting of NF2.
- Ophthalmoplegic migraine is characterized by transient, self-limited headaches and oculomotor dysfunction.
- Miller-Fisher syndrome is thought to represent a variant of GBS with ophthalmoplegia, ataxia, and areflexia.

Suggested Reading

Mark AS, Casselman J, Brown D et al. Ophthalmoplegic migraine: reversible enhancement and thickening of the cisternal segment of the oculomotor nerve on contrast-enhanced MR images. Am J Neuroradiol 1998; 19: 1887–1891

Case 101

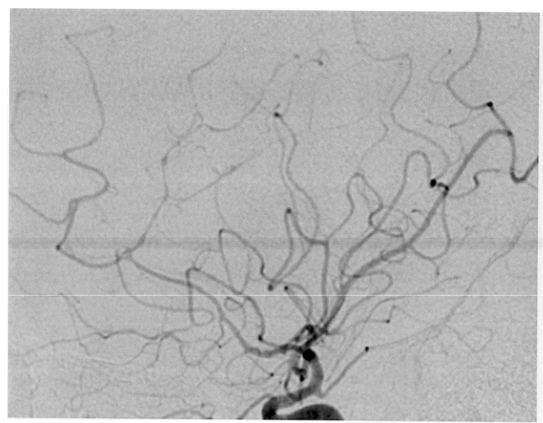

Fig. 101.1 Lateral projection from a digital subtraction angiogram with selective internal carotid artery injection demonstrates multifocal regions of alternating stenosis and mild dilatation involving the anterior cerebral artery branch vessels; visualized portions of the middle cerebral artery branch vessels appear normal. (Courtesy of Aaron Betts, MD and Todd Abruzzo, MD.)

▦ Clinical Presentation

An adult man with headaches; history otherwise withheld (▶ Fig. 101.1)

■ Key Imaging Finding

Multifocal regions of vascular stenosis

■ Top 3 Differential Diagnoses

- **Vasculitis.** Vasculitis results in inflammatory infiltration of arterial walls. Although it may occur at any age, young adults are most often affected. Within the central nervous system (CNS), it may be characterized as primary (primary CNS angiitis) or secondary. Secondary etiologies include autoimmune, infectious or granulomatous disease, radiation, and illicit drugs. Magnetic resonance imaging (MRI) demonstrates bilateral regions of superficial and deep gray and white matter signal abnormality (increased T2/fluid-attenuated inversion recovery signal intensity). Gradient echo and susceptibility-weighted imaging commonly reveal multifocal regions of microhemorrhage. Patchy enhancement may be seen. There may be involvement of small, medium, and large arteries. Angiography is often necessary to visualize alternating regions of stenosis and dilatation because MR angiography (MRA) and computed tomography angiography (CTA) are less sensitive. Biopsy is diagnostic. Treatment includes steroid and immunosuppressive therapy.
- **Vasospasm.** Vasospasm refers to reversible narrowing of the arterial lumen and most often occurs in the setting of subarachnoid hemorrhage (SAH) secondary to a ruptured intracranial aneurysm or trauma. The typical onset is between 4 and 14 days after the inciting event. Patients may be asymptomatic (most common) or present with symptoms related to vascular stenosis; most are identified during screening with transcranial Doppler, which shows increased velocities in the involved vasculature. CTA, MRA, or digital subtraction angiography may be useful in evaluating patients; CTA and MRA are often limited in evaluating distal, small caliber vessels. However, CTA has proven beneficial in detecting clinically significant regions of stenosis. Imaging reveals multifocal regions of smooth, relatively long segments of vascular narrowing. Clinically, patients are treated with "triple H" therapy, which includes hypertension, hypervolemia, and hemodilution, to maintain perfusion pressures. Endovascular therapeutic options include angioplasty and intraarterial chemical vasodilatation (calcium channel blockers).
- **Reversible cerebral vasoconstriction syndrome (RCVS).** RCVS, also referred to as Call-Fleming syndrome, is a transient syndrome characterized by multifocal regions of vascular stenosis and dilatation involving the cerebral arterial vasculature. Patients often present with episodic "thunderclap" headaches; young to middle-aged adult women are more often affected than men. There is an increased incidence with vasoactive drugs, a history of migraines, pregnancy, hypertension, and nonaneurysmal SAH. Imaging demonstrates multifocal regions of alternating stenoses and dilatations within the involved vasculature, which may appear similar to both vasculitis and posthemorrhagic vasospasm. Treatment options depend upon the duration and severity of symptoms, as they are usually transient. Medical options include discontinuance of the offending drug or chemical vasodilatation in severe cases.

■ Additional Differential Diagnoses

- **Atherosclerosis.** Atherosclerosis is common in middle-age and elderly patients and may be more advanced with comorbidities, such as diabetes, hypertension, and hyperlipidemia. It results in thickening and calcification of the arterial wall with associated luminal narrowing, which is often irregular and eccentric. Common intracranial locations include the internal carotid, basilar, and proximal portions of the cerebral arteries. CTA and MRA are useful in evaluating involved segments. Complications include decreased cerebrovascular perfusion, emboli, and vessel thrombosis, all of which may result in transient ischemic attacks or strokes.

■ Diagnosis

RCVS (secondary to vasoactive drug use)

✓ Pearls

- Vasculitis results in inflammatory infiltration of arterial walls; it may involve small, medium, and large arteries.
- Vasculitis results in multifocal regions of gray and white matter signal abnormality and microhemorrhage.
- Vasospasm causes reversible arterial narrowing; common causes include ruptured aneurysms and trauma.
- RCVS has an increased incidence with vasoactive drugs, migraines, pregnancy, and nonaneurysmal SAH.

Suggested Readings

Küker W. Cerebral vasculitis: imaging signs revisited. Neuroradiology 2007; 49: 471–479

Yoon DY, Choi CS, Kim KH, Cho BM. Multidetector-row CT angiography of cerebral vasospasm after aneurysmal subarachnoid hemorrhage: comparison of volume-rendered images and digital subtraction angiography. Am J Neuroradiol 2006; 27: 370–377

Case 102

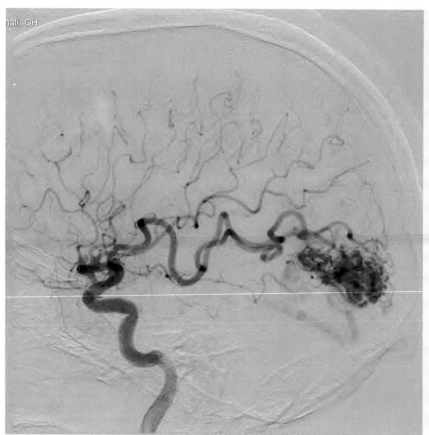

Fig. 102.1 Lateral DSA image of an internal carotid artery injection during late arterial phase demonstrates a large hypervascular mass in the occipital region supplied by enlarged arterial feeders. There is early venous drainage along the inferior aspect of the mass, consistent with arteriovenous shunting.

■ Clinical Presentation

A 40-year-old man with headaches for 2 months (▶ Fig. 102.1)

Key Imaging Finding

Hypervascular cerebral mass/abnormality on digital subtraction angiography (DSA)

Top 3 Differential Diagnoses

- **Arteriovenous malformation (AVM).** AVM is a form of arteriovenous shunting with no intervening capillary network. Most AVMs become symptomatic during the patient's lifetime. The peak age of presentation is 20 to 40 years of age. Hemorrhage, seizures, and headaches represent the most common clinical presentations. The vast majority are supratentorial and solitary. The best diagnostic clue is a cluster or tangle of flow voids on magnetic resonance imaging (MRI) with minimal or no mass effect, unless underlying hemorrhage occurs. There is little or no intervening brain tissue. Fluid-attenuated inversion recovery imaging often shows hyperintensity due to adjacent gliosis. AVMs demonstrate avid enhancement with enlarged arterial feeders and draining vein(s). Complete characterization is obtained with DSA, which will define the arterial supply, size of the nidus, and location of venous drainage. The Spetzler-Martin classification determines the operative risk and is based upon the AVM's size (< 3 cm, 3 to 6 cm, > 6 cm), location (eloquent vs. noneloquent), and venous drainage pattern (deep or superficial). Treatment options include transarterial embolization, stereotaxic radiosurgery, and/or microvascular surgery.
- **Aneurysm.** Aneurysms occur in ~2 to 4% of the population; they are multiple in 20 to 25% of cases. The average risk of rupture is 1 to 2% per year, in the absence of prior hemorrhage. On computed tomography (CT), aneurysms may be slightly hyperdense to brain parenchyma, particularly if partially thrombosed or calcified. They show strong enhancement when patent. MRI typically demonstrates a flow void or heterogeneous signal, especially with thrombus. Pulsation artifact, when present, is a useful discriminator. CT angiography, MR angiography, and DSA can be used to identify and characterize aneurysms.;90 to 95% arise from the Circle of Willis. The most common locations include the anterior communicating artery (ACOM), posterior communicating artery (PCOM), middle cerebral artery (MCA) bifurcation/trifurcation, and basilar tip. Giant aneurysms (> 2.5 cm) commonly involve the cavernous carotid and basilar arteries. Treatment options include endovascular coiling or craniotomy with aneurysm clipping.
- **Hypervascular tumor.** Hypervascular tumors, such as a glioblastoma multiforme (GBM) or meningioma, demonstrate a characteristic tumor blush, as opposed to an enhancing vascular nidus, as is seen with AVMs. On DSA, meningiomas show a "sunburst" or radial appearance with a prolonged vascular stain. Enlarged arterial feeders may be seen, especially with GBMs that demonstrate neovascularity. Occasionally, GBMs will also demonstrate intralesional shunting with early filling of draining veins; on DSA, this may mimic an arteriovenous shunt lesion. On MRI, GBMs will show tumoral enhancement, mass effect, vasogenic edema, and central necrosis. Meningiomas present as circumscribed extraaxial masses with a broad dural base and a dural tail. Enlarged vasculature presents as serpentine flow voids on T2 sequences. CT is useful in evaluating meningiomas, as they are typically hyperdense with calcification. Overlying bony changes are commonly seen.

Additional Differential Diagnoses

- **Moyamoya.** Moyamoya refers to an idiopathic, progressive narrowing of the distal internal carotid artery and proximal circle of Willis with secondary formation of multiple collaterals. The moyamoya or "puff of smoke" appearance of cloudlike perforating collaterals (lenticulostriate and thalamostriate) is seen on MRI and angiography. There is a bimodal age distribution with peaks in the first and fourth decades of life. Secondary causes include neurofibromatosis type 1, sickle cell disease, Down syndrome, radiation therapy, and progressive atherosclerotic disease. Patients present clinically with sequelae of chronic ischemia.

Diagnosis

Arteriovenous malformation

✓ Pearls

- AVMs have an arterial supply, a vascular nidus, and enlarged draining veins without a capillary network.
- The most common aneurysm locations include the ACOM, PCOM, MCA bi/trifurcation, and basilar tip.
- GBMs/meningiomas may have flow voids from neovascularity; GBMs may also have arteriovenous shunting.
- Moyamoya ("puff of smoke") results in numerous collateral vessels secondary to internal carotid artery occlusion.

Suggested Readings

Geibprasert S, Pongpech S, Jiarakongmun P, Shroff MM, Armstrong DC, Krings T. Radiologic assessment of brain arteriovenous malformations: what clinicians need to know. Radiographics 2010; 30: 483–501

O'Brien WT, Vagal A, Cornelius R. Applications of CT angiography in neuroimaging. Semin Roentgenol 2010; 45: 107–115

Case 103

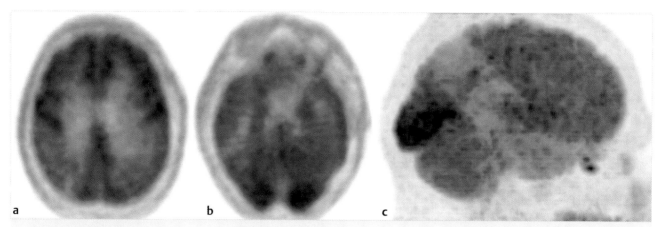

Fig. 103.1 Attenuation corrected axial FDG-PET images of the brain demonstrate decreased activity within the bilateral parietal **(a)** and temporal **(b)** lobes with intact normal activity within the bilateral frontal and occipital lobes. Attenuation corrected FDG-PET maximum intensity projection image, in sagittal projection **(c)**, demonstrates decreased activity in both the parietal and temporal lobes with intact normal activity within the cerebellum, frontal, and occipital lobes. (Case courtesy of Cameron C. Foster, MD.)

■ Clinical Presentation

A 62-year-old man with a 6-year history of cognitive decline (▶ Fig. 103.1)

▩ Key Imaging Finding

Decreased cortical 18F-fluorodeoxyglucose (FDG) activity in the setting of dementia

▩ Top 3 Differential Diagnoses

- **Alzheimer disease (AD).** AD is the most common dementia affecting adults. Presentation is typically after age 65 and incidence increases with age. Initial imaging findings demonstrate decreased metabolism (FDG-PET [positron emission tomography]) and blood flow (single-photon emission computed tomography [SPECT]) in the temporal and parietal lobes with relative sparing of the primary motor, somatosensory, and visual (occipital) cortices. Hypometabolic activity in the posterior cingulate gyri is one of the earliest findings. Early-stage AD may show hemispheric asymmetry. More advanced AD will begin to show decreased metabolic activity in the frontal lobes at a faster rate than normal aging dementia. In general, the amount of decreased metabolism directly correlates with the degree of symptoms. Studies have shown FDG-PET to have > 90% sensitivity and 70 to 75% specificity for AD.
- **Pick disease.** Pick disease is the classic—although rare—form of frontotemporal dementia (FTD). It is characterized by decreased metabolism in the bilateral frontal and anterior temporal lobes on FDG-PET. Differentiation from other disorders, such as AD, is based on symptoms; memory impairment in Pick disease is a secondary or absent feature, whereas it is a primary feature in AD. Differential considerations for isolated decreased metabolism in the frontotemporal regions include multi-infarct dementia (MID), depression, schizophrenia, amyotrophic lateral sclerosis (ALS), and drug abuse; this distribution is rarely seen in AD.
- **Multi-infarct dementia (MID).** MID is the most common cause of vascular dementia and is the second most common cause of dementia in adults over 65 years of age (AD is the most common). Whereas MID is usually identified via computed tomography or magnetic resonance imaging (MRI), FDG-PET and SPECT imaging show similar patterns of decreased activity in a diffuse or multifocal distribution. The clinical symptoms and imaging findings progress over time. Occasionally, the imaging appearance of MID may mimic FTD (frontotemporal distribution) or AD (diffuse temporoparietal distribution) on FDG-PET. MRI is useful in suggesting the correct diagnosis, demonstrating multifocal regions of microvascular ischemic disease and prior infarcts.

▩ Additional Differential Diagnoses

- **Parkinson disease.** Parkinson disease is associated with Lewy body dementia. It is largely a clinical diagnosis that typically has a normal appearance on FDG-PET, especially in its early stages. In later stages, decreased activity may be seen in the cortices, which is generally proportional to the severity of symptoms and disease progression. The appearance can be similar to AD with less sparing of the occipital (visual) cortices. Use of serial 18F-fluorodopa (FDOPA)-PET scans in patients with PD will initially show decreased activity within the posterior putamina with sparing of the caudate; over time, decreased activity will involve more of the putamina and eventually include the posterior caudate.

▩ Diagnosis

Alzheimer disease

✓ Pearls

- AD shows bilateral temporoparietal hypometabolism with sparing of the occipital lobes (visual cortices).
- Frontal lobe hypometabolism can be seen in frontotemporal dementias, depression, schizophrenia, and ALS.
- MID presents as diffuse or multifocal regions of decreased activity; MRI is useful in suggesting the diagnosis.
- Dementia associated with Parkinson disease may appear similar to AD with less sparing of the occipital lobes.

Suggested Readings

Hoffman JM, Welsh-Bohmer KA, Hanson M et al. FDG PET imaging in patients with pathologically verified dementia. J Nucl Med 2000; 41: 1920–1928

Van Heertum RL, Tikofsky RS. Positron emission tomography and single-photon emission computed tomography brain imaging in the evaluation of dementia. Semin Nucl Med 2003; 33: 77–85

Case 104

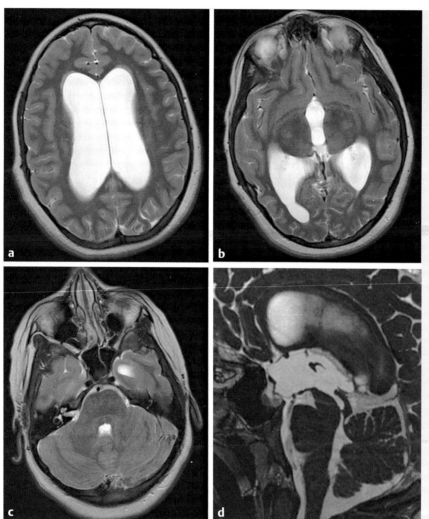

Fig. 104.1 Serial axial T2 magnetic resonance images demonstrate moderate-to-marked enlargement of the lateral (a) and third (b) ventricles with a normal-sized fourth ventricle (c). High-resolution sagittal T2 FIESTA (fast imaging employing steady state acquisition) image (d) reveals focal narrowing of the inferior cerebral aqueduct with a small web. The proximal aqueduct is dilated.

■ Clinical Presentation

A 13-year-old girl with progressively worsening headaches (▶ Fig. 104.1)

■ Key Imaging Finding

Narrowing of the cerebral aqueduct with lateral and third ventriculomegaly

■ Diagnosis

Aqueductal stenosis. The cerebral aqueduct is the conduit for cerebrospinal fluid (CSF) flow from the third to the fourth ventricle. It is situated between the tegmentum and the tectal plate. Narrowing results in aqueductal stenosis, which may be congenital or acquired. Congenital stenosis is most often due to membranes or webs within the cerebral aqueduct. Acquired causes include prior hemorrhage, infection, or obstruction secondary to adjacent masses.

Clinical presentation varies based upon the cause and duration of stenosis or obstruction. Patients may present in utero or well into adulthood. In infants and young children, the most common presentation is a bulging fontanelle with macrocrania secondary to increased intracranial pressure. Older children and adults tend to present with headaches, which are often insidious in nature.

Noncontrast computed tomography (CT) demonstrates enlargement of the third and lateral ventricles with a normal-sized fourth ventricle. The ventricular enlargement results in relative effacement of CSF within the sulci of the cerebral convexities. With acute, uncompensated hydrocephalus, a rind of hypoattenuation is seen along the margins of the lateral ventricles, corresponding to transependymal flow of CSF. It is important to evaluate the pineal region for an obstructing mass. Congenital webs or posthemorrhagic/inflammatory causes of stenosis are not typically seen on CT, unless there is significant dilatation of the cerebral aqueduct proximal to the region of stenosis.

Magnetic resonance imaging findings are similar with third and lateral ventriculomegaly, a normal-sized fourth ventricle, and transependymal flow of CSF in the setting of uncompensated hydrocephalus. The transependymal flow manifests as a rind of increased T2/fluid-attenuated inversion recovery signal intensity along the margins of the lateral ventricles. T2 sequences will show hyperdynamic CSF flow in the third and lateral ventricles. Sagittal T2 or cine images demonstrate absence of the normal CSF flow through the aqueduct. High-resolution, thin sagittal T2 sequences are useful in identifying congenital webs. These are more conspicuous with dilatation of the aqueduct proximal to the site of stenosis or obstruction. Posthemorrhagic and inflammatory exudative obstruction is more difficult to identify. It is important to evaluate the pineal region, to include the tectal plate and tegmentum. Periaqueductal signal abnormality may represent gliosis from an inflammatory process or abnormal signal associated with a low-grade tectal plate glioma. Larger pineal region masses are readily identified and do not represent a diagnostic dilemma.

Treatment is geared toward the causative etiology and/or diversion of CSF flow. A third ventriculostomy is the most common diverting procedure and has proven effective in managing symptoms related to obstructive hydrocephalus. High-resolution, thin sagittal T2 and cine sequences are useful for post-treatment follow-up imaging, demonstrating a flow void through the ventriculostomy site when patent.

✓ Pearls

- Aqueductal stenosis may be congenital (webs) or acquired (posthemorrhagic/infectious or obstructing mass).
- Imaging demonstrates third and lateral ventriculomegaly with a normal sized fourth ventricle.
- High-resolution, thin sagittal T2 sequences are useful in identifying the stenosis and possible etiologies.
- Treatment of aqueductal stenosis is geared toward the causative etiology and/or diversion of CSF flow.

Suggested Reading

Stoquart-El Sankari S, Lehmann P, Gondry-Jouet C et al. Phase-contrast MR imaging support for the diagnosis of aqueductal stenosis. Am J Neuroradiol 2009; 30: 209–214

Case 105

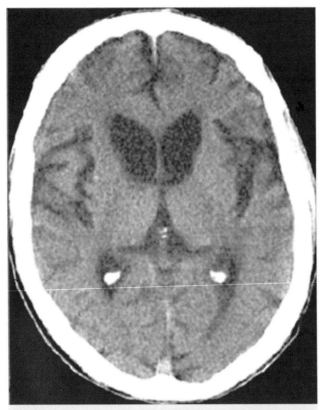

Fig. 105.1 Axial computed tomography image reveals prominent, symmetric volume loss involving the caudate heads with compensatory enlargement of the frontal horns of the lateral ventricles. The intercaudate distance is significantly enlarged. (Courtesy of Paul M. Sherman, MD.)

■ Clinical Presentation

A 44-year-old man with progressive dementia (▶ Fig. 105.1)

■ Key Imaging Finding

Preferential caudate volume loss in an adult

■ Diagnosis

Huntington disease. Huntington disease (HD) is an autosomal dominant neurodegenerative disorder that most often presents in early to mid-adulthood (fourth and fifth decades) with dementia, psychosis, and choreoathetosis; chorea is the dominant clinical feature. A juvenile variant is less common, presents prior to 20 years of age, and clinically manifests with rigidity as a dominant feature rather than chorea.

The most common imaging feature in the adult variant is preferential atrophy of the caudate nuclei with associated dilatation of the frontal horns of the lateral ventricles. Atrophic changes result in an increased intercaudate distance, which refers to the distance between the medial aspects of the caudate heads. In normal individuals, the distance is typically 10 to 14 mm, whereas in Huntington chorea it is > 20 mm. There is often diffuse parenchymal volume loss; however, the caudate nuclei are disproportionately involved to a greater degree. Signal abnormality of the deep gray matter structures is not a characteristic feature of the adult variant.

In the juvenile form of HD, symmetric hyperintense T2/fluid-attenuated inversion recovery signal is visualized in the basal ganglia, particularly the caudate nuclei and putamina. The signal abnormality is nonspecific and may be seen in additional neurodegenerative processes, metabolic diseases, and with ischemic, toxic, or infectious injury. Preferential caudate atrophy is a useful secondary finding to suggest HD.

HD is incurable and progressive. Treatment strategies are geared toward mitigating the clinical manifestations (chorea, rigidity, psychosis, etc.).

✓ Pearls

- HD is an autosomal dominant neurodegenerative disorder that most often affects adults; chorea is the main clinical feature.

- The most common imaging feature in the adult variant is preferential atrophy of the caudate nuclei.
- Juvenile HD presents prior to 20 years of age with rigidity and hyperintense T2 signal in the basal ganglia.

Suggested Readings

Ho VB, Chuang HS, Rovira MJ, Koo B. Juvenile Huntington disease: CT and MR features. Am J Neuroradiol 1995; 16: 1405–1412

Stober T, Wussow W, Schimrigk K. Bicaudate diameter—the most specific and simple CT parameter in the diagnosis of Huntington's disease. Neuroradiology 1984; 26: 25–28

Case 106

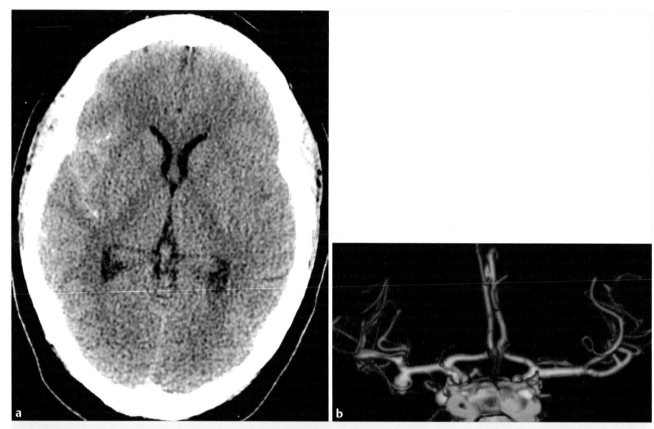

Fig. 106.1 Unenhanced axial CT image (a) demonstrates subarachnoid hemorrhage within the Sylvian fissure on the right. Three-dimensional volume rendered reformatted image from a CTA (b) reveals a saccular right middle cerebral artery aneurysm (M1-M2 junction) pointing inferiorly with an M2 branch originating from its base.

■ Clinical Presentation

A young adult man with acute onset headache; no history of trauma (▶ Fig. 106.1)

▓ Key Imaging Finding

Subarachnoid hemorrhage (SAH) with adjacent aneurysm

▓ Diagnosis

Ruptured aneurysm. A ruptured intracranial aneurysm is the most common nontraumatic cause of acute SAH, accounting for ~85% of cases. Intracranial aneurysms occur in ≈2 to 4% of the general population; multiple aneurysms are seen in ≈20 to 25% of cases. Although the vast majority occur sporadically, there is an increased incidence in the setting of hypertension, aortic coarctation, autosomal dominant polycystic kidney disease, connective tissue disorders, vasculitis, fibromuscular dysplasia, and neurofibromatosis type 1. They may also occur in association with trauma (pseudoaneurysm), infection (mycotic), and vascular malformations. Pseudoaneurysms and mycotic aneurysms are more likely to involve peripheral vasculature and have a higher incidence of rapid growth and rupture if left untreated.

The risk of rupture varies based upon the size of the aneurysm; however, the average risk of rupture is ≈1 to 2% per year in the absence of prior hemorrhage. After rupture, the risk of re-bleeding in the first 6 months is more than 50% if left untreated. The risk then drops down to 3% per year 6 months after hemorrhage. Patients who survive large hemorrhages often have residual neurological deficits, especially those with intraparenchymal hemorrhage.

Patients with hemorrhage often present with the "worst headache of life." Noncontrast computed tomography (CT) is the initial modality of choice to evaluate for SAH. In early stages, the SAH is centered in the region of the aneurysm. Over time, the hemorrhage becomes more diffuse, making it more difficult to localize or predict the site of rupture, especially when multiple aneurysms are present.

CT angiography (CTA) or MR angiography (MRA) may be used to evaluate for the presence of intracranial aneurysms. CTA is typically preferred due to its rapid acquisition time and widespread availability in the emergency room setting. MRA lacks ionizing radiation; however, it takes longer to obtain the study and is more susceptible to motion artifact compared with CTA. With advanced postprocessing, CTA can detect aneurysms <3 mm in size. A digital subtraction angiogram is typically performed to further evaluate and potentially treat the aneurysm.

Important descriptors for aneurysms include location, size of the aneurysm and its neck, shape, orientation, and relationship to branch and parent vessels. The most common locations in decreasing order of frequency include the anterior communicating artery, posterior communicating artery, middle cerebral artery bifurcation/trifurcation, and basilar terminus. Additional locations include the cavernous segment of the internal carotid artery, vertebrobasilar junction, ophthalmic artery, and posterior inferior cerebellar artery. Giant aneurysms are described as ≥2.5 cm and commonly occur within the cavernous segment of the internal carotid artery and basilar terminus.

Identifying which aneurysm bled may be difficult in the setting of multiple aneurysms. An irregular shape or excrescence is suggestive of rupture. The orientation of the aneurysm and its relationship to branch and parent vessels are important factors in determining surgical versus endovascular management. Endovascular treatment consists of aneurysm coiling; occasionally, stent or balloon-assisted techniques are required, especially in aneurysms with a wide neck. Post-treatment follow-up is essential to evaluate for recurrence.

✓ Pearls

- A ruptured intracranial aneurysm is the most common nontraumatic cause of acute SAH.
- Risk of rupture varies based upon size of aneurysm; average risk is 1 to 2% per year in absence of prior bleed.
- Early on, SAH is centered in the region of the aneurysm; over time, the hemorrhage becomes more diffuse.
- Important descriptors for aneurysms include location, size, shape, orientation, and relationship to vessels.

Suggested Reading

O'Brien WT, Vagal AS, Cornelius RS. Applications of CTA in neuroimaging. Semin Roentgenol 2010; 45: 107–115

Case 107

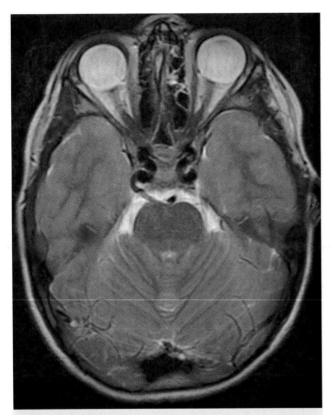

Fig. 107.1 Axial T2 magnetic resonance image reveals an anomalous artery originating from the posterior cavernous segment of the right internal carotid artery and extending posteriorly to the midbasilar artery.

▧ Clinical Presentation

A young boy with an incidental finding on workup for headaches (▶ Fig. 107.1)

■ Key Imaging Finding

Anomalous carotid-vertebrobasilar anastomosis

■ Diagnosis

Persistent fetal carotid-vertebrobasilar anastomoses (persistent trigeminal artery). During early fetal development, anastomoses exist between the developing carotid arteries and the vertebrobasilar system. Failure of these connections to regress results in persistent vascular communications. The arteries are named with respect to adjacent structures. The most common persistent vessels from superior to inferior include the trigeminal, otic, hypoglossal, and proatlantal arteries.

A persistent trigeminal artery is the most common of the fetal carotid-vertebrobasilar anastomoses. It originates anteriorly just after the carotid artery exits the carotid canal and extends posteriorly to the midbasilar artery. The inferior aspect of the basilar artery proximal to the anastomosis is relatively hypoplastic, whereas the portion distal to the anastomosis is prominent in caliber. The persistent trigeminal artery may course laterally along the trigeminal nerve or medially through the sellar or suprasellar regions. The most important reason for identifying this normal variant is to avoid inadvertent injury in patients requiring transsphenoidal or other skull-base surgeries. As with other anomalies that alter hemodynamics, there is an increased incidence of intracranial aneurysms.

A persistent hypoglossal artery is the second most common of the fetal carotid-vertebrobasilar anastomoses. It originates from the distal cervical internal carotid artery, passes through an enlarged hypoglossal canal, and connects with the basilar artery. The vertebral arteries and inferior aspect of the basilar artery proximal to the anastomosis are typically hypoplastic. Given its location within the hypoglossal canal, patients may present with hypoglossal nerve dysfunction.

The proatlantal artery originates from the distal common carotid or proximal internal/external carotid arteries and anastomoses with the suboccipital vertebral artery. The vertebral artery proximal to the anastomosis may be hypoplastic or absent. Additional intracranial vascular variants and intracranial aneurysms have been reported.

A persistent otic artery is the rarest of the fetal carotid-vertebrobasilar anastomoses. It arises from the petrous segment of the internal carotid artery, extends posteriorly and laterally through the internal auditory canal, and connects with the proximal basilar artery. The inferior aspect of the basilar artery proximal to the anastomosis is typically hypoplastic.

✓ Pearls

- Persistent fetal carotid-vertebrobasilar anastomoses are uncommon but important anomalies.
- Persistent arteries are named based upon adjacent structures: trigeminal, otic, hypoglossal, and proatlantal.
- The persistent trigeminal artery is the most common and is important to identify prior to skull-base surgery.
- A persistent hypoglossal artery extends through the hypoglossal canal and may result in cranial neuropathy.

Suggested Reading

Dimmick SJ, Faulder KC. Normal variants of the cerebral circulation at multidetector CT angiography. Radiographics 2009; 29: 1027–1043

Case 108

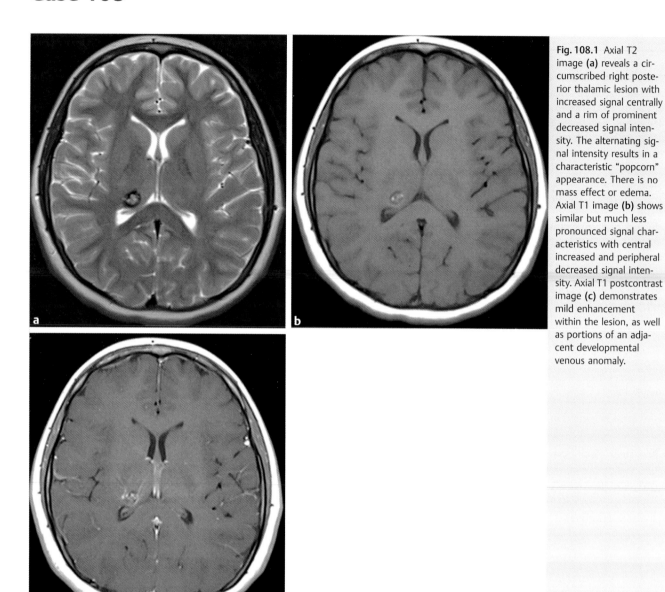

Fig. 108.1 Axial T2 image **(a)** reveals a circumscribed right posterior thalamic lesion with increased signal centrally and a rim of prominent decreased signal intensity. The alternating signal intensity results in a characteristic "popcorn" appearance. There is no mass effect or edema. Axial T1 image **(b)** shows similar but much less pronounced signal characteristics with central increased and peripheral decreased signal intensity. Axial T1 postcontrast image **(c)** demonstrates mild enhancement within the lesion, as well as portions of an adjacent developmental venous anomaly.

▧ Clinical Presentation

A 16-year-old boy with chronic headaches (▶ Fig. 108.1)

▧ Key Imaging Finding

Circumscribed lesion with central increased and peripheral decreased signal with a "popcorn" appearance

▧ Diagnosis

Cavernous malformation (CM). CMs are slow-flow lesions that are composed of dilated sinusoids, intercapillary spaces, and cavernous spaces without intervening brain parenchyma. They are filled with blood of various stages and surrounded by a hemosiderin capsule. CMs represent the second most common vascular malformation (VM) after developmental venous anomalies (DVAs) and commonly occur in association with DVAs.

The vast majority of CMs are sporadic and solitary. They may be multiple in ~10 to 20% of cases, especially in familial cases (autosomal dominant) or in the setting of prior radiation therapy. Most lesions are asymptomatic. When present, common symptoms include acute intracranial hemorrhage, seizures, or focal neurological deficits. The location of the lesion(s) often corresponds with symptoms; lesions in the posterior fossa have a higher incidence of hemorrhage, whereas superficial supratentorial lesions more often result in seizures or focal neurological deficits. The average annual risk of hemorrhage is < 1%. After an episode of acute hemorrhage, the risk of re-bleeding increases to ~4.5% per year for the next 2 to 3 years and then returns to baseline.

On unenhanced computed tomography (CT), large lesions present as relatively well-defined regions of subtle increased attenuation. Calcification may be seen in ≈60% of cases. Small lesions are often isodense to surrounding brain parenchyma and difficult to identify. In the absence of acute hemorrhage, there is typically no mass effect or surrounding edema. Acute hemorrhage extending through the capsule will typically result in surrounding edema and mass effect, as well as acute onset of symptoms.

The magnetic resonance imaging (MRI) appearance of CMs is characteristic. On T2 sequences, the lesions have a peripheral hypointense hemosiderin rim. Centrally, there are alternating regions of increased and decreased signal intensity on both T1 and T2 sequences due to blood products of various stages; this is termed the *"popcorn" appearance*. The lesions "bloom" on gradient echo and susceptibility-weighted imaging. Enhancement is variable and seen in ≈15% of cases. As with CT, there is typically no mass effect or edema unless complicated by acute hemorrhage.

If asymptomatic, CMs are usually followed to ensure stability. In the setting of acute hemorrhage, conservative therapy is ideal, unless the clinical picture requires intervention. Treatment options include surgical resection or radiosurgery, depending upon the lesion size, lesion location, and clinical setting.

✓ Pearls

- CMs are slow-flow lesions without intervening brain tissue; they are the second most common VM after DVAs.
- The vast majority of CMs are sporadic and solitary; they may be multiple in familial cases or prior radiation therapy.

- On MRI, CMs have a peripheral hypointense hemosiderin rim with a central "popcorn" appearance.
- CMs are typically followed for stability unless lesion size, location, or clinical setting requires intervention.

Suggested Reading

Smith AB. Vascular malformations of the brain: radiologic and pathologic correlation. J Am Osteopath Coll Radiol. 2012; 1: 10–22

Case 109

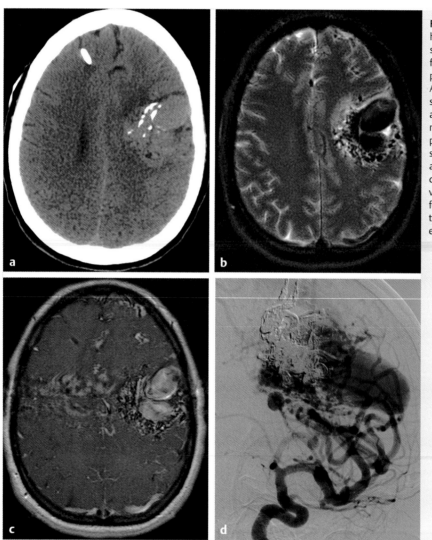

Fig. 109.1 Axial CT image (**a**) demonstrates a hyperdense mass with calcifications and mild surrounding edema within the posterior left frontal lobe. A ventricular drainage catheter is partially visualized within the right frontal lobe. Axial T2 MR image (**b**) reveals a nidus of enlarged serpentine flow voids with a large venous aneurysm laterally. There is prominent enhancement and flow-related artifact on the axial T1 postcontrast image (**c**). Lateral oblique digital subtraction angiogram of the left internal carotid artery (**d**) demonstrates early venous filling during the arterial phase, including the large venous aneurysm, as well as enlarged vessels feeding, draining, and within the nidus. Serpentine subtraction artifact corresponds to partial embolization.

■ Clinical Presentation

A 44-year-old woman with headaches and seizures (▶ Fig. 109.1)

Key Imaging Finding

Parenchymal mass with a vascular nidus and enlarged feeding and draining vessels

Diagnosis

Arteriovenous malformation (AVM). AVMs are high-flow lesions characterized by abnormal arteriovenous communications with an intervening vascular nidus, which is composed of arteriovenous shunts and dysplastic vessels. The majority are supratentorial and present in young adults. Common presentations include headaches, seizures, and parenchymal hemorrhage; the risk of hemorrhage is ~2 to 4% per year. AVMs are the most common cause of spontaneous intraparenchymal hemorrhage in this age group.

In the absence of hemorrhage, large AVMs are typically slightly hyperdense to surrounding brain parenchyma on unenhanced computed tomography (CT) due to the presence of flowing blood. Calcifications are noted in ≈30% of cases. Small lesions may be isodense and difficult to visualize. CT angiography is useful in demonstrating enlarged feeding arteries and draining veins. On magnetic resonance imaging (MRI), AVMs demonstrate a tangle of T2 flow voids that correspond to the vascular nidus and feeding/draining vessels; the appearance is often described as a "bag of worms." There is typically blooming on gradient echo sequences due to the presence of blood products and/or calcification. MR angiography is useful in identifying enlarged feeding arteries and draining veins, as well as intranidal or venous aneurysms, which are a common source of hemorrhage. Vascular shunting often results in localized gliosis within surrounding brain parenchyma.

The presence of hemorrhage complicates the imaging appearance and may even obscure an underlying AVM. In the setting of spontaneous intraparenchymal hemorrhage, it is important to perform a contrast-enhanced study to evaluate for an underlying mass, such as an AVM or neoplasm.

Table 109.1 The Spetzler Martin grading system

Size	Small (< 3 cm) = 1
	Medium (3–6 cm) = 2
	Large (> 6 cm) = 3
Location	Noneloquent = 0
	Eloquent = 1
Venous Drainage	Superficial = 0
	Deep = 1

Reprinted with permission, J Am Osteopath Coll Radiol 2012;1:10–22.

Conventional angiography remains the gold standard for characterizing AVMs, especially with regards to identifying vascular contributions and associated aneurysms, if present. It is important to evaluate the internal carotid, external carotid, and vertebral arteries because multiple vascular supplies are not uncommon. Angiography reveals vascular shunting with visualization of venous drainage in the arterial phase, enlarged feeding arteries and draining veins, and an intervening vascular nidus.

Treatment options for AVMs include endovascular embolization, surgery, and/or radiosurgery. The Spetzler Martin grading system helps predict the risk of surgical morbidity and mortality. The grading system criteria include size, location, and the pattern of venous drainage. Lesions with a higher score have a higher surgical morbidity and mortality. The Spetzler Martin grading system is listed in ▶ Table 109.1.

✓ Pearls

- AVMs are high flow and characterized by arteriovenous communications with an intervening vascular nidus.
- AVMs are most common in young adults; typical presentations include headaches, seizures, and hemorrhage.

- Imaging demonstrates a vascular nidus with enlarged feeding arteries and draining veins.
- The Spetzler Martin grading system (size, location, and venous drainage) predicts surgical morbidity/mortality.

Suggested Reading

Smith AB. Vascular malformations of the brain: radiologic and pathologic correlation. J Am Osteopath Coll Radiol. 2012; 1: 10–22

Case 110

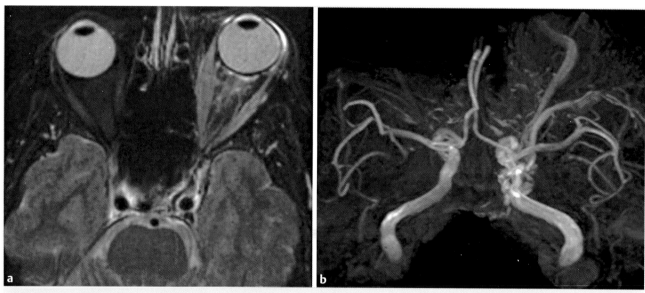

Fig. 110.1 Coned-down axial T2 image with fat suppression **(a)** demonstrates a convex lateral border and increased flow voids within the left cavernous sinus, enlargement and edema involving the left EOMs, inflammation of the intraorbital and periorbital fat, and proptosis. Three-dimensional volume rendered reformation from a magnetic resonance angiogram **(b)** reveals increased signal/flow within the left cavernous sinus and the left superior ophthalmic vein (coursing superiorly on the image). (Reprinted with permission: Smith AB. J Am Osteopath Coll Radiol 2012;1 [1]:10–22.)

■ Clinical Presentation

An adult patient with orbital pain, visual loss, and bruit (▶ Fig. 110.1)

■ Key Imaging Finding

Enlarged cavernous sinus with early venous filling on arterial phase imaging

■ Diagnosis

Carotid-cavernous fistula (CCF). CCFs refer to abnormal communications between the carotid artery and cavernous sinus. They are classified as direct or indirect. Direct CCFs result in high-flow arteriovenous shunting between the cavernous internal carotid artery (ICA) and the cavernous sinus with a relatively rapid onset of symptoms, which include pulsatile exophthalmos, orbital bruit, chemosis, and occasionally intracranial hemorrhage. The vast majority of direct CCFs result from trauma; rupture of a cavernous carotid aneurysm is a much less common cause. Indirect CCFs are slow-flow shunts between dural branches of the ICA or the external carotid artery (ECA) and the cavernous sinus. They most often occur spontaneously and have a more insidious onset of symptoms.

CCFs result in increased venous and orbital pressures. There is enlargement of the cavernous sinus and diversion of venous drainage through the ipsilateral superior ophthalmic vein (SOV). Magnetic resonance imaging demonstrates a convex lateral border of the cavernous sinus on the involved side (it is typically flat or concave), increased T2 flow voids within the cavernous sinus, enlarged ipsilateral SOV and extraocular muscles (EOMs), and proptosis. Cavernous sinus enlargement may be bilateral because there are communications with the contralateral side within the cavernous sinus.

Angiography demonstrates early venous filling (cavernous sinus and superior ophthalmic vein) in the arterial phase. Endovascular treatment options are favored and include glue or coil embolization.

✓ Pearls

- CCFs (direct or indirect) are abnormal communications between the carotid artery and cavernous sinus.
- Direct CCFs result from trauma and have a rapid onset of pulsatile exophthalmos, orbital bruit, and chemosis.
- Imaging findings include enlargement of the cavernous sinus (with flow voids), SOV, EOMs, and proptosis.
- Endovascular treatment options for CCFs are favored and include glue or coil embolization.

Suggested Reading

Smith AB. Vascular malformations of the brain: radiologic and pathologic correlation. J Am Osteopath Coll Radiol. 2012; 1: 10–22

Case 111

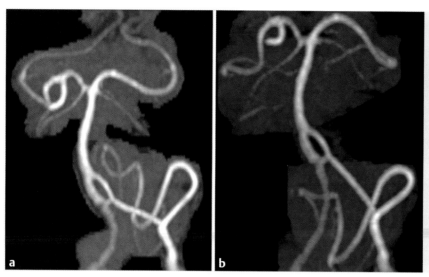

Fig. 111.1 Three-dimensional volume rendered magnetic resonance angiography reformations (a,b) demonstrate two separate lumens at the vertebrobasilar junction. The lumens converge proximally and distally. Slight loss of flow signal intensity at the origin of the fenestration on the right corresponds to a region of focal arterial stenosis.

■ **Clinical Presentation**

A 77-year-old man with transient ischemic attacks and vertigo (▶ Fig. 111.1)

■ Key Imaging Finding

Separate arterial lumens that converge proximal and distally

■ Diagnosis

Arterial fenestration. A fenestration refers to two separate vascular channels composed of independent endothelium and muscular walls but shared adventitia. They typically occur in short segments with a normal caliber parent artery or arteries proximally and distally. Because fenestrations alter hemodynamic flow, there is an increased association with aneurysm formation compared with the general population.

Within the circle of Willis, the most common locations include the anterior communicating and basilar arteries. In the case of basilar artery fenestrations, they are thought to result from incomplete fusion of paired fetal longitudinal neural arteries. Most basilar artery fenestrations occur near the vertebrobasilar junction. Involvement of the cerebral and vertebral arteries is less common but does occur.

✓ Pearls

- Fenestrations refer to distinct arterial channels with their own endothelium/muscularis but a shared adventitia.
- Because fenestrations alter hemodynamic flow, there is an increased association with aneurysm formation.

- The most common locations of fenestrations include the anterior communicating and basilar arteries.

Suggested Reading

Dimmick SJ, Faulder KC. Normal variants of the cerebral circulation at multidetector CT angiography. Radiographics 2009; 29: 1027–1043

Case 112

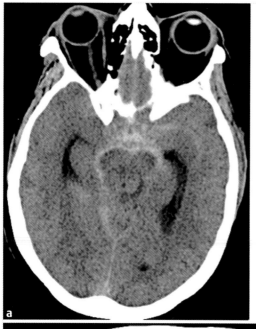

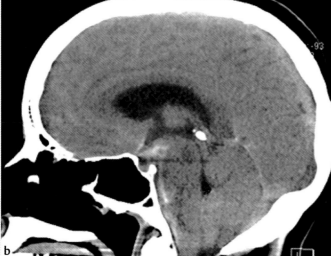

Fig. 112.1 Axial unenhanced CT image (**a**) demonstrates SAH centered within the perimesencephalic cisterns. Sagittal reformatted image (**b**) shows the hemorrhage within the prepontine, premedullary, and perimesencephalic cisterns.

▦ Clinical Presentation

A young adult man with postcoital headache; no recent trauma. Digital subtraction angiogram (DSA) was normal initially and 2 weeks following initial presentation (▶ Fig. 112.1).

■ Key Imaging Finding

Nontraumatic subarachnoid hemorrhage (SAH) centered within prepontine and perimesencephalic cisterns

■ Diagnosis

Nonaneurysmal perimesencephalic hemorrhage (PMH). Nonaneurysmal PMH refers to SAH centered within the perimesencephalic cisterns anterior to the brain stem. It is postulated that the nonaneurysmal hemorrhage results from a venous origin, which accounts for the lack of visualization of an aneurysm on imaging and low rate/risk of re-bleeding.

Patients with nonaneurysmal PMH typically present with headache after an exertional episode. Compared with those with a ruptured aneurysm, the onset of headache is more insidious and less severe. Additionally, there is typically no loss of consciousness or neurological deficits. The long-term prognosis is very good because the risks of immediate complications and re-bleeding are low.

Computed tomography (CT) findings include hyperdense SAH centered within the cisterns anterior to the brain stem, particularly the prepontine and perimesencephalic cisterns. There may be extension into the ambient cisterns, basal portions of the Sylvian fissures, and proximal aspect of the anterior interhemispheric fissure. However, there typically is no extension into the lateral portions of the Sylvian fissures, distal portion of the anterior interhemispheric fissure, or within the ventricles.

Current guidelines recommend CT angiography (CTA) in the setting of suspected nonaneurysmal PMH. With a negative CTA and the appropriate clinical setting, no further workup is necessary. That being said, many institutions still perform initial and follow-up DSAs as a precautionary measure to exclude an underlying occult or thrombosed aneurysm.

✓ Pearls

- Nonaneurysmal PMH refers to SAH centered within the perimesencephalic cisterns anterior to the brain stem.
- Nonaneurysmal PMH is thought to be of venous origin, accounting for the low rate/risk of re-bleeding.

- Workup of nonaneurysmal PMH typically includes noncontrast CT, followed by CTA or DSA.

Suggested Reading

Agid R, Andersson T, Almqvist H et al. Negative CT angiography findings in patients with spontaneous subarachnoid hemorrhage: when is digital subtraction angiography still needed? Am J Neuroradiol 2010; 31: 696–705

Case 113

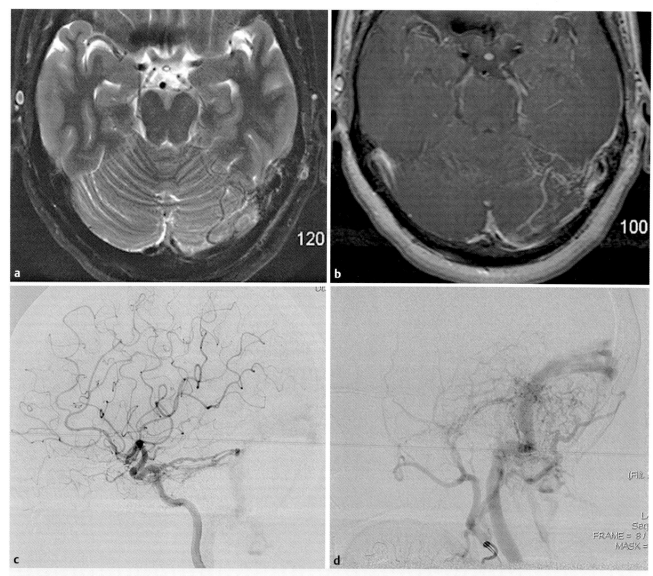

Fig. 113.1 Axial T2 MR image **(a)** demonstrates increased flow voids extending along the tentorium on the left, extending to the distal transverse sinus. Axial T1 postcontrast image **(b)** reveals corresponding vascular enhancement. Lateral images from a digital subtraction angiogram with selective injection of the left internal **(c)** and external **(d)** carotid arteries shows early filling of the left transverse and sigmoid sinuses during arterial phase imaging. Additional imaging revealed the primary arterial vascular supply from the meningohypophyseal trunk, middle meningeal, ascending pharyngeal, and occipital arteries. (Courtesy of Aaron Betts, MD and Andrew Ringer, MD.)

■ **Clinical Presentation**

A 51-year-old woman with left retroauricular headache (▶ Fig. 113.1)

▨ Key Imaging Finding

Dural-based arteriovenous shunt

▨ Diagnosis

Dural arteriovenous fistula (AVF). AVFs differ from arteriovenous malformations (AVMs) in that AVFs have a direct arterial to venous communication without an intervening vascular nidus, as is seen with AVMs. Otherwise, both are high-flow shunt lesions.

Dural AVFs (dAVFs) are classified as infantile or adult lesions. The infantile form is rare and is characterized by multiple dAVFs in response to venous sinus thrombosis. Magnetic resonance imaging (MRI) is useful in identifying the venous sinus thrombosis, as well as identifying the vascular lesion, which is typically centered in the torcula.

The adult form is thought to be acquired also as a result of dural venous sinus thrombosis. It typically presents in middle-aged adults. The dAVFs consist of small shunts in the wall of a thrombosed venous sinus; the most common locations include the junction of the transverse and sigmoid sinuses and the cavernous sinus. Symptoms are variable and based upon location. Those located at the transverse-sigmoid junction often present with tinnitus and vertigo. Focal neurological deficits and hemorrhage are potential complications and are thought to result from venous congestion.

dAVFs are characterized as benign or aggressive based upon the pattern of venous drainage. The presence of retrograde leptomeningeal venous drainage is an indicator of a more aggressive lesion and should prompt early intervention.

Noncontrast computed tomography (CT) is often normal in the setting of an uncomplicated dAVF. CT angiography may reveal enlarged arteries or draining veins along a dural venous sinus. CT venography may reveal flow-limiting stenosis or occlusion of the adjacent dural venous sinus. On MRI, there are often multiple flow voids on T2 sequences corresponding to the dAVF; these may be subtle. A thrombosed sinus will have absence of the normal T2 flow void and is better depicted on MR venography. Venous congestion results in gliosis within the adjacent brain parenchyma.

Digital subtraction angiography best depicts dAVFs with multiple arterial feeders and venous filling during arterial phase imaging. The majority of lesions have arterial supply from dural and transosseous branches of the external carotid artery; however, dural and tentorial branches of the internal carotid and/or vertebral arteries may also be involved. Therefore, it is important to interrogate all arterial vessels during a cerebral angiogram. More aggressive lesions will demonstrate reversal of flow within the dural venous sinus and leptomeningeal/cortical veins with a characteristic "pseudophlebitic" pattern.

Treatment options include endovascular embolization, surgical resection, or radiosurgery.

✓ Pearls

- AVFs have a direct arterial to venous communication without an intervening vascular nidus.
- dAVFs are thought to be acquired due to dural venous sinus thrombosis; there are adult and infantile forms.

- Treatment options for dAVFs include endovascular embolization, surgical resection, or radiosurgery.

Suggested Reading

Smith AB. Vascular malformations of the brain: radiologic and pathologic correlation. J Am Osteopath Coll Radiol 2012; 1: 10–22

Case 114

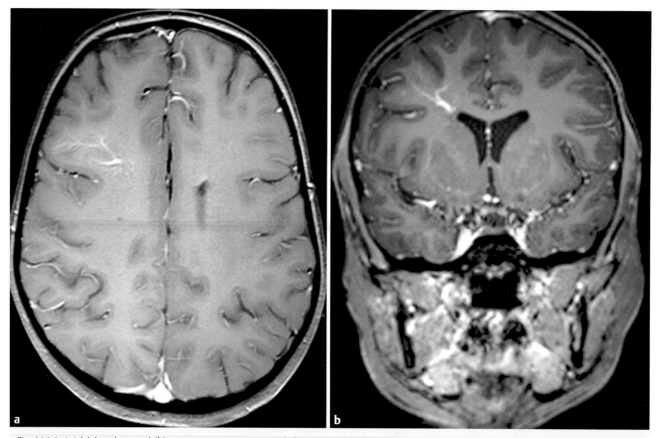

Fig. 114.1 Axial **(a)** and coronal **(b)** postcontrast T1 images with fat suppression demonstrate branching regions of enhancement within the right frontal lobe with a common trunk that drains into an enlarged deep ependymal vein, rendering the characteristic "caput medusa" sign.

■ Clinical Presentation

An 8-year-old girl with headaches (▶ Fig. 114.1)

▨ Key Imaging Finding

Branching regions of enhancement extending into a dilated venous trunk ("caput medusa" sign)

▨ Diagnosis

Developmental venous anomaly (DVA). DVAs are the most common vascular malformations of the brain. They are considered normal variants and provide venous drainage for surrounding brain parenchyma. Therefore, they are considered "do not touch" lesions. DVAs are composed of dilated medullary veins that drain into a common venous trunk. They are typically asymptomatic, except in cases of acute thrombosis, which is relatively uncommon. They are commonly seen in association with adjacent cavernous malformations.

On unenhanced computed tomography (CT), DVAs may be isodense or slightly hyperdense to brain parenchyma. If acutely thrombosed, the thrombus will be hyperdense with surrounding hypodense edema. Routine magnetic resonance imaging (MRI) sequences demonstrate branching flow voids extending into a venous trunk, producing the characteristic "caput medusa" sign; this is best seen on T2 sequences. Enhanced studies (CT or MRI) better depict the dilated medullary veins and venous trunk that drain into a dural venous sinus or ependymal vein.

✓ Pearls

- DVAs are the most common vascular malformations of the brain; they are considered normal variants.
- DVAs are composed of dilated medullary veins that drain into a common venous trunk.
- MRI demonstrates branching flow voids extending into a venous trunk, producing the "caput medusa" sign.

Suggested Reading

Smith AB. Vascular malformations of the brain: radiologic and pathologic correlation. J Am Osteopath Coll Radiol. 2012; 1: 10–22

Case 115

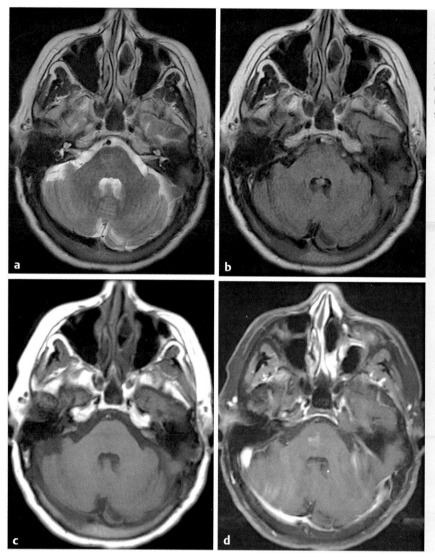

Fig. 115.1 Axial T2 **(a)** and FLAIR **(b)** images demonstrate a very subtle region of increased signal intensity within the central pons, slightly eccentric to the right. There is no appreciable signal abnormality on precontrast T1 sequences **(c)**. A fat-suppressed postcontrast T1 image **(d)** reveals ill-defined enhancement in the region of subtle T2 signal abnormality.

■ Clinical Presentation

A 74-year-old woman with memory loss (▶ Fig. 115.1)

■ Key Imaging Finding

Faint region of brain stem signal abnormality with ill-defined enhancement

▨ Diagnosis

Capillary telangiectasia. Capillary telangiectases represent dilated vessels that are interspersed between normal brain parenchyma. Although their etiology is uncertain, they are thought to be acquired lesions associated with venous drainage or venous anomalies. The majority are located within the pons; additional locations include the temporal lobes, basal ganglia, and other portions of the brain stem. They are typically small (< 1 cm), incidental, and asymptomatic.

Telangiectases are not visible on computed tomography. Magnetic resonance imaging (MRI) often shows a region of normal or subtly increased T2/fluid-attenuated inversion recovery (FLAIR) signal intensity with ill-defined "brush-like" enhancement. On gradient echo (GRE) or susceptibility-weighted (SWI) sequences, there is hypointense signal due to deoxyhemoglobin within the lesions. There is no mass effect, gliosis, or calcification associated with the lesions. In many cases, there may be a prominent draining vein or associated developmental venous anomaly. If characteristic in appearance, no further imaging workup or follow-up is necessary.

✓ Pearls

- Telangiectases represent dilated capillary-like vessels interspersed between normal brain parenchyma.
- Capillary telangiectases are thought to be acquired lesions; the majority are located within the pons.

- MRI shows subtle increased T2/FLAIR signal, decreased signal on GRE/SWI, and "brush-like" enhancement.

Suggested Reading

Smith AB. Vascular malformations of the brain: radiologic and pathologic correlation. J Am Osteopath Coll Radiol. 2012; 1: 10–22

Case 116

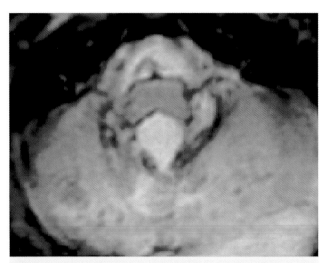

Fig. 116.1 Axial T2* GRE image reveals decreased signal intensity along the surface of the brain stem and cerebellum, as well as along the ependymal surface of the fourth ventricle.

▨ Clinical Presentation

A young boy with headache, hearing loss, and ataxia (▶ Fig. 116.1)

▦ Key Imaging Finding

Decreased gradient echo (GRE) signal along surface of brain and brain stem

▦ Diagnosis

Superficial siderosis. Superficial siderosis refers to subpial and leptomeningeal hemosiderin deposition along the surface of the brain, brain stem, and spinal cord. The hemosiderin results from persistent and repeated bouts of subarachnoid hemorrhage (SAH). Common etiologies include trauma, prior surgery, dural tears, vascular malformations, and neoplasms. Clinically, patients often present with insidious onset of progressive sensorineural hearing loss, ataxia, and dysarthria. In some cases, patients may be asymptomatic. Treatment is geared toward the cause of hemorrhage.

Magnetic resonance imaging (MRI) is the imaging modality of choice for superficial siderosis. T2 GRE and susceptibility-weighted imaging sequences demonstrate pathognomonic hypointensity along the surface of the brain, brain stem, and spinal cord, as well as along the ependymal surface of the ventricles. The brain stem, cerebellum, and spinal cord are most commonly involved, accounting for the presence of cranial neuropathies and cerebellar signs clinically. There is often associated cerebellar atrophy and gliosis.

It is important to not only recognize the presence of superficial siderosis but also to look for the underlying cause. This requires evaluation of the entire neuroaxis and frequently includes angiography to exclude occult vascular malformations.

✓ Pearls

- Superficial siderosis refers to subpial and leptomeningeal hemosiderin from persistent and recurrent SAH.
- Patients often present with insidious onset of progressive sensorineural hearing loss, ataxia, and dysarthria.

- MRI reveals pathognomonic subpial T2/GRE hypointensity along the surface of the brain, brain stem, and cord.
- It is critical to evaluate the entire neuroaxis to look for the underlying cause of hemorrhage.

Suggested Reading

Kumar N. Neuroimaging in superficial siderosis: an in-depth look. Am J Neuroradiol 2010; 31: 5–14

Case 117

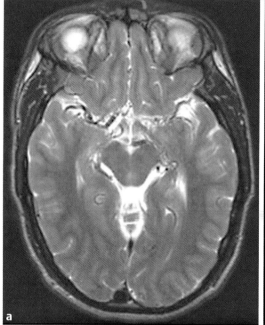

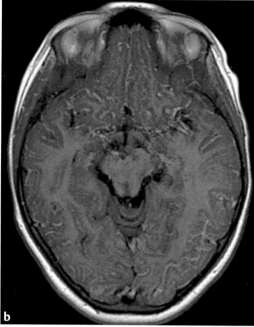

Fig. 117.1 Axial T2 image **(a)** reveals occlusion of the left and severe stenosis of the right carotid terminus with multiple small basal collateral flow voids. Axial T1 postcontrast image **(b)** demonstrates enhancement of the deep perforating (basal) collateral vessels, as well as enhancement of leptomeningeal collateral vessels along the cerebral convexities. Maximum intensity projection image from an MR angiogram **(c)** shows terminal occlusion of the intracranial carotid arteries and proximal M1 segments with multiple small collateral vessels, demonstrating a characteristic smudgy or "puff of smoke" appearance on the left. There is filling of the distal MCA vasculature secondary to corticocortical anastomoses.

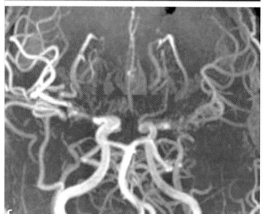

▩ Clinical Presentation

A 16-year-old boy with chronic headaches (▸ Fig. 117.1)

▨ Key Imaging Finding

Carotid terminus occlusion with numerous basal collateral vessels

▨ Diagnosis

Moyamoya. Moyamoya is a relatively rare, progressive, occlusive cerebrovascular disease that primarily involves the intracranial internal carotid and proximal cerebral arteries. The term *"moyamoya"* means "puff of smoke" in Japanese and corresponds to the appearance of abnormal collateral vessels on angiography when first described. The idiopathic variant is commonly seen in Asia. Moyamoya syndrome may be associated with neurofibromatosis type 1 (NF1), sickle cell disease (SCD), Down syndrome, collagen vascular disease (CVD), and prior radiation therapy.

There is a bimodal age distribution involving children within the first decade of life and young adults within the third and fourth decades of life. Children often present with headaches, multiple transient ischemic attacks or infarcts, and seizures. Hemorrhage is more common in adults. Treatment is geared toward the underlying etiology and prevention and management of complications. Depending upon the severity of the disease and symptoms, anticoagulation and vascular bypass procedures, such as superficial temporal artery (STA)–middle cerebral artery (MCA) bypass, may be beneficial.

Unenhanced computed tomography (CT) is useful to evaluate for parenchymal hemorrhage and may also show signs of chronic ischemia, often in a watershed distribution. Magnetic resonance imaging (MRI) is the imaging modality of choice to identify the disease and its complications. T2 sequences reveal stenosis or occlusion of the carotid terminus and portions of the proximal cerebral arteries. Bilateral involvement is common. Multiple enlarged T2 flow voids are seen involving the perforating parenchymal (basilar) vessels near the carotid terminus. Enhanced sequences demonstrate enhancement of the basilar collateral vessels, as well as enhancement of enlarged collateral leptomeningeal veins. The appearance of leptomeningeal collaterals along the cerebral convexities has been described as the "climbing ivy" sign. Dural collaterals are not as well seen on MRI but are readily identified on conventional angiography.

MR angiography demonstrates loss of flow signal at the carotid terminus and proximal cerebral arteries. The enlarged basilar collaterals demonstrate a smudgy or "puff of smoke" appearance. With an appropriate field of view, enlarged leptomeningeal collaterals are well depicted along the cerebral convexities. Findings are similar to those noted on conventional angiography. Conventional angiography offers real-time evaluation and better depiction of dural collaterals. However, given that angiography is an invasive procedure, diagnostic findings on MRI/MR angiography are often sufficient.

CT and MR perfusion may be utilized to monitor disease progression and identify potential candidates for bypass procedures. CT angiography is especially useful because it allows for better visualization of external carotid artery branches (STA) used for bypass. After bypass treatment, perfusion imaging is used to determine if there is improved/adequate reserve in the affected vascular distribution, as well as to directly visualize patency of the STA–MCA anastomosis.

✓ Pearls

- Moyamoya results in progressive occlusion of the intracranial internal carotid and proximal cerebral arteries.
- Moyamoya may be idiopathic or associated with NF1, SCD, Down syndrome, CVD, or prior radiation therapy.

- MR angiography demonstrates occlusion of the carotid terminus and proximal cerebral arteries with multiple collaterals.
- Enlarged basilar collaterals demonstrate a "puff of smoke" appearance on MR and conventional angiography.

Suggested Readings

Burke GM, Burke AM, Sherma AK, Hurley MC, Batjer HH, Bendok BR. Moyamoya disease: a summary. Neurosurg Focus 2009; 26: E11

Geibprasert S, Pongpech S, Jiarakongmun P, Shroff MM, Armstrong DC, Krings T. Radiologic assessment of brain arteriovenous malformations: what clinicians need to know. Radiographics 2010; 30: 483–501

Case 118

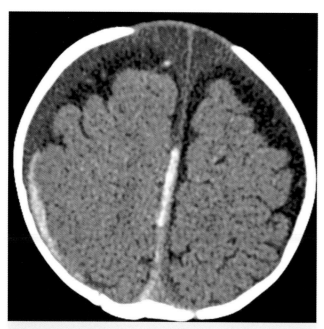

Fig. 118.1 Noncontrast head CT demonstrates acute extraaxial hemorrhages within the interhemispheric fissure/parafalcine region and right posterior convexity, as well as subacute to chronic bilateral frontoparietal subdural hematomas.

■ Clinical Presentation

A 6-month-old female infant brought to the emergency room by her mother, having lost consciousness after rolling off the bed (▶ Fig. 118.1)

■ **Key Imaging Finding**

Subdural hemorrhages of various ages

■ **Diagnosis**

Nonaccidental trauma (NAT). Central nervous system (CNS) injury is the leading cause of morbidity and mortality in NAT and may be seen in up to 40% of cases. CNS injury may result from direct trauma, aggressive shaking, suffocation, or strangulation. Direct trauma and shaking injury often cause regions of intracranial hemorrhage. Ischemic injury occurs with severe trauma (direct or shaking injury), suffocation, and strangulation. Calvarial fractures are seen with direct blunt trauma.

The most common type of intracranial hemorrhage in the setting of NAT is subdural hemorrhage, which may cross sutures but does not cross midline unless it occurs within the posterior fossa. Extension of subdural hemorrhage into the interhemispheric fissure(s) is common in NAT. Subarachnoid hemorrhage is the second most common type of intracranial hemorrhage and may be diffuse or focal. Epidural hemorrhages are often associated with overlying calvarial fractures. Because the infant skull is relatively soft, significant force is required to produce a calvarial fracture. The presence of multiple or depressed calvarial fractures in the absence of an appropriate history is highly suspect of NAT. Parenchymal hemorrhage and shear/diffuse axonal injury may be seen and correspond to severe head injury.

It is important to describe the location, size, and mass effect/complications of extraaxial hemorrhages. Hemorrhages of varying ages are highly suspicious for NAT and present as regions of alternating density (computed tomography, CT) or signal intensity (magnetic resonance imaging, MRI). The presence of septations within a subdural hemorrhage corresponds to chronicity. Aside from identifying hemorrhages of varying ages, radiologists should use caution when asked to "date" hemorrhages. Unlike parenchymal hemorrhages, extraaxial hemorrhages do not follow a predictable pattern of evolution, and the signal intensity on MRI may be multifactorial.

Ischemia is common in severe direct head trauma, aggressive shaking, suffocation, and strangulation. Ischemic changes may be focal, diffuse, or occur in a watershed distribution depending upon the type and severity of the insult, as well as the degree of brain maturation at the time of injury. Infants and young children are prone to brain and neck injury from shaking due to the relatively large head size, prominent subarachnoid spaces, and weak neck musculature. The acceleration and deceleration may result in tearing of cortical bridging veins, cerebral edema, shear/diffuse axonal injury, and, occasionally, cervical vasculature or cord injury.

Retinal hemorrhages are a specific clinical finding for NAT, especially when bilateral. Otherwise, the clinical presentation of NAT is variable and often nonspecific. Therefore, the radiologist plays a critical role in suggesting the diagnosis. The presence of subdural hemorrhage, ischemia, and calvarial fracture(s) in the absence of an appropriate mechanism is highly suspect of NAT. Once NAT is suspected, appropriate notification and imaging needs to be performed. CT better depicts acute intracranial hemorrhage and calvarial fractures. MRI is more sensitive for subtle hemorrhage, ischemia, and focal parenchymal injuries. A skeletal survey should be performed to evaluate for other characteristic injuries associated with NAT. If the patient has siblings, they often warrant a workup for NAT as well.

✓ **Pearls**

• CNS injury associated with NAT may result from direct trauma, violent shaking, suffocation, or strangulation.
• Subdural hemorrhage, ischemia, and skull fractures without appropriate history are highly suggestive of NAT.

• Aside from identifying hemorrhages of varying ages, use caution when asked to "date" hemorrhages.

Suggested Readings

Demaerel P, Casteels I, Wilms G. Cranial imaging in child abuse. Eur Radiol 2002; 12: 849–857

Dias MS. Traumatic brain and spinal cord injury. Pediatr Clin North Am 2004; 51: 271–303

Case 119

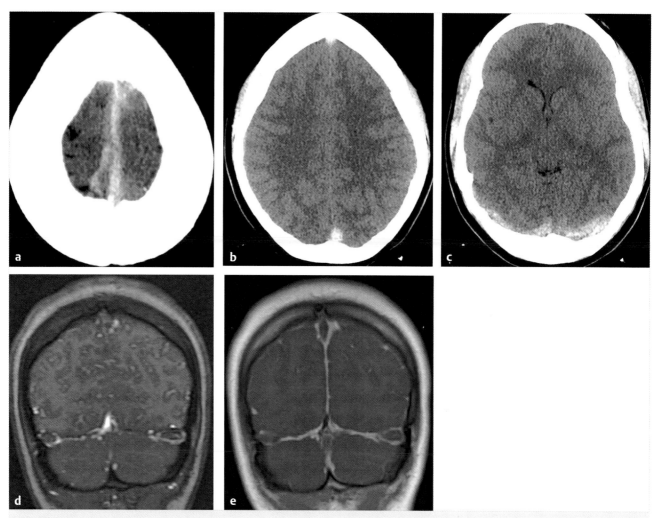

Fig. 119.1 Axial unenhanced CT images **(a–c)** demonstrate hyperattenuation involving the superior sagittal sinus **(a,b)**, cortical veins along the cranial vertex **(a)**, and the transverse sinuses **(c)**. Coronal 2-D TOF MR image **(d)** reveals iso- to hypointense filling defects within the superior sagittal and bilateral transverse sinuses. Minimal hyperintense flow can be seen along the periphery of the filling defects. Corresponding coronal T1 postcontrast image **(e)** shows the "empty delta sign" with enhancement around nonenhancing filling defects within the superior sagittal and transverse sinuses.

■ Clinical Presentation

A 19-year-old woman with persistent, worsening headaches (▶ Fig. 119.1)

▤ Key Imaging Finding

Hyperdense dural venous sinuses (computed tomography, CT) with loss of flow signal (magnetic resonance venography, MRV) and filling defects (postcontrast)

▤ Diagnosis

Venous sinus thrombosis. Venous sinus thrombosis most often occurs in patients with an underlying hypercoagulable state related to trauma, regional or systemic infection, malignancy, pregnancy, medications (including oral contraceptives), dehydration, or inherited coagulopathies. In ~25% of cases, however, a causative factor is not identified. The clinical presentation of venous sinus thrombosis is variable; therefore, imaging plays a critical role in reaching the correct diagnosis. The most common clinical presentation is headaches. Focal neurological deficits and seizures typically result when there are parenchymal abnormalities associated with the venous sinus thrombosis. Treatment consists of anticoagulation and correction of the underlying hypercoagulable state.

Venous sinus thrombosis most often involves the sagittal, transverse, and sigmoid sinuses. At times, congenital variability in sinus development may complicate evaluation for stenosis or occlusion. In some patients, the anterior portion of the superior sagittal sinus is hypoplastic or atretic. Also, most patients have a dominant transverse and sigmoid sinus on one side with variable degrees of hypoplasia on the contralateral side. An additional pitfall is the presence of arachnoid granulations that project into the dural sinuses, most often the distal transverse sinus. A useful discriminator is that arachnoid granulations typically follow cerebrospinal fluid density and signal intensity, whereas thrombus does not.

On unenhanced CT, a thrombosed sinus is typically hyperdense compared with the remaining vascular structures. One caveat is that in the setting of dehydration or increased hematocrit, all vascular structures may be hyperdense. To distinguish between the two, it is helpful to compare arterial and venous density. In the setting of venous thrombosis, the thrombosed venous structure will have increased density compared with the arteries of the circle of Willis. On contrast-enhanced CT,

there is contrast outlining a central hypodense clot, which is referred to as the "empty delta" sign.

On unenhanced MR imaging, routine sequences demonstrate variable signal intensity depending upon the age of the clot secondary to the paramagnetic effects of hemoglobin breakdown products. Acutely (within the first 5 days), thrombus is typically isointense on T1 and hypointense on T2 images, which may mimic a patent flow void on T2. In the subacute stage (6 to 15 days), thrombus is more conspicuous and hyperintense on both T1 and T2. Chronically, the appearance is heterogeneous and variable based upon the degree of recanalization and hemosiderin. Gradient echo or susceptibility-weighted images often demonstrate blooming artifact in the region of thrombus.

MRV is useful for evaluating venous thrombosis. Typically two-dimensional (2-D) time-of-flight (TOF) or contrast-enhanced MRV are utilized. It is important to perform TOF imaging in two planes because in-plane flow may result in loss of signal, which may be mistaken for absent flow. Contrast-enhanced MRV is helpful, especially in the acute phase where decreased T2 signal in the thrombus may mimic patent flow. Findings are similar to CTV with contrast outlining an intraluminal filling defect. In the chronic stage, enhanced MRV is less useful because enhancement may be seen within an organized thrombus or partially recanalized clot, which can be mistaken for a patent sinus.

Parenchymal abnormalities associated with venous thrombosis most often occur when there is venous hypertension or when thrombus extends into superficial veins. Parenchymal complications include cytotoxic or vasogenic edema, infarct, and hemorrhage. One of the more commonly involved superficial veins is the vein of Labbe; occlusion of the vessel often results in characteristic temporal lobe hemorrhage.

✓ Pearls

- Venous thrombosis is hyperdense on unenhanced CT; the "empty delta sign" is seen on enhanced CTV.
- MR signal of thrombus varies based upon chronicity; 2-D TOF MRV is most often used for venous thrombosis.

- Parenchymal findings (edema, infarct, or hemorrhage) typically occur with clot extension into superficial veins.

Suggested Reading

Leach JL, Fortuna RB, Jones BV, Gaskill-Shipley MF. Imaging of cerebral venous thrombosis: current techniques, spectrum of findings, and diagnostic pitfalls. Radiographics 2006; 26 Suppl 1: S19–S41, discussion S42–S43

Case 120

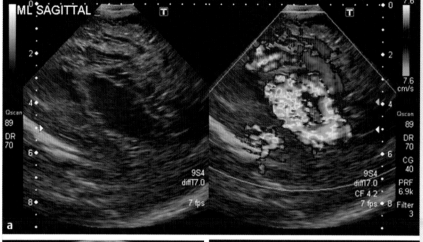

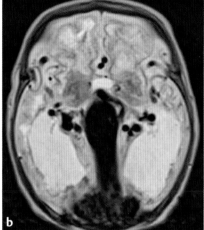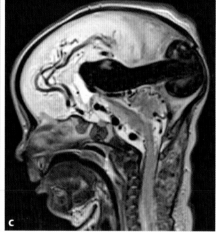

Fig. 120.1 Midline sagittal US images (a) demonstrate a large tubular hypoechoic mass with pronounced vascularity. Axial (b) and sagittal (c) T2 images reveal a large vascular malformation in the region of the vein of Galen, as well as numerous additional enlarged cerebral vessels. The malformation drains into the superior sagittal sinus via a persistent falcine sinus. There is ventriculomegaly with parenchymal volume loss. The sagittal image shows enlargement of the cervical cord and volume loss within the brain stem.

■ Clinical Presentation

A 2-day-old boy with congestive heart failure (▶ Fig. 120.1)

■ Key Imaging Finding

Large vascular malformation draining from the tectal region to the superior sagittal sinus in a neonate

■ Diagnosis

Vein of Galen malformation (VOGM). VOGMs are rare congenital vascular anomalies that result in intracranial arteriovenous (AV) shunting. Patients often present in the neonatal period with congestive heart failure; lesions with a lesser degree of shunting present in early childhood with symptoms related to venous hypertension and ischemia. Due to increased availability and utilization of fetal ultrasound (US) and magnetic resonance imaging (MRI), more and more cases are being detected prenatally, allowing for appropriate care at the time of birth.

VOGMs consist of abnormal connections between choroidal and deep midbrain arteries and the fetal median prosencephalic vein, which normally involutes in the fetal period with development of the vein of Galen. Increased flow within the median prosencephalic vein prevents its involution, and the vein of Galen fails to form. The enlarged median prosencephalic vein drains into the superior sagittal sinus via an enlarged persistent falcine vein/sinus. The straight sinus is typically absent. Additional venous abnormalities include regions of venous stenosis and anomalous venous drainage.

There are two types of VOGM: choroidal and mural. The choroidal type is most common and consists of multiple choroidal and deep midbrain arteries feeding into the anterior aspect of the median prosencephalic vein. The mural variant differs in that the feeding arteries are fewer in number, more lateral in location, and insert into the wall of the median prosencephalic vein. Clinically, the choroidal variant typically presents in the neonatal period with congestive heart failure (CHF); the mural variant is more insidious with a later presentation.

Prior to the availability of endovascular embolization, treatment of VOGMs was limited to surgery, which carried a mortality rate of close to 90%. Embolization has significantly decreased mortality and improved clinical outcomes associated with VOGMs. Liquid embolic agents are preferred, and treatment is directed to the site of fistulization and feeding arteries.

Many patients with VOGMs also have hydrocephalus, which is likely due to decreased cerebrospinal fluid (CSF) resorption related to increased venous pressures. Management of hydrocephalus is controversial because CSF shunting prior to treatment of the VOGM may result in increased AV shunting and worsening of symptoms.

✓ Pearls

- VOGMs result in AV shunting between choroidal arteries and a persistent median prosencephalic vein.
- Patients often present in the neonatal period with CHF; lesions may also be detected during prenatal US or MRI.

- Endovascular treatment directed at the fistula and feeding arteries has greatly improved clinical outcomes.

Suggested Reading

Jones BV, Ball WS, Tomsick TA, Millard J, Crone KR. Vein of Galen aneurysmal malformation: diagnosis and treatment of 13 children with extended clinical follow-up. Am J Neuroradiol 2002; 23: 1717–1724

Case 121

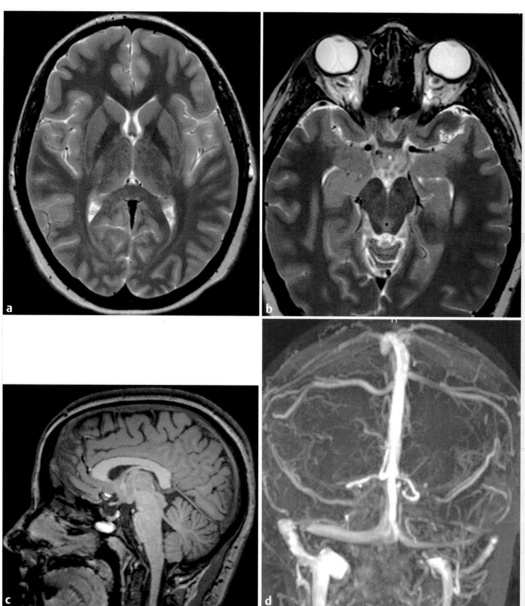

Fig. 121.1 Axial T2 image (a) reveals normal to slightly small ventricles with normal brain parenchyma. Axial T2 image through the orbits (b) shows enlargement of the optic nerve-sheath complexes with flattening and reverse cupping at the optic nerve insertion onto the globes. Sagittal T1 image (c) demonstrates increased cerebrospinal fluid in the sella with flattening of the pituitary gland inferiorly. Increased T1 signal in the sphenoid sinus corresponds to a mucous retention cyst. Maximum intensity projection image from an MR venogram (d) shows narrowing of the distal left transverse sinus.

▪ Clinical Presentation

A young adult woman with progressive headaches (▶ Fig. 121.1)

■ Key Imaging Finding

Small ventricles, partially empty sella, reverse cupping of the globes, and venous sinus stenosis

■ Diagnosis

Pseudotumor cerebri. Pseudotumor cerebri, also known as intracranial hypertension, typically occurs in overweight women of childbearing age. Common presenting symptoms include headache and visual changes. Physical examination findings may include loss of visual acuity and papilledema. The precise etiology remains unknown and is controversial. Although the vast majority of patients with idiopathic intracranial hypertension have stenosis of the transverse sinus, it is debatable whether the stenosis is the cause or result of intracranial hypertension.

Classic imaging findings include decreased size of ventricles, a partially empty sella, increased cerebrospinal fluid within the optic nerve-sheath complex, and flattening or reverse cupping of the globes at the optic nerve insertions. Occasionally, there may be enhancement of the optic nerves, which is thought to represent a combination of venous congestion and breakdown of the blood–nerve barrier. On magnetic resonance (MR) venography, there is narrowing of the transverse sinus in more than 90% of cases.

Many cases of pseudotumor cerebri are self-limited. Treatment options for cases with more severe visual symptoms include carbonic anhydrase inhibitors, steroids, and therapeutic lumbar puncture or lumbar shunts.

✓ Pearls

- Pseudotumor cerebri presents in overweight women of childbearing age with headaches and visual changes.
- MR findings include small ventricles, partially empty sella, flattening of the globes, and venous sinus stenosis.
- Treatment options include carbonic anhydrase inhibitors, steroids, and therapeutic lumbar puncture/shunts.

Suggested Reading

Degnan AJ, Levy LM. Pseudotumor cerebri: brief review of clinical syndrome and imaging findings. Am J Neuroradiol 2011; 32: 1986–1993

Case 122

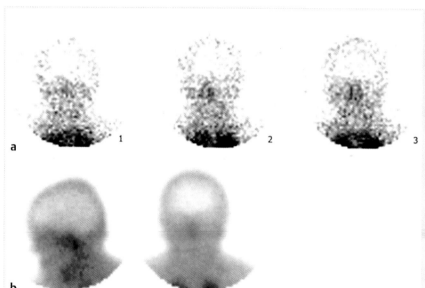

Fig. 122.1 Brain death study with Tc99m-HMPAO. Selected images from dynamic flow (1 second per frame for 1 minute) **(a)** demonstrate absence of intracranial flow. Blood pool imaging in anterior and lateral projections **(b)** reveals absent cerebral or cerebellar uptake and physiological faint scalp activity, along with increased activity in the nasal region ("hot nose" sign). These findings were confirmed on delayed single-photon emission computed tomography imaging of the head (not included). (Case courtesy of Kamal D. Singh, M.D.)

■ Clinical Presentation

A 57-year-old male unresponsive after a motor vehicle accident (▶ Fig. 122.1)

▦ Key Imaging Finding

Absent intracranial activity on technetium 99 m hexamethyl-propyleneamine oxime (Tc99m-HMPAO) scan

▦ Diagnosis

Brain death. Brain death is a clinical diagnosis utilizing a combination of physical examination, electroencephalogram (EEG), and imaging findings. Brain death scan has a high specificity as a confirmatory study for absent intracranial perfusion. Scintigraphic imaging can be performed at the patient's bedside with a portable gamma camera. Imaging may be performed with a nonspecific flow agent (Tc99 m diethylene-triamine-pentaacetate [Tc99m-DTPA]) or with lipophilic brain perfusion agents (Tc99m-HMPAO or Tc99 m ethyl cysteinate dimer [Tc99m-ECD]), which are extracted by viable brain tissue proportional to cerebral flow. A scalp band or tourniquet may be placed around the head to avoid interfering activity from extracranial vessels. The scalp band, however, is contraindicated in pediatric patients due to increased intracranial pressure.

First minute dynamic flow imaging is performed in an anterior projection with subsequent static blood pool images in both anterior and lateral projections. Delayed single-photon emission computed tomography imaging may improve sensitivity in cases where brain perfusion agents are utilized. Normal imaging reveals symmetric flow within the anterior and middle cerebral arteries ("trident sign") on anterior view with visualization of dural venous sinuses on blood pool imaging. In brain death, there is termination of carotid activity at the skull base due to increased intracranial pressure overcoming perfusion pressure, thereby shunting blood through the external carotid artery branches projecting over nasal region ("hot nose" sign).

Appropriate quality control is necessary to prevent mistakenly calling brain death in the setting of a poor radiopharmaceutical bolus. Peripheral intravenous injection of the radiotracer is performed as a rapid/tight bolus. A proper bolus is confirmed by visualizing distinct activity within the proximal common carotid arteries. Dose infiltration, slow radiotracer injection, or missed bolus can result in false-positive studies, especially when flow agents (such as Tc99m-DTPA, which does not cross the blood–brain barrier) are utilized. Tc99m-DTPA is rapidly cleared through renal excretion, which allows for re-injection and re-imaging in the setting of equivocal or technically limited studies.

✓ Pearls

- Brain death scan has a high specificity as a confirmatory study for absent intracranial perfusion.
- Scintigraphic imaging can be performed with a nonspecific flow agent or lipophilic brain perfusion agents.
- A normal study shows cerebral artery flow on anterior view and dural venous sinuses on blood pool imaging.
- Absent intracranial flow with the presence of the "hot nose" sign confirms brain death.

Suggested Reading

Conrad GR, Sinha P. Scintigraphy as a confirmatory test of brain death. Semin Nucl Med 2003; 33: 312–323

Case 123

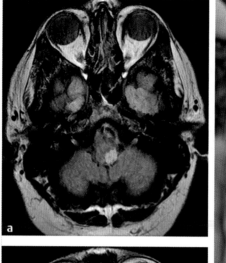
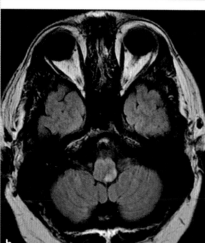
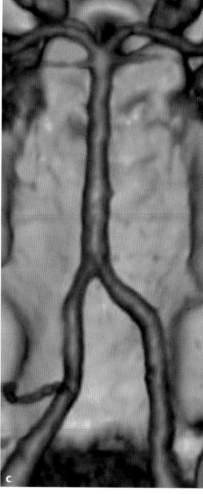

Fig. 123.1 Axial FLAIR images **(a,b)** demonstrate abnormal increased signal intensity within the posterolateral medulla on the left. Three-dimensional volume rendered image from a computed tomography angiogram (CTA) **(c)** reveals absence of the left PICA; a portion of the proximal right PICA is visualized on the contralateral side. Although visualization of PICA on CTA is variable, occlusion was confirmed on conventional angiogram (not shown).

■ Clinical Presentation

A 42-year-old man with left facial and contralateral body sensory loss, left-sided ptosis, hoarseness, and vertigo (► Fig. 123.1)

■ Key Imaging Finding

Abnormal increased fluid-attenuated inversion recovery (FLAIR) signal along the posterolateral medulla

■ Diagnosis

Lateral medullary syndrome (LMS). LMS or Wallenberg syndrome classically results from occlusion of the posterior inferior cerebellar artery (PICA) with associated infarct of the posterolateral medulla. Similar findings may be seen with involvement of the vertebral artery as well. The majority of cases occur in older patients secondary to thromboembolic disease; in younger patients, vertebral artery dissection associated with trauma or vasculopathies are the most common etiologies.

Clinically, patients present acutely with loss of pain and temperature sensation involving the ipsilateral face and contralateral body, ipsilateral Horner syndrome, ipsilateral limb ataxia, and vertigo. Hoarseness and difficulty swallowing commonly occur secondary to cranial nerve involvement. The clinical symptoms and prognosis correlate well with the overall size of the infarct; patients with larger infarcts have a worse prognosis. The majority of patients, however, have a relatively good outcome with improvement of symptoms over time.

Computed tomography is often normal due to the inherent difficulty in evaluating posterior fossa structures. Magnetic resonance imaging (MRI) is more sensitive, demonstrating regions of increased T2/FLAIR signal along the posterolateral medulla. Isolated medullary lesions may be subtle and only visualized on the inferior-most axial images. Larger infarcts may also involve the inferior cerebellum and are more conspicuous. Restricted diffusion and mass effect/edema is seen acutely. Subtle enhancement may be seen in the subacute phase. Chronically, there is volume loss of the involved segments.

✓ Pearls

- LMS classically results from occlusion of PICA with associated infarct of the posterolateral medulla.
- Symptoms include loss of pain/temperature sensation, Horner syndrome, limb ataxia, hoarseness, and vertigo.

- MRI reveals increased T2/FLAIR signal and restricted diffusion (acutely) along the posterolateral medulla.
- Isolated medullary lesions may be subtle and only visualized on the inferior-most axial MR images.

Suggested Reading

Kim JS, Lee JH, Suh DC, Lee MC. Spectrum of lateral medullary syndrome. Correlation between clinical findings and magnetic resonance imaging in 33 subjects. Stroke 1994; 25: 1405–1410

Case 124

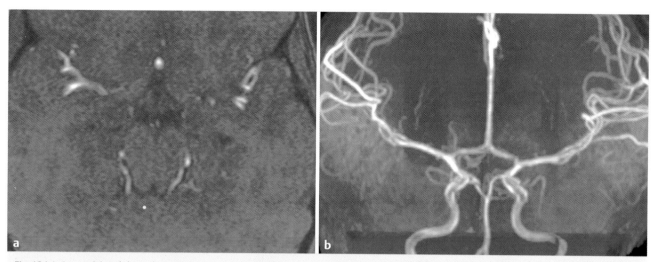

Fig. 124.1 Source **(a)** and three-dimensional volume rendered **(b)** magnetic resonance angiography images through the circle of Willis demonstrate a solitary vertical A2 segment of the ACA and absence of the ACOM.

■ Clinical Presentation

A young girl with a known congenital brain malformation (▶ Fig. 124.1)

■ Key Imaging Finding

Solitary vertical A2 segment of the anterior cerebral artery (ACA)

■ Diagnosis

Azygous anterior cerebral artery (ACA). The ACA represents the anterior branch of the internal carotid artery after its bifurcation into the anterior and middle cerebral arteries. The horizontal or A1 segment extends anteriorly for a short distance, communicates with the contralateral A1 segment via the anterior communicating artery (ACOM), and then extends vertically into the A2 segment within the interhemispheric fissure. The dominant branches of the A2 segment include the callosomarginal and pericallosal arteries.

A solitary or azygous vertical A2 segment of the ACA is a relatively uncommon vascular variant that may occur sporadically or in association with syndromes such as holoprosencephaly. A more common anatomic variant is bihemispheric ACAs where there are two vertical A2 segments, one of which is dominant and the second of which is diminutive. A true azygous ACA presents an underlying risk for both ischemic disease of the bilateral ACA territories with underlying stenosis, occlusion, or arterial injury, as well as an increased risk for aneurysms within the distal ACA vascular distribution due to altered hemodynamic flow. An azygous ACA is in the differential for patients who present with bilateral ACA territory infarcts, along with more common entities such as bilateral ACA injury due to trauma or subfalcine herniation and thromboembolic disease involving portions of both ACAs.

On cross-sectional imaging or angiography, an azygous ACA presents as a solitary, midline A2 segment that originates directly from the bilateral A1 segments. There is typically absence of an ACOM. It is important to look for additional findings or anomalies involving development of the prosencephalon (e.g., holoprosencephaly variants), as well as the presence of aneurysms.

✓ Pearls

- An azygous ACA may occur sporadically or in association with syndromes such as holoprosencephaly.
- An azygous ACA presents a risk for bilateral ACA territory infarcts and an increased risk of distal aneurysms.

- Cross-sectional imaging or angiography shows a solitary midline A2 segment and absence of the ACOM.

Suggested Reading

LeMay M, Gooding CA. The clinical significance of the azygos anterior cerebral artery (A.C.A.). Am J Roentgenol Radium Ther Nucl Med 1966; 98: 602–610

Case 125

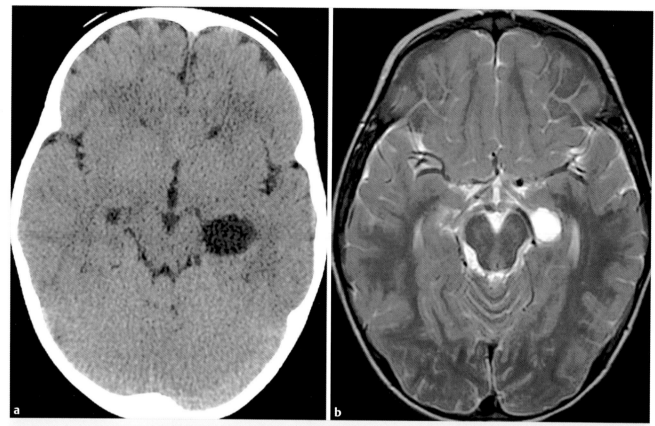

Fig. 125.1 Axial computed tomography image **(a)** demonstrates a well-circumscribed CSF density mass in the left choroidal fissure. Axal T2 magnetic resonance image **(b)** at a sequential level reveals similar findings with the lesion in the choroidal fissure following CSF signal intensity.

■ Clinical Presentation

A young man with chronic headaches (▶ Fig. 125.1)

◼ Key Imaging Finding

Cerebrospinal fluid (CSF) cyst within the choroidal fissure

◼ Diagnosis

Choroidal fissure cyst. A choroidal fissure cyst is a type of neuroepithelial/neuroglial or arachnoid cyst that occurs within the choroidal fissure. The choroidal fissure anatomically represents a cleft along the wall of the lateral ventricle, thalamus, fornix, and hippocampus. It is the site of attachment of the choroid plexus. Other common locations of neuroepithelial or neuroglial cysts include the cerebral hemispheres (frontal lobes most common), thalami, and brain stem. These congenital cysts are relatively uncommon. The neuroepithelial or neuroglial variant represents sequestered neural tube elements that do not communicate with the ventricles and are lined by ependymal or choroid plexus cells. On imaging, the cysts are smooth, unilocular, nonenhancing, and follow CSF signal on all sequences. There is typically no (or minimal) surrounding parenchymal signal abnormality.

✓ Pearls

- A choroidal fissure cyst is a type of neuroepithelial or arachnoid cyst that occurs within the choroidal fissure.
- Congenital variants represent sequestered neural tube elements that do not communicate with the ventricles.

- Choroidal fissure cysts are smooth, unilocular, nonenhancing, and follow CSF signal on all sequences.

Suggested Readings

Osborn AG, Preece MT. Intracranial cysts: radiologic-pathologic correlation and imaging approach. Radiology 2006; 239: 650–664

Sherman JL, Camponovo E, Citrin CM. MR imaging of CSF-like choroidal fissure and parenchymal cysts of the brain. Am J Roentgenol 1990; 155: 1069–1075

Case 126

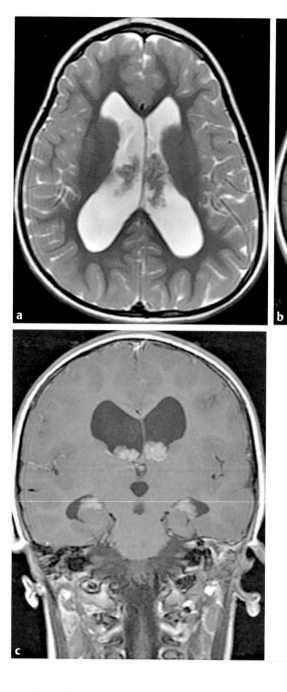

Fig. 126.1 Axial T2-weighted image **(a)** reveals diffuse enlargement of the choroid plexus within the lateral ventricles, as well as lateral ventricular enlargement. Axial **(b)** and coronal **(c)** contrast-enhanced T1-weighted images show avid, symmetric enhancement and enlargement of the choroid plexus without a focal mass. Both the lateral and third ventricles are enlarged on the coronal image.

■ Clinical Presentation

A 4-year-old girl with headaches (▶ Fig. 126.1)

▒ Key Imaging Finding

Diffuse, symmetric choroid plexus enlargement without focal mass

▒ Diagnosis

Villous hyperplasia of the choroid plexus. Villous hyperplasia of the choroid plexus is a rare congenital abnormality characterized by diffuse, symmetric enlargement of the choroid plexus. Patients present with communicating hydrocephalus due to overproduction of cerebrospinal fluid (CSF). On pathological examination, the choroid plexus cells have a normal appearance but are increased in number. Magnetic resonance imaging (MRI) and computed tomography (CT) demonstrate diffuse, symmetric choroid plexus enlargement and enhancement without focal mass, which distinguishes this entity from focal lesions such as choroid plexus papilloma or carcinoma. Treatment options include CSF shunting versus choroid plexus resection or coagulation.

✓ Pearls

- Villous hyperplasia is characterized by diffuse, symmetric choroid plexus enlargement.
- Patients present with communicating hydrocephalus due to overproduction of CSF.
- MRI and CT demonstrate diffuse choroid plexus enlargement and enhancement without focal mass.
- Treatment options for hydrocephalus include CSF shunting versus choroid plexus resection/coagulation.

Suggested Reading

Naeini RM, Yoo JH, Hunter JV. Spectrum of choroid plexus lesions in children. Am J Roentgenol 2009; 192: 32–40

Case 127

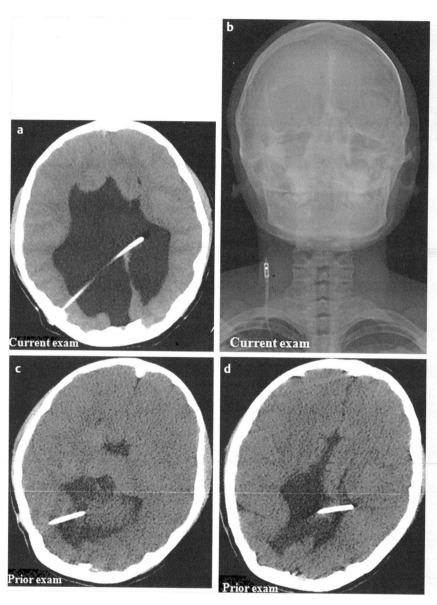

Fig. 127.1 Unenhanced axial CT image (**a**) demonstrates significant ventricular enlargement compared with the baseline examination (**c,d**). A right posterior approach ventricular drainage catheter is identified. Frontal radiograph of the skull and neck from a shunt series (**b**) shows discontinuity of the VP shunt within the soft tissues of the neck on the right. (Courtesy of Michael Zapadka, DO.)

■ Clinical Presentation

A 12-year-old boy with altered mental status and a history of Chiari II malformation with ventriculoperitoneal (VP) shunting (▶ Fig. 127.1)

■ **Key Imaging Finding**

Interval dilatation of ventricles and clinical decline in a patient with a VP shunt

■ **Diagnosis**

Shunt catheter malfunction. Hydrocephalus may result from obstruction, overproduction, or reduced resorption of cerebrospinal fluid (CSF). Communicating hydrocephalus occurs secondary to decreased resorption of CSF at the arachnoid villi and may be due to hemorrhage, infection, carcinomatosis, or arachnoid villi immaturity. Noncommunicating hydrocephalus is caused by a congenital or acquired obstruction of CSF at the ventricular level. Overproduction of CSF is seen in the setting of tumors or villous hypertrophy of the choroid plexus.

VP shunting remains the most common treatment for chronic hydrocephalus. VP shunts consist of the intraventricular drainage catheter, an extracranial valve and reservoir, and a catheter that extends throughout the superficial soft tissues and into the peritoneum. Shunt malfunctions are unfortunately common in chronically shunted patients. Malfunction may be mechanical (most common) or due to an underlying infection. Common presenting symptoms include headache, irritability, lethargy, nausea, and vomiting. Additional symptoms include fever and localizing pain. Young children with open sutures often present with increasing head size. Clinically, slowed filling of the shunt reservoir is suggestive of malfunction.

Mechanical failure may result from obstruction of the shunt catheter, disconnections or breaks in the catheter tubing system, and migration. Obstruction is most common at the intraventricular end of the shunt catheter and may be caused by proteinaceous material (hemorrhage, infection, tumor), brain parenchyma, or choroid plexus obstructing the inflow of CSF. Distal obstruction at the peritoneal end is less common and typically results from peritoneal adhesions near the catheter tip. Occasionally, an intraventricular cyst or abdominal pseudocyst may obstruct CSF flow. Nuclear medicine radioisotope or contrast-enhanced computed tomography (CT) or fluoroscopic shunt studies can be used to evaluate for obstruction within the VP shunt system.

Disconnection of shunt components most often occurs where catheter tubing connects to the reservoir. Breaks occur in regions of increased mobility, such as the neck. Migration typically affects the proximal or distal end of the VP shunt catheter. When interpreting a plain film shunt study, it is important to know the type of catheter used, particularly with respect to the portions that are normally radio-opaque and radiolucent, to avoid mistaking normal radiolucent portions of the tubing as regions of discontinuity. If needed, cross-sectional imaging can be used for problem solving. A focal fluid collection may be identified at the site of malfunction.

CT or magnetic resonance imaging (MRI) (preferred) of the brain most often demonstrates ventricular enlargement with shunt malfunction; however, this finding is not entirely sensitive or specific. False-negatives occur with scarring along the ventricles or decreased parenchymal compliance. Conversely, ventricular enlargement may be seen with normally functioning shunts. Secondary findings of shunt malfunction include sulcal and cisternal effacement and transependymal flow of CSF, which suggest uncompensated, acute hydrocephalus. Complications of VP shunting also include slit ventricle syndrome and subdural fluid collections. Etiologies of slit ventricle syndrome include overshunting, fibrosis, decreased parenchymal compliance, and intracranial hypotension. Overdrainage may result in subdural hematomas or hygromas. Typically, subdural collections are self-limited.

Shunt infections most often occur within the first few months of catheter placement. Patients present with signs of shunt malfunction, as well as fever. Imaging may be normal or demonstrate findings associated with ventriculitis or meningitis, to include abnormal T2/fluid-attenuated inversion recovery signal intensity and enhancement along the margins of the ventricles and meninges. Replacement of the infected shunt is often necessary.

✓ **Pearls**

- Shunt malfunction is common in chronically shunted patients and may be mechanical or related to infection.
- It is important to know the type of catheter used and which portions are normally radio-opaque and radiolucent.
- CT or MRI (preferred) most often demonstrate ventricular enlargement in the setting of shunt failure.
- Overshunting may result in slit ventricle syndrome and subdural hematomas or hygromas.

Suggested Reading

Goeser CD, McLeary MS, Young LW. Diagnostic imaging of ventriculoperitoneal shunt malfunctions and complications. Radiographics 1998; 18: 635–651

Case 128

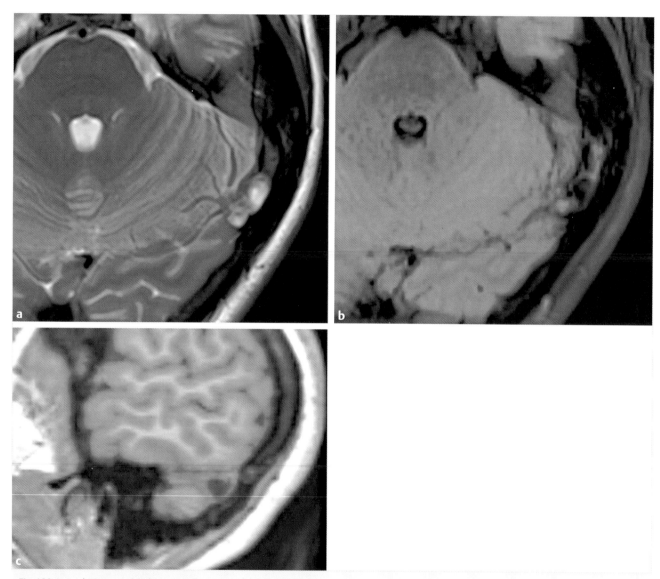

Fig. 128.1 Axial T2 image **(a)** shows a well-circumscribed ovoid hyperintense lesion within the distal left transverse sinus at a venous entry site. The majority of the lesion follows CSF signal intensity on fluid-attenuated inversion recovery **(b)** with signal loss. Off-midline sagittal T1 image through the distal left transverse sinus **(c)** reveals hypointense signal intensity, similar to that of CSF, within the lesion.

▪ Clinical Presentation

A 19-year-old woman with headaches (▸ Fig. 128.1)

■ Key Imaging Finding

Well-circumscribed T1 hypointense, T2 hyperintense lesion within a dural sinus

■ Diagnosis

Arachnoid granulation. Arachnoid granulations represent protuberances of the leptomeninges that extend into the lumen of dural venous sinuses, particularly the sagittal, transverse, and sigmoid sinuses. They are normal, incidental structures but may be mistaken for dural sinus pathology, such as thrombus, on cross-sectional imaging studies.

Arachnoid granulations are similar to arachnoid villi but are exponentially larger (villi are microscopic) and more complex. Their precise function remains unclear; however, they are thought to play a role in cerebrospinal fluid (CSF) resorption, similar to arachnoid villi. They are commonly seen at venous entry sites and have increased incidence and conspicuity with age. Although anatomically they are most frequently seen in the sagittal sinus, on imaging studies, they are most commonly identified in the distal transverse sinus.

On contrast-enhanced computed tomography (CT), arachnoid granulations present as focal, well-circumscribed filling defects within the dural venous sinus, surrounded by enhancing portions of the dural sinus. They are typically hypodense, similar in attenuation to CSF, but they may occasionally be isodense relative to brain parenchyma. On magnetic resonance imaging (MRI), arachnoid granulations are hypointense on T1 and hyperintense on T2 sequences with variable signal intensity on proton density and fluid-attenuated inversion recovery sequences. Lesions do not demonstrate contrast enhancement.

The characteristic locations and imaging appearance of arachnoid granulations are helpful in distinguishing them from venous thrombosis, which typically involves an entire segment of a dural venous sinus or multiple segments with extension into cortical veins. Thrombus is often hyperdense on CT and hyperintense on unenhanced T1-weighted MR sequences, especially with acute or subacute thrombus. Secondary signs of venous hypertension, such as collateralization, meningeal enhancement, parenchymal edema, and hemorrhage, may be seen with venous sinus thrombosis, especially with extension of thrombus into cortical veins. These are never seen in the setting of arachnoid granulations.

As normal structures, arachnoid granulations are incidental, asymptomatic lesions that require no treatment or follow-up.

✓ Pearls

- Arachnoid granulations represent protuberances of leptomeninges that extend into a dural venous sinus lumen.
- Functionally, arachnoid granulations are similar to arachnoid villi but are much larger and more complex.

- Arachnoid granulations are most common in the sagittal, transverse, and sigmoid sinuses at venous entry points.
- Arachnoid granulations are normal structures that are well-circumscribed, T1 hypo-, and T2 hyperintense.

Suggested Reading

Leach JL, Jones BV, Tomsick TA, Stewart CA, Balko MG. Normal appearance of arachnoid granulations on contrast-enhanced CT and MR of the brain: differentiation from dural sinus disease. Am J Neuroradiol 1996; 17: 1523–1532

Section II

Head and Neck

Case 129

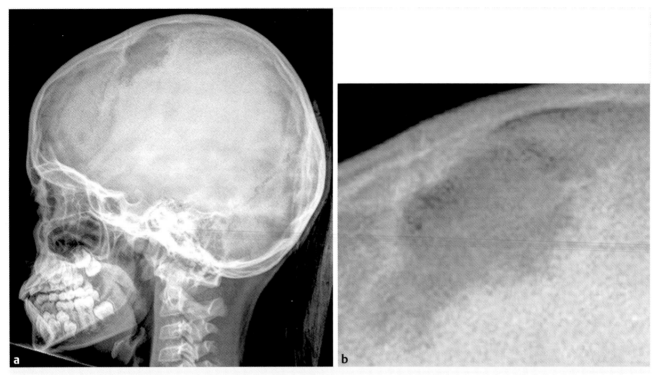

Fig. 129.1 Lateral radiograph of the skull **(a)** demonstrates a solitary lytic lesion with lobulated margins and well-defined borders involving the parietal bone just posterior to the coronal suture. Coned-down view **(b)** reveals a "beveled edge" appearance without sclerotic margins.

▧ Clinical Presentation

A 9-year-old girl with headaches (▶ Fig. 129.1)

■ Key Imaging Finding

Lytic skull lesion in a child

■ Top 3 Differential Diagnoses

- **Langerhans cell histiocytosis (LCH).** The skull is the most common location for osseous involvement in LCH. The classic radiological description is a well-defined lytic lesion without sclerotic borders. A "beveled" edge appearance often results from greater involvement of the inner than outer table of the skull. LCH may also present as a round, radiolucent skull defect with a central dense nidus or sequestrum of intact bone, referred to as a "button sequestrum." The most common clinical symptoms include pain, palpable mass, and/or systemic symptoms. Magnetic resonance imaging (MRI) reveals a T1 hypointense and T2 intermediate to hyperintense soft-tissue mass with moderate enhancement associated with an osseous defect.
- **Epidermoid cyst.** Epidermoid cysts result from abnormal deposition of epithelial rests within the diploic space during development. They are a relatively common cause of solitary lytic skull lesions in the pediatric population and tend to occur along sutural lines. When an epidermoid cyst involves the diploic space, the radiographical appearance may overlap

that of LCH. Epidermoid cysts are generally well-defined expansile lesions without a central matrix. They may or may not have a sclerotic rim. On MRI, epidermoid cysts are iso- to hypointense to cerebrospinal fluid (CSF) on T1 and iso- to hyperintense on T2 with characteristic increased signal on diffusion-weighted imaging.
- **Malignancy.** The most common malignancies to involve the calvarium in children include lymphoma, leukemia, Ewing sarcoma, and metastatic neuroblastoma. Rhabdomyosarcoma may also invade the calvarium via direct spread. Malignancies often result in bony expansion and destruction, which manifests as poorly defined lucencies. Aggressive periosteal reaction may be noted, especially with Ewing sarcoma. Lesions may be solitary or multiple; multiple lesions are suggestive of hematogenous spread. On MRI, malignancies demonstrate marrow infiltration or bony expansion and destruction with a soft-tissue mass. The soft-tissue component is typically hypointense on T1 and hyperintense on T2 with avid but heterogeneous enhancement.

■ Additional Differential Diagnoses

- **Infection.** Osteomyelitis has a variety of imaging manifestations, which range from a normal appearance to an aggressive appearance that mimics a neoplastic process. Bony destruction from osteomyelitis commonly results in lytic calvarial lesions that often have poorly defined, infiltrating margins. There may be overlying soft-tissue swelling. Subacute and chronic infections may present radiographically as a round, radiolucent skull defect with a central dense nidus or sequestrum of intact bone, referred to as a "button sequestrum." On MRI, osteomyelitis presents as regions of marrow infiltration or bony destruction with variable enhancement.

- **Leptomeningeal cyst.** The term *leptomeningeal cyst* (growing skull fracture) refers to a well-defined bony defect that arises when traumatic laceration of the dura exposes the bone to the pulsations of CSF within the subarachnoid space. Pulsatile pressure erosion gradually widens the fracture line. Leptomeningeal cysts are an uncommon complication of skull fractures and are most common in children < 3 years of age. Cross-sectional imaging demonstrates CSF attenuation or signal without an underlying soft-tissue component.

■ Diagnosis

Langerhans cell histiocytosis

✓ Pearls

- LCH classically presents as a lytic skull lesion with nonsclerotic, "beveled" margins.
- LCH and osteomyelitis can have "button sequestra" and systemic symptoms.

- Common malignant skull lesions in children include lymphoma, leukemia, Ewing sarcoma, and neuroblastoma.
- A leptomeningeal cyst (growing skull fracture) is caused by CSF pulsations from disruption of the dura.

Suggested Readings

Gibson SE, Prayson RA. Primary skull lesions in the pediatric population: a 25-year experience. Arch Pathol Lab Med 2007; 131: 761–766

Glass RBJ, Fernbach SK, Norton KI, Choi PS, Naidich TP. The infant skull: a vault of information. Radiographics 2004; 24: 507–522

Krasnokutsky MV. The button sequestrum sign. Radiology 2005; 236: 1026–1027

Yalçin O, Yildirim T, Kizilkiliç O et al. CT and MRI findings in calvarial non-infectious lesions. Diagn Interv Radiol 2007; 13: 68–74

Case 130

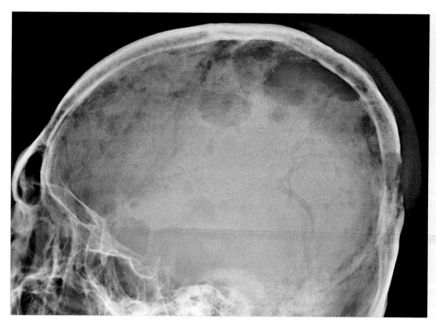

Fig. 130.1 Lateral skull radiograph reveals multiple circumscribed calvarial lucencies of various sizes without sclerotic margins. Many of the lesions have a "punched out" appearance. (Courtesy of Eva Escobedo, MD.)

■ Clinical Presentation

A 42-year-old man with generalized aches and pain (► Fig. 130.1)

■ Key Imaging Finding

Lytic skull lesion(s) in an adult

■ Top 3 Differential Diagnoses

- **Malignancy.** Metastases, multiple myeloma, and lymphoma are common causes of solitary or multiple (more common) lytic calvarial lesions in adults. Primary sites of metastatic disease include lung, breast, prostate, renal, and thyroid carcinomas. Lung metastases are lytic; prostate lesions are sclerotic; and breast metastases may be lytic or sclerotic. Renal and thyroid lesions are often solitary, hypervascular, and may also be lytic or sclerotic. Metastatic disease may appear as enhancing regions of marrow infiltration or soft-tissue masses with bony destruction. Multiple myeloma is the most common primary bone tumor in adults; plasmacytoma is the solitary form. Myeloma lesions appear as well-defined "punched out" lesions with involvement of both the inner and outer tables of the calvarium. The soft-tissue component is hypointense on T1 and hyperintense on T2 images with enhancement. A skeletal survey should be performed to identify additional areas of involvement. Lymphoma is similar in appearance to metastatic disease with an enhancing lytic calvarial lesion.
- **Fibrous dysplasia (FD).** FD occurs most often in young adults and is more common in women. The calvarium and facial bones are most often affected in the head and neck. The classic appearance on computed tomography (CT) is focal bony expansion with "ground glass" attenuation of the diploic space. However, sclerotic and cystic variants due occur; the cystic variant may mimic a lytic lesion. On magnetic resonance imaging (MRI), FD is typically hypointense on both T1 and T2 sequences and demonstrates avid enhancement. Regions of cystic involvement are less characteristic because they are often hyperintense on T2 sequences. The MRI appearance can mimic aggressive lesions; therefore, CT is preferred in suspected cases of FD.
- **Paget disease.** Paget disease occurs in elderly patients and consists of three stages: lytic, sclerotic, and mixed. Calvarial involvement during the lytic phase results in a characteristic large lytic lesion with erosion of the outer table, referred to as osteoporosis circumscripta. During the sclerotic phase, there is expansion and sclerosis of the cortex and diploic spaces, which may be diffuse or focal. In the mixed phase, a combination of lytic and sclerotic lesions results in the characteristic "cotton wool" appearance of the skull.

■ Additional Differential Diagnoses

- **Surgical defect.** Surgical defects may be secondary to burr holes or craniotomy; craniotomy changes are typically obvious. Bur holes are well-circumscribed and most often located over the frontal lobes (right > left). There is no associated soft-tissue component, unless portions of the meninges and/or parenchyma extend into the defect. Occasionally, a hypodense (CT) or T2 hyperintense (MRI) tract may be seen in cases of prior shunt catheter or intracranial monitor placement.
- **Epidermoid cyst.** Epidermoid cysts result from abnormal deposition of epithelial rests within the diploic space during development. They are generally well-defined expansile lesions without a central matrix. They may or may not have a sclerotic rim. On MRI, epidermoid cysts are iso- to hypointense to CSF on T1 and iso- to hyperintense on T2 with characteristic increased signal on diffusion-weighted imaging.
- **Metabolic disease.** Hyperparathyroidism (HPT) may be primary due to hyperfunctioning parathyroid glands, secondary due to vitamin D deficiency or chronic renal failure, or tertiary due to hyperplasia from long-standing secondary HPT. Increased parathormone results in systemic calcium/bony resorption. In the skull, this manifests as alternating regions of lucency and sclerosis, referred to as the "salt and pepper" appearance. In advanced cases, focal Brown tumors may occur, presenting as well-circumscribed lytic lesions that are often multiple.

■ Diagnosis

Malignancy (multiple myeloma)

✓ Pearls

- Metastases, multiple myeloma, and lymphoma often involve the skull; myeloma has "punched out" lesions.
- Paget disease of the skull may result in osteoporosis circumscripta, sclerosis, or a "cotton wool" appearance.
- HPT manifests as alternating regions of lucency and sclerosis, referred to as a "salt and pepper" appearance.

Suggested Reading

Yalçin O, Yildirim T, Kizilkiliç O et al. CT and MRI findings in calvarial non-infectious lesions. Diagn Interv Radiol 2007; 13: 68–74

Case 131

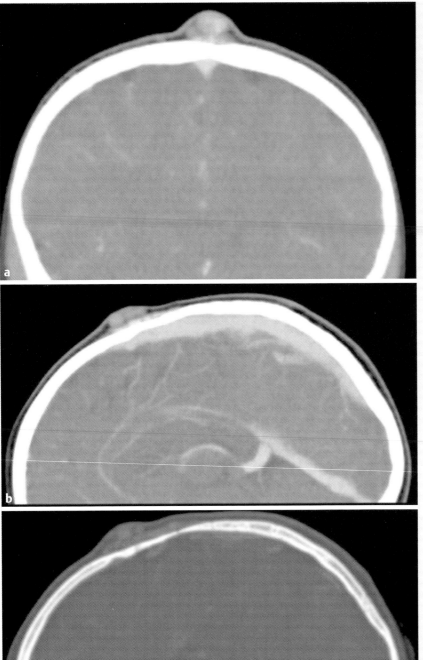

Fig. 131.1 Coronal **(a)** and sagittal **(b)** reformatted postcontrast CT images reveal a circumscribed, avidly enhancing, midline scalp mass with tubular components **(b)**. The sagittal reformatted image in bone window **(c)** shows an intact calvarium and absence of intracranial communication/extension.

Clinical Presentation

A 6-year-old girl with a soft "bump" on the head (▶ Fig. 131.1)

▨ Key Imaging Finding

Enhancing scalp lesion in a child

■ Top 3 Differential Diagnoses

- **Hemangioma.** Hemangiomas are benign lesions composed of endothelial cells and commonly occur in the head and neck (~60%). They are often solitary and sporadic; however, they may be multiple in the setting of PHACES syndrome (posterior fossa malformations, hemangiomas, arterial anomalies, cardiac defects, eye abnormalities, and sternal cleft and supra-umbilical raphe syndrome). Lesions are categorized as infantile (most common), which typically occur within the first few weeks of life, proliferate in infancy and early childhood, and involute within the first decade of life with fatty replacement; or congenital, which are present at birth and either involute shortly thereafter (rapidly involuting congenital hemangioma [RICH]) or do not involute (noninvoluting congenital hemangioma [NICH]). On computed tomography (CT) and magnetic resonance imaging (MRI), lesions are well-defined, lobulated, and avidly enhance. They are characteristically hyperintense on T2 sequences. They are typically located within superficial soft tissues but may extend into multiple compartments. Treatment is reserved for symptomatic lesions with mass effect on vital structures.
- **Venolymphatic malformation (VM).** VMs are congenital anomalies that are part of the spectrum of low-flow venolymphatic malformations. They commonly occur in the head and neck region (~40%), and the majority are solitary and sporadic; however, multiple lesions may be seen in the setting of

Klippel-Trenaunay-Weber (bony overgrowth/hypertrophy), Maffucci (multiple enchondromatosis), and blue rubber bleb nevus (superficial and visceral hemangiomas) syndromes. Unlike infantile hemangiomas, they are present at birth and do not undergo involution. Growth is seen in childhood proportional to somatic growth. On imaging, lesions are typically circumscribed and may be multicystic with avid enhancement. Thrombosis may complicate the imaging findings. Phleboliths are characteristic and are hyperdense on CT and hypointense on MRI.
- **Sinus pericranii.** Sinus pericranii refers to anomalous transosseous communication between extracranial and intracranial venous structures, typically a dural venous sinus. It most often presents in childhood as a blue or purplish soft scalp mass that increases in size when lying flat or with Valsalva maneuvers. Ultrasound reveals a superficial vascular scalp mass that extends intracranially via a dilated transdiploic vein. The extracranial component may be circumscribed or consist of a single or multiple dilated veins. CT is ideal for identifying the underlying osseous defect, which may be subtle; the venous communication is best depicted on CT or MR venography. MR venography is often preferred due to the lack of ionizing radiation. On routine MR sequences, the scalp mass is T1 iso- to hypointense and T2 hyperintense with avid enhancement. Treatment is surgical.

■ Additional Differential Diagnoses

- **Langerhans cell histiocytosis (LCH).** The skull is the most common location for osseous involvement in LCH. The classic radiological description is a well-defined lytic lesion without sclerotic borders. A "beveled" edge appearance often results from greater involvement of the inner than outer table of the skull. LCH may also present as a round, radiolucent skull defect with a central dense nidus or sequestrum of intact bone, referred to as a "button sequestrum." The most common clinical symptoms include pain, palpable mass, and/or systemic symptoms. MRI reveals a T1 hypointense and T2

intermediate to hyperintense soft-tissue mass with moderate enhancement associated with an osseous defect.
- **Malignancy.** Superficial scalp neoplasms are uncommon in children and most often result from spread of an underlying bony malignancy, such as lymphoma, leukemia, Ewing sarcoma, or metastases (neuroblastoma being most common); a primary sarcoma is less common. Malignancies are typically aggressive with soft-tissue infiltration and bony destruction, T2 intermediate to hyperintense, and avid but heterogeneous enhancement.

■ Diagnosis

Scalp venous malformation

✓ Pearls

- Infantile hemangiomas occur after birth, proliferate in infancy/childhood, and involute within the first decade.
- VMs are congenital anomalies, are present at birth, grow proportional to somatic growth, and do not involute.

- Sinus pericranii refers to anomalous transosseous communication between extracranial and intracranial veins.

Suggested Reading

Morón FE, Morriss MC, Jones JJ, Hunter JV. Lumps and bumps on the head in children: use of CT and MR imaging in solving the clinical diagnostic dilemma. Radiographics 2004; 24: 1655–1674

Case 132

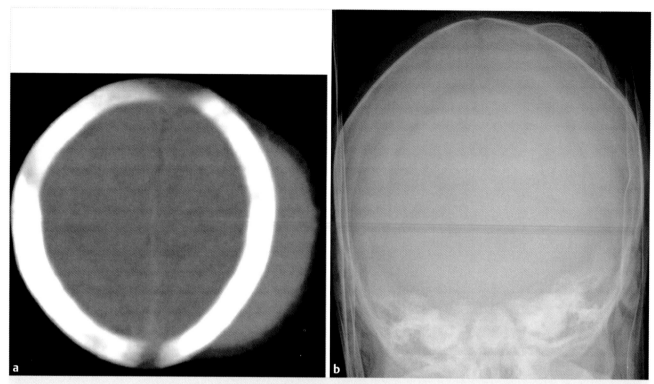

Fig. 132.1 Axial computed tomography image **(a)** reveals a hyperdense hematoma overlying the left parietal bone. The hematoma is well demarcated and confined by the sutures. Follow-up frontal radiograph years later **(b)** demonstrates a residual skull deformity deep to the outer periosteum of the calvarium.

■ Clinical Presentation

A newborn with a superficial hematoma after prolonged labor with vacuum-assisted delivery (▶ Fig. 132.1)

■ Key Imaging Finding

Superficial hematoma in a neonate

■ Top 3 Differential Diagnoses

- **Subgaleal hematoma.** A subgaleal hemorrhage occurs when blood accumulates superficial to the periosteum of the calvarium and beneath the galeal aponeurosis. It most often occurs in the setting of instrumentation during labor, typically with suction devices. The instrumentation results in rupture of small, bridging emissary veins. It is important to look for underlying calvarial fracture, which occurs relatively frequently. Given its location and source of bleeding, a subgaleal hematoma may spread diffusely through the cranium. Although the majority of cases are self-limited, subgaleal hemorrhage may occasionally be extensive and symptomatic.
- **Cephalohematoma.** A cephalohematoma refers to hemorrhage between the calvarium and periosteum. It most often results from birth trauma with rupture of venous structures traversing the periosteum. There is an increased incidence

with prolonged labor and instrumentation (forceps, suction devices, etc.) during delivery. Given the subperiosteal location, the hemorrhage does not cross sutures. It is important to evaluate for the presence of underlying fracture or intracranial hemorrhage. The hematoma may persist for several months; in a minority of cases, the hemorrhage may calcify, resulting in a focal region of calvarial thickening and sclerosis.
- **Caput succedaneum.** Caput succedaneum refers to scalp hemorrhage superficial to both the periosteum of the skull and the epicranial aponeurosis. Given its location, it is not bound by sutures; therefore, it may spread diffusely throughout the scalp, even across midline. Most cases present with a scalp contour abnormality, are self-limited, and resolve fairly quickly.

■ Diagnosis

Cephalohematoma

✓ Pearls

- With subgaleal hemorrhage, blood accumulates superficial to the periosteum and beneath the aponeurosis.
- Subgaleal hemorrhage may spread diffusely and occasionally result in extensive, symptomatic hemorrhage.

- Cephalohematomas occur between the calvarium and periosteum and are bound by sutures.
- Caput succedaneum refers to scalp hemorrhage superficial to both the skull periosteum and galeal aponeurosis.

Suggested Reading

Glass RBF, Fernbach SK, Norton KI, Choi PS, Naidich TP. The infant skull: a vault of information. Radiographics 2004; 24: 507–522

Case 133

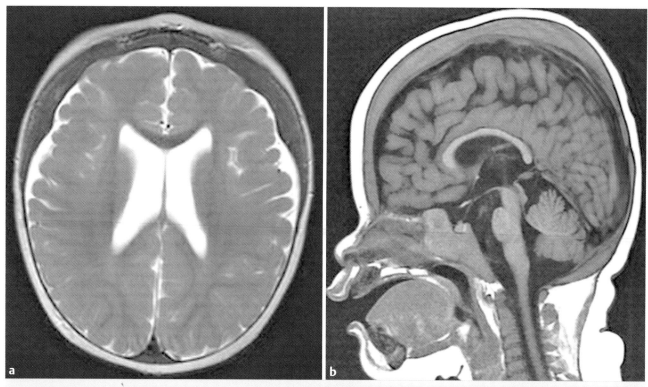

Fig. 133.1 Axial T2 **(a)** and sagittal T1 **(b)** images reveal symmetric enlargement of the parietal and frontal bones with decreased marrow signal intensity throughout.

▪ Clinical Presentation

A 2-year-old boy with chronic illness and "large head" (▶ Fig. 133.1)

Key Imaging Finding

Diffuse calvarial thickening in a child

Top 3 Differential Diagnoses

- **Normal variant.** Most cases of mild or equivocal calvarial thickening are within the range of normal variation and are found incidentally. In cases of normal variation, there is symmetric expansion of the diploic space, which is otherwise normal in density (computed tomography) and signal intensity (magnetic resonance imaging, MRI), and the cortices are normal in appearance. Focal osseous lesions, abnormalities in density or signal intensity, or a history of metabolic or hematologic disorder should warrant further workup.
- **Chronic anemias/hemoglobinopathies.** Chronic anemia or hemoglobinopathies result in increased hematopoietic marrow, which manifests as enlargement of the diploic space with conversion of yellow marrow to red marrow. The calvarial enlargement is typically symmetric with the parietal and frontal bones most commonly involved; the occipital bones are often relatively spared. β-thalassemia has a characteristic appearance on radiographs where the expansion of the diploic space resembles a "hair on end" appearance. On MRI, red marrow conversion results in decreased signal intensity on both T1 and T2 sequences.
- **Bony dysplasia.** Fibrous dysplasia is the most common bony dysplasia to involve the calvarium, skull base, and facial bones; however, it is typically a focal rather than diffuse process. The characteristic finding is focal enlargement of the diploic space with a "ground glass" matrix. Osteopetrosis is an inherited disorder that is caused by ineffective osteoclastic activity and results in increased bony deposition and sclerosis. Although sclerotic, the bones are relatively fragile. Calvarial involvement presents with diffuse skull thickening and sclerosis. Gigantism is the pediatric form of acromegaly and is caused by increased growth hormone.

Additional Differential Diagnoses

- **Phenytoin therapy.** Phenytoin is a common antiepileptic medication used in treatment of most types of seizures. Chronic usage may lead to numerous adverse effects, the most common of which is gingival hyperplasia. Central nervous system abnormalities include cerebellar hypoplasia with associated neurological deficits and diffuse calvarial thickening. Calvarial thickening occurs in approximately one-third of epilepsy patients on long-term phenytoin treatment, is thought to result from osteoblast stimulation, and is primarily cosmetic.
- **Hyperparathyroidism (HPT).** HPT may be primary due to hyperfunctioning parathyroid glands, secondary due to vitamin D deficiency or chronic renal failure, or tertiary due to hyperplasia from long-standing secondary HPT. Increased parathormone results in systemic calcium/bony resorption. In the skull, this manifests as alternating regions of lucency and sclerosis within the diploic space, referred to as a granular or "salt and pepper" appearance. There is also thinning of the inner and outer tables of the calvarium. In advanced cases, focal Brown tumors may occur, presenting as well-circumscribed lytic lesions that are often multiple. Characteristic loss of the lamina dura (thin region of sclerosis) surrounding dentition may be identified.
- **Chronic shunted hydrocephalus.** The growth of the brain parenchyma and its coverings stimulates growth of the overlying calvarium during skeletal development and maturity. Patients with successful, chronic shunted hydrocephalus often have relative intracranial hypotension and decreased intracranial volume, which decreases the growth stimulus on the calvarium. Without the stimulus for outward growth, there is diffuse endosteal calvarial thickening to fill the vacated space. Ventricle size is variable but often small in caliber.

Diagnosis

Chronic anemia

✓ Pearls

- Chronic anemia/hemoglobinopathies result in enlargement of the diploic space and decreased marrow signal.
- β-thalassemia has a characteristic "hair on end" appearance on plain films due to diploic space expansion.
- Calvarial thickening with chronic shunted hydrocephalus is due to decreased stimulus for skull growth.
- Chronic phenytoin antiepileptic therapy may result in diffuse calvarial thickening and cerebellar hypoplasia.

Suggested Readings

Chow KM, Szeto CC. Cerebral atrophy and skull thickening due to chronic phenytoin therapy. Canadian Med Assoc J 2007; 176: 321–323

Georgy BA, Snow RD, Brogdon BG et al. Value of bone window images in routine brain CT: examinations beyond trauma. Appl Radiol 1997; 2: 26–38

Case 134

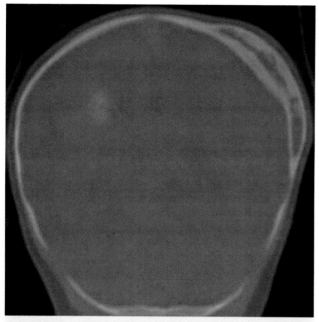

Fig. 134.1 Coronal CT reformatted image demonstrates focal, smooth calvarial thickening with central lucency involving the left parietal bone.

■ Clinical Presentation

A hard, palpable scalp abnormality (► Fig. 134.1)

■ **Key Imaging Finding**

Focal calvarial thickening

■ **Top 3 Differential Diagnoses**

- **Fibrous dysplasia.** FD occurs most often in young adults and is more common in women. The calvarium, skull base, and facial bones are most often affected in the head and neck. The classic appearance on computed tomography (CT) is focal bony expansion with "ground glass" attenuation of the diploic space; sclerotic and cystic or lytic variants are less common. On magnetic resonance imaging (MRI), FD is typically hypointense on both T1 and T2 sequences and demonstrates avid enhancement; regions of cystic involvement, however, are T2 hyperintense. The MRI appearance can mimic aggressive lesions; therefore, CT is preferred in suspected cases of FD.
- **Malignancy.** Metastatic disease commonly involves the calvarium. Typically, metastatic lesions present as soft-tissue infiltration or soft-tissue masses with bony destruction; focal sclerosis is less common. Malignancies prone to sclerotic metastases include prostate and breast carcinoma, as well as lymphoma. Primary bone tumors are less common and include Ewing sarcoma in children and osteosarcoma in young adults or the elderly with a history of Paget disease or prior radiation therapy. Both Ewing and osteosarcoma present as focal, aggressive bone-forming tumors on CT; lytic lesions are less common. MRI most often reveals intermediate T1 and T2 signal intensity with avid but heterogeneous enhancement; calcified portions are hypointense.
- **Paget disease.** Paget disease occurs in elderly patients and consists of three stages: lytic, sclerotic, and mixed. Calvarial involvement during the lytic phase results in a characteristic large lytic lesion with erosion of the outer table, referred to as osteoporosis circumscripta. During the sclerotic phase, there is expansion and sclerosis of the cortex and diploic spaces, which may be diffuse or focal. In the mixed phase, a combination of lytic and sclerotic lesions results in the characteristic "cotton wool" appearance of the skull.

■ **Additional Differential Diagnoses**

- **Meningioma.** Meningiomas are benign dural-based masses and represent the most common extraaxial masses. Common locations include parasagittal, convexities, middle cranial fossa, and planum sphenoidale. Less common locations include the sellar/suprasellar region and cerebellopontine angle. Extradural meningiomas are rare, accounting for fewer than 2% of cases. Intraosseous meningiomas are a subset of extradural meningiomas that typically occur in adults; most often involve the calvarium, skull base, or facial bones; and are centered within the diploic space. They present with expansion of the diploic space, cortical thickening, and mixed sclerosis and lucency, often mimicking fibrous dysplasia or a malignant lesion, especially on MRI.
- **Calcified cephalohematoma.** A cephalohematoma refers to hemorrhage between the calvarium and periosteum. It most often results from birth trauma with rupture of venous structures traversing the periosteum. There is an increased incidence with prolonged labor and instrumentation (forceps, suction devices, etc.) during delivery. Given the subperiosteal location, the hemorrhage does not cross sutures. The hematoma may persist for several months; in a minority of cases, the hemorrhage may calcify, resulting in a focal region of calvarial thickening and sclerosis that persists into adulthood.

■ **Diagnosis**

Calcified cephalohematoma

✓ **Pearls**

- FD occurs in young adults; the classic CT appearance is focal bony expansion with "ground glass" attenuation.
- Malignant calvarial lesions include metastases, lymphoma, osteosarcoma, and Ewing sarcoma (in a child).
- Paget disease occurs in elderly patients; the sclerotic phase results in cortical/diploic thickening and sclerosis.
- Meningiomas may result in calvarial thickening due to primary bony involvement or reactive hyperostosis.

Suggested Reading

Georgy BA, Snow RD, Brogdon BG et al. Value of bone window images in routine brain CT: examinations beyond trauma. Appl Radiol 1997; 2: 26–38

Case 135

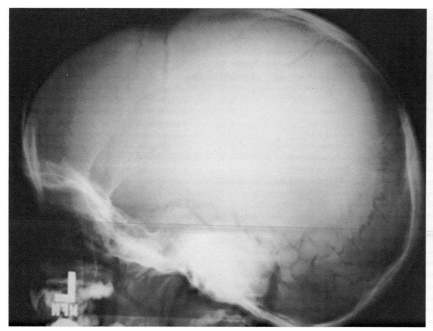

Fig. 135.1 Lateral skull radiograph reveals intra-sutural ossification (Wormian bones) involving the squamosal and lambdoid sutures. (Case courtesy of University of California, Davis, Pediatric Imaging.)

▨ Clinical Presentation

A child with facial abnormalities (▶ Fig. 135.1)

▧ Key Imaging Finding

Wormian bones

▧ Top 3 Differential Diagnoses

- **Idiopathic.** Wormian bones are irregular ossicles located within the sutures of the calvarium (intrasutural bones). Idiopathic or incidental Wormian bones are reported to be smaller and less numerous (usually < 10) than those associated with skeletal dysplasias; however, there are no definitive criteria to distinguish between benign and pathological causes. Most commonly located within the lambdoid suture (50%), Wormian bones may also occur in the coronal suture (25%) and have been identified in all cranial sutures and fontanelles. A large intrasutural bone located at the junction of the lambdoid and sagittal sutures is termed an *"Inca bone."* Arriving at a definitive diagnosis radiographically often requires additional studies to assess for the wide spectrum of pathological entities that may be associated with Wormian bones.
- **Osteogenesis imperfecta.** Osteogenesis imperfecta (OI) is a genetic disorder (typically autosomal dominant), which results in abnormal type 1 collagen formation. Type 1 collagen is found in osseous structures and the sclera of the eyes; hence, patients present with fragile bones, multiple fractures, and blue sclera. There are four major types of OI with types 1 and 4 being the most common. Type 1 presents in childhood with multiple fractures and Wormian bones. Wormian bones in OI are often numerous and demonstrate a mosaic ("crazy paving") pattern. Musculoskeletal imaging findings include diffuse demineralization, bowing deformities, multiple fractures, vertebra plana, kyphoscoliosis, enlarged epiphyses, characteristic "popcorn" metaphyseal calcifications, and cortical thinning.
- **Cleidocranial dysostosis.** Cleidocranial dysostosis is a genetic disorder characterized by a defect in the formation of membranous bones. Clinical findings include macrocephaly, hypertelorism, facial hypoplasia, and absence or hypoplasia of the clavicles. Central nervous system imaging reveals these findings, along with Wormian bones and delayed closure of fontanelles and sutures. Systemic musculoskeletal abnormalities include a widened symphysis pubis and dysplasia of the femoral neck with a coxa vara deformity.

▧ Additional Differential Diagnoses

- **Down syndrome.** Down syndrome (trisomy 21) is the most common genetic cause of mental impairment in children and has been associated with an increased incidence with advanced maternal age (> 35 years of age). A host of radiographic findings are associated with Down syndrome, including Wormian bones. Additional musculoskeletal findings include a hypoplastic arch of C1 with craniocervical stenosis, atlantoaxial subluxation, absent 12th ribs, short tubular bones of the hands (including clinodactyly of the middle phalanx of the little finger), wide iliac wings, hip dysplasia, and patellar dislocation. There is an increased incidence of early onset Alzheimer disease in patients with Down syndrome.
- **Metabolic disease (rickets, hypothyroidism).** Wormian bones may be found in patients with multiple metabolic deficiencies, including rickets, hypothyroidism, and hypophosphatasia (genetic cause of rickets). In rickets, there is demineralization and softening of bones due to Vitamin D (most common), calcium, or phosphorous deficiencies. Early systemic musculoskeletal findings include frayed physes and flaring (cupping) of the metaphyses. Wormian bones are associated with the healing phase of the disorder. Hypothyroidism is characterized by markedly delayed skeletal maturity, "bullet" vertebrae at the thoracolumbar junction, epiphyseal fragmentation, and Wormian bones.

▧ Diagnosis

Cleidocranial dysostosis

✓ Pearls

- Wormian bones may be idiopathic or incidental in etiology; the lambdoid suture is most commonly involved.
- Wormian bones in osteogenesis imperfecta may be numerous and demonstrate a mosaic pattern.
- Cleidocranial dysostosis presents with Wormian bones and absence or hypoplasia of the clavicles.
- Wormian bones may be found in patients with metabolic deficiencies, including rickets and hypothyroidism.

Suggested Readings

Jeanty P, Silva SR, Turner C. Prenatal diagnosis of wormian bones. J Ultrasound Med 2000; 19: 863–869

Paterson CR. Radiological features of the brittle bone diseases J Diagn Radiogr Imaging. 2003; 5: 39–45

Case 136

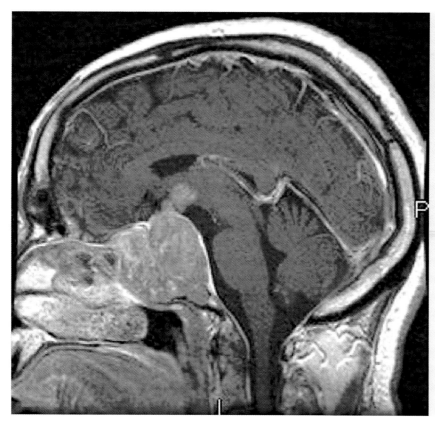

Fig. 136.1 Contrast-enhanced sagittal T1 midline image through the brain demonstrates a large, expansile, enhancing soft-tissue mass centered over the clivus. There is intracranial extension with involvement of the sella/suprasellar region. A pituitary gland was not identified separate from the mass.

■ **Clinical Presentation**

A 53-year-old man with visual disturbances (▶ Fig. 136.1)

■ Key Imaging Finding

Clival mass

■ Top 3 Differential Diagnoses

- **Metastases.** Metastatic disease commonly involves the skull base. Common primary neoplasms include breast, lung, and prostate carcinoma; lymphoma may be primary or secondary. Breast and lung carcinoma are most often lytic, along with renal and thyroid carcinomas. Prostate (and occasionally breast) carcinoma produces sclerotic metastases. Computed tomography (CT) demonstrates bony involvement in better detail than magnetic resonance imaging (MRI), especially along the skull base. MRI is superior in evaluating the soft-tissue component, as well as intracranial involvement. Metastases are hypointense on T1 and hyperintense on T2 with avid enhancement; lymphoma may be T2 hypointense.
- **Chordoma.** Chordoma is a malignant tumor that arises from notochordal remnants. It most commonly affects the clivus and sacrum in young to middle-aged adults and is more common in men; vertebral body involvement is less common.

Patients with clival involvement often present with headache and ophthalmoplegia due to cranial nerve involvement. CT reveals a midline, expansile, lytic mass with hyperdense foci centrally. Chordomas are classically hyperintense on T2 sequences with hypointense fibrous septations. They are typically hypo- to isointense on T1 sequences with heterogeneous but avid enhancement.
- **Chondrosarcoma.** Chondrosarcoma is a malignant primary bone lesion that may involve the skull base where it is typically off-midline. They may occur at any age but are most common in middle-aged patients who present with cranial nerve deficits. CT demonstrates an expansile lesion with internal chondroid matrix in an "arcs and swirls" pattern. The soft-tissue component is commonly hyperdense. On MRI, the chondroid matrix is hyperintense on T2 sequences; internal calcifications are hypointense. Heterogeneous enhancement is typical.

■ Additional Differential Diagnoses

- **Invasive pituitary macroadenoma.** Pituitary adenomas are common benign neoplasms of the pituitary gland. They are characterized as microadenomas (< 10 mm) or macroadenomas (≥ 10 mm). As a general rule, microadenomas are hormonally active, whereas macroadenomas are inactive but exert local mass effect. Occasionally, a macroadenoma can display infiltrative characteristics, invading the cavernous sinus, paranasal sinuses, clivus/skull base, and brain parenchyma. Imaging findings include a large, expansile soft-tissue mass with decreased T1 and increased T2 signal; avid enhancement is typical. The normal pituitary gland is obliterated by the mass, which is a key differentiating feature.
- **Plasmacytoma.** Plasmacytoma is the result of abnormal proliferation of plasma cells; it is the solitary form of multiple myeloma. Patients are often ≥ 40 years of age. Presentation depends upon the location of the mass; pain, headache, and

cranial neuropathies are common. CT demonstrates a poorly defined, expansile lytic lesion. On MRI, they are typically isointense to gray matter on T1 and T2 sequences; homogeneous enhancement is typical. Flow voids may be present. Patients must be followed to exclude multiple myeloma.
- **Meningioma.** Extradural meningiomas are relatively rare, accounting for fewer than 2% of cases. Intraosseous meningiomas are a subset of extradural meningiomas; most often involve the calvarium, skull base, or facial bones; and are centered within the diploic space. They typically present in adults. CT reveals bony expansion and smooth or irregular sclerosis; they may mimic fibrous dysplasia or malignancies. There may be an associated soft-tissue component. Sclerotic components are hypointense on both T1 and T2 MR sequences; avid enhancement is typical.

■ Diagnosis

Invasive pituitary macroadenoma

✓ Pearls

- Metastases and lymphoma often involve the clivus; breast, lung, and prostate carcinomas are most common.
- Chordomas arise from notochord remnants; they are midline and characteristically bright on T2 sequences.

- Chondrosarcoma demonstrates a chondroid matrix with "arcs and swirls" calcifications and bright T2 signal.
- Invasive macroadenomas may involve the clivus; absence of the pituitary gland is a differentiating feature.

Suggested Reading

Kimura F, Kim KS, Friedman H, Russell EJ, Breit R. MR imaging of the normal and abnormal clivus. Am J Roentgenol 1990; 155: 1285–1291

Case 137

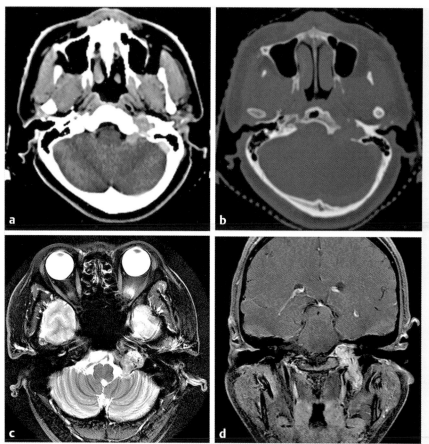

Fig. 137.1 Contrast-enhanced axial CT images in soft-tissue **(a)** and bone **(b)** windows demonstrate an enhancing soft-tissue mass with expansion and irregular erosion of the jugular foramen. T2-weighted axial image **(c)** reveals the presence of multiple flow voids within an intermediate to hyperintense left jugular foramen mass. Coronal T1 postcontrast MR image with fat suppression **(d)** shows the extent of the avidly enhancing mass centered within the jugular foramen and extending intracranially, into the internal auditory canal, and inferiorly into the upper cervical region.

■ Clinical Presentation

A 46-year-old woman with dysphagia and tinnitus (▶ Fig. 137.1)

■ Key Imaging Finding

Jugular foramen mass

■ Top 3 Differential Diagnoses

- **Paraganglioma.** Jugular foramen paragangliomas (glomus jugulare) are highly vascular lesions that enlarge the jugular foramen, often with associated irregular, permeative bone destruction. The infiltrative osseous pattern is best appreciated on computed tomography (CT) bone windows. These aggressive lesions are associated with jugular vein invasion and intraluminal growth. On magnetic resonance imaging (MRI), glomus jugulare tumors often demonstrate the classic "salt and pepper" appearance, characterized by multiple T2 hypointense flow voids and occasional intralesional calcifications. The solid components of the mass are isointense on T1, iso- to hyperintense on T2, and avidly enhance. The tumors commonly extend intracranially, as well as inferiorly into the cervical region. Tumors that also involve the middle ear cavity are termed *glomus jugulotympanicum.*
- **Schwannoma.** Schwannomas of the jugular foramen are fairly uncommon and most often arise along the glossopharyngeal nerve. Clinical symptoms are related to local mass effect; unilateral hearing loss and dysphagia are the most common presenting symptoms. The benign, slow-growing nature of schwannomas causes smooth osseous expansion/remodeling of the jugular foramen. Larger lesions may compress the ipsilateral jugular vein and/or sigmoid sinus. On CT, schwannomas tend to be isodense to brain parenchyma and avidly enhance. On MRI, they most often appear hypointense on T1 and hyperintense on T2 sequences with marked enhancement; cystic degeneration may occasionally occur.
- **Meningioma.** Meningiomas are the most common extraaxial tumors and may occasionally arise within or adjacent to the jugular foramen. On CT, meningiomas typically appear iso- to slightly hyperdense relative to brain parenchyma and may contain internal calcifications. The presence of adjacent bony hyperostosis is a useful discriminator, when present. On MRI, lesions appear relatively isointense with respect to gray matter on T1- and T2-weighted sequences with diffuse homogeneous enhancement, a broad dural base, and a dural tail.

■ Additional Differential Diagnoses

- **Metastases.** Metastatic involvement of the jugular foramen may have a variety of imaging appearances, ranging from a nonaggressive pattern with osseous remodeling to an aggressive pattern with erosive, destructive osseous changes. Breast, lung, and prostate carcinoma are the most common primary tumors associated with skull-base metastases. The lesions have variable soft-tissue attenuation (CT) and signal intensity (MRI), as well as variable enhancement patterns based upon the origin and cell type of the primary tumor. Metastatic foci may be multifocal, so it is important to search for additional osseous, meningeal, or parenchymal lesions.
- **Jugular bulb variants.** The most common jugular bulb variant is asymmetric prominence, which is seen on most brain MR images. The increased prominence may cause variable signal intensity at the junction of the sigmoid sinus and internal jugular vein, resulting in a pseudolesion. When in doubt, a pseudolesion can be confirmed on CT or MR venography. A dehiscent or high-riding (far more common) jugular bulb has a prevalence of ~6% in the general population and may occasionally be a cause of tinnitus. When the jugular bulb is seen above the inferior margin of the round window, it is considered high-riding. High-resolution CT can evaluate for the presence of bony dehiscence of the petrous septum between the middle ear and jugular bulb. CT venography may also be helpful in confirming the diagnosis.

■ Diagnosis

Paraganglioma (glomus jugulare)

✓ Pearls

- Paragangliomas are highly vascular tumors that may demonstrate a "salt and pepper" appearance on MRI.
- Jugular foramen schwannomas are sharply demarcated and result in smooth osseous expansion/remodeling.
- Jugular foramen meningiomas may be hyperdense on CT with calcification and avid enhancement.
- Skull-base metastases are most often from breast, lung, and prostate carcinoma; look for additional lesions.

Suggested Reading

Caldemeyer KS, Mathews VP, Azzarelli B, Smith RR. The jugular foramen: a review of anatomy, masses, and imaging characteristics. Radiographics 1997; 17: 1123–1139

Case 138

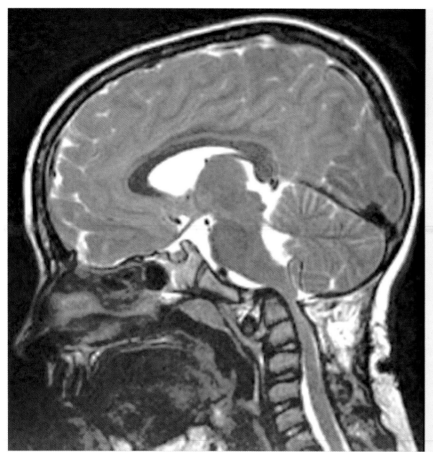

Fig. 138.1 Sagittal T2 magnetic resonance image reveals upward migration of the dens through the foramen magnum with associated severe compression of the cervicomedullary junction and upper cervical cord.

■ Clinical Presentation

A 10-year-old boy with hypochondroplasia and neurological deficits (▶ Fig. 138.1)

■ Key Imaging Finding

Extension of dens through foramen magnum with compression of the craniocervical junction

■ Top 3 Differential Diagnoses

- **Basilar invagination.** Basilar invagination refers to abnormal protrusion of the vertebral column through the foramen magnum due to a congenital or developmental defect. There are numerous causes, including hypoplasia of the osseous components of the skull base, atlantooccipital assimilation, bony and cartilaginous dysplasias, Klippel-Feil syndrome, Down syndrome, and Chiari craniocervical junctions. Clinically, patients may be asymptomatic or present with insidious onset of cerebellar, brain stem, or cervical cord neurological deficits. On imaging, the tip of the odontoid projects through the foramen magnum with indentation or compression of the cervicomedullary junction. There is typically normal orientation of C1 with respect to C2. The Chamberlain line is used to evaluate for abnormal positioning of the vertebral column with respect to the skull base. It is drawn from the posterior margin of the hard palate to the opisthion, which is the posterior margin of the foramen magnum. In the majority of normal cases, the tip of the odontoid process is at or below the Chamberlain line. In some cases, it may extend a few millimeters above the line. Extension 5 mm or more above the Chamberlain line is abnormal and consistent with basilar invagination or basilar impression (see below). Both may be associated with platybasia or flattening of the skull base.

- **Basilar impression.** The clinical and imaging manifestations of basilar invagination and basilar impression are identical. The key distinction between the two is that basilar invagination is a congenital or developmental abnormality, whereas basilar impression is acquired. Because basilar impression is acquired, the underlying bony development is normal. Common acquired causes of basilar impression include Paget disease, osteogenesis imperfecta, rickets, metabolic abnormalities involving calcium and phosphate, and trauma.

- **Cranial settling.** Cranial setting also results in upward extension of the dens through the foramen magnum; however, it is due to disruption of the occipitoatlantal and atlantoaxial articulations and subsequent inferior migration of the atlas and skull base with respect to C2. The key imaging distinction is that the anterior arch of C1 articulates with the base of C2 rather than with the dens. Rheumatoid arthritis (RA) is the most common cause of cranial settling and most often involves middle-aged women.

■ Diagnosis

Basilar invagination

✓ Pearls

- Basilar invagination/basilar impression results in upward migration of the dens through the foramen magnum.
- Basilar invagination is primary or congenital, whereas basilar impression is acquired.

- The Chamberlain line is used to diagnose basilar invagination; it extends from the posterior hard palate to the opisthion.
- Cranial setting refers to inferior migration of C1 and the skull base with respect to C2, most often due to RA.

Suggested Reading

Smoker WRK. Craniovertebral junction: normal anatomy, craniometry, and congenital anomalies. Radiographics 1994; 14: 255–277

Case 139

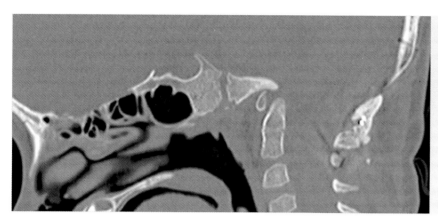

Fig. 139.1 Sagittal reformatted computed tomography image reveals flattening of the skull base with the clivus nearly parallel to the foramen magnum. Postoperative changes are noted at the craniocervical junction posteriorly.

■ Clinical Presentation

A 5-year-old boy with bony dysplasia and a history of headaches and neurological deficits (▶ Fig. 139.1)

■ Key Imaging Finding

Abnormal flattening of skull base

■ Diagnosis

Platybasia. Platybasia refers to flattening of the skull base. The causes of platybasia are similar to congenital causes of basilar invagination (hypoplasia of the osseous components of the skull base, atlantooccipital assimilation, bony and cartilaginous dysplasias, Chiari craniocervical junctions, etc.) and acquired causes of basilar impression (Paget disease, osteogenesis imperfecta, rickets, metabolic abnormalities involving calcium and phosphate, and trauma). In most cases, there is associated basilar invagination/impression; however, isolated cases of platybasia do occur.

The Welcher basal angle is used to evaluate for platybasia. The first line is drawn from the nasion to the tuberculum sellae; the second line is drawn from the tuberculum to the basion (anterior margin of the foramen magnum). The average angle in normal individuals is ~132 degrees. An angle > 140 degrees is consistent with platybasia.

Treatment is generally reserved for cases of brain stem and/or cervical cord compression and consists of posterior decompression and craniocervical fusion.

✓ Pearls

- Platybasia refers to flattening of the skull base; the causes are similar to basilar invagination/impression.
- The Welcher basal angle is used to evaluate for platybasia; an angle > 140 degrees is consistent with platybasia.

- Treatment is reserved for neurological compression and consists of posterior decompression with fusion.

Suggested Reading

Smoker WRK. Craniovertebral junction: normal anatomy, craniometry, and congenital anomalies. Radiographics 1994; 14: 255–277

Case 140

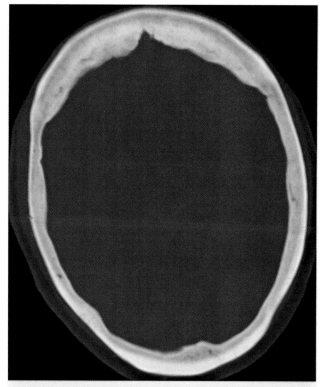

Fig. 140.1 Axial computed tomography image in bone window reveals symmetric calvarial thickening involving the inner tables of the frontal bones.

■ Clinical Presentation

An 82-year-old woman with chronic headaches (▶ Fig. 140.1)

◼ Key Imaging Finding

Symmetric calvarial thickening involving the inner tables of the frontal bones

◼ Diagnosis

Hyperostosis frontalis interna (HFI). HFI refers to calvarial thickening due to bony overgrowth along the inner table. It occurs in adults and is far more common in women. HFI characteristically involves the frontal bones and is typically bilateral and symmetric. In some cases, it may extend to the orbital roofs or, occasionally, beyond the coronal sutures to involve the parietal bones. The exact etiology remains unknown; however, there have been reported associations with endocrinopathies. HFI is an asymptomatic incidental finding that requires no further workup or imaging.

✓ Pearls

- Hyperostosis frontalis interna refers to calvarial thickening due to bony overgrowth along the inner table.
- HFI is more common in women, characteristically involves the frontal bones, and is bilateral and symmetric.
- HFI is an asymptomatic incidental finding that requires no further workup or imaging.

Suggested Reading

She R, Szakacs J. Hyperostosis frontalis interna: case report and review of literature. Ann Clin Lab Sci 2004; 34: 206–208

Case 141

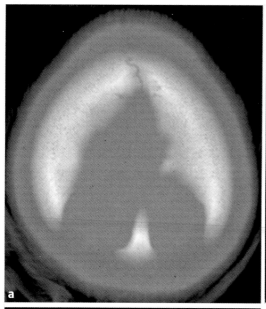

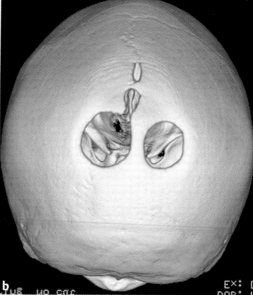

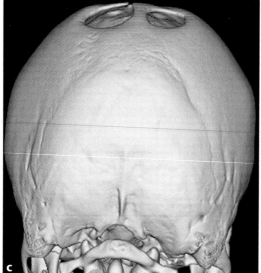

Fig. 141.1 Axial **(a)** and three-dimensional reformatted computed tomography images with a posterior view **(b,c)** reveal paired, circumscribed ossification defects of the parietal bones separated by a midline region of ossification.

▨ Clinical Presentation

A 10-year-old girl with "soft spots" (▶ Fig. 141.1)

■ **Key Imaging Finding**

Circumscribed, symmetric parietal calvarial defects

■ **Diagnosis**

Parietal foramina. Parietal foramina refer to hereditary ossification defects involving the parietal bone. They are most often isolated abnormalities but may be associated with syndromes. On clinical exam, parietal foramina present with "soft spots" in addition to the normal open sutures. Imaging reveals either paired, circumscribed parietal defects separated by a midline region of ossification or a large, single ossification defect that extends across the midline. The defects may persist into adulthood.

✓ **Pearls**

- Parietal foramina are hereditary ossification defects that occur in isolation or in association with syndromes.
- Clinically, parietal foramina present with "soft spots" in addition to the normal open sutures.

- Imaging shows paired parietal ossification defects or a solitary defect that may persist into adulthood.

Suggested Reading

Glass RBF, Fernbach SK, Norton KI, Choi PS, Naidich TP. The infant skull: a vault of information. Radiographics 2004; 24: 507–522

Case 142

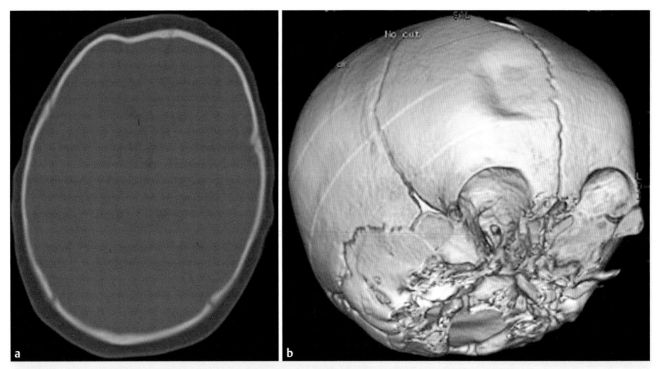

Fig. 142.1 Axial computed tomography (CT) image in bone window **(a)** reveals a concave deformity of the frontal bone on the right. There was no intracranial injury. Three-dimensional volume reformatted CT image **(b)** better depicts the deformity adjacent to the metopic suture, which mimics a dented ping pong ball.

■ Clinical Presentation

A 6-month-old girl with head injury (▶ Fig. 142.1)

▨ Key Imaging Finding

Concave skull deformity in an infant

▨ Diagnosis

Ping Pong fracture. "Ping pong" fractures refer to specific depressed skull fractures in infants that result in a concave deformity, similar to a dented ping pong ball. Oftentimes, there is no associated lucency because the infant skull is malleable. Ping pong fractures are relatively rare and may be congenital or secondary to external injury; instrumentation during delivery is one of the more common causes. Treatment options depend upon the severity of the deformity and presence or absence of associated injuries, including intracranial hemorrhage. Mild forms may resolve spontaneously or be treated with suction devices. More severe deformities may require surgical correction.

✓ Pearls

- "Ping pong" fractures occur in infants and result in a concave deformity, similar to a dented ping pong ball.
- Ping pong fractures are rare; instrumentation during delivery is one of the more common causes.

- Treatment options depend upon the severity of the deformity and presence or absence of associated injuries.

Suggested Readings

Basaldella L, Marton E, Bekelis K, Longatti P. Spontaneous resolution of atraumatic intrauterine ping-pong fractures in newborns delivered by cesarean section. J Child Neurol 2011; 26: 1449–1451

Brittain C, Muthukumar P, Job S, et al. "Ping pong" fracture in a term infant. BMJ Case Reports. 2012

Case 143

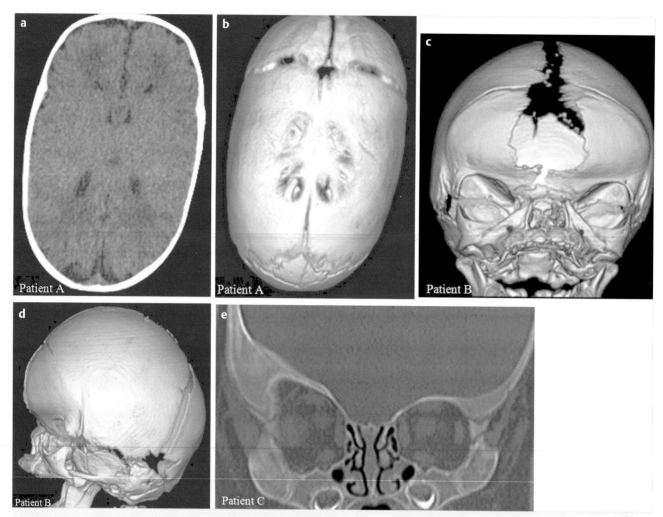

Fig. 143.1 Axial (a) and three-dimensional (3-D) reformatted (b) computed tomography (CT) images in a 4-month-old boy reveal scaphocephaly and premature closure of the sagittal suture. Frontal (c) and lateral (d) 3-D reformatted CT images in a 5-day-old girl demonstrate premature closure of the coronal sutures with brachycephaly, a prominent forehead, and midface hypoplasia. Coronal CT image (e) in a 4-month-old boy shows uplifting of the right orbit with a "harlequin eye" from unilateral coronal suture craniosynostosis.

▮ Clinical Presentation

Three newborns and infants with head deformities (▶ Fig. 143.1)

■ Key Imaging Finding

Premature closure of sutures with head deformities

■ Diagnosis

Craniosynostoses. Craniosyntostosis refers to premature closure of sutures, resulting in head deformities with or without associated facial abnormalities. Patients present at birth, infancy, or early childhood with asymmetric cranial development. Craniosynostosis is more common in boys and may be sporadic (~85%) or associated with numerous syndromes (≈15%), including Apert (hand/foot anomalies, midface hypoplasia, hearing loss) and Crouzon (craniofacial dysostosis, external auditory canal atresia) syndromes, as well as thanatophoric dwarfism (pansynostosis). Syndromic causes are more severe, more likely to involve multiple sutures, and present earlier in life. Treatment depends on the degree of deformity and age at diagnosis. Moderate to severe deformities are treated with surgical distraction and/or reconstruction.

Premature closure of a suture causes increased growth parallel to the suture and decreased growth perpendicular to the suture. Therefore, characteristic head deformities occur based upon which sutures are involved:

○ Sagittal suture—increased anteroposterior (AP) and decreased transverse diameter, referred to as scaphocephaly or dolichocephaly.
○ Metopic suture—triangular-shaped forehead, referred to as trigonocephaly.
○ Unilateral coronal or lambdoid suture—asymmetric unilateral growth, referred to as plagiocephaly; unilateral coronal suture synostosis results in uplifting of the ipsilateral orbit causing a "harlequin eye" deformity.
○ Bilateral coronal or lambdoid sutures—increased transverse and decreased AP diameter, referred to as brachycephaly.
○ Bilateral coronal and lambdoid sutures—increased transverse and decreased AP diameter with a "towering" appearance, referred to as turricephaly.
○ Sagittal, bilateral coronal, and bilateral lambdoid sutures—cloverleaf configuration of the skull, referred to as kleeblattschädel.

The sagittal suture is by far the most commonly involved suture in craniosynostosis, followed by the coronal, metopic, and lambdoid sutures. Sutures normally remain open during skeletal growth with the exception of the metopic suture, which typically closes in the first year of life (usually 6 to 9 months of age). The sagittal suture is the last to close under normal conditions.

Low dose computed tomography with three-dimensional reformats/volume rendering is best for initial and follow-up evaluation for craniosynostosis. The region of synostosis may be fibrous or osseous and may involve all or only a portion of the suture to result in head deformity. It is important to evaluate for associated malformations of the temporal and facial bones.

✓ Pearls

• Craniosyntostosis refers to premature closure of sutures, resulting in head and possibly facial deformities.
• Craniosynostosis is most often sporadic but may also occur in association with numerous syndromes.

• Characteristic head deformities occur based upon which suture(s) prematurely close.
• Sagittal suture is by far most commonly involved, followed by the coronal, metopic, and lambdoid sutures.

Suggested Reading

Glass RBF, Fernbach SK, Norton KI, Choi PS, Naidich TP. The infant skull: a vault of information. Radiographics 2004; 24: 507–522

Case 144

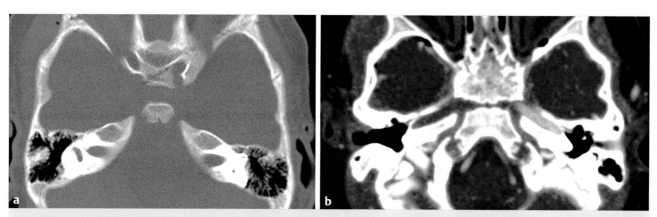

Fig. 144.1 Axial CT image in bone window **(a)** shows a fracture through the sphenoid/central skull base with extension into the right carotid canal and left orbital apex. Superficial soft-tissue swelling overlying the right temporal bone is partially seen. CTA **(b)** demonstrates occlusion of the petrous segment of the right internal carotid artery. Additional findings include subtle pneumocephalus within the right middle cranial fossa, as well as orbital emphysema on the left (near the orbital apex).

■ **Clinical Presentation**

A 16-year-old boy post–motor vehicle crash (▶ Fig. 144.1)

■ Key Imaging Finding

Central skull-base fracture with vascular injury

■ Diagnosis

Skull-base fracture with carotid occlusion. Fractures involving the central skull base are typically the result of blunt trauma with extension of associated calvarial or facial fractures. With the configuration of the cranial vault, the vectors and fractures caused by blunt trauma extend inferiorly and centrally to involve the skull base.

In the setting of significant trauma, such as a motor vehicle crash, the vast majority of trauma centers perform panscan computed tomography (CT), which includes unenhanced scans of the head and cervical spine, followed by a CT angiogram (CTA) of the head and neck and contrast-enhanced studies of the chest, abdomen, and pelvis. Dedicated studies or reformatted images of the orbits, facial bones, and temporal bones may be performed based upon the clinical setting and associated findings. Central skull-base/sphenoid fractures may be subtle because they are typically nondisplaced and may occur in the plane of imaging; therefore, multiplanar reformats are helpful. CTA is recommended and necessary to evaluate the integrity of vascular structures in the setting of a skull-base fracture.

It is important to evaluate and describe the extent of fractures and structures involved. Sphenoid fractures will commonly involve the carotid canals and orbital apices. Carotid canal extension may result in vascular injury, including dissection, emboli, occlusion, and carotid-cavernous fistula (CCF). Extension into the orbital apex may result in optic nerve injury or compression. An uncommon but important complication of skull-base fractures is a cerebrospinal fluid (CSF) leak. Most leaks resolve spontaneously. If persistent, there is a significant risk of infection. A nuclear medicine or CT myelogram may be performed to evaluate a persistent CSF leak.

✓ Pearls

- Central skull-base fractures typically result from blunt trauma with extension of calvarial or facial fractures.
- Sphenoid fractures may involve the carotid canal with internal carotid artery injury or the orbital apex, or they may cause a CSF leak.
- Vascular injuries associated with central skull-base fractures include dissection, emboli, occlusion, and CCF.

Suggested Reading

Sliker CW. Blunt cerebrovascular injuries: imaging with multidetector CT angiography. Radiographics 2008; 28: 1689–1708, discussion 1709–1710

Case 145

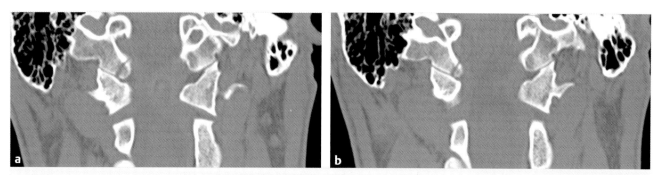

Fig. 145.1 Coronal reformatted computed tomography images **(a,b)** demonstrate a vertically oriented lucency/medial avulsion fracture of the occipital condyle on the right with minimal displacement of the fracture fragment.

▓ Clinical Presentation

A 28-year-old man involved in a motor vehicle crash (▶ Fig. 145.1)

■ Key Imaging Finding

Vertically oriented lucency through the occipital condyle

■ Diagnosis

Occipital condyle fracture (OCF). The occipital condyles are paired extensions of the occipital bone that form portions of the foramen magnum and articulate with C1. They are integral components of the craniocervical junction (CCJ), along with the atlas (C1) and axis (C2). Ligamentous structures provide stability of the CCJ. Structures intimately related to the occipital condyles include the medulla, vertebral arteries, spinal arteries, hypoglossal canals, and jugular foramina.

OCFs have become more evident as imaging technology and resolution have improved. The fractures most often result from high-speed deceleration injuries, such as those seen with motor vehicle collisions, falls, or direct trauma.

OCFs are categorized into three main types based upon their overall morphology and mechanism of injury. A type I fracture refers to a comminuted impaction fracture of the occipital condyle with no or minimal displacement of fracture fragments. It is thought to occur from axial loading and is considered a stable fracture if unilateral because the major stabilizing ligaments of the CCJ (tectorial membrane and alar ligaments) typically remain intact. If bilateral, however, there may be some degree of instability. A type II fracture consists of a more complex basilar skull-base fracture that extends into one or both occipital condyles. It most often occurs secondary to a direct blow to the skull and is considered stable. A type III fracture represents an avulsion fracture along the medial aspect of the occipital condyle at the insertion of the alar ligament. The fracture fragment is typically displaced medially into the foramen magnum. The mechanism of injury consists of forced rotation and side bending. The fracture is potentially unstable due to strain or disruption of the stabilizing ligaments.

Occipital condyle fractures are often occult on conventional radiographs, especially if nondisplaced. Computed tomography with sagittal and coronal reformats is the imaging modality of choice to identify bony injuries, which may be subtle. Magnetic resonance imaging allows for evaluation of underlying ligamentous structures, which ultimately determines stability of the injury. Additional findings associated with high-velocity trauma include multiple bony fractures, soft-tissue injury, vascular injury, cord injury, as well as injury to intracranial structures.

Treatment options depend upon the stability of the injury. Stable fractures are managed conservatively with immobilization. Unstable fractures may require surgical fixation.

✓ Pearls

- Type I OCF refers to a comminuted impaction fracture with no or minimal displacement of fracture fragments.
- Type II OCF consists of a basilar skull-base fracture that extends into one or both occipital condyles.
- Type III OCF represents a medial avulsion fracture of the occipital condyle at the insertion of the alar ligament.
- Type II and unilateral type I OCFs are usually stable; type III and bilateral type I OCFs are potentially unstable.

Suggested Reading

Leone A, Cerase A, Colosimo C, Lauro L, Puca A, Marano P. Occipital condylar fractures: a review. Radiology 2000; 216: 635–644

Case 146

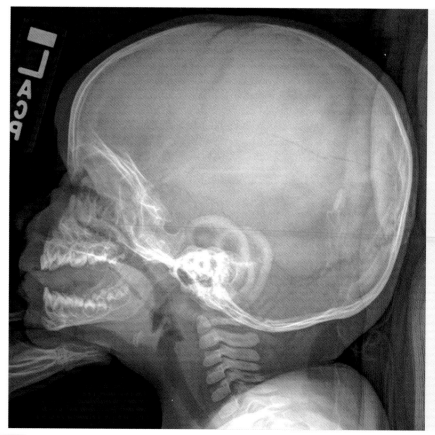

Fig. 146.1 Lateral radiograph of the skull demonstrates a linear lucency traversing the parietal bone in the anterior-posterior plane.

Clinical Presentation

A 6-month-old girl with irritability and "normal" head computed tomography (CT) (▶ Fig. 146.1)

▪ Key Imaging Finding

Linear skull lucency

▪ Diagnosis

Linear skull fracture. Linear fractures are the most common type of skull fracture and result from blunt injury. In most cases, the fractures are clinically insignificant, unless there is depression of fracture fragments (depressed skull fracture), involvement of vascular structures (e.g., middle meningeal artery), or extension into and diastasis of a cranial suture. Prognosis is more dependent upon the presence or absence of associated intracranial injuries (e.g., intracranial hemorrhage, parenchymal shear injury, cerebral edema, etc.).

CT is the imaging modality of choice for head injury because it is readily available, allows for rapid acquisition, and best depicts acute intracranial abnormalities, especially intracranial hemorrhage. In most cases, skull fractures are readily visualized on bone windows. However, when the fracture is parallel to the plane of imaging, nondisplaced skull fractures may be overlooked. In these cases, linear fractures are best seen on coronal reformatted images, three-dimensional volume rendered images, or on the scout view or plain radiographs.

Linear skull fractures may be differentiated from sutures by their linear rather than serrated or interdigitating contour. Additionally, fractures are more lucent compared with sutures. Fractures may also be distinguished from vascular grooves because fractures involve both the inner and outer tables of the skull, whereas vascular grooves only involve the inner table.

When presented with a skull fracture in a child, it is important to consult with the ordering provider to ensure that the history is appropriate and corresponds with the imaging findings. In cases where the history or proposed mechanism of injury is not consistent with the imaging findings, nonaccidental trauma should be considered.

✓ Pearls

- Linear fractures are the most common type of skull fracture and result from blunt injury.
- In the absence of depressed fracture fragments, vascular injury, or sutural diastasis, they are often self-limited.

- Linear fractures may be differentiated from sutures by their linear contour and increased lucency.
- CT is the modality of choice for head injury; it is readily available and best depicts acute intracranial injuries.

Suggested Reading

Glass RBF, Fernbach SK, Norton KI, Choi PS, Naidich TP. The infant skull: a vault of information. Radiographics 2004; 24: 507–522

Case 147

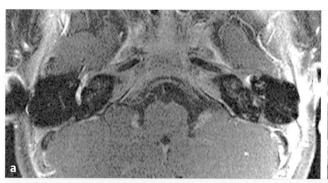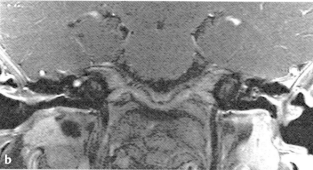

Fig. 147.1 Axial **(a)** and coronal **(b)** T1 postcontrast MR images with fat suppression reveal abnormal asymmetric enhancement and enlargement of the tympanic segment of the right facial nerve. The coronal image **(b)** shows the normal nonenhancing labyrinthine segments bilaterally (medially above the cochlea) and normal size and enhancement of the tympanic segment (just lateral to the labyrinthine segment) of the left facial nerve.

■ **Clinical Presentation**

A young adult man with facial asymmetry (▶ Fig. 147.1)

■ Key Imaging Finding

Facial nerve enhancement

■ Top 3 Differential Diagnoses

- **Normal facial nerve enhancement.** The proximal portions of the facial nerve that are surrounded by cerebrospinal fluid (the cisternal, canalicular, and labyrinthine segments) should not enhance; enhancement of these segments is considered abnormal. Beginning at the geniculate ganglion and extending distally into the horizontal (tympanic) and vertical (mastoid) segments, the facial nerve may enhance normally. Normal enhancement is typically symmetric or mildly asymmetric.
- **Bell palsy.** Bell palsy refers to acute onset infectious or postinfectious ipsilateral facial nerve palsy. Most cases are self-limiting and thought to result from the herpes simplex virus type 1, the same virus that causes cold sores. Imaging is reserved for atypical or nonresolving cases. On magnetic resonance imaging (MRI), the geniculate ganglion, tympanic segment, and mastoid segment of the facial nerve may enhance in normal patients. With Bell palsy, there is often smooth asymmet-

ric enhancement of the involved tympanic and/or mastoid segments, as well as abnormal enhancement of the portions of the facial nerve that are usually protected by the blood–nerve barrier, to include the intracanalicular and labyrinthine segments. The distal intracanalicular and labyrinthine segments are most commonly involved.
- **Nerve sheath tumor.** Schwannomas arise from perineural Schwann cells. They are composed of two tissue types: Antoni A (densely packed) and Antoni B (loosely packed, T2 hyperintense). The majority of patients with facial nerve schwannomas present with hearing loss or facial neuropathy. Temporal bone computed tomography (CT) reveals smooth enlargement of the involved segments of the facial nerve canal. The region of the geniculate ganglion is the most common site with extension into adjacent segments of the facial nerve. MRI demonstrates abnormal signal, tubular or fusiform enlargement, and abnormal enhancement of the involved segments.

■ Additional Differential Diagnoses

- **Facial nerve hemangioma.** Facial nerve hemangioma is a vascular tumor that occurs along the course of the facial nerve. It most often occurs in the region of the geniculate ganglion, followed by the distal internal auditory canal and junction of the horizontal (tympanic) and vertical (mastoid) segments of the facial nerve. CT reveals a characteristic "honeycomb" bony matrix. On MRI, lesions are T2 hyperintense with avid enhancement, corresponding to the vascular nature of the tumor.
- **Perineural spread of tumor.** Perineural spread of tumor along the facial nerve most often results from parotid malignancies, specifically adenoid cystic carcinoma, which has a propensity for perineural spread. Facial nerve involvement from primary head and neck or skin neoplasms is much less common. On CT, perineural spread most often manifests as abnormal enlargement of the bony facial nerve canal within the involved segments, typically extending proximally from the

stylomastoid foramen. MRI demonstrates abnormal enlargement, signal intensity, and enhancement of the involved portions of the facial nerve. When perineural spread of tumor is suspected, imaging should extend through the neck to evaluate for a primary origin.
- **Ramsey Hunt syndrome.** Ramsey Hunt syndrome is caused by reactivation of the varicella-zoster virus, which lies dormant in the geniculate ganglion. Patients are often elderly or immunocompromised and present with ipsilateral otalgia, a vesicular rash involving the external auditory canal and auricle, and facial neuropathy. MRI reveals abnormal enhancement within the involved segments of the facial nerve; abnormal enhancement of the vestibulocochlear nerve and labyrinthine structures is also commonly seen. Patients are typically treated with steroids and antiviral medications (e.g., acyclovir). There is a good prognosis/recovery in ~50 to 70% of cases.

■ Diagnosis

Facial nerve schwannoma

✓ Pearls

- Bell palsy most often involves the distal intracanalicular and labyrinthine segments; it is usually self-limiting.
- Tumors (schwannoma and perineural spread) result in abnormal signal, enhancement, and nerve enlargement.

- Hemangiomas are vascular tumors that result in a "honeycomb" matrix on CT and avid enhancement on MRI.

Suggested Reading

Saremi F, Helmy M, Farzin S, Zee CS, Go JL. MRI of cranial nerve enhancement. Am J Roentgenol 2005; 185: 1487–1497

Case 148

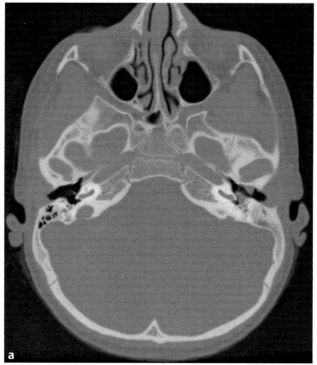

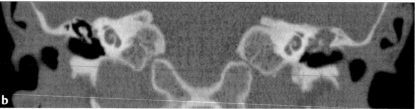

Fig. 148.1 Axial image from a noncontrast head computed tomography (CT) (a) demonstrates a lobulated soft-tissue density within the left middle ear. There is sclerosis and opacification within the left mastoid air cells, suggestive of chronic inflammation. Coronal reformatted CT image through the temporal bone (b) shows the mass within the epitympanum and lateral attic (Prussak's space) with blunting of the scutum and erosion/demineralization of the ossicles.

▣ Clinical Presentation

A young boy with chronic ear pain and conductive hearing loss (▶ Fig. 148.1)

■ Key Imaging Finding

Middle ear mass

■ Top 3 Differential Diagnoses

- **Acquired cholesteatoma.** Cholesteatomas are epidermoid cysts composed of keratinized squamous epithelium. Within the middle ear, the vast majority result from chronic otitis media. Patients suffer from multiple ear infections with perforation of a retracted tympanic membrane and conductive hearing loss. On imaging, cholesteatomas appear as soft-tissue masses within Prussak's space within the lateral attic. There is often blunting of the scutum (lateral wall of the attic) and erosion of the ossicles. When large, cholesteatomas may extend into the mastoid air cells. It is important to identify the bony margin of the facial nerve and integrity of the tegmen tympani (roof of the tympanic cavity) for presurgical planning, as well as to define the full extent of the mass for the surgeon. On magnetic resonance imaging (MRI), cholesteatomas commonly show increased signal on diffusion-weighted imaging. Complications include coalescent mastoiditis, meningitis, epidural abscesses, and venous sinus thrombosis.
- **Facial nerve schwannoma.** Facial nerve schwannomas may occur anywhere along the course of the facial nerve. When they occur within the tympanic segment within the middle ear, there is often enlargement of the bony facial nerve canal. Postcontrast images will demonstrate tubular enlargement and enhancement of the involved segment; involvement of the labyrinthine segment is a helpful finding to distinguish this entity from other middle ear masses. As small lesions can be subtle, it is important to look for asymmetry with the contralateral side.
- **Glomus tympanicum.** Glomus tympanicum is a paraganglioma that occurs within the middle ear along the cochlear promontory and course of Jacobson nerve. It arises from neural crest origin and is highly vascular with avid enhancement. As the mass grows, it may fill the middle ear and encroach on the ossicles. Bony erosion may be seen. When large, glomus tumors may contain calcifications and flow voids, resulting in a "salt and pepper" appearance on MRI. Clinically, patients present with conductive hearing loss and pulsatile tinnitus.

■ Additional Differential Diagnoses

- **Normal variant vasculature.** An aberrant internal carotid artery (ICA) is a developmental abnormality that likely results from regression of the cervical and proximal petrous ICA and the development of alternate anastomoses. Imaging findings include deviation and narrowing of the ICA within the temporal bone (extending into the middle ear), along with absence of the cervical and proximal portion of the petrous ICA. A dehiscent jugular bulb occurs when the sigmoid plate of the jugular bulb is absent, allowing for extension of the jugular bulb into the middle ear cavity. Imaging findings are diagnostic and typically straightforward.
- **Cholesterol granuloma.** Cholesterol granulomas occur secondary to nonspecific chronic inflammatory changes and are seen most commonly in the temporal bone (middle ear and petrous apex). Computed tomography reveals a soft-tissue mass within the middle ear without osseous erosion. On physical examination, there is a bluish or purplish coloration of the tympanic membrane. The lesions are hyperintense on both T1- and T2-weighted MRI sequences due to hemorrhage within the lesions. There may be peripheral rim enhancement.

■ Diagnosis

Acquired cholesteatoma

✓ Pearls

- Acquired cholesteatomas originate in Prussak's space and cause blunting of the scutum and ossicular erosion.
- Facial nerve schwannoma presents as an enhancing mass within an expanded facial nerve canal.
- Glomus tympanicum is a highly vascular paraganglioma that occurs along the cochlear promontory.
- Normal variant vasculature (aberrant ICA, dehiscent jugular bulb) may present clinically as a middle ear mass.

Suggested Readings

Betts A, Esquivel C, O'Brien WT. Vascular retrotympanic mass. J Am Osteopath Coll Radiol. 2012; 1: 31–33

Remley KB, Coit WE, Harnsberger HR, Smoker WR, Jacobs JM, McIff EB. Pulsatile tinnitus and the vascular tympanic membrane: CT, MR, and angiographic findings. Radiology 1990; 174: 383–389

Swartz JD, Harnsberger HR, Mukherji SK. The temporal bone. Contemporary diagnostic dilemmas. Radiol Clin North Am 1998; 36: 819–853, vi

Case 149

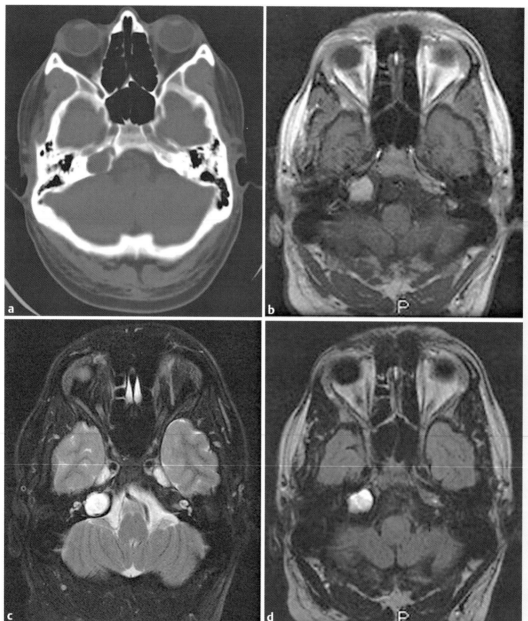

Fig. 149.1 Axial CT image in bone windows **(a)** demonstrates an expansile lucent lesion within the right petrous apex. The lesion is hyperintense on unenhanced T1 **(b)**, T2 with fat suppression **(c)**, and fluid-attenuated inversion recovery **(d)** weighted images. The lesion did not enhance on postcontrast sequences (not shown). (Courtesy of Rebecca Cornelius, MD.)

▪ Clinical Presentation

A 37-year-old man with headaches and hearing loss (▶ Fig. 149.1)

▨ Key Imaging Finding

Petrous apex mass

▨ Top 3 Differential Diagnoses

- **Cholesterol granuloma.** Cholesterol granulomas occur secondary to nonspecific chronic inflammatory changes and are seen most commonly in the temporal bone (petrous apex and middle ear cavity). They represent the most common primary lesion of the petrous apex. Computed tomography (CT) reveals a hypodense mass, which is often expansile with benign bony remodeling; bony erosion is less commonly seen. On magnetic resonance imaging (MRI), the lesions are characteristically hyperintense on both unenhanced T1 and T2 sequences due to hemorrhage within the lesions. Occasionally, a T2 hypointense hemosiderin ring is seen. There may be peripheral rim enhancement, but the lesions themselves will not enhance.
- **Mucous retention cyst or Mucocele.** Mucous retention cysts and mucoceles are typically seen in the paranasal sinuses but may also occur within a pneumatized petrous apex. They occur secondary to entrapped secretions in an aerated petrous apex. They are hypodense and often expansile (more common with mucoceles) on CT. On MRI, lesions are typically hypointense on T1 and hyperintense on T2 sequences. With inspissated, proteinaceous secretions, they may be slightly hyperintense on T1; however, not to the same degree as cholesterol granulomas. The lesions do not enhance, although peripheral inflammatory enhancement may be seen.
- **Congenital cholesteatoma.** Congenital cholesteatomas are epidermoids that most commonly occur within the middle ear and petrous apex, similar to cholesterol granulomas. On CT, the lesions are hypodense and expansile. MRI demonstrates increased T2 signal intensity secondary to internal cystic components. The lesions are commonly hypointense to slightly hyperintense on T1-weighted sequences. As with other epidermoids, there is typically increased signal on diffusion-weighted imaged, which is fairly characteristic. Thin peripheral enhancement may be seen, but the lesions themselves do not enhance.

▨ Additional Differential Diagnoses

- **Apical petrositis.** Serous or reactive fluid within a pneumatized petrous apex is a common finding in asymptomatic patients and is of little clinical significance. Apical petrositis, however, refers to superimposed infection of a pneumatized petrous apex, often in association with otomastoiditis. CT reveals fluid density within the petrous apex, as well as possible adjacent bony erosion. The fluid is hypointense on T1-weighted and hyperintense on T2-weighted MR sequences. Inflammatory changes result in prominent enhancement, which often extends along the overlying dura. Gradenigo syndrome refers to retroorbital pain and diplopia secondary to cranial nerve (CN) VI (abducens) deficits as a result of petrous apicitis; the infectious process compresses the nerve as it extends through the dural reflection of the Dorello canal. Prompt diagnosis and treatment is necessary to reduce morbidity associated with this entity.
- **Neoplasm.** Metastases commonly involve the skull base secondary to direct or hematogenous spread. Direct spread may result from nasopharyngeal or sinonasal primary neoplasms (squamous cell carcinoma). Lung, breast, renal cell, and prostate cancer disseminate via hematogenous spread. Primary involvement can be seen with chondrosarcoma, multiple myeloma, or plasmacytoma. Chondrosarcomas are expansile, off-midline, and characteristically bright on T2-weighted sequences due to a chondroid matrix; on CT there are internal calcifications in an "arcs and swirls" pattern. Bony destruction is often irregular and aggressive with tumors. Enhancement is prominent and best seen on fat-suppressed sequences.

▨ Diagnosis

Cholesterol granuloma

✓ Pearls

- Cholesterol granuloma is the most common primary petrous apex lesion and is bright on T1- and T2-weighted images.
- Mucous retention cysts and mucoceles may occur within a pneumatized petrous apex with entrapped secretions.
- Apical petrositis may lead to Gradenigo syndrome (apical petrositis, retroorbital pain, and CN VI deficits).
- Chondrosarcomas may arise from the petrous bone, are bright on T2 sequences, and contain "arcs and swirls" calcifications.

Suggested Readings

Chapman PR, Shah R, Curé JK, Bag AK. Petrous apex lesions: pictorial review. Am J Roentgenol 2011; 196 Suppl: WS26–WS37, Quiz S40–S43

Connor SEJ, Leung R, Natas S. Imaging of the petrous apex: a pictorial review. Br J Radiol 2008; 81: 427–435

Case 150

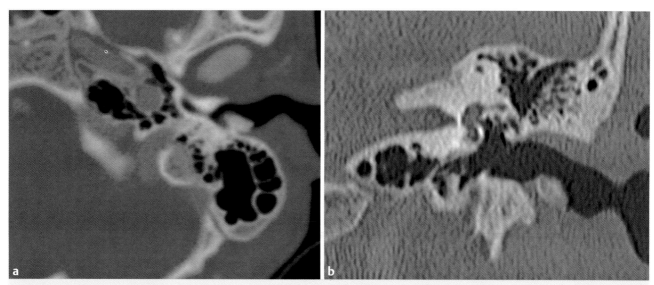

Fig. 150.1 Axial computed tomography (CT) image **(a)** demonstrates focal calcification and narrowing of the left EAC. Coronal reformatted CT image of the left temporal bone **(b)** reveals the calcification at the junction of the cartilaginous and bony EAC. A pedunculated morphology was seen on sequential images (stalk out of plane).

▒ Clinical Presentation

A 14-year-old boy with abnormality on physical exam (▶ Fig. 150.1)

▨ Key Imaging Finding

Circumscribed external auditory canal (EAC) calcification/ossification

▨ Top 2 Differential Diagnoses

- **EAC exostosis.** EAC exostoses are benign overgrowths that result from chronic inflammation. They occur most often in young adults and have a disproportionate involvement in surfers, as well as divers and swimmers; hence, the term *"surfer's ear."* Chronic exposure to cold water leads to repeated bouts of otitis externa, most often due to *Staphylococcus aureus* or *Pseudomonas aeruginosa.* This entity differs from malignant otitis externa, which is an aggressive infection that occurs in immunocompromised patients, most often elderly diabetics. Acutely, patients may present with otalgia, pruritis, EAC drainage, and conductive hearing loss. Chronically, there is bony overgrowth of the EAC that is characteristically bilateral, circumferential, and sessile. Treatment is often not necessary; when needed, it consists of surgical correction of the EAC stenosis.

- **EAC osteoma.** Osteomas are benign bony overgrowths that rarely involve the temporal bone. They occur sporadically and are typically asymptomatic and incidental. On computed tomography, they appear as unilateral, circumscribed, pedunculated bony lesions that occur at the junction of the bony and cartilaginous portion of the EAC. The overlying soft-tissue portion of the EAC is normal. Lesions are typically not treated unless there is significant, symptomatic EAC stenosis.

▨ Diagnosis

EAC osteoma

✓ Pearls

- EAC exostoses are a complication of "surfer's ear"; bony lesions are often bilateral, circumferential, and sessile.
- Osteomas are bony overgrowths that are unilateral, pedunculated, and occur at the bony-cartilaginous junction.
- In the vast majority of cases, neither EAC exostoses nor osteomas require treatment.

Suggested Reading

Tran LP, Grundfast KM, Selesnick SH. Benign lesions of the external auditory canal. Otolaryngol Clin North Am 1996; 29: 807–825

Case 151

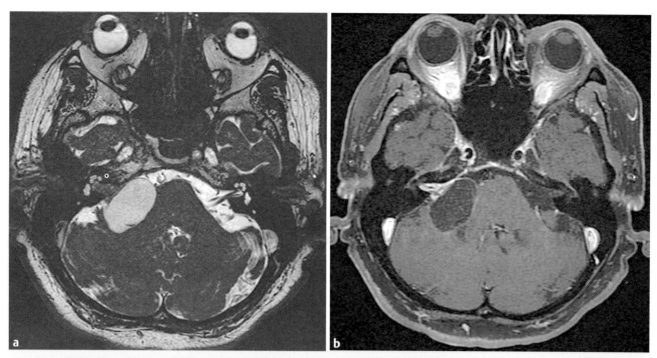

Fig. 151.1 High-resolution axial fast imaging employing steady state acquisition (FIESTA) image **(a)** reveals a cystic mass in the right CPA with soft-tissue signal within the right IAC. Postcontrast axial T1 image with fat suppression **(b)** shows avid enhancement of the solid component within the IAC and extending through the porous acousticus.

▨ Clinical Presentation

A 32-year-old man with sensorineural hearing loss (▶ Fig. 151.1)

■ Key Imaging Finding

Cerebellopontine angle (CPA) mass

■ Top 3 Differential Diagnoses

- **Vestibular schwannoma.** Vestibular schwannomas arise from perineural Schwann cells. They are composed of two tissue types: Antoni A and B. Antoni A tissue is densely packed, which results in relatively darker signal on T2 sequences; Antoni B tissue is loosely packed and hyperintense on T2 sequences. Vestibular schwannomas may involve the superior or inferior divisions of the vestibular nerve within the posterior internal auditory canal (IAC). There is typically expansion of the IAC and flaring of the porus acousticus. The border of a schwannoma typically makes an acute angle with the petrous temporal bone. Lesions are variable in signal but typically hyperintense on T2 sequences. Cystic change and hemorrhage may occur; calcification is uncommon. Enhancement is heterogeneous but avid. Bilateral vestibular schwannomas are diagnostic of neurofibromatosis type 2 (NF2).
- **Meningioma.** Meningiomas arise from meningothelial arachnoid cells and are the most common extraaxial tumors. They typically occur in adult women; they may also be seen in children with NF2 or a history of prior cranial radiation. CPA

meningiomas may be circumscribed or plaque-like. They often have a broad dural base along the petrous temporal bone and avidly enhance with a dural tail. An isolated intracanalicular meningioma is rare. On unenhanced computed tomography (CT), meningiomas are iso- to hyperdense compared with brain parenchyma with adjacent bony remodeling or hyperostosis. Calcification is common.
- **Arachnoid cyst.** Arachnoid cysts are cerebrospinal fluid (CSF) collections contained within the arachnoid. The vast majority are developmental due to embryonic failure of meningeal fusion; acquired cases have also been described. The most common locations include the middle cranial fossa, followed by the posterior fossa. The cysts are hypodense on CT and follow CSF signal on magnetic resonance imaging. Slight increased signal may be seen on proton density and T2 sequences due to lack of normal CSF pulsations. There is no restricted diffusion, which is a key discriminator from epidermoid cysts, and no enhancement. Larger cysts exert mass effect on the adjacent parenchyma.

■ Additional Differential Diagnoses

- **Epidermoid.** Epidermoid cysts are tumors of ectodermal origin, composed of keratinaceous debris, and lined by stratified squamous epithelium. The most common intracranial location is the CPA. Epidermoids are hypointense on T1 and hyperintense on T2 sequences. There is typically heterogeneous hypointensity on fluid-attenuated inversion recovery imaging. The key distinction from arachnoid cysts is the presence of restricted diffusion, which is characteristic of epidermoid cysts. In addition, epidermoid cysts have irregular margins and engulf vessels and nerves rather than displace them, in contradistinction to arachnoid cysts.

- **Lipoma.** Intracranial lipomas result from persistence of the meninx primitiva, which is a precursor to the pia and arachnoid. They are typically midline and supratentorial in location; however, the CPA is the most common location in the posterior fossa. Lipomas are characteristically hypodense on CT and follow fat signal intensity on all pulse sequences. The presence of chemical shift artifact and suppression on fat-saturated sequences are key to making the diagnosis. The vast majority are asymptomatic; however, cranial neuropathies may occasionally occur. Treatment is reserved for symptomatic lesions. Gross total resection is difficult.

■ Diagnosis

Vestibular schwannoma

✓ Pearls

- Vestibular schwannomas are the most common CPA masses; bilateral lesions are diagnostic of NF2.
- Meningiomas are hyperdense on CT, may have calcification, intensely enhance, and have a dural tail.

- Arachnoid cysts follow CSF signal on all pulse sequences and may exert local mass effect.
- Epidermoids mimic arachnoid cysts with the exception of restricted diffusion, which is characteristic.

Suggested Readings

Bonneville F, Savatovsky J, Chiras J. Imaging of cerebellopontine angle lesions: an update. Part 1: enhancing extra-axial lesions. Eur Radiol 2007; 17: 2472–2482

Bonneville F, Savatovsky J, Chiras J. Imaging of cerebellopontine angle lesions: an update. Part 2: intra-axial lesions, skull base lesions that may invade the CPA region, and non-enhancing extra-axial lesions. Eur Radiol 2007; 17: 2908–2920

Case 152

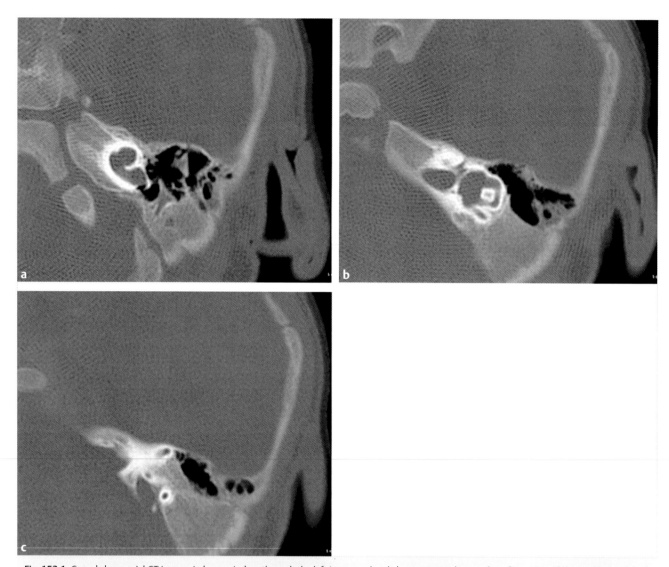

Fig. 152.1 Coned-down axial CT images in bone window through the left inner ear **(a–c)** demonstrate abnormal configuration of the cochlea with lack of visualization of the normal 2½ turns **(a)**, an enlarged vestibule **(b)**, and enlargement of the vestibular aqueduct **(c)**.

▨ Clinical Presentation

A 6-year-old boy with hearing loss (▶ Fig. 152.1)

▦ Key Imaging Finding

Congenital inner ear malformation

▦ Top 3 Differential Diagnoses

- **Large vestibular aqueduct syndrome (LVAS).** LVAS is a common cause of sensorineural deafness in early childhood. Affected patients hear normally at birth with bilateral sensorineural hearing loss progressing over the first few months to years of life. Unenhanced computed tomography (CT) reveals enlargement of the vestibular aqueducts (bilateral in > 90% of cases), measuring > 1.5 mm in diameter at its midpoint. The size of the semicircular canals can also be used as an internal rough estimate of the expected size of the vestibular aqueduct. Associated abnormalities of cochlea and vestibule are common but may be subtle.
- **Cystic cochleovestibular anomaly.** Cystic cochleovestibular anomaly is a result of arrested inner ear development, resulting in cystic dilatation of the cochlea and vestibule. No internal architecture or features can be identified. Patients have sensorineural hearing loss at birth. On unenhanced axial CT and T2 magnetic resonance imaging, the dilated cochlea and vestibule demonstrate a "figure 8" appearance. Semicircular canals are commonly dilated as well. The vestibular aqueduct is typically normal.
- **Cystic common cavity.** Cystic common cavity refers to lack of development of the cochlea and vestibule. The semicircular canals are variably affected and are most often absent; occasionally, they may be dysplastic or even normal. As with cystic cochleovestibular anomaly, patients present with sensorineural hearing loss at birth. Imaging findings include a single cystic cavity in place of normal inner ear structures (cochlea, vestibule, and, commonly, semicircular canals). Middle ear structures and the vestibular aqueduct are typically normal.

▦ Additional Differential Diagnoses

- **Cochlear aplasia.** Cochlear aplasia results from arrest of normal development of the cochlea during embryogenesis. It may be unilateral or bilateral depending upon the type and timing of insult, and patients present with sensorineural hearing loss at birth. Imaging findings include an absent cochlea. Remaining inner ear structures, including the vestibule and semicircular canals, may be dysplastic or normal. The middle ear structures and vestibular aqueduct are typically normal.

▦ Diagnosis

Large vestibular aqueduct with associated cochlear and vestibular abnormalities

✓ Pearls

- LVAS presents with vestibular aqueducts > 1.5 mm in diameter; hearing loss is bilateral and progressive.
- Cystic cochleovestibular anomaly has a characteristic "figure 8" appearance of the cochlea and vestibule.
- Cystic common cavity refers to a single cavity in place of normal inner ear structures.

Suggested Reading

Joshi VM, Navlekar SK, Kishore GR, Reddy KJ, Kumar EC. CT and MR imaging of the inner ear and brain in children with congenital sensorineural hearing loss. Radiographics 2012; 32: 683–698

Case 153

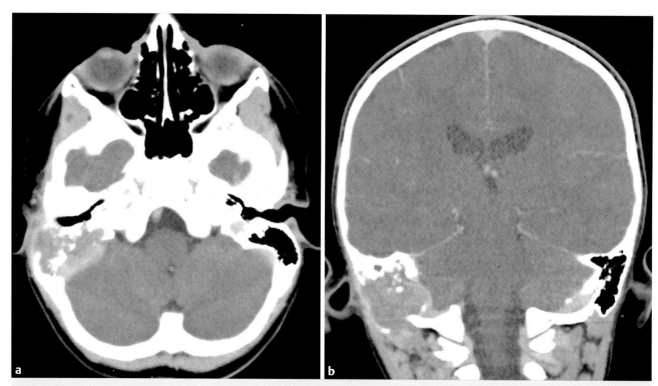

Fig. 153.1 Axial **(a)** and reformatted coronal **(b)** contrast-enhanced CT images demonstrate opacification, bony destruction, and enhancement centered on the mastoid portion of the right temporal bone. There is bony dehiscence medially with intracranial extension along the lateral aspect of the right cerebellar hemisphere.

▧ Clinical Presentation

A 6-year-old boy with severe otalgia (▶ Fig. 153.1)

■ Key Imaging Finding

Aggressive temporal bone mass in a child

■ Top 3 Differential Diagnoses

- **Coalescent otomastoiditis.** Coalescent mastoiditis refers to an acute infectious process of the middle ear cavity and mastoids with destruction of the bony mastoid septae and overlying cortex. It may occur as a primary infection or in association with an acquired cholesteatoma. Patients present clinically with fever, hearing loss, and otalgia. Computed tomography (CT) demonstrates opacification of the middle ear cavity and mastoids with erosion of the mastoid septae and mastoid cortex; the ossicles may also be involved. On magnetic resonance imaging (MRI), the inflammatory process is T2 hyperintense with relatively diffuse enhancement. Focal abscesses or an underlying cholesteatoma may be hyperintense on diffusion-weighted imaging. Complications include subperiosteal, Bezold (mastoid tip into sternocleidomastoid muscle), epidural, or brain parenchymal abscesses; meningitis; and dural venous sinus thrombosis.

- **Langerhans cell histiocytosis (LCH).** LCH refers to abnormal proliferation of histiocytes. It may be localized (formerly eosinophilic granuloma), multifocal (formerly Hand-Schüller-Christian disease), or disseminated (formerly Letterer-Siwe disease). The localized form is the most common and mildest form. The calvarium is most often involved, followed by the spine. The classic radiological description is a well-defined lytic lesion without sclerotic borders. A "beveled" edge appearance can result from greater involvement of the inner than outer table of the skull. MRI will show marrow replacement and avid soft-tissue enhancement. Temporal bone involvement typically occurs within the petrous apex or otic capsule. Temporal bone LCH may also present with diffuse bony destruction, mimicking a neoplastic or aggressive infectious/inflammatory process. The most common clinical symptoms include pain, palpable mass, and/or systemic symptoms.

- **Rhabdomyosarcoma.** Rhabdomyosarcoma is a rare, aggressive malignancy of childhood that commonly involves the head and neck region. With temporal bone involvement, the mass often originates within the middle ear and extends into the mastoids and external auditory canal. More aggressive lesions extend intracranially, into the skull base, and/or into the extracranial soft tissues of the upper neck. Cervical nodal metastases may rarely be seen. CT demonstrates a soft-tissue mass centered within the middle ear cavity and mastoids with aggressive bony destruction. The mass is typically hypointense on T1 and hyperintense on T2 MRI sequences, nonspecific. There is heterogeneous but avid contrast enhancement; enhancement of the dura is indicative of intracranial extension. Perineural spread along cranial nerves VII and VIII may also be seen. Clinically, patients present in the first or second decades of life with symptoms mimicking recurrent, chronic otomastoiditis.

■ Diagnosis

Langerhans cell histiocytosis

✓ Pearls

- Coalescent mastoiditis refers to acute infectious bony destruction of the mastoid septae and overlying cortex.
- LCH classically presents as a well-defined lytic lesion with "beveled" edges; Temporal bone involvement may be diffuse.

- Rhabdomyosarcoma is a childhood malignancy; the destructive mass is centered in the middle ear and mastoids.
- LCH and rhabdomyosarcoma demonstrate soft-tissue rather than inflammatory (otomastoiditis) enhancement.

Suggested Readings

Connor SEJ, Leung R, Natas S. Imaging of the petrous apex: a pictorial review. Br J Radiol 2008; 81: 427–435

Razek AA, Huang BY. Lesions of the petrous apex: classification and findings at CT and MR imaging. Radiographics 2012; 32: 151–173

Case 154

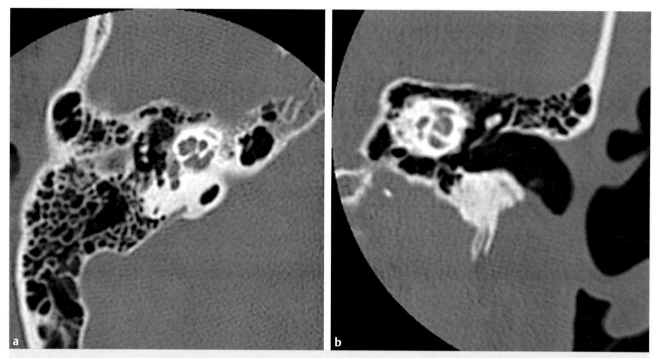

Fig. 154.1 Axial **(a)** and coronal **(b)** CT images of the temporal bone reveal abnormal fenesteral **(a)** (adjacent to the oval window along the anterolateral aspect of the vestibule) and pericochlear **(a,b)** lucencies.

▦ Clinical Presentation

An adult man with mixed hearing loss (▶ Fig. 154.1)

▨ Key Imaging Finding

Otic capsule lucencies

▨ Top 3 Differential Diagnoses in Older Adults

- **Otosclerosis.** Otosclerosis results in abnormal bony development and growth that characteristically involves the region of the stapes and oval window. Approximately 60% of cases are thought to be hereditary, whereas the remainder appear sporadic. Although patients may present anytime from adolescence to adulthood, most present as young adults with progressive, mixed hearing loss. Computed tomography (CT) is ideal for identifying the regions of abnormal mineralization that appear as otic capsule lucencies (of various morphologies), but the findings may be subtle. Approximately 85% of cases are termed *fenesteral* with abnormal otic lucencies in the region of the oval and round windows. Approximately 15% of cases are termed *cochlear* with abnormal pericochlear lucencies. Often times, there are components of both fenesteral and cochlear otosclerosis. Treatment options include hearing aids for more mild cases and stapedectomy and prosthesis placement for more severe cases.

- **Paget disease.** Paget disease affects the elderly population and is more common in men. It results in bony expansion with cortical thickening and thickened trabeculae. Common locations include the axial skeleton, pelvis, long bones, and calvarium. The most common forms of calvarial involvement consist of osteoporosis circumscripta, which presents as a prominent lucency, and the more diffuse "cotton wool" appearance, which refers to the radiographic appearance of the bony and trabeculae thickening. Otic capsule involvement most often consists of bony thickening with diffuse lucency. The bony involvement extends beyond the otic capsule, which in conjunction with patient age, is a useful discriminator.

- **Osteoradionecrosis.** Radiation necrosis is a late complication that may be seen months or years after radiation therapy. It is thought to be caused by vascular injury and resultant ischemia. The severity is dependent upon the region treated, the dose of treatment, length of time between treatments, and the duration of treatments. Imaging findings include demineralization, manifested as abnormal lucencies that are typically diffuse. In severe cases, there may be frank bony destruction. Common primary neoplasms to involve the otic capsule in the radiation field include skull base, nasopharyngeal, and brain neoplasms.

▨ Top 3 Differential Diagnoses in Children and Young Adults

- **Otosclerosis.** See above.

- **Normal variation of mineralization.** High-resolution CT in infants and young children may occasionally demonstrate otic capsule lucencies in otherwise asymptomatic patients. On follow-up studies, many patients demonstrate interval ossification of the regions in question, suggesting a form of normal variation or delayed cartilaginous ossification. When presented with a case of suspected otosclerosis in a young, asymptomatic child, correlation with symptoms, audiometric testing, and possibly follow-up imaging may help distinguish normal variant ossification from otosclerosis.

- **Osteogenesis imperfect tarda.** Osteogenesis imperfect (OI) is a connective tissue disorder that results in fragile bones, as well as other connective tissue abnormalities. Type 1 is referred to as OI tarda, is the mildest form, and may present with otic capsule lucencies, in addition to nondeforming fragile bones and blue sclera. The disorder is clinically evident but may appear identical to otosclerosis on CT imaging with otic capsule lucencies predominantly in the pericochlear regions. The diagnosis of OI should only be suggested in the appropriate clinical setting due to its rarity.

▨ Diagnosis

Otosclerosis

✓ Pearls

- Otosclerosis results in mixed hearing loss with fenesteral (most common) and/or pericochlear lucencies on CT.
- Paget disease causes bony expansion in elderly patients; calvarial involvement extends beyond the otic capsule.

- Osteoradionecrosis occurs in the treatment field and results from vascular injury and resultant bony ischemia.
- OI tarda results in otic capsule lucencies similar to otosclerosis, nondeformed fragile bones, and blue sclera.

Suggested Reading

Pekkola J, Pitkaranta A, Jappel A et al. Localized pericochlear hypoattenuating foci at temporal-bone thin-section CT in pediatric patients: nonpathologic differential diagnostic entity? Radiology 2004; 230: 88–92

Case 155

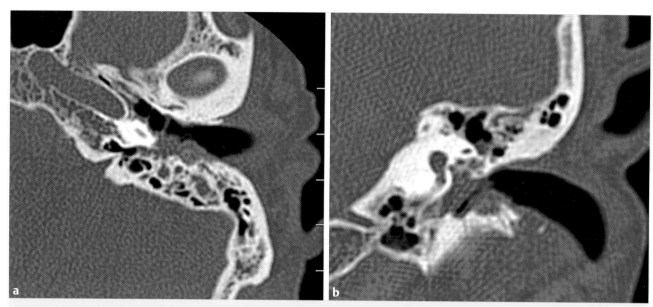

Fig. 155.1 Axial CT image of the left temporal bone **(a)** demonstrates a soft-tissue mass along the posterior aspect of the EAC with underlying bony erosion. Coronal image **(b)** shows similar findings along the posteroinferior EAC, as well as opacification of the visualized portions of the mesotympanum and hypotympanum.

▨ Clinical Presentation

A 59-year-old man with otalgia and otorrhea (▸ Fig. 155.1)

▦ Key Imaging Finding

External auditory canal (EAC) soft-tissue mass with bony erosion

▦ Top 3 Differential Diagnoses

- **Necrotizing otitis externa (NOE).** NOE most often results from pseudomonas infection in elderly diabetic or immunosuppressed patients. Patients present with otalgia, hearing loss, external ear drainage (otorrhea), and adjacent soft-tissue swelling. Unenhanced computed tomography (CT) reveals soft-tissue opacification of the EAC with superficial soft-tissue swelling. As the infection progresses, there is underlying bony destruction and soft-tissue abscess formation. Magnetic resonance imaging (MRI) reveals diffuse intermediate to hyperintense T2 signal and enhancement within the EAC and soft tissues due to phlegmonous inflammatory tissue. Focal abscesses will demonstrate rim enhancement. Treatment consists of appropriate antibiotic therapy with or without surgical debridement. Complications include skull-base and intracranial spread of the infectious process.

- **EAC squamous cell carcinoma (SCC).** SCC typically occurs in elderly patients as a result of local spread from an auricle carcinoma. The primary site presents as an ulcerating skin lesion. With EAC spread, patients present with otalgia, hearing loss, and otorrhea. Unenhanced CT findings vary based upon the stage and extent of disease. Early findings include soft-tissue opacification and narrowing of the EAC. In later stages, there is bony destruction and lymphadenopathy, which commonly involves the periauricular and ipsilateral parotid lymph nodes. MRI better depicts the extent of involvement and may identify intracranial or perineural spread. The regions of tumor involvement are hyperintense on T2 with variable patterns of enhancement. Treatment options include surgical resection or debridement with adjuvant radiation and/or chemotherapy depending upon the extent of tumor and presence of regional or distant spread.

- **EAC cholesteatoma.** EAC cholesteatomas most often occur in middle-aged and elderly patients and are composed of keratinized squamous epithelium. Although benign, the lesions are locally aggressive. Patients often present with otalgia, hearing loss, and otorrhea. Unenhanced CT reveals soft-tissue filling and narrowing of the EAC with underlying bony erosion/fragmentation. There may mastoid and/or middle ear involvement as well. MRI reveals T2 intermediate soft-tissue signal intensity with peripheral inflammatory enhancement. Increased signal is commonly seen on diffusion-weighted imaging. Treatment consists of surgical resection.

▦ Diagnosis

Necrotizing otitis externa

✓ Pearls

- Clinical and imaging findings of NOE, EAC SCC, and EAC cholesteatomas have significant overlap.
- NOE most often results from pseudomonas infection in elderly diabetic or immunosuppressed patients.

- EAC SCC typically occurs in elderly patients as a result of local spread from an ulcerated auricle carcinoma.
- Cholesteatoma is composed of keratinized squamous epithelium; although benign, it is locally aggressive.

Suggested Readings

Grandis JR, Curtin HD, Yu VL. Necrotizing (malignant) external otitis: prospective comparison of CT and MR imaging in diagnosis and follow-up. Radiology 1995; 196: 499–504

Heilbrun ME, Salzman KL, Glastonbury CM, Harnsberger HR, Kennedy RJ, Shelton C. External auditory canal cholesteatoma: clinical and imaging spectrum. Am J Neuroradiol 2003; 24: 751–756

Case 156

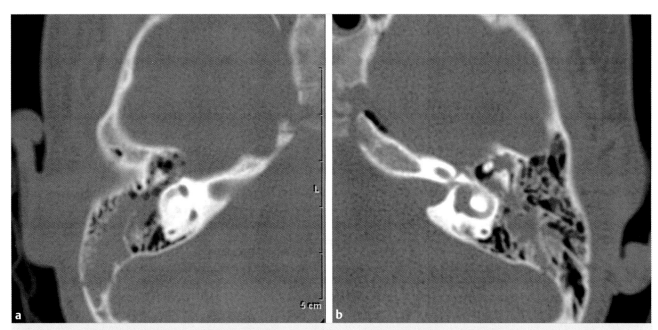

Fig. 156.1 Bilateral axial images of the temporal bones **(a,b)** demonstrate longitudinally oriented temporal bone fractures with dislocation of the incudomalleal joints with the "ice cream" falling off the "cone." There is associated fluid within the middle ear cavities and mastoids. Transverse-oriented fractures are also seen bilaterally extending through the posterior aspect of the mastoids. The otic capsule structures were spared. A small amount of pneumocephalus is seen within the left middle cranial fossa **(b)**.

■ Clinical Presentation

A young man involved in a motor vehicle accident (▶ Fig. 156.1)

▦ Key Imaging Finding

Temporal bone fracture

▦ Diagnosis

Temporal bone fracture. Temporal bone fractures typically occur in the setting of significant trauma. Patients may present with hearing loss (typically conductive), facial nerve deficits, or otorrhea; inner ear involvement may also lead to vertigo. From a clinical standpoint, temporal bone fractures are managed based upon whether or not there is otic capsule involvement. On imaging, temporal bone fractures have been historically characterized based upon their orientation relative to the temporal bone and described as longitudinal, transverse, or mixed.

Longitudinal fractures are the most common subtype (75%) and are oriented along the long axis of the temporal bone, affecting the squamous portion of the temporal bone and extending into the mastoid portion. Nondisplaced fractures can be subtle on computed tomography examinations, especially in the absence of dedicated temporal bone imaging or reformats. Secondary findings include blood products within the mastoid air cells, middle ear cavity, or external auditory canal. Complications of longitudinal fractures include ossicular dislocation (most common) and facial nerve injury (less common than with transverse fractures). Ossicular dislocation commonly presents as the "ice cream" (head of the malleus) falling off of the "cone" (short process of the incus) and/or dislocation of the incudostapedial joint. The orientation of the fracture may extend into the carotid canal and central skull base.

Transverse temporal bone fractures are less common than longitudinal fractures and are oriented perpendicular to the long axis of the temporal bone. Due to their orientation, they commonly involve the facial nerve canal and may extend into the otic capsule with involvement of inner ear structures. Clinically, patients present with symptoms similar to longitudinal fractures with the addition of sensorineural hearing loss and vertigo, depending upon the structures involved. Facial nerve injury is more common with transverse temporal bone fractures than longitudinal fractures; approximately 50% of all transverse fractures will involve the facial nerve. Once a transverse fracture is identified, care should be taken to evaluate for involvement of the facial nerve canal, inner ear structures, and jugular fossa.

In many instances, there will be variants of both longitudinal and transverse temporal bone fractures in the setting of trauma, which are referred to as mixed temporal bone fractures. When this occurs, it is important to evaluate all segments of the fracture, paying close attention to involvement of vascular channels (including the jugular canal and petrous segment of the internal carotid artery [ICA]), inner ear structures, the facial nerve, and ossicles.

✓ Pearls

- Clinically, temporal bone fractures are characterized based upon involvement or sparing of the otic capsule.
- Longitudinal temporal bone fractures commonly result in ossicular dislocation and conductive hearing loss.
- Transverse temporal bone fractures more commonly affect the facial nerve and inner ear structures.
- Vascular injury may occur when fractures extend into the jugular canal and/or petrous segments of the ICA.

Suggested Readings

Fatterpekar GM, Doshi AH, Dugar M, Delman BN, Naidich TP, Som PM. Role of 3D CT in the evaluation of the temporal bone. Radiographics 2006; 26 Suppl 1: S117–S132

Zayas JO, Feliciano YZ, Hadley CR, Gomez AA, Vidal JA. Temporal bone trauma and the role of multidetector CT in the emergency department. Radiographics 2011; 31: 1741–1755

Case 157

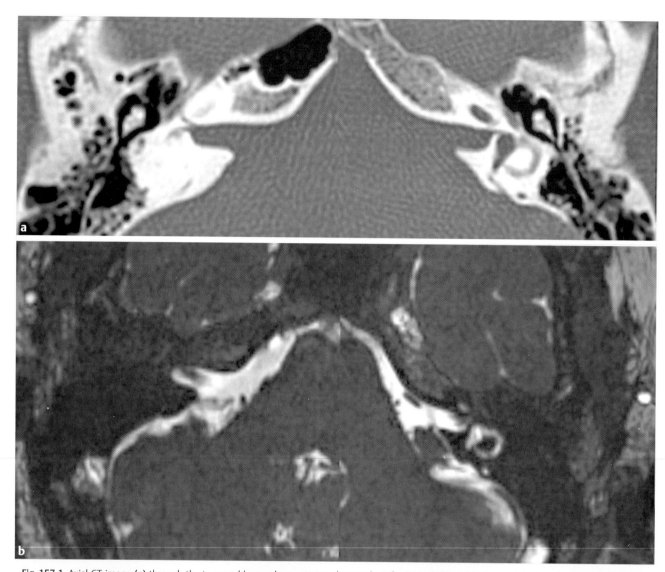

Fig. 157.1 Axial CT image **(a)** through the temporal bones demonstrates abnormal ossification of the vestibule, semicircular canals, and cochlea on the right. Corresponding high-resolution T2 image **(b)** reveals absence of the normal T2 hyperintense endolymph within the inner structures on the right. Normal T2 signal is seen within the vestibule and lateral semicircular canal on the left.

◼ Clinical Presentation

A 28-year-old woman with severe unilateral hearing loss and vertigo (▶ Fig. 157.1)

▧ Key Imaging Finding

Abnormal mineralization (computed tomography, CT) and loss of signal intensity (magnetic resonance imaging, MRI) within labyrinthine structures

▧ Diagnosis

Labyrinthitis ossificans (LO). LO refers to ossification of the membranous labyrinth (vestibule, semicircular canals, and/or cochlea) due to some form of insult, typically infectious or inflammatory. Meningitis and otitis media represent the most common infectious etiologies. Post-traumatic hemorrhage is a less common cause. Findings may be unilateral or bilateral, depending upon the etiology and extent of insult.

LO occurs in three stages: acute, fibrous, and ossifying. The acute stage is characterized by focal or diffuse labyrinthine inflammation. Imaging in this stage may be normal or demonstrate enhancement of labyrinthine structures on MRI. There is preservation of normal T2 hyperintense labyrinthine fluid (MRI) initially and normal inner ear attenuation on CT. As the disease progresses into the fibrous stage, there is partial loss of signal intensity within the labyrinthine structures on T2-weighted MRI sequences and corresponding hazy increased attenuation on CT. During this phase, there may be residual labyrinthine enhancement on postcontrast T1 sequences. In the ossifying stage, mineralization results in loss of the normal T2 signal intensity on MRI and increased attenuation of the labyrinthine structures on CT.

Patients with LO present with sensorineural hearing loss up to a year after an antecedent insult. Vertigo may also be seen clinically and can be severe. Cochlear implantation is the treatment of choice for cochlear involvement, especially with bilateral disease. It is important to describe fibrous or ossifying changes within the cochlea because these findings affect surgical management and prognosis.

✓ Pearls

- LO refers to ossification of the membranous labyrinth and often results from infectious or inflammatory insults.
- Imaging reveals mineralization of inner structures on CT and loss of the normal T2 signal on MRI.
- Patients present with sensorineural hearing loss and vertigo, which can be debilitating.

Suggested Reading

Phillips GS, LoGerfo SE, Richardson ML, Anzai Y. Interactive Web-based learning module on CT of the temporal bone: anatomy and pathology. Radiographics 2012; 32: E85–E105

Case 158

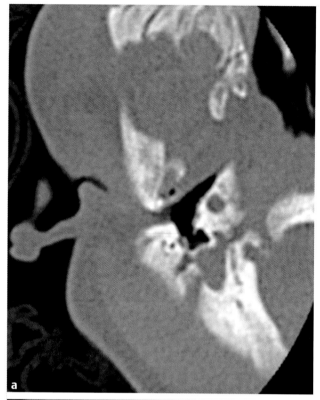

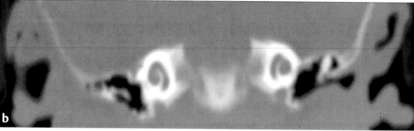

Fig. 158.1 Axial **(a)** and reformatted coronal **(b)** computed tomography images demonstrate bony stenosis and soft-tissue atresia of the right EAC. The coronal image shows hypoplasia of the visualized portions of the malleus and incus on the right with fusion along the lateral wall of the middle ear cavity. The right pinna is slightly maldeveloped and hypoplastic but not optimally seen on the selected images.

▪ Clinical Presentation

A 3-day-old girl with abnormal neonatal physical exam (▶ Fig. 158.1)

■ Key Imaging Finding

Underdevelopment of the external auditory canal (EAC)

■ Diagnosis

External auditory canal (EAC) atresia. EAC atresia comprises a spectrum of anomalies that result from underdevelopment of the EAC and pinna. The genetic deformity involves the first and second branchial arches (malleus and incus) and the first pharyngeal pouch (EAC).

Unenhanced computed tomography is the modality of choice for identifying and characterizing the associated anomalies. EAC stenosis or atresia may be bony, soft tissue, or a combination of both. More mild forms consist of a narrowed EAC and small or dysmorphic pinna. More severe forms consist of complete bony atresia with significant deformity of the pinna. The mastoids and middle ear structures are commonly involved with under-pneumatization and hypoplastic or absent ossicles, particularly the malleus and incus, which originate from the first and second branchial arches. Portions of the ossicles that are formed may be fused to the walls of the middle ear cavity.

There may also be atresia of the oval window. It is important to identify the course of the facial nerve as it is commonly altered and its location will be important for surgical planning. Inner ear structures are typically spared, although malformations of labyrinthine structures may be seen in approximately 10% of cases.

Patients present clinically with a deformed pinna and conductive hearing loss. The EAC may be stenotic or completely atretic on physical exam. In terms of genetics, EAC atresia may be sporadic, inherited, or associated with syndromes, including Pierre Robin, Treacher Collins, Crouzon, and Goldenhar. In unilateral disease, treatment typically consists of cosmetic reconstruction and a bone conduction hearing aid. Bilateral disease requires more extensive surgical intervention for hearing preservation, including middle ear/ossicular reconstruction.

✓ Pearls

- EAC atresia comprises a spectrum of anomalies that result from underdevelopment of the EAC and pinna.
- EAC atresia commonly involves the EAC, pinna, and middle ear structures, particularly the malleus and incus.

- EAC atresia may be sporadic, inherited, or syndromic (Pierre Robin, Treacher Collins, Crouzon, and Goldenhar).

Suggested Reading

Gassner EM, Mallouhi A, Jaschke WR. Preoperative evaluation of external auditory canal atresia on high-resolution CT. Am J Roentgenol 2004; 182: 1305–1312

Case 159

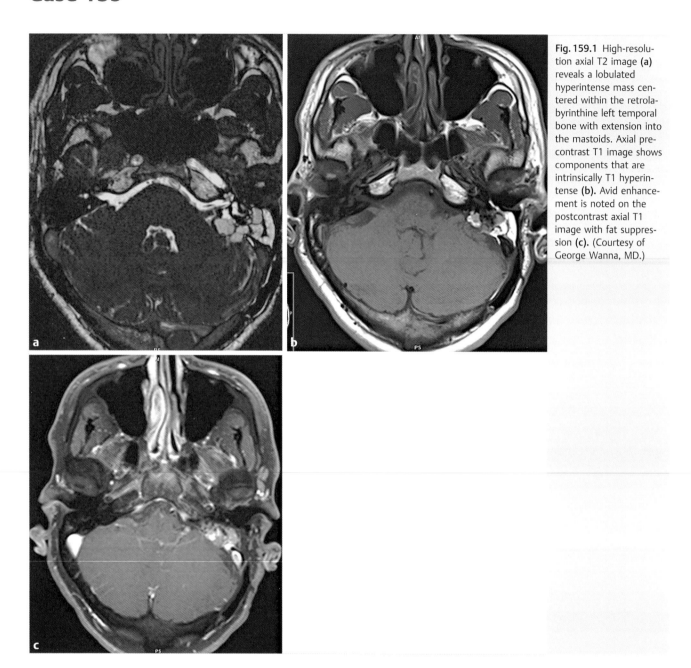

Fig. 159.1 High-resolution axial T2 image **(a)** reveals a lobulated hyperintense mass centered within the retrolabyrinthine left temporal bone with extension into the mastoids. Axial precontrast T1 image shows components that are intrinsically T1 hyperintense **(b).** Avid enhancement is noted on the postcontrast axial T1 image with fat suppression **(c).** (Courtesy of George Wanna, MD.)

■ Clinical Presentation

A young adult man with long-standing hearing loss and occasional vertigo (▶ Fig. 159.1)

■ Key Imaging Finding

Enhancing mass with intrinsic T1 hyperintensity centered within the retrolabyrinthine temporal bone

■ Diagnosis

Endolymphatic sac tumor. Endolymphatic sac tumor is a papillary adenomatous tumor that originates from the endolymphatic duct/sac. Most cases are sporadic, although there is an increased incidence and association with von Hippel-Lindau (VHL) syndrome. Patients typically present with insidious onset of hearing loss, tinnitus, and vertigo; acute onset of symptoms may occasionally occur in the setting of intralesional hemorrhage.

The tumor originates within the endolymphatic duct/sac along the retrolabyrinthine temporal bone and most often spreads medially and posteriorly into the cerebellopontine angle. Less common patterns of spread include lateral extension into the mastoids, middle ear cavity, and external auditory canal or anteriorly along the petrous ridge and into the clivus/central skull base.

On computed tomography (CT), endolymphatic sac tumors present as soft-tissue masses with amorphous calcifications and aggressive bony destruction. On magnetic resonance imaging (MRI), lesions are T2 hyperintense with regions of increased T1 signal intensity due to intralesional hemorrhage; the intrinsic T1 hyperintensity and location is fairly characteristic. The tumors are hypervascular with intense nodular enhancement. Larger lesions may demonstrate prominent flow voids.

Surgical resection with wide surgical margins is the treatment of choice.

✓ Pearls

- Endolymphatic sac tumor is a papillary adenomatous tumor that originates from the endolymphatic duct/sac.
- Most cases are sporadic, although there is an increased incidence and association with VHL syndrome.
- On CT, endolymphatic sac tumors demonstrate amorphous calcifications and aggressive bony destruction
- On MRI, lesions are T2 bright with regions of increased T1 signal due to hemorrhage; they intensely enhance.

Suggested Readings

Chapman PR, Shah R, Curé JK, Bag AK. Petrous apex lesions: pictorial review. Am J Roentgenol 2011; 196 Suppl: WS26–WS37, Quiz S40–S43

Connor SEJ, Leung R, Natas S. Imaging of the petrous apex: a pictorial review. Br J Radiol 2008; 81: 427–435

Razek AA, Huang BY. Lesions of the petrous apex: classification and findings at CT and MR imaging. Radiographics 2012; 32: 151–173

Case 160

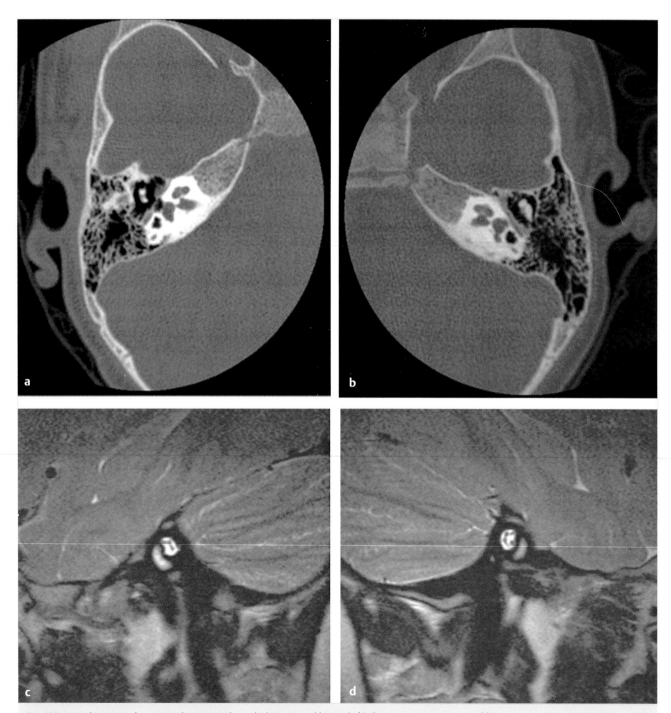

Fig. 160.1 Axial computed tomography images through the temporal bones **(a,b)** demonstrate a narrow cochlear aperture (opening for the cochlear nerve) on the right **(a)** with relative hypoplasia of the cochlea compared with the normal left side **(b).** Oblique sagittal high-resolution T2 MR images through the IACs **(c,d)** demonstrate deficiency of the cochlear nerve on the right along the anteroinferior aspect of the IAC **(c)** with a normal appearance on the left **(d).** The facial (anterosuperior) and superior and inferior divisions of the vestibular (posterior) nerves are normal bilaterally.

■ **Clinical Presentation**

A young child with unilateral sensorineural hearing loss (▶ Fig. 160.1)

▓ Key Imaging Finding

Deficiency of the cochlear nerve with a narrow cochlear aperture

▓ Diagnosis

Cochlear nerve deficiency. Cochlear nerve deficiency may be congenital (far more common) or acquired and results in sensorineural hearing loss. On magnetic resonance imaging (MRI), the cochlear nerve is best visualized on oblique sagittal high-resolution T2 sequences oriented perpendicular to the internal auditory canal (IAC). In this plane, the four "quadrants" of the IAC are seen and anatomically divided into superior and inferior by the horizontally oriented crista falciformis and divided into anterior and posterior above the level of the crista falciformis at the IAC fundus by the vertically oriented Bill's bar. The facial nerve is the largest and is seen within the anterosuperior aspect of the IAC. The cochlear nerve is located anteriorly in the IAC inferior to the facial nerve (hence the mnemonic "7Up, Coke down"). Under normal circumstances, the cochlear nerve is smaller than the facial nerve but larger than the superior and inferior divisions of the vestibular nerve, which are located posteriorly within the IAC.

With cochlear nerve deficiency, the nerve is either imperceptible or significantly decreased in caliber compared with the facial and vestibular nerves. With congenital causes of cochlear deficiency, there are associated osseous abnormalities because the bony development of the IAC and cochlea are affected by development of the underlying nerves. In isolated cochlear nerve deficiency, the IAC and cochlear aperture (opening from the IAC into the cochlea) are small in caliber. With vestibulocochlear deficiency, the IAC is nearly aplastic because it is only slightly larger than the facial nerve traversing through it. Some degree of cochlear dysplasia may be seen in a minority of congenital cases with modiolar deficiency being the most common abnormality. Acquired cases of cochlear nerve deficiency result from some form of insult (typically ischemic or traumatic) that occurs after normal development; therefore, the IAC and cochlear aperture will be normal in size.

Treatment of cochlear nerve deficiency consists of cochlear implantation. Although complete absence of the cochlear nerve is a contraindication to cochlear implantation, it is best to describe the entity on MRI as cochlear nerve deficiency rather than aplasia because the presence of even small nerve fibers that may be beyond imaging resolution may lead to successful surgical treatment. This is especially important in cases with bilateral findings. As is the case with many disease processes, the imaging findings must be correlated with clinical findings and evaluations, including nerve stimulation.

✓ Pearls

- Cochlear nerve deficiency is most often congenital and results in sensorineural hearing loss.
- The cochlear nerve is seen along the anteroinferior IAC and is best visualized on oblique sagittal T2 sequences.
- Congenital cochlear nerve deficiency commonly results in hypoplasia of the IAC and cochlear aperture.
- Cochlear implantation is the treatment of choice for congenital cochlear nerve deficiency.

Suggested Reading

Glastonbury CM, Davidson HC, Harnsberger HR, Butler J, Kertesz TR, Shelton C. Imaging findings of cochlear nerve deficiency. Am J Neuroradiol 2002; 23: 635–643

Case 161

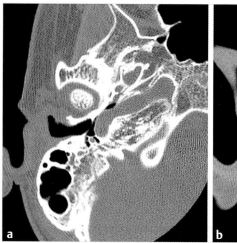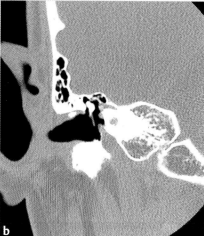

Fig. 161.1 Axial **(a)** and coronal **(b)** computed tomography images reveal narrowing and posterolateral deviation of the right ICA into the middle ear cavity.

▓ Clinical Presentation

A young adult man with pulsatile tinnitus and a retrotympanic mass (▶ Fig. 161.1)

▨ Key Imaging Finding

Posterolateral deviation of the internal carotid artery (ICA) into the middle ear cavity

▨ Diagnosis

Aberrant internal carotid artery (ICA). An aberrant ICA is a developmental abnormality that results from agenesis of the cervical and proximal petrous portions of the ICA. As a result, alternate anastomoses form via the external carotid artery. There is collateralization through the inferior tympanic artery (a branch of the ascending pharyngeal artery) to the caroticotympanic branch of the petrous ICA, both of which traverse the middle ear cavity. The enlarged caroticotympanic branch then forms anastomoses with the horizontal segment of the petrous ICA.

Cross-sectional imaging demonstrates narrowing and posterolateral deviation of the ICA into the middle ear cavity, along with absence of the cervical and proximal portion of the petrous ICA. The ICA skull-base foramen is absent. A persistent stapedial artery may coexist with an aberrant ICA in approximately one-third of cases. With a persistent stapedial artery, there is absence of the ipsilateral foramen spinosum.

Clinically, patients present with pulsatile tinnitus and a vascular retrotympanic mass, similar to a glomus tympanicum. It is critical to confirm or exclude this diagnosis prior to inadvertent clinical biopsy of a vascular retrotympanic mass.

✓ Pearls

- An aberrant ICA results from agenesis of the cervical and proximal petrous portions of the ICA.
- Computed tomography demonstrates narrowing and posterolateral deviation of the ICA into the middle ear cavity.
- Occasionally, a persistent stapedial artery may coexist with an aberrant ICA.
- Patients present clinically with pulsatile tinnitus and a vascular retrotympanic mass on physical exam.

Suggested Readings

Betts A, Esquivel C, O'Brien WT. Vascular retrotympanic mass. J Am Osteopath Coll Radiol. 2012; 1: 28–30

Sauvaget E, Paris J, Kici S et al. Aberrant internal carotid artery in the temporal bone: imaging findings and management. Arch Otolaryngol Head Neck Surg 2006; 132: 86–91

Case 162

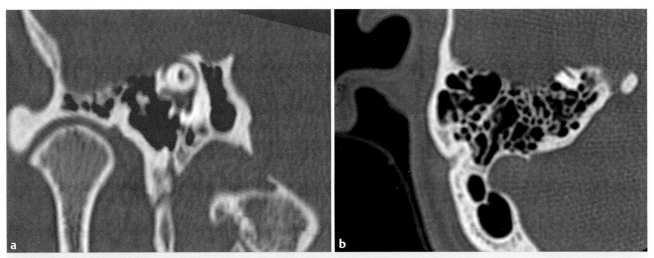

Fig. 162.1 Reformatted CT image through the plane of the superior semicircular canal **(a)** demonstrates dehiscence of the overlying superior bony margin of the semicircular canal. Corresponding axial CT image **(b)** shows uncovering of the superior semicircular canal along its anterosuperior margin.

■ Clinical Presentation

An adult man with episodic "dizziness" associated with loud noises (▶ Fig. 162.1)

▓ Key Imaging Finding

Bony dehiscence involving the superior semicircular canal

▓ Diagnosis

Superior semicircular canal dehiscence. Tullio phenomenon refers to a clinical entity in which patients experience vestibular symptoms and/or nystagmus in the setting of auditory stimuli or changes in intracranial or middle ear pressure. It may be caused by several middle and inner ear pathologies, including superior semicircular canal dehiscence, perilymphatic fistulas, trauma, and Méniére disease. Under normal circumstances, the semicircular canals remain in a closed system that is unaffected by auditory or pressure stimuli; however, dehiscence or fenestration of the bony canal surrounding the semicircular canals allows for transmission of auditory or pressure-related inputs into the endolymph of the semicircular canals, resulting in clinical symptoms. Treatment options include avoidance of provoking stimuli and surgical covering of the region of dehiscence.

The diagnosis of superior semicircular canal dehiscence is made based upon clinical symptoms, vestibular functions tests, and characteristic imaging findings. High-resolution computed tomography (CT) imaging of the temporal bones demonstrates a bony defect or dehiscence overlying the superior semicircular canal. Although the findings are often seen on routine axial and coronal series, reformatted images in the plane of the superior semicircular canal can be helpful in demonstrating the abnormality. High-resolution T2-weighted three-dimensional magnetic resonance imaging sequences may also demonstrate the characteristic findings.

✓ Pearls

- Tullio phenomenon refers to vertigo or nystagmus in the setting of auditory stimuli or pressure-related changes.
- Temporal bone CT demonstrates a bony defect or dehiscence overlying the superior semicircular canal.
- Reformations in the plane of the superior semicircular canal can be helpful in identifying the abnormality.

Suggested Readings

Belden CJ, Weg N, Minor LB, Zinreich SJ. CT evaluation of bone dehiscence of the superior semicircular canal as a cause of sound- and/or pressure-induced vertigo. Radiology 2003; 226: 337–343

Offiah CE, Ramsden RT, Gillespie JE. Imaging appearances of unusual conditions of the middle and inner ear. Br J Radiol 2008; 81: 504–514

Case 163

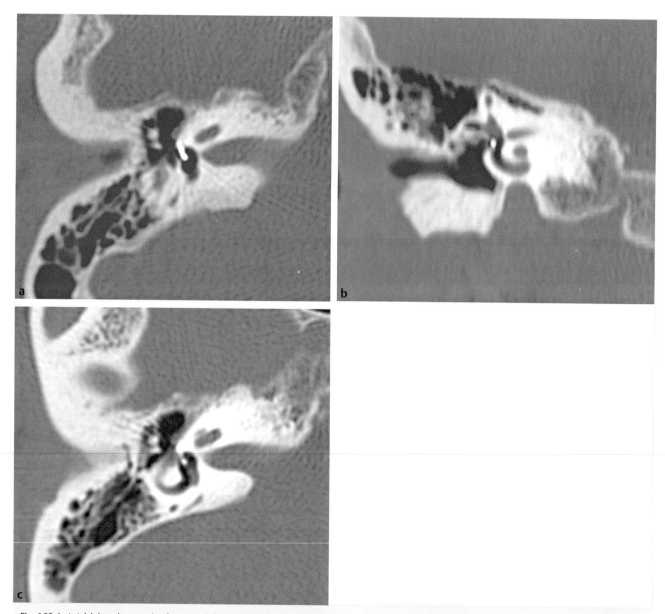

Fig. 163.1 Axial **(a)** and coronal reformatted **(b)** computed tomography images of the right temporal bone demonstrate an ossicular prosthesis extending through the oval window, consistent with vestibular perforation. The presence of pneumolabyrinth is best depicted on sequential axial images **(a,c).**

■ **Clinical Presentation**

An adult man with recurrent conductive hearing loss following corrective surgery (▶ Fig. 163.1)

▓ Key Imaging Finding

Extension of an ossicular prosthesis through the oval window with pneumolabyrinth

▓ Diagnosis

Middle ear ossicular prosthesis malpositioning. A variety of ossicular prostheses are available for the operative treatment of conductive hearing loss. Common indications include ossicular erosion secondary to chronic inflammation or cholesteatoma, otosclerosis, and congenital anomalies involving the ossicular chain. Although the type of material and imaging appearance of prostheses vary widely, their function is similar, with restoration of sound wave transmission from the tympanic membrane to the oval window. In normal circumstances, sound waves travel through the external auditory canal to the tympanic membrane and then along the ossicular chain, which includes the malleus, incus, and stapes; the stapes articulates with the oval window and allows for transmission of sound waves into the vestibule. Prostheses may replace all or a portion of the ossicular chain.

Common complications associated with prostheses include malpositioning, subluxation, dislocation, and fracture. Loss of function may also occur in a well-placed prosthesis in the setting of recurrent middle ear disease or with the formation of granulation tissue along the prosthesis.

The most common cause of ossicular failure is subluxation or dislocation. In evaluating a prosthesis, it is important to follow the ossicles and prosthesis from the articulation with the tympanic membrane to the footplate at the oval window. Loss of articulation along the ossicular chain or lack of articulation with the oval window is indicative of subluxation or dislocation. Occasionally, a prosthesis may extend through the oval window, resulting in vestibular perforation and a perilymphatic fistula. A perilymphatic fistula is suggested in the setting of pneumolabyrinth or with a combination of fluid within the middle ear cavity and a malpositioned stapes prosthesis. It is also important to evaluate for recurrent disease (e.g., cholesteatoma) and the formation of granulation tissue along the prosthesis, as these may result in conductive hearing loss despite appropriate alignment of the ossicular-prosthesis chain.

✓ Pearls

- Common indications for ossicular prostheses include cholesteatoma, otosclerosis, and congenital anomalies.
- The ossicular-prosthesis chain should extend from the tympanic membrane to the oval window.
- Common prosthesis complications include malpositioning, subluxation, dislocation, and fracture.
- Prosthesis extension through the oval window may result in vestibular perforation with a perilymphatic fistula.

Suggested Reading

Stone JA, Mukherji SK, Jewett BS, Carrasco VN, Castillo M. CT evaluation of prosthetic ossicular reconstruction procedures: what the otologist needs to know. Radiographics 2000; 20: 593–605

Case 164

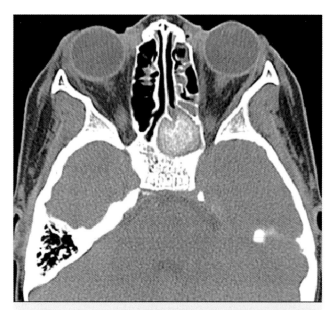

Fig. 164.1 Axial CT image reveals hyperdense opacification of the left sphenoid sinus with extension through and obstruction of the sphenoethmoidal recess. There is also mild mucosal thickening involving the left ethmoid sinus.

■ Clinical Presentation

An adolescent with headaches (▶ Fig. 164.1)

■ Key Imaging Finding

Hyperdense sinus opacification

■ Top 3 Differential Diagnoses

- **Inspissated secretions.** Inspissated secretions are seen in the setting of chronic sinusitis where sinus opacification becomes concentrated with increased proteinaceous and decreased water content. There is often chronic obstruction of the sinus outlet with or without underlying mucous retention cyst or mucocele; occasionally, superimposed sinonasal polyposis syndromes are seen. On computed tomography (CT), as the protein content increases and the water content decreases, there is increased density of the sinus opacification. Rarely, the sinus disease may begin to calcify and form a sinolith. Chronic sinus wall thickening with osteitis may be seen. On magnetic resonance imaging (MRI), as protein content initially increases, there is a corresponding increase in T1 signal intensity; T2 signal intensity remains hyperintense. As the protein content continues to increase, there is gradual decrease in the T2 signal intensity.
- **Fungal sinusitis.** Noninvasive fungal sinusitis occurs predominantly in immunocompetent patients and may present as a mycetoma in a solitary (usually) nonexpanded sinus or as allergic fungal sinusitis (AFS) with multiple expanded sinuses. AFS often occurs in patients with polyposis and/or multiple allergies. Both processes result in hyperdense sinus opacification on CT due to the presence of fungal elements with or without superimposed inspissated secretions. Calcifications and chronic sinus wall thickening with osteitis may be seen. On MRI, the fungal elements may result in decreased signal on both T1 and T2 sequences, which may mimic an aerated sinus. Chronic invasive fungal sinusitis may also present with hyperdense sinus opacification, as well as bony destruction and extension beyond the sinus margins. It is far less common and occurs most often in elderly patients with diabetes.
- **Trauma/Hemorrhage.** Fractures of the paranasal sinuses may result from direct facial trauma or orbital trauma or indirect trauma with extension of calvarial or skull-base fractures into the paranasal sinuses. Resultant hemorrhage occurs, which typically manifests as hyperdense air-fluid levels in a fractured sinus. At times, the fracture may not be readily seen but should be suspected in the appropriate clinical setting with hyperdense air-fluid levels. The maxillary and ethmoid sinuses are most often involved with direct orbital or facial trauma. The sphenoid sinus is most commonly involved with extension of skull-base fractures.

■ Diagnosis

Inspissated secretions

✓ Pearls

- Inspissated secretions are seen in chronic sinusitis and have increased protein and decreased water content.
- Fungal sinusitis results in hyperdense sinus opacification on CT due to the presence of fungal elements.
- On MRI, fungal elements may show decreased T1 and T2 signal intensity, mimicking an aerated sinus.
- Fractures of the paranasal sinuses may result in hyperdense hemorrhagic air-fluid levels in the involved sinus.

Suggested Reading

Aribandi M, McCoy VA, Bazan C, III. Imaging features of invasive and noninvasive fungal sinusitis: a review. Radiographics 2007; 27: 1283–1296

Case 165

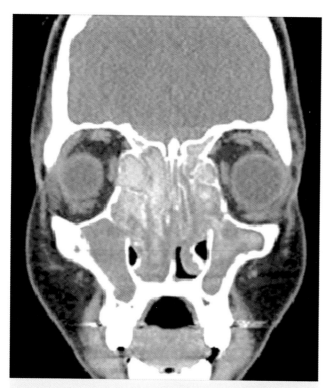

Fig. 165.1 Coronal reformatted CT image reveals pansinusitis with additional opacification of the ostiomeatal complexes, nasal cavity, and olfactory recesses bilaterally. Portions of the sinus opacification within the bilateral ethmoid and left maxillary sinuses are hyperdense. The ethmoid sinuses and maxillary sinus ostia are expanded; there is bony thinning of the lateral ethmoid sinus walls with dehiscence on the right. Sinus expansion results in hypertelorism.

Clinical Presentation

A young adult man with chronic congestion and facial pain (▶ Fig. 165.1)

Key Imaging Finding

Opacified expanded sinuses

Top 3 Differential Diagnoses

- **Allergic fungal sinusitis (AFS).** AFS is a noninvasive fungal sinusitis that occurs predominantly in immunocompetent patients. It represents the most common form of fungal sinusitis; is more prevalent in warm, humid climates; and is thought to represent a hypersensitivity reaction to fungal elements. There is an increased incidence in patients with multiple allergies, atopy, asthma, and polyposis. The disease occurs bilaterally with involvement of multiple—if not all—sinuses; involved sinuses are typically expanded. On computed tomography (CT), sinus opacification is hyperdense due to the presence of fungal elements with or without superimposed inspissated secretions. Calcifications and chronic sinus wall thickening with osteitis may be seen. On magnetic resonance imaging (MRI), the most common appearance is intermediate T1 and decreased T2 signal intensity; the decreased T2 signal is thought to result from manganese, iron, and magnesium content. Fungal elements may also result in decreased signal on both T1 and T2 sequences, which may mimic an aerated sinus.
- **Sinonasal polyposis.** Sinonasal polyps result from hyperplasia of inflamed mucosa. They are associated with chronic inflammation and may occur in isolation or in association with allergic sinusitis or asthma. There is also an increased incidence in children with cystic fibrosis and Kartagener syndrome (ciliary dysmotility and situs inversus). One or more sinuses may be involved. Polyps often extend through and expand sinus ostia or outlets. On CT, polyps present as rounded lesions or complete sinus opacification. There may be extension into the nasal cavity, characteristic of an antrochoanal polyp. Bony findings include osteitis with sinus wall thickening due to chronic inflammation, bony expansion with thinning of the sinus walls, or a more aggressive appearance with bony destruction and dehiscence. MRI reveals decreased T1 and increased T2 signal with surrounding mucosal enhancement. The lack of central enhancement distinguishes polyposis from sinonasal carcinoma.
- **Mucocele.** Mucoceles are cystic lesions that result in chronic sinus opacification and expansion due to sinus outlet obstruction. Typically, one or two adjacent sinuses are affected with the frontal, ethmoid, and sphenoid sinuses most often involved (in decreasing order of frequency). Due to slow growth and indolent nature, patients often remain asymptomatic; when symptoms are present, pain or visual disturbances are most common. The CT appearance depends upon the protein content within the obstructed sinus. As the protein content increases, there is associated increase in density. There is often bony thinning without destruction. On MRI, as protein content initially increases, there is a corresponding increase in T1 signal intensity; T2 signal intensity remains hyperintense. As the protein content continues to increase, there is gradual decrease in the T2 signal intensity.

Additional Differential Diagnoses

- **Sinonasal neoplasm.** Squamous cell carcinoma (SSC) accounts for approximately 90% of sinus malignancies. The maxillary sinus is most commonly involved, followed by the ethmoid sinus. Patients present relatively late in the disease process with obstructive sinus symptoms. On CT, SCC presents as a soft-tissue mass with bony destruction; extension beyond the sinus margins may be seen. Involvement of the pterygopalatine fossa allows for communication with the orbit and middle cranial fossa, most commonly through perineural spread of tumor. The tumor is hypointense on T1 and intermediate to hypointense on T2 sequences with heterogeneous enhancement. Less common sinonasal neoplasms include sinonasal undifferentiated carcinoma, adenocarcinoma, rhabdomyosarcoma (most common in children), and lymphoma.

Diagnosis

Allergic fungal sinusitis

✓ Pearls

- AFS occurs bilaterally with involvement of multiple sinuses; involved sinuses are typically expanded.
- Sinonasal polyps result from hyperplasia of inflamed mucosa; they expand involved sinuses and ostia.
- Mucoceles are cystic lesions that result in sinus opacification and expansion due to sinus outlet obstruction.

Suggested Readings

Aribandi M, McCoy VA, Bazan C, III. Imaging features of invasive and noninvasive fungal sinusitis: a review. Radiographics 2007; 27: 1283–1296

Yousem DM. Imaging of sinonasal inflammatory disease. Radiology 1993; 188: 303–314

Case 166

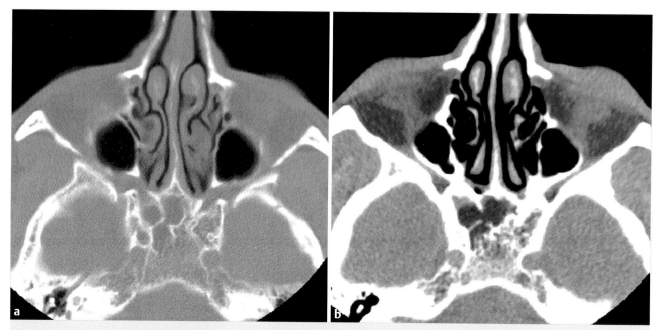

Fig. 166.1 Axial CT image through the skull base in bone window **(a)** reveals a nonexpansile multiloculated lytic lesion involving the skull base. Corresponding image in soft-tissue window **(b)** demonstrates central fatty attenuation.

■ Clinical Presentation

An adult woman with symptoms of chronic sinusitis (▶ Fig. 166.1)

▦ Key Imaging Finding

Lytic skull-base lesion

▦ Top 3 Differential Diagnoses

- **Fibrous dysplasia (FD)**. FD occurs most often in young adults and is more common in women. In the head and neck the calvarium, skull base, and facial bones are most often affected. The classic appearance on computed tomography (CT) is focal bony expansion with "ground glass" attenuation of the diploic space; sclerotic and cystic or lytic variants are less common. On magnetic resonance imaging (MRI), FD is typically hypointense on both T1 and T2 sequences and demonstrates avid enhancement; regions of cystic involvement, however, are T2 hyperintense. The MRI appearance can mimic aggressive lesions; therefore, CT is preferred in suspected cases of FD.
- **Malignancy.** Metastatic and primary bone tumors may involve the skull base and are often overlooked on imaging, especially when small. Breast, lung, and prostate carcinomas are the most common primary tumors to metastasize to the skull base and may result in expansile lytic or sclerotic (prostate and occasionally breast) lesions on CT. Common primary tumors to involve the skull base include chordomas, chondrosarcomas, lymphoma, and plasmacytoma. The key distinctions for malignant lesions are bony expansion or erosion with enhancing soft-tissue components. The MRI appearance varies by tumor type with most malignancies being intermediate in signal on T1 and T2 sequences. Chordomas (midline) and chondrosarcomas (off-midline) are characteristically T2 hyperintense. Heterogeneous enhancement is most often seen.
- **Arrested pneumatization.** During sinus development, there is initially conversion of red marrow to fatty marrow with subsequent pneumatization. When this process is arrested prior to pneumatization, regions of heterogeneous fatty marrow are seen, which may mimic pathological skull-base processes. Although arrested pneumatization may occur adjacent to any sinus or the mastoids, the sphenoid sinus is by far the most common location. On CT, arrested pneumatization presents as a nonexpansile region of heterogeneous density with thin sclerotic margins and central fatty attenuation along the margin of a relatively underdeveloped sinus. On MRI, arrested pneumatization is seen as a region of nonexpansile and nonenhancing fatty signal intensity along the margins of the involved sinus.

▦ Additional Differential Diagnoses

- **Osteomyelitis.** Osteomyelitis has a variety of imaging manifestations, which range from a normal appearance to an aggressive appearance that mimics a neoplastic process. Bony destruction from osteomyelitis commonly results in lytic skull-base lesions that often have poorly defined, infiltrating margins. Subacute and chronic infections may have a lytic defect with a central dense nidus or sequestrum of intact bone, referred to as a "button sequestrum." On MRI, osteomyelitis presents as regions of marrow infiltration or bony destruction with decreased T1 and intermediate to hyperintense T2 signal intensity, as well as variable enhancement.

▦ Diagnosis

Arrested pneumatization

✓ Pearls

- Fibrous dysplasia classically presents with focal bony expansion and "ground glass" attenuation.
- Skull-base malignancies present with focal bony expansion or erosion and enhancing soft-tissue components.
- Arrested pneumatization presents as a nonexpansile region with thin sclerotic margins and central fat.
- Skull-base osteomyelitis most often presents as a lytic lesion with poorly defined, infiltrating margins.

Suggested Readings

Georgy BA, Snow RD, Brogdon BG et al. Value of bone window images in routine brain CT: examinations beyond trauma. Appl Radiol 1997; 2: 26–38

Welker KM, DeLone DR, Lane JI, Gilbertson JR. Arrested pneumatization of the skull base: imaging characteristics. Am J Roentgenol 2008; 190: 1691–1696

Case 167

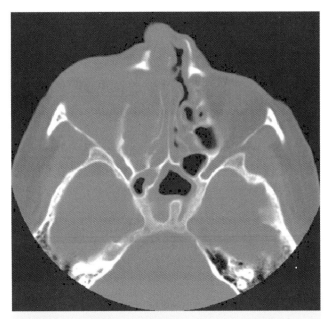

Fig. 167.1 Axial CT image through the paranasal sinuses in bone window reveals complete opacification of the right ethmoid sinus with bony erosion and overlying cartilage deformity. Soft-tissue attenuation replaces the normal fat in the right orbit. There is mucosal thickening involving the left ethmoid and sphenoid sinuses.

▓ Clinical Presentation

A 32-year-old woman with chronic, progressive nasal congestion and cough (▶ Fig. 167.1)

▓ Key Imaging Finding

Aggressive sinus disease/mass with bony destruction

■ Top 3 Differential Diagnoses

- **Invasive fungal sinusitis (IFS).** IFS most commonly occurs in immunosuppressed patients, especially elderly patients with diabetes. Mucormycosis and Aspergillus are the most common causative agents, with aspergilosis also occurring in otherwise healthy individuals. Mucormycosis has a tendency to spread through the cavernous sinus and orbits, resulting in a life-threatening infection. Aspergilosis invades vasculature, which results in mycotic aneurysm formation and vessel spasm or thrombosis. Fungal secretions are often hyperdense on computed tomography (CT) scans; calcifications are common. Hypointensity on both T1 and T2 (more so on T2) is characteristic of fungal infection. Bony erosion and extension beyond sinus margins are suggestive of an aggressive infection.
- **Granulomatous disease (Wegener/sarcoid).** Wegner granulomatosis is a systemic vasculitis that primarily affects the kidneys and respiratory tract. Patients commonly present with recurrent sinonasal "infections," respiratory symptoms, and renal insufficiency. The necrotizing vasculitis of small and medium-size vessels results in sinus disease (usually within the maxillary sinus) with locally erosive features. Early in the disease, the nasal septum is most involved. As the disease progresses, there is formation of a sinus mass with extensive bony erosion and involvement of adjacent compartments, including the orbits. The soft-tissue mass is hypointense on T1- and T2-weighted sequences and enhances. Sarcoid has a similar appearance on imaging and nearly always has associated pulmonary disease, which manifests as hilar/mediastinal adenopathy and/or interstitial lung disease.
- **Sinonasal carcinoma.** Squamous cell carcinoma (SSC) accounts for approximately 90% of sinus malignancies. The maxillary sinus is most commonly involved, followed by the ethmoid sinus. Patients present relatively late in the disease process with obstructive sinus symptoms. On CT, SCC presents as a soft-tissue mass with bony destruction; extension beyond the sinus margins may be seen. Involvement of the pterygopalatine fossa allows for communication with the orbit and middle cranial fossa, most commonly through perineural spread of tumor. The tumor is hypointense on T1 and intermediate to hypointense on T2 sequences with heterogeneous enhancement. Less common sinonasal neoplasms include sinonasal undifferentiated carcinoma, adenocarcinoma (associated with wood working and chemical exposures), and rhabdomyosarcoma (most common in children).

■ Additional Differential Diagnoses

- **Lymphoma.** Lymphoma of the paranasal sinuses is of the non-Hodgkin variant. The imaging appearance is nearly identical to that of SSC with typically a unilateral sinus mass that invades bone and is intermediate to hypointense on T2 sequences. A key distinguishing feature is the presence of lymphadenopathy within the neck and involvement of the Waldeyer tonsillar ring (a pharyngeal ring of lymphoid tissue composed of the adenoids, tubal tonsils, palatine tonsils, and lingual tonsils).
- **Cocaine nose.** Chronic use of cocaine results in a granulomatous response with a soft-tissue mass and cartilaginous erosion. The local granulomatous response combined with the vasoconstrictive properties of cocaine results in necrosis of the nasal septum. Continued insults lead to expansion of the septal perforation.

▓ Diagnosis

Granulomatous disease (Wegener granulomatosis)

✓ Pearls

- IFS most often occurs in immunosuppressed patients and may be hyperdense (CT) and hypointense (magnetic resonance imaging).
- Wegner granulomatosis results in aggressive sinus disease, pulmonary symptoms, and renal insufficiency.
- SCC (by far the most common) and lymphoma commonly involve the sinuses.
- Chronic cocaine abuse can lead to ischemic necrosis with bony and cartilaginous destruction.

Suggested Readings

Allbery SM, Chaljub G, Cho NL, Rassekh CH, John SD, Guinto FC. MR imaging of nasal masses. Radiographics 1995; 15: 1311–1327

Valencia MP, Castillo M. Congenital and acquired lesions of the nasal septum: a practical guide for differential diagnosis. Radiographics 2008; 28: 205–224, quiz 326

Case 168

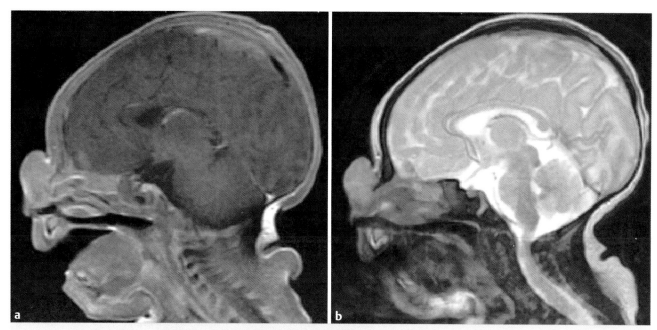

Fig. 168.1 Sagittal T1 postcontrast image with fat suppression **(a)** reveals a lobulated mass along the nasal dorsum. The mass is iso- to hyperintense to brain parenchyma on the sagittal T2 image **(b).** There was no visualized connection with intracranial contents.

■ Clinical Presentation

A newborn with a nasal mass (▶ Fig. 168.1)

▨ Key Imaging Finding

Superficial nasal mass in a newborn

▨ Top 3 Differential Diagnoses

- **Nasal glioma.** Nasal glioma is a misnomer because it represents ectopic glial tissue, rather than a neoplasm. In most cases, they are extranasal along the dorsum of the nasal bone near the glabella; a medial canthal location is less common. Approximately 30% of cases are intranasal and present with a nasal mass or nasal obstruction. Up to 15% of cases have a fibrous band of tissue that extends to the intracranial compartment. On clinical exam, the extranasal masses are often misdiagnosed as hemangiomas due to their discoloration. The masses tend to increase in size with somatic growth. On magnetic resonance imaging (MRI), nasal gliomas are typically well-circumscribed and slightly lobulated. Gliosis usually results in T1 hypointensity and T2 hyperintensity compared with gray matter.

- **Nasal dermal sinus.** Nasal dermal sinus anomalies result from incomplete separation of the neuroectoderm (dura) from the skin during fetal development. As a result, dermal elements remain along a regressing tract, forming a dermal sinus and/or inclusion cysts (dermoid or epidermoid). The dermal sinus or inclusion cyst may occur anywhere from the prenasal subcutaneous tissues to the foramen cecum, which is adjacent to the crista galli. Patients often present with a nasal pit (dermal sinus) or a palpable soft-tissue mass (inclusion cyst). Epidermoid cysts are composed of desquamatized epithelium; dermoids also contain keratin debris and skin appendages. Dermal sinuses form linear tracts with fluid signal intensity (MRI) extending to and occasionally through an enlarged foramen cecum. Dermoid cysts typically have fatty components that are hyperintense on T1 and variable in T2 signal

intensity. Epidermoid cysts follow fluid signal intensity on MRI but demonstrate characteristic increased signal on diffusion-weighted imaging. Peripheral enhancement may be seen surrounding nasal dermal sinus anomalies. It is critical to assess for intracranial extension. Helpful secondary findings include a bifid crista galli, enlarged foramen cecum, hypertelorism (50% of cases), and additional craniofacial malformations.

- **Cephalocele.** Cephaloceles refer to extrusion of central nervous system contents through a dural and skull defect due to improper separation of neural and surface ectoderm. *Cephalocele* is a broad term that encompasses meningoceles and encephaloceles. Nasofrontal cephaloceles are less common than posterior cephaloceles, are not associated with neural tube defects, and are more common in Southeast Asian populations. Sincipital cephaloceles are clinically visible and characterized as nasofrontal, nasoethmoidal, or nasoorbital based upon the location of the bony defect. Basal encephaloceles (transethmoidal, transsphenoidal, sphenoethmoidal) occur at the skull base and are clinically occult, often presenting as an intranasal mass or with a history of cerebrospinal fluid (CSF) leak or episodes of meningitis. Many cases of anterior cephaloceles also have hypertelorism. MRI is the modality of choice in evaluation of cephaloceles. Continuity of the mass with intracranial contents is the key distinguishing feature. Nasofrontal masses occur at the glabella; nasoethmoidal masses extend through the foramen cecum. CSF follows fluid signal intensity; brain parenchyma typically follows gray matter signal with regions of gliosis.

▨ Additional Differential Diagnoses

- **Hemangioma.** Hemangiomas are unencapsulated, proliferative vascular neoplasms and represent the most common benign tumors of infancy. The proliferative growth phase typically occurs in the first year of life; infantile and rapidly involuting congenital variants then undergo involution with fatty

replacement. Treatment is typically conservative, unless there is mass effect on adjacent vital structures. Clinically, patients present with a superficial mass that is bluish or scarlet in color. MRI reveals a lobulated hyperintense T2 and slightly hyperintense T1 mass with avid enhancement.

▨ Diagnosis

Nasal glioma

✓ Pearls

- Nasal glioma refers to ectopic glial tissue that may be extranasal (most common) or intranasal.
- Nasal dermal sinus anomalies (sinus or cyst) often present with a bifid crista galli and enlarged foramen cecum.

- Cephaloceles may be sincipital (visible) or basal (occult); continuity with intracranial contents is a key feature.
- Infantile hemangiomas (T2 bright with avid enhancement) proliferate during the first year of life, then involute.

Suggested Reading

Hedlund G. Congenital frontonasal masses: developmental anatomy, malformations, and MR imaging. Pediatr Radiol 2006; 36: 647–662, quiz 726–727

Case 169

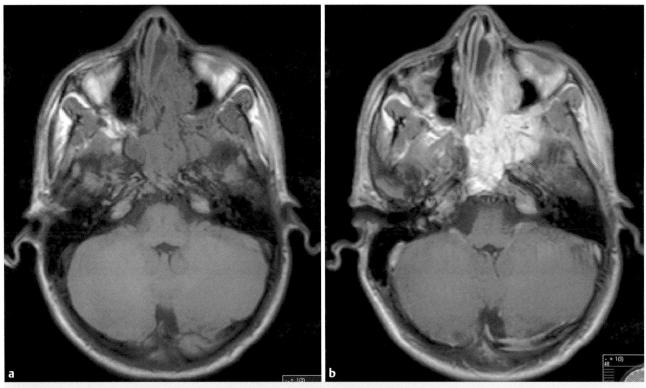

Fig. 169.1 Pre- **(a)** and postcontrast **(b)** T1-weighted MR images demonstrate a large T1 hypointense mass that demonstrates intense homogeneous enhancement. The mass involves the left nasopharynx, nasal cavity, and pterygopalatine fossa with extension through the sphenopalatine foramen. There is involvement of the maxillary sinus medially and anterior displacement of the posterior wall of the maxillary sinus. There is skull-base involvement without intracranial or intraorbital extension (images not shown). (Courtesy of Children's Hospital and Research Center Oakland.)

▦ Clinical Presentation

A 17-year-old male with chronic "stuffy nose" and intermittent epistaxis (▶ Fig. 169.1)

▥ Key Imaging Finding

Enhancing nasal mass in an adolescent

■ Top 3 Differential Diagnoses

- **Juvenile nasopharyngeal angiofibroma (JNA).** JNAs are benign but locally aggressive lesions that occur in adolescent boys. They originate in the nasopharynx adjacent to the sphenopalatine foramen and pterygopalatine fossa. The lesions commonly extend into multiple compartments, including the infratemporal, intracranial, and intraorbital, as well as into the paranasal sinuses. Anterior bowing of the posterior maxillary sinus wall is commonly seen. Patients present with nasal obstruction and epistaxis. JNAs are hypointense to intermediate on T1 and intermediate to hyperintense on T2 sequences. They avidly enhance and flow voids are commonly seen. The lesions are commonly resected with preoperative embolization to minimize intraoperative bleeding.
- **Esthesioneuroblastoma (ENB).** ENB is a malignant neuroendocrine tumor that arises from olfactory endothelium within the superior nasal cavity. It most commonly occurs in adolescents and middle-aged patients who present with nasal obstruction and epistaxis. Imaging findings include an enhancing mass that is hypointense to intermediate on T1 and hyperintense on T2 sequences. Intracranial extension through the cribriform plate is common. The classic finding is a dumbbell-shaped mass in the nasal cavity/nasopharynx and anterior cranial fossa with a narrowed waist at the level of the cribriform plate. Intracranial portions of the tumor often demonstrate cystic components.
- **Rhabdomyosarcoma.** Rhabdomyosarcoma represents a malignant tumor composed of striated musculature and is the most common nasal sarcoma in adolescents. It may involve the sinuses, nasal cavity, and nasopharynx with bony destruction. Intracranial extension is common. The mass is relatively homogeneous, iso- to hypointense on T1 and hyperintense on T2 compared with musculature, and avidly enhances.

■ Additional Differential Diagnoses

- **Hemangioma.** Hemangiomas are benign tumors that may occur within the nasal cavity at any age but most often present in the pediatric population or during pregnancy. The may be capillary (more common) or cavernous and typically occur along the nasal septum or turbinates. Presenting symptoms include nasal obstruction and epistaxis. Imaging findings include a well-circumscribed, lobulated, avidly enhancing nasal soft-tissue mass that is hyperintense on T2 sequences.
- **Sinonasal lymphoma.** Non-Hodgkin lymphoma (NHL) commonly involves the head and neck, most often with cervical lymphadenopathy. Paranasal sinus involvement is less common and may present as a well-defined or infiltrative soft-tissue mass. On magnetic resonance imaging (MRI), NHL is variable but most often intermediate to hypointense in signal intensity with relatively homogeneous enhancement.
- **Inverted papilloma (IP).** IPs are benign, locally aggressive neoplasms that may occur in adolescents but are most common in adult men who present with nasal obstruction. They originate along the middle meatus and extend into the paranasal sinuses. Calcifications may be seen on computed tomography. They are isointense on T1 and hyperintense on T2 MRI sequences with characteristic linear striations. There is heterogeneous enhancement.

▥ Diagnosis

Juvenile nasopharyngeal angiofibroma

✓ Pearls

- JNAs occur in adolescent boys, avidly enhance, and commonly extend into multiple compartments.
- ENBs are malignant neuroendocrine tumors that may extend intracranially through the cribriform plate.
- Hemangiomas most commonly occur along the septum and turbinates in children or during pregnancy.
- IPs are locally aggressive, may have calcifications, and have a characteristic striated appearance on MRI.

Suggested Reading

Valencia MP, Castillo M. Congenital and acquired lesions of the nasal septum: a practical guide for differential diagnosis. Radiographics 2008; 28: 205–224, quiz 326

Case 170

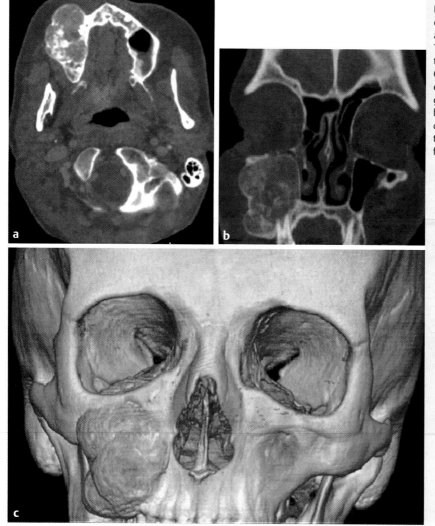

Fig. 170.1 Axial CT image **(a)** demonstrates an expansile lesion with central "ground glass" attenuation involving the maxilla on the right. The roots of maxillary teeth can be seen within the lesion as regions of round, increased density. Coronal reformatted CT image **(b)** shows an expanded and thinned cortex with central ground glass attenuation, as well as the degree of bony expansion into the maxillary sinus. Three-dimensional volume rendered image **(c)** reveals the external contour, bony enlargement, and facial asymmetry.

■ Clinical Presentation

A young adult woman with facial asymmetry (▶ Fig. 170.1)

▥ Key Imaging Finding

Expansile bony lesion

▥ Top 3 Differential Diagnoses

- **Fibrous dysplasia (FD).** FD results in replacement of normal compact bone with fibrous connective tissue and disorganized lamellar bone. The craniofacial bones are commonly involved (maxilla > mandible). FD occurs most frequently in young adults and is often asymptomatic unless bony enlargement results in impingement of adjacent structures. Approximately 80% of cases are monostotic with the remainder being polyostotic. Monostotic cases have a relatively equal incidence in men and women. McCune-Albright syndrome consists of polyostotic FD, café-au-lait spots, and precocious puberty and is more common in women. The appearance on computed tomography (CT) is variable with most cases demonstrating characteristic bony expansion and "ground glass" attenuation. Cystic and sclerotic variants are less specific and are more often associated with mandibular involvement. On magnetic resonance imaging (MRI), FD may mimic an aggressive lesion with decreased T1 and T2 signal and moderate enhancement.

- **Ossifying fibroma.** Ossifying fibroma is in the spectrum of benign fibroosseous lesions and consists of a combination of mature bone and fibrous tissue. As with FD, ossifying fibromas commonly involve the maxillofacial bones (mandible more often than maxilla), are more common in young to middle-aged adults with a female predominance, and are typically asymptomatic unless there is impingement on adjacent structures, especially sinus drainage pathways. Classically, ossifying fibromas appear as well-circumscribed, expansile bony lesions with a thick peripheral rim of ossified bone and a central fibrous matrix that may have a ground glass appearance on CT. Less common imaging patterns include central regions of ossified bone surrounded by fibrous tissue or central fibrous tissue with a thin rim of ossified bone. On MRI, lesions are hypo- to isointense on T1 and have variable signal on T2 sequences; typically, the fibrous components are intermediate, whereas ossified components are more hypointense on T2. Heterogeneous enhancement is often seen.

- **Osteoma.** Osteomas are benign tumors characterized by proliferation of compact or cancellous bone. The vast majority are solitary and isolated lesions; multiple osteomas may also be sporadic or associated with Gardner syndrome. In the maxillofacial region, they are far more common in the paranasal sinuses compared with the maxilla and mandible; the mandible is more often involved than the maxilla. Most lesions are asymptomatic, unless they interfere with mechanics of the jaw or compress adjacent neurovascular structures. Osteomas are characterized as peripheral, extending from the periosteum, or central, originating along the endosteal surface. On CT, peripheral osteomas appear as exophytic pedunculated or sessile, densely calcified masses extending from the surface of the periosteum. Endosteal osteomas reveal focal bony sclerosis with or without bony expansion. Osteomas may be distinguished from regions of exostoses by the presence of compact bone and the absence of a contiguous medullary cavity extending into the lesion. However, the two lesions may be indistinguishable in some cases where characteristic features are not present.

▥ Additional Differential Diagnoses

- **Osteomyelitis.** Osteomyelitis most often results from spread of an underlying dental infection; postprocedural infection is less common. Susceptible patients have poor dentition, diabetes, immunosuppression, or are undergoing bisphosphonate therapy. The CT appearance of osteomyelitis is variable and based upon the nature and duration of the infection. Lytic, sclerotic, and mixed variants may be seen. Chronic infections may have an underlying bony sequestrum. The presence of periosteal reaction is commonly seen and is a useful secondary finding to suggest osteomyelitis, although it is not specific to infection.

▥ Diagnosis

Fibrous dysplasia

✓ Pearls

- FD characteristically presents as an expansile bony lesion with central "ground glass" attenuation.
- Ossifying fibromas often present with thick peripheral ossified bone and central ground glass fibrous tissue.

- Osteomas are benign expansile bony tumors that may occur along the periosteum (exophytic) or endosteum.
- On CT, osteomyelitis may appear lytic, sclerotic, or mixed; periosteal reaction is commonly seen.

Suggested Reading

Yonetsu K, Nakamura T. CT of calcifying jaw bone diseases. Am J Roentgenol 2001; 177: 937–943

Case 171

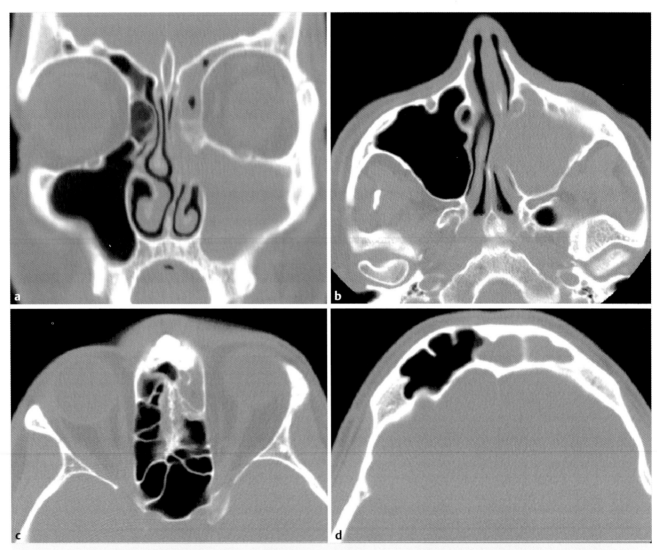

Fig. 171.1 Coronal CT image **(a)** reveals opacification of the left OMC and visualized portions of the left maxillary, anterior ethmoid, and frontal sinuses. There is demineralization of the bony uncinate process and middle turbinate. Axial CT images **(b–d)** demonstrate corresponding complete opacification of the left maxillary **(b)**, anterior ethmoid **(c)**, and frontal **(d)** sinuses.

■ Clinical Presentation

A young adult man with facial pain and headaches (▶ Fig. 171.1)

■ Key Imaging Finding

Opacification of the ostiomeatal complex (OMC), and maxillary, anterior ethmoid, and frontal sinuses

■ Diagnosis

Ostiomeatal complex (OMC) sinus disease. The OMC is the primary drainage pathway for the maxillary, anterior ethmoid, and frontal sinuses. It is best evaluated on coronal computed tomography (CT) images, and its outflow tract includes the maxillary antrum, infundibulum, hiatus semilunaris, and middle meatus. The bony and soft-tissue borders of the OMC include the uncinate process and middle turbinate medially and the inferior and medial orbital walls laterally. Anatomic variants that may narrow the outflow tract of the OMC include Haller cells (ethmoidal air cells along the orbital floor), pneumatized middle turbinate (concha bullosa), paradoxical rotation of the middle turbinate, and a deviated nasal septum.

Patients with chronic sinusitis or complications related to recurrent sinusitis may require functional endoscopic sinus surgery (FESS) to alleviate symptoms and restore the natural physiological drainage pathways. The OMC is the primary focus of FESS. Preoperative CT imaging provides important landmarks for surgical planning and also affords the opportunity to identify anatomic variants that may predispose to surgical complications. Important structures to evaluate on the preoperative sinus CT may be recalled with the mnemonic CLOSE: cribriform plate, lamina papyracea, presence of an Onodi cell, sphenoid sinus pneumatization variants and relationship to the carotid canal, and location of the anterior ethmoidal artery.

In evaluating the cribriform plate, the Keros classification is used to determine the depth of the olfactory fossa. A deeper fossa or asymmetry between right and left side places the patient at risk for penetration of the lateral lamella into the anterior cranial fossa. Medial orbital wall fractures cause medial deviation of the lamina papyracea into the ethmoid sinus. Inadvertent penetration through the lamina papyracea may result in injury to intraorbital contents. An Onodi cell refers to an anatomic variant with superior and posterior positioning of an ethmoid air cell above the sphenoid sinus. The optic nerve is typically located within an Onodi cell and is often dehiscent, making it susceptible to injury. In evaluating the sphenoid sinus, it is important to comment on pneumatization extending inferior and posterior to the sella because this pattern increases the risk for surgical penetration through the clivus. Additionally, it is important to identify sphenoid sinus pneumatization that extends to and around the margins of the internal carotid artery because this places the artery at risk for injury. Finally, the anterior ethmoidal artery is identified by the notch along the medial orbital wall. When the notch abuts the lateral lamella or fovea ethmoidalis, it is typically well protected. However, the presence of pneumatized supraorbital ethmoid air cells surrounding the anterior ethmoidal artery notch renders the artery susceptible to intraoperative injury.

✓ Pearls

- The OMC is the primary drainage pathway for the maxillary, anterior ethmoid, and frontal sinuses.
- FESS is designed to restore the natural physiological drainage pathways and is primarily directed at the OMC.

- Preoperative CT imaging provides surgical landmarks and identifies potential risks for surgical complications.

Suggested Reading

Hoang JK, Eastwood JD, Tebbit CL, Glastonbury CM. Multiplanar sinus CT: a systematic approach to imaging before functional endoscopic sinus surgery. Am J Roentgenol 2010; 194: W527–36

Case 172

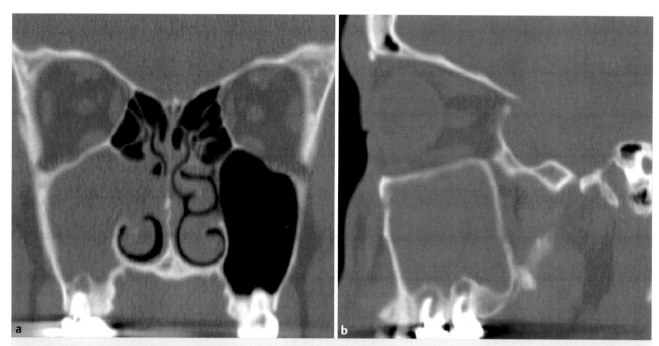

Fig. 172.1 Coronal CT image **(a)** shows complete opacification of the right maxillary sinus and ostiomeatal complex, including the maxillary antrum, infundibulum, hiatus semilunaris, and middle meatus. Bony portions of the right uncinate process and turbinates are not appreciable. Incidental paradoxical rotation of the left middle turbinate is identified. Periapical lucencies are seen involving the maxillary teeth on the right on the coronal and sagittal reformatted **(b)** ▶ CT images with overlying bony expansion and demineralization, as well as small regions of dehiscence along the maxillary sinus floor.

■ Clinical Presentation

A 24-year-old man with refractory sinusitis and persistent right-sided facial pain (▶ Fig. 172.1)

■ Key Imaging Finding

Periapical dental lucencies, overlying bony demineralization, and maxillary sinus disease

■ Diagnosis

Odontogenic sinus disease. Odontogenic sinusitis represents ~10% of cases of maxillary sinusitis. It may result from significant dental caries or periodontal disease or as a result of dental intervention. Patients present with recurrent or persistent sinusitis despite what is assumed to be appropriate medical treatment. However, typical antibiotic coverage for sinusitis is often inadequate because odontogenic sinusitis tends to be polymicrobial with both aerobic and anaerobic organisms.

Panoramic radiographs or sinus computed tomography (CT) are the modalities of choice in evaluating for suspected odontogenic sinusitis. Imaging reveals prominent dental caries or periapical lucencies along the floor of the maxillary sinus with overlying bony thinning or dehiscence. There is associated maxillary sinus mucosal thickening or opacification. With a region of large bony dehiscence, the involved tooth may herniate into the sinus.

Treatment includes broad spectrum antibiotic therapy, tooth extraction, and repair of the odontogenic-maxillary fistula, if present.

✓ Pearls

- Odontogenic sinusitis may result from dental caries, periodontal disease, or as a result of dental intervention.
- CT reveals dental caries or periapical lucencies with bony thinning or dehiscence of the maxillary sinus floor.
- Treatment includes broad spectrum antibiotics, tooth extraction, and repair of the odontogenic-maxillary fistula.

Suggested Reading

Mehra P, Murad H. Maxillary sinus disease of odontogenic origin. Otolaryngol Clin North Am 2004; 37: 347–364

Case 173

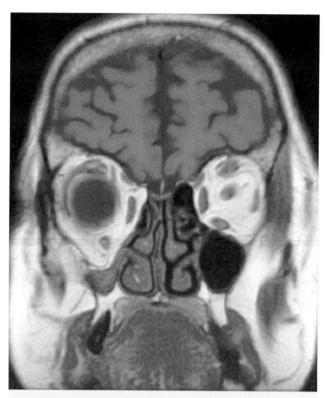

Fig. 173.1 Coronal T1-weighted magnetic resonance image shows asymmetry of the maxillary sinuses with a completely opacified right maxillary sinus that is significantly smaller in size compared with the left. There is volume loss within the right maxillary sinus with inferior displacement of the right orbital floor and lateral deviation of the right uncinate process that contacts the inferomedial orbital wall. The inferior extent of maxillary sinus pneumatization is symmetric on both sides. (Courtesy of Rocky Saenz, DO.)

▧ Clinical Presentation

A young adult woman with progressive facial deformity (▶ Fig. 173.1)

■ Key Imaging Finding

Atelectatic maxillary sinus

■ Diagnosis

Silent sinus syndrome. Silent sinus syndrome refers to atelectasis of a completely (most common) or partially opacified maxillary sinus. Although the pathophysiology is not entirely understood, it is believed that obstruction of the maxillary sinus outlet results in negative pressure within the maxillary sinus and subsequent inward displacement of the sinus walls. Patients often present with an acquired facial deformity and progressive enophthalmos on the involved side.

The imaging findings are fairly characteristic in the appropriate clinical setting. The maxillary sinus, antrum, and infundibulum are typically opacified, and there is inward displacement of the maxillary sinus walls, particularly the medial wall and roof (orbital floor) of the maxillary sinus. There is lateral deviation of the uncinate process, which may contact the medial orbital floor. The thickness of the walls of the maxillary sinus is variable; they may be normal, thinned, or thickened. Chronic sinus opacification may lead to inspissated secretions,

which are hyperdense on CT, hyperintense on T1, and relatively hypointense on T2 magnetic resonance imaging sequences.

The main differential diagnosis for silent sinus syndrome is an opacified hypoplastic maxillary sinus, which is more common and does not present with a developing facial deformity. Although it may be difficult to distinguish between the two based solely upon imaging, a useful criterion is the location of the maxillary sinus floor. With a hypoplastic maxillary sinus, there is incomplete development or pneumatization of the maxillary sinus; therefore, the floor of the maxillary sinus is thicker and more cephalad on the involved side. In silent sinus syndrome, there is relatively symmetric development of the maxillary sinuses with subsequent atelectasis on the involved side; therefore, inferior pneumatization of the maxillary sinuses is similar. Occasionally, the two conditions may coexist with acquired sinus atelectasis superimposed upon underlying developmental hypoplasia.

✓ Pearls

- Silent sinus syndrome refers to atelectasis of a completely (usually) or partially opacified maxillary sinus.
- Patients present most often as young adults with a progressive, acquired facial deformity and enophthalmos.

- Imaging reveals inward displacement of the maxillary sinus walls, particularly the medial wall and orbital floor.
- The main differential diagnosis for silent sinus syndrome is an opacified hypoplastic maxillary sinus

Suggested Reading

Hourany R, Aygun N, Della Santina CC, Zinreich SJ. Silent sinus syndrome: an acquired condition. Am J Neuroradiol 2005; 26: 2390–2392

Case 174

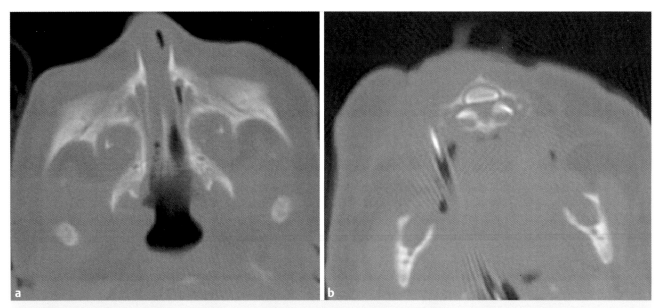

Fig. 174.1 Axial CT image through the inlet of the nasal cavity **(a)** demonstrates stenosis of the piriform aperature with soft tissue filling the anterior nasal cavity. The posterior choanae are normal in size. Axial CT image at the level of the maxilla **(b)** reveals a triangular-shaped palate with a single central mega incisor.

■ Clinical Presentation

A newborn with respiratory distress and inability to pass nasogastric tube (▶ Fig. 174.1)

▦ Key Imaging Finding

Narrowing of the piriform aperature with a single mega incisor

■ Diagnosis

Piriform aperature stenosis. The piriform aperature constitutes the anterior bony opening or inlet of the nasal cavity and is formed by the nasal and maxillary bones. Piriform aperature stenosis is relatively rare and results in respiratory distress in neonates, especially during feeding because they are obligate nasal breathers. The anomaly may occur in isolation or in association with syndromes, including holoprosencephaly. Common presentations include cyanosis, respiratory distress, and/or the inability to pass a nasogastric tube in a neonate.

Computed tomography (CT) is the modality of choice in evaluating for piriform aperature stenosis. Characteristic findings include inward bowing of the maxillary spines, resulting in a transverse piriform aperature measurement < 11 mm; a triangular-shaped palate; and in some cases, a single mega central maxillary incisor. The presence of a single mega incisor has a high association with additional anomalies.

Treatment is typically conservative with respiratory symptoms resolving after appropriate growth of the nasal inlet.

✓ Pearls

- The piriform aperature constitutes the anterior bony opening or inlet of the nasal cavity.
- Piriform aperature stenosis is a rare cause of respiratory distress in neonates.

- CT findings include a narrowed piriform aperature, a triangular-shaped palate, and a central mega incisor.

Suggested Readings

Belden CJ, Mancuso AA, Schmalfuss IM. CT features of congenital nasal piriform aperture stenosis: initial experience. Radiology 1999; 213: 495–501

Lowe LH, Booth TN, Joglar JM, Rollins NK. Midface anomalies in children. Radiographics 2000; 20: 907–922, quiz 1106–1107, 1112

Case 175

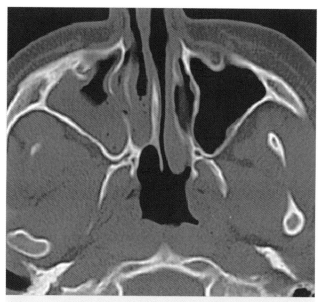

Fig. 175.1 Axial CT image demonstrates bony obstruction of the right choana with an air-fluid level in the nasal cavity. There is mild thickening and rightward deviation of the nasal septum. Right maxillary sinus opacification is also noted with an air-fluid level.

■ Clinical Presentation

A young child with chronic nasal congestion and rhinorrhea (▶ Fig. 175.1)

■ Key Imaging Finding

Obstruction of the posterior nasal cavity/choana

■ Diagnosis

Choanal atresia. Choanal atresia refers to congenital or developmental obstruction of the posterior nasal cavity and is the most common cause of nasal obstruction in neonates. The obstruction may be bony or membranous with bony atresia accounting for ~90% of cases. The abnormality is most often unilateral and typically associated with additional anomalies or syndromes. Approximately one-fourth of cases are isolated abnormalities.

Age and symptoms at the time of presentation depend upon whether the atresia is unilateral or bilateral. Bilateral choanal atresia may be life-threatening and presents in the neonatal period or early infancy with respiratory distress, which is more evident during feeding and relieved by crying. An additional common presentation is the inability to pass a nasogastric tube. Respiratory distress during feedings results from the fact that newborns and young infants are obligate nasal breathers; feeding prevents mouth breathing, and the choanal obstruction prevents nasal breathing. Crying relieves the symptoms because it forces mouth breathing. With unilateral atresia, symptoms are less severe, and patients often present later in childhood with a history of nasal stuffiness and chronic, unilateral rhinorrhea on the involved side.

Computed tomography (CT) is the modality of choice in evaluating for choanal atresia. Findings include narrowing and bony or soft-tissue obstruction of the posterior nasal cavity/choana, often with soft tissue or fluid superficial to the level of obstruction. Additional findings include thickening of the vomer and medial bowing of the posterior maxilla. In neonates and infants, a quantitative measurement for choanal atresia includes a choanal opening < 3.4 mm.

Membranous choanal atresia may be treated with perforation of the membrane; bony atresia requires surgical correction with occasional reconstruction.

✓ Pearls

- Choanal atresia refers to congenital or developmental obstruction of the posterior nasal cavity.
- Choanal atresia may be bony (more common) or membranous, as well as unilateral (more common) or bilateral.
- CT demonstrates bony or membranous obstruction of the posterior nasal cavity with thickening of the vomer.

Suggested Reading

Lowe LH, Booth TN, Joglar JM, Rollins NK. Midface anomalies in children. Radiographics 2000; 20: 907–922, quiz 1106–1107, 1112

Case 176

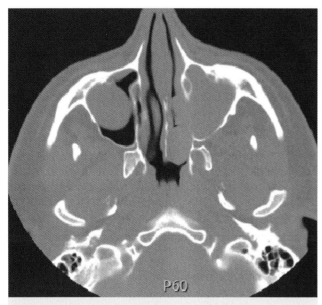

Fig. 176.1 Axial CT image in bone windows demonstrates complete opacification of the left maxillary sinus with polypoid soft-tissue attenuation extending through an expanded maxillary sinus ostia into the posterior nasal cavity/choana. The lateral wall of the left maxillary sinus is slightly thickened and sclerotic compared with the contralateral side secondary to chronic inflammation. A mucous retention cyst with surrounding mucosal thickening is seen in the right maxillary sinus.

▒ Clinical Presentation

A young adult man with unilateral nasal congestion/obstruction (▶ Fig. 176.1)

▥ Key Imaging Finding

Dumbbell-shaped polypoid mass involving the maxillary sinus and nasal cavity/choana

▥ Diagnosis

Antrochoanal polyp. An antrochoanal polyp refers to an inflammatory polyp located within the maxillary sinus with extension through an expanded primary or accessory maxillary sinus ostium/antrum and into the nasal cavity (choana) and/or nasopharynx. A spehnochoanal polyp is a less common variant that extends from the sphenoid sinus into the nasal cavity and/or nasopharynx. Patients often present in adolescence or early adulthood with symptoms related to unilateral nasal obstruction; bilateral involvement is rare.

Unenhanced computed tomography (CT) demonstrates a well-circumscribed, dumbbell-shaped, polypoid mass with its waist located at the maxillary sinus ostium and expanded components within the maxillary sinus and nasal cavity and/or nasopharynx. On occasion, the stalk at the maxillary ostium may be small and can be overlooked. Antrochoanal polyps are most often hypodense; increased density may be seen with inspissated secretions or superimposed fungal colonization. On contrast-enhanced studies, there is mild peripheral inflammatory mucosal enhancement, but there should be no enhancement of the polyp itself.

On magnetic resonance imaging, the vast majority of lesions are hypointense on T1 and hyperintense on T2 sequences with mild peripheral inflammatory mucosal enhancement. As protein concentration increases, there may be slight increase of signal on T1 sequences. As with CT, antrochoanal polyps are dumbbell-shaped with their waist at the maxillary sinus ostium.

Treatment consists of complete endoscopic surgical resection, which is considered curative; partial resection leads to a high rate of recurrence.

✓ Pearls

- Antrochoanal polyp is a polypoid mass that involves the maxillary sinus with extension into the nasal cavity.
- Antrochoanal polyp is dumbbell-shaped with its waist at an enlarged primary or accessory maxillary ostia.
- Treatment consists of complete endoscopic surgical resection; partial resection leads to recurrence.

Suggested Reading

Yaman H, Yilmaz S, Karali E, Guclu E, Ozturk O. Evaluation and management of antrochoanal polyps. Clin Exp Otorhinolaryngol 2010; 3: 110–114

Case 177

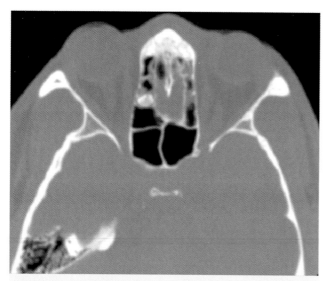

Fig. 177.1 Axial CT image reveals a well-circumscribed sclerotic/calcified lesion in the right ethmoid sinus. Minimal ethmoid sinus mucosal thickening is also identified.

▨ Clinical Presentation

A 33-year-old man with intermittent sinusitis and headaches (▶ Fig. 177.1)

■ Key Imaging Finding

Sclerotic/calcified paranasal sinus mass

■ Diagnosis

Osteoma. Osteomas are slow-growing bone-forming tumors that represent the most common benign tumors of the paranasal sinuses. They are classified as compact (most common), cancellous, or mixed. They may occur at any age but are most common in middle-aged adults. The vast majority (>95%) are asymptomatic and found incidentally. Those with symptoms often present with pain or sinusitis due to sinus outlet obstruction. A classic description is pain associated with air travel due to a frontal sinus osteoma. Rarely, osteomas may extend into the orbit or even intracranially, resulting in orbital emphysema or pneumocephalus, respectively, due to communication with the paranasal sinuses.

On computed tomography (CT), osteomas present as well-circumscribed sclerotic or calcified lesions within the paranasal sinuses. The frontal and ethmoid sinuses are by far the most commonly involved, followed by the maxillary and sphenoid sinuses. Most are small, measuring <1 cm. Lesions >3 cm are referred to as giant osteomas and are more likely to be symptomatic. On magnetic resonance imaging, osteomas are typically hypointense on all sequences, mimicking an aerated sinus.

If asymptomatic, no treatment is necessary. Symptomatic lesions are treated with open or endoscopic surgical resection.

✓ Pearls

- Osteomas are bone-forming tumors that represent the most common benign tumors of the paranasal sinuses.
- Frontal/ethmoid sinuses are by far most commonly involved, followed by the maxillary and sphenoid sinuses.

- On CT, osteomas present as well-circumscribed sclerotic or calcified lesions within the paranasal sinuses.

Suggested Reading

Price HI, Batnitzky S, Karlin CA et al. Computed tomography of benign disease of the paranasal sinuses. Radiographics 1983; 3: 107–140

Case 178

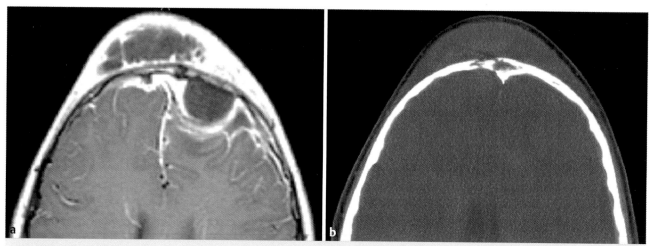

Fig. 178.1 Contrast-enhanced axial T1-weighted magnetic resonance (MR) image **(a)** demonstrates pronounced soft-tissue swelling, inflammatory changes, and a rim-enhancing abscess within the superficial soft tissues overlying the frontal bone. An underlying epidural abscess with abnormal dural and leptomeningeal enhancement is noted with mass effect on the left frontal lobe. Axial CT image in bone windows **(b)** shows frontal sinus opacification with bony disruption of its anterior and posterior walls/cortical margins. (Courtesy of Richard Latchaw, MD.)

■ Clinical Presentation

An adolescent with fever, sinus congestion, headache, and "facial swelling" (► Fig. 178.1)

■ Key Imaging Finding

Soft-tissue swelling overlying opacified frontal sinus

■ Diagnosis

Pott puffy tumor. Pott puffy tumor is a relatively uncommon complication of frontal sinusitis and, less frequently, trauma. Focal infection spreads through emissary veins, resulting in thrombophlebitis, frontal bone osteomyelitis, and subperiosteal abscess formation. Patients present with signs and symptoms related to sinusitis, as well as focal induration and swelling overlying the frontal bone.

Cross-sectional imaging demonstrates frontal sinus opacification, ill-defined lucency of the surrounding inner and/or outer tables of the frontal bone, and superficial or deep subperiosteal phlegmon or abscess formation. Scalp soft-tissue swelling and inflammatory fatty infiltration is typically seen. Enhancement is ill-defined with phlegmonous change and rim enhancing with abscess formation. It is important to closely evaluate intracranial structures for evidence of intracranial spread, which is commonly seen with inner table involvement.

Complications of Pott puffy tumor include intracranial spread with subsequent epidural abscess, subdural empyema, cerebritis or parenchymal abscess, and dural venous sinus or cavernous sinus thrombosis. Treatment consists of focal drainage of infectious collections and prolonged intravenous antibiotic therapy.

✓ Pearls

- Pott puffy tumor refers to subperiosteal abscess formation as a complication of frontal sinusitis.
- Imaging demonstrates frontal sinusitis, osteomyelitis, subperiosteal abscess, and superficial soft-tissue swelling.
- Complications include underlying parenchymal and/or extra-axial infection and dural venous sinus thrombosis.

Suggested Reading

Ludwig BJ, Foster BR, Saito N, Nadgir RN, Castro-Aragon I, Sakai O. Diagnostic imaging in nontraumatic pediatric head and neck emergencies. Radiographics 2010; 30: 781–799

Case 179

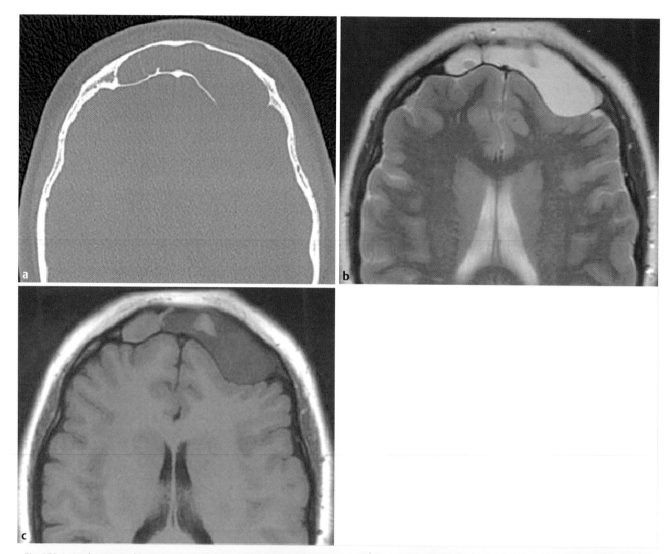

Fig. 179.1 Axial computed tomography image **(a)** demonstrates complete opacification and expansion of the frontal sinus with demineralization and dehiscence of the posterior sinus wall on the left. Axial T2 **(b)** and T1 **(c)** magnetic resonance images reveal fluid signal intensity filling the expanded frontal sinus with focal regions of intermediate T2 and hyperintense T1 signal, consistent with inspissated or proteinaceous sinus disease. There is mass effect on the underlying left frontal lobe without parenchymal edema.

Clinical Presentation

An adolescent boy with chronic headaches (▶ Fig. 179.1)

■ Key Imaging Finding

Opacified, expanded sinus with bony demineralization

■ Diagnosis

• **Mucocele.** Mucoceles are mucosal-lined lesions that result from chronic obstruction of a sinus outlet or ostium. They most commonly involve the frontal sinus (roughly two-thirds of cases), followed by the ethmoid, maxillary, and sphenoid sinuses. Cross-sectional imaging reveals a completely opacified, expanded sinus with benign bony remodeling and demineralization. Regions of bony dehiscence may be seen. Portions of the sinus opacification may demonstrate increased density or T1 signal intensity due to inspissated or proteinaceous secretions. Contrast-enhanced studies often demonstrate peripheral mucosal enhancement. Infected mucoceles are referred to as mucopyoceles.

✓ Pearls

• Mucoceles are mucosal-lined lesions that result from chronic obstruction of a sinus outlet or ostium.
• Imaging reveals a completely opacified, expanded sinus with benign bony remodeling and demineralization.

• Inspissated or proteinaceous secretions demonstrate increased density or T1 signal intensity.

Suggested Reading

Van Tassel P, Lee YY, Jing BS, DePena CA. Mucoceles of the paranasal sinuses: MR imaging with CT correlation Am J Roentgenol 1989; 153: 407–412

Case 180

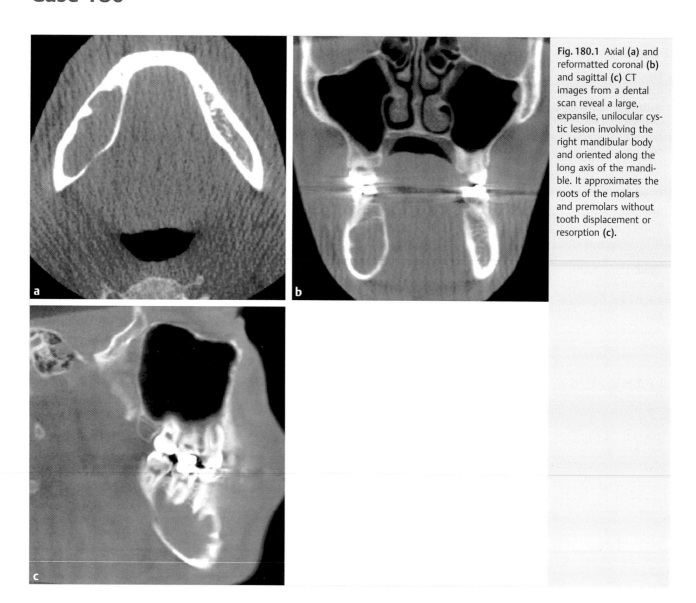

Fig. 180.1 Axial (a) and reformatted coronal (b) and sagittal (c) CT images from a dental scan reveal a large, expansile, unilocular cystic lesion involving the right mandibular body and oriented along the long axis of the mandible. It approximates the roots of the molars and premolars without tooth displacement or resorption (c).

▨ Clinical Presentation

An 18-year-old man for dental evaluation (▶ Fig. 180.1)

▥ Key Imaging Finding

Circumscribed cystic lesion of the mandible

▥ Top 3 Differential Diagnoses

- **Periapical (radicular) cyst.** A periapical cyst is the most common odontogenic cystic lesion. It typically occurs in adults with a history of dental caries or prior trauma. Inflammatory changes spread along the tooth to the apex with resultant periodontitis. Acutely, a periapical abscess may form; chronically, granulomatous changes result in a periapical cyst. On computed tomography (CT), periapical cysts present as well-circumscribed lucencies involving the apex of the involved tooth. Bony expansion, displacement of adjacent structures, and root absorption may occasionally be seen. Cortical disruption with overlying soft-tissue inflammatory changes suggests abscess formation rather than a simple cyst. Treatment options include tooth extraction or apical surgery.
- **Dentigerous (follicular) cyst.** A dentigerous cyst is the second most common mandibular cystic lesion and forms along the crown of an unerupted tooth. They can grow quite large and may cause bony expansion. The vast majority of lesions occur sporadically; bilateral lesions are rare and may be seen with cleidocranial dysostosis or mucopolysaccharidosis. On CT, a dentingerous cyst presents as a well-circumscribed, unilocular cystic lesion surrounding an unerupted crown, typically the third molar. The roots are usually outside of the cystic lesion. Cortical expansion and thinning is common, especially with large lesions. The larger the lesion, the less characteristic the imaging findings and the more overlap with odontogenic tumors.
- **Keratocystic odontogenic tumor (KOT).** A KOT is a benign cystic neoplasm that may appear locally aggressive and has a high recurrence rate. It most often occurs in the mandibular body or ramus and is oriented along the long axis of the bone. The vast majority are solitary lesions; multiple lesions may be seen in the setting of Gorlin (basal cell nevus) syndrome. On CT, keratocystic odontogenic tumors may be unilocular (more common) or multilocular and have lobulated, corticated margins. There is often bony expansion with overlying bony thinning or erosion. Displacement of adjacent teeth and root resorption may be seen.

▥ Additional Differential Diagnoses

- **Ameloblastoma.** Ameloblastoma is a benign but locally aggressive cystic and solid tumor that may involve the mandible (80%) or maxilla. They are most often large and multicystic (85%) with solid components. On CT, there is bony expansion, bony erosion, and characteristic pronounced root absorption of adjacent teeth. The less common unilocular cystic variant may mimic a dentigerous cyst when associated with an unerupted tooth. The more common multicystic variant has a relatively high recurrence rate.
- **Odontogenic myxoma.** Odontogenic myxoma is a benign, slow-growing tumor that may appear locally aggressive. It involves the mandible (most often the ramus) and maxilla equally. On CT, myxomas appear as poorly defined cystic lesions with thin bony septations. There may be tooth displacement and resorption.
- **Nonodontogenic processes.** Unicameral bone cysts are unilocular medullary lesions without tooth displacement or resorption. Aneurysmal bone cysts are multiloculated, expansile, and present with blood-fluid levels. Osteomyelitis is typically of dental origin and has a variety of appearances from lucent to sclerotic; periosteal reaction is a useful finding. Non-odontogenic tumors, such as metastases, multiple myeloma (or plasmacytoma), lymphoma, and leukemia, rarely affect the mandible. These lesions demonstrate soft-tissue enhancement with bony destruction. Occasionally, fibrous dysplasia may appear cystic with bony expansion.

▥ Diagnosis

Keratocystic odontogenic tumor (formerly odontogenic keratocyst)

✓ Pearls

- Periapical cysts are the most common odontogenic cysts; they are caused by dental caries or prior trauma.
- Dentigerous cysts form along the crown of an unerupted tooth, typically the third molar.
- KOT is a benign tumor of the mandibular body and/or ramus; it is oriented along the long axis of the bone.
- Ameloblastoma is often multicystic with solid components and characteristic root absorption of adjacent teeth.

Suggested Reading

Devenney-Cakir B, Subramaniam RM, Reddy SM, Imsande H, Gohel A, Sakai O. Cystic and cystic-appearing lesions of the mandible: review. Am J Roentgenol 2011; 196 Suppl: WS66–WS77

Case 181

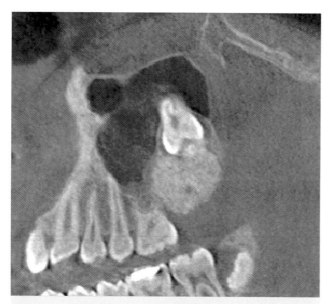

Fig. 181.1 Oblique sagittal reformatted image from a facial CT demonstrates a circumscribed region of sclerosis adjacent to the crown of a superior displaced, unerupted maxillary molar.

■ Clinical Presentation

A young adult man with tooth pain and an unerupted molar on clinical examination (▶ Fig. 181.1)

■ Key Imaging Finding

Sclerotic mass associated with dentition

■ Top 3 Differential Diagnoses

- **Cementoosseous dysplasia.** Cementoosseous dysplasia is a non-neoplastic process that involves the periapical region of dentition. It may occur as a solitary lesion or involve multiple teeth. The entity is asymptomatic and self-limiting. Computed tomography (CT) typically reveals well-circumscribed, lobular regions of homogeneous calcification surrounding the apex of one or more teeth. Lesions are often small, measuring less than 1 cm. Florid cementoosseous dysplasia is a less common subtype and is more advanced, resulting in numerous calcified periapical lesions that may grow quite large and cause bony expansion; simple bone cysts may be associated with the florid variant. Despite the more aggressive appearance, the florid variant is also self-limiting.

- **Fibrous dysplasia (FD).** FD results in replacement of normal compact bone with fibrous connective tissue and disorganized lamellar bone. The craniofacial bones are commonly involved (maxilla > mandible). FD occurs most frequently in young adults and is often asymptomatic unless extensive. Approximately 80% of cases are monostotic with the remainder being polyostotic. McCune-Albright syndrome consists of polyostotic FD, café-au-lait spots, and precocious puberty. The appearance on CT is variable with most cases demonstrating characteristic bony expansion and "ground glass" attenuation. Smaller lesions may lack bony expansion. Cystic and sclerotic variants are less specific and are more often associated with mandibular involvement. On magnetic resonance imaging, FD may mimic an aggressive lesion with decreased T1 and T2 signal and moderate enhancement.

- **Odontoma.** Odontomas are congenital malformations involving hard or dense dental tissue (e.g., dentin, cementum, enamel); they are characterized as complex or compound based upon morphology. Complex odontomas are more disorganized and result in a densely and homogeneously calcified mass involving the maxilla or mandible. The mass often results in bony expansion and lacks resemblance to a tooth. Compound odontomas, on the other hand, are more organized, resulting in a calcified mass that nearly resembles a tooth.

■ Additional Differential Diagnoses

- **Osteomyelitis.** Osteomyelitis most often results from spread of an underlying dental infection; postprocedural infection is less common. Susceptible patients have poor dentition, diabetes, immunosuppression, or are undergoing bisphosphonate therapy. The CT appearance of osteomyelitis is variable and based upon the nature and duration of the infection. Lytic, sclerotic, and mixed variants may be seen. Chronic infections may have an underlying bony sequestrum. The presence of periosteal reaction is commonly seen and is a useful secondary finding to suggest osteomyelitis, although it is not specific to infection.

- **Condensing osteitis.** Condensing osteitis occurs in the setting of periodontitis associated with periapical spread of infection from dental caries. The chronic periapical inflammatory response leads to bony sclerosis. CT reveals ill-defined periapical regions of bony sclerosis without bony expansion; a periapical cyst or abscess may be seen. When extensive, the inciting dental cavity may be identified.

- **Cementoblastoma.** Cementoblastoma is a benign tumor that involves the cementum of a tooth and presents most often in young adults. It occurs along the root of the tooth (typically the first mandibular molar) and often causes root resorption. Patients may be asymptomatic or present with pain. On CT, cementoblastoma presents as lobulated, bulbous, expansile hyperdense mass (cementum) with a circumferential lucency along the periphery. Lesions may grow quite large.

■ Diagnosis

Odontoma (complex)

✓ Pearls

- Cementoosseous dysplasia results in well-circumscribed, lobular regions of periapical calcification.
- Odontomas are malformations involving hard or dense dental tissue; they may be complex or resemble a tooth.
- Condensing osteitis results from periodontitis and results in ill-defined periapical regions of bony sclerosis.
- Cementoblastomas present as lobulated, expansile hyperdense masses with circumferential peripheral lucency.

Suggested Reading

Yonetsu K, Nakamura T. CT of calcifying jaw bone diseases. Am J Roentgenol 2001; 177: 937–943

Case 182

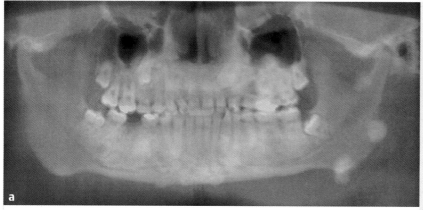

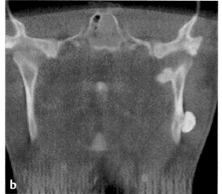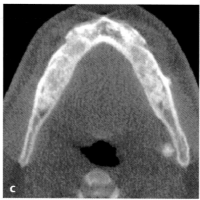

Fig. 182.1 Panoramic reformation **(a)** demonstrates multiple exophytic, pedunculated calcified masses along the surface of the mandible, sclerosis of the alveolar ridge, and supernumerary teeth. Coronal reformatted **(b)** and axial **(c)** CT images from a dental scan better depict the exophytic, pedunculated calcified mandibular masses. The axial image **(c)** also shows diffuse endosteal sclerosis with some bony expansion.

■ Clinical Presentation

A young adult man with jaw pain that is worse when eating (▶ Fig. 182.1)

■ Key Imaging Finding

Multiple osteomas and supernumerary teeth

■ Diagnosis

Gardner syndrome/multiple osteomas. Osteomas are benign tumors that are characterized by proliferation of compact or cancellous bone. The vast majority are solitary and isolated lesions; multiple osteomas may also be sporadic or associated with Gardner syndrome. In the maxillofacial region, they are far more common in the paranasal sinuses compared with the maxilla and mandible; the mandible is more often involved than the maxilla. Most lesions are asymptomatic, unless they interfere with the mechanics of the jaw or compress adjacent neurovascular structures.

Osteomas are characterized as peripheral, extending from the periosteum, or central, originating along the endosteal surface. On computed tomography (CT), peripheral osteomas appear as exophytic pedunculated or sessile, densely calcified masses extending from the surface of the periosteum. Endosteal osteomas reveal focal bony sclerosis with or without bony expansion. Osteomas may be distinguished from regions of exostoses by the presence of compact bone and the absence of a contiguous medullary cavity extending into the lesion. However, the two lesions may be indistinguishable in some cases where characteristic features are not present.

Gardner syndrome is an autosomal dominant syndrome characterized by colorectal polyps, bone tumors, and soft-tissue tumors (e.g., abdominal desmoid tumors). It typically affects young to middle-aged adults. Characteristic maxillofacial findings include multiple osteomas, supernumerary teeth, dental impaction, and bone cysts. Because sporadic cases of multiple osteomas are rare, patients found to have multiple craniofacial osteomas should undergo colorectal screening to exclude Gardner syndrome.

✓ Pearls

- Osteomas are benign tumors characterized by proliferation of compact or cancellous bone.
- Osteomas may be peripheral, extending from the periosteum, or central, originating along the endosteal surface.
- Supernumerary teeth, tooth impaction, and bone cysts are additional craniofacial findings of Gardner syndrome.
- Patients with multiple craniofacial osteomas should undergo colorectal screening to exclude Gardner syndrome.

Suggested Readings

Woldenberg Y, Nash M, Bodner L. Peripheral osteoma of the maxillofacial region. Diagnosis and management: a study of 14 cases. Med Oral Patol Oral Cir Bucal 2005; 10 Suppl 2: E139–E142

Case 183

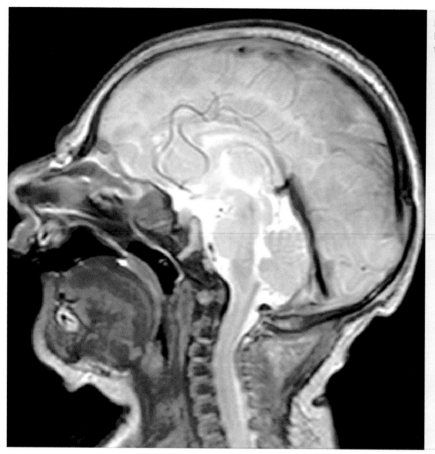

Fig. 183.1 Sagittal T2 image reveals marked hypoplasia and posterior positioning (retrognathia) of the mandible.

▥ Clinical Presentation

A 5-day-old boy with respiratory and feeding difficulties (▶ Fig. 183.1)

■ Key Imaging Finding

Mandibular hypoplasia

■ Diagnosis

Micrognathia. Micrognathia refers to underdevelopment or hypoplasia of the mandible. It is clinically important due to the potential for airway compromise and difficulty with feeding. Micrognathia may occur as an isolated abnormality or in association with multiple syndromes. Associated syndromes include Pierre Robin (cleft soft palate, high-arched palate, glossoptosis, natal teeth, and multiple ear infections), Treacher Collins (mandibulofacial dysostosis), Goldenhar (hemifacial microsomia, developmental delay, cleft lip/palate, optic/orbital abnormalities, microtia, hearing loss, vertebral anomalies, and cardiac and visceral anomalies), Cornelia de Lange (short stature dwarfism, microcephaly, mental retardation, low-set ears, facial anomalies, and cardiac and visceral anomalies), trisomy 13 (Patau syndrome—central nervous system malformations, mental retardation, cleft lip/palate, cardiac and visceral anomalies, and polydactyly), and trisomy 18 (Edward syndrome—cranial malformations, mental retardation, optic/orbital abnormalities, low-set ears, deafness, and cardiac and gastrointestinal anomalies).

Micrognathia may be identified objectively in utero. On fetal ultrasound, micrognathia is suggested on the sagittal profile by a small mandible and measured using the jaw index, which is calculated by dividing the anterior-posterior diameter of the mandible by the biparietal diameter × 100; a value < 23 is sensitive and specific for micrognathia. Alternatively, micrognathia may be suggested by measuring the frontal nasomental angle on the profile view; a measurement below the fifth percentile (142 degrees) is suggestive of micrognathia/retrognathia.

✓ Pearls

- Micrognathia refers to mandibular hypoplasia; it may occur in isolation or in association with syndromes.
- Micrognathia is clinically important due to the potential for airway compromise and difficulty with feeding.
- Micrognathia may be suggested objectively in utero using the jaw index or frontal nasomental angle.

Suggested Readings

Paladini D, Morra T, Teodoro A, Lamberti A, Tremolaterra F, Martinelli P. Objective diagnosis of micrognathia in the fetus: the jaw index. Obstet Gynecol 1999; 93: 382–386

Palit G, Jacquemyn Y, Kerremans M. An objective measurement to diagnose micrognathia on prenatal ultrasound. Clin Exp Obstet Gynecol 2008; 35: 121–123

Case 184

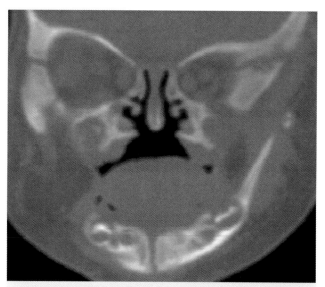

Fig. 184.1 Coronal CT image reveals a large midline defect involving the hard palate with direct communication between the oral and nasal cavities. The appearance of the mandible is age appropriate.

■ Clinical Presentation

A 3-week-old boy with feeding difficulty (▶ Fig. 184.1)

▓ Key Imaging Finding

Bony defect involving the hard palate

▓ Diagnosis

Cleft palate. Cleft lip and/or palate are caused by failure of fusion of paired structures. They are among the most common craniofacial congenital anomalies and may occur in isolation or in association with numerous syndromes. There is an increased incidence in those with a first-degree relative with a cleft lip and/or palate. Most cases involve both a cleft lip and cleft palate with unilateral abnormalities being more common than bilateral. A cleft lip results from nonfusion of the medial nasal processes; it may be unilateral or bilateral. A cleft palate results from nonfusion of the lateral palatine processes, nasal septum, and/or the median palatine processes and may affect the hard and/or soft palate. Cleft palates allow for direct communication between the oral and nasal cavity and pharynx, resulting in feeding difficulties for neonates.

Clefts may be found in utero during a fetal anatomy scan or identified clinically at birth. Prenatal anatomic imaging is performed around the 20th week of gestation. Part of the routine anatomy scan includes dedicated coronal views of the nose and lips to evaluate for a facial cleft. The hard palate may be evaluated in the axial plane. Cases of cleft lip and palate may be very subtle on ultrasound, especially when unilateral. In cases of bilateral cleft lip and cleft palate, a paranasal echogenic premaxillary protrusion may be seen. The use of three-dimensional ultrasound further increases the sensitivity for identifying clefts. Fetal magnetic resonance imaging (MRI) is useful to confirm or further evaluate suspected clefts because it provides superior soft-tissue detail.

Postnatal computed tomography (CT) imaging readily identifies a cleft palate as bony (hard palate) and/or soft-tissue (soft palate) defects, which are best visualized on coronal reformats. A cleft lip is seen as a soft-tissue defect overlying the maxilla and may be unilateral (more common) or bilateral.

Clefts are treated surgically. Unilateral cleft lips often require a single surgery in the neonatal period. More severe clefts often require multiple surgeries to complete the repair.

✓ Pearls

- Cleft lip and/or palate are common craniofacial anomalies caused by failure of fusion of paired structures.
- Cleft palate allows for direct communication between the oral and nasal cavity, resulting in feeding difficulties.
- Clefts may be found during a fetal anatomy scan or MRI, noted clinically at birth, or evaluated on postnatal CT.

Suggested Reading

Stroustrup Smith A, Estroff JA, Barnewolt CE, Mulliken JB, Levine D. Prenatal diagnosis of cleft lip and cleft palate using MRI. Am J Roentgenol 2004; 183: 229–235

Case 185

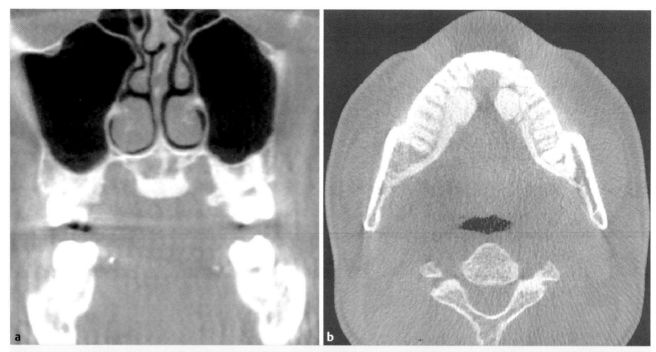

Fig. 185.1 Coronal reformatted image from cone beam (dental) computed tomography (CT) examination **(a)** reveals a focal bony protuberance along the midline hard palate extending into the oral cavity. An additional small bony outgrowth is seen along the lateral aspect of the maxilla on the left. Axial CT image through the floor of the mouth **(b)** demonstrates sclerotic bony protuberances along the inner margin of the mandible. (Courtesy of Giovanni Millare, MD.)

Clinical Presentation

An adult woman for orthodontic evaluation (▶ Fig. 185.1)

■ Key Imaging Finding

Bony protuberances along the hard palate/roof and floor of mouth

■ Diagnosis

Torus palatinus and mandibularis. Torus palatinus refers to a localized bony protuberance or outgrowth along the surface of the maxilla. It most often occurs midline in the hard palate along the roof of the mouth. Torus mandibularis represents a localized bony protuberance or outgrowth along the inner surface of the mandible. It is most often bilateral and occurs along the floor of the mouth.

Tori are composed of compact bone, which differentiate them from osteochondromas that maintain marrow continuity with the parent bone. They are incidental findings but may interfere with denture fabrication and placement.

✓ Pearls

- Torus palatinus is a localized bony protuberance or outgrowth of the hard palate within the roof of the mouth.
- Torus mandibularis is a localized bony protuberance/outgrowth of the mandible within the floor of the mouth.

- Tori are composed of compact bone, whereas osteochondromas maintain marrow continuity with the parent bone.
- Tori are typically incidental findings but may interfere with denture fabrication and placement.

Suggested Reading

Yonetsu K, Nakamura T. CT of calcifying jaw bone diseases. Am J Roentgenol 2001; 177: 937–943

Case 186

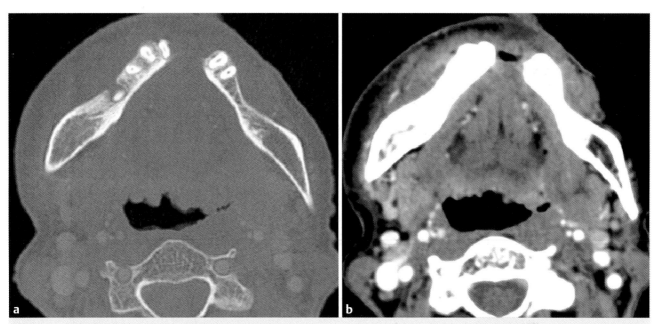

Fig. 186.1 Axial CT images in bone **(a)** and soft-tissue **(b)** windows reveal a periapical lucency surrounding a right mandibular premolar with adjacent bony sclerosis medially and cortical disruption laterally **(a)**. Soft-tissue swelling and a tiny, rim-enhancing abscess is noted within the superficial soft tissues **(b)**.

▧ Clinical Presentation

A young adult man with acute onset tooth and facial pain (▶ Fig. 186.1)

■ Key Imaging Finding

Periapical lucency with cortical disruption

■ Diagnosis

Periapical abscess. Periodontitis typically results from periapical spread of infectious and inflammatory components of a dental cavity. If the body's immune response effectively walls off the infection, a periapical granuloma occurs in the subacute setting with subsequent formation of a chronic periapical cyst. In the absence of an organized cavity, a periapical abscess may result. Continued spread of the infectious process beyond the periapical region may result in acute osteomyelitis or an intra-alveolar abscess.

On computed tomography (CT), periapical disease, including granulomas, cysts, and abscesses, may be indistinguishable. All demonstrate periapical lucencies; cysts and granulomas are well-circumscribed, whereas abscesses may be well-circumscribed or ill defined. In the first 1 to 2 weeks of infection, a periapical lucency may be absent due to the lack of bony resorption. Local spread of a periapical abscess may result in resorption of medullary and cortical bone, reactive bony sclerosis, or a combination of both. These findings are typically not seen with periapical granulomas or cysts. Further spread beyond the cortical margin may result in overlying soft-tissue inflammation and soft-tissue abscess formation.

Periapical cysts are typically asymptomatic and found incidentally. Periapical abscesses, on the other hand, are painful. Treatment may consist of tooth extraction with evacuation of the abscess and cosmetic restoration or root canal therapy.

✓ Pearls

- Periodontitis results from periapical spread of infectious and inflammatory components of a dental cavity.
- On CT, periapical disease, including granulomas, cysts, and abscesses, may be indistinguishable.

- Periapical cysts and granulomas are circumscribed, whereas abscesses may be circumscribed or ill defined.
- Spread of a periapical abscess may result in bony lucency and/or sclerosis, as well as soft-tissue involvement.

Suggested Readings

Devenney-Cakir B, Subramaniam RM, Reddy SM, Imsande H, Gohel A, Sakai O. Cystic and cystic-appearing lesions of the mandible: review. Am J Roentgenol 2011; 196 Suppl: WS66–WS77

Scheinfeld MH, Shifteh K, Avery LL, Dym H, Dym RJ. Teeth: what radiologists should know. Radiographics 2012; 32: 1927–1944

Case 187

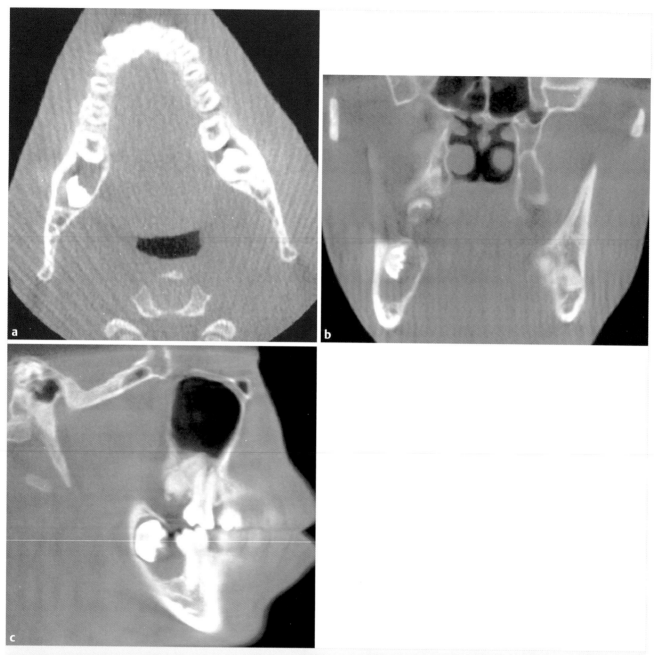

Fig. 187.1 Axial (**a**), coronal (**b**), and sagittal (**c**) CT images from a dental scan reveal a circumscribed lucent lesion associated with the crown of an unerupted right third molar, which is also impacted.

▪ Clinical Presentation

A 22-year-old man for dental evaluation (▶ Fig. 187.1)

▩ Key Imaging Finding

Cystic lesion associated with the crown of an unerupted molar

■ Diagnosis

Dentigerous cyst. A dentigerous or follicular cyst is the second most common odontogenic cyst following a periapical cyst. It is associated with the crown of an unerupted tooth, typically the third molars. The roots are usually outside of the lesion. Approximately 75% occur in the mandible; 25% involve the maxilla.

Dentigerous cysts may be found at any age but are most often detected during adolescence and young adulthood. Lesions may grow quite large and cause bony expansion, although they are typically asymptomatic. The vast majority of lesions occur spo-radically; bilateral lesions are rare and may be seen with clei-docranial dysostosis or mucopolysaccharidosis.

On computed tomography (CT), dentigerous cysts present as well-circumscribed, unilocular cystic lesions surrounding the crown of an unerupted tooth, typically the third molar. There may be displacement and root resorption of adjacent teeth. On magnetic resonance imaging (MRI), lesions appear cystic (T1 hypointense and T2 hyperintense) without enhancement.

✓ Pearls

- Dentigerous cysts are the second most common odontogenic cysts, following periapical cysts.
- Dentigerous cysts are associated with the crown of an unerupted tooth, typically the third mandibular molar.

- On CT, dentigerous cysts are well-circumscribed and unilocular cystic lesions; they follow fluid signal on MRI.

Suggested Reading

Devenney-Cakir B, Subramaniam RM, Reddy SM, Imsande H, Gohel A, Sakai O. Cystic and cystic-appearing lesions of the mandible: review. Am J Roentgenol 2011; 196 Suppl: WS66–WS77

Case 188

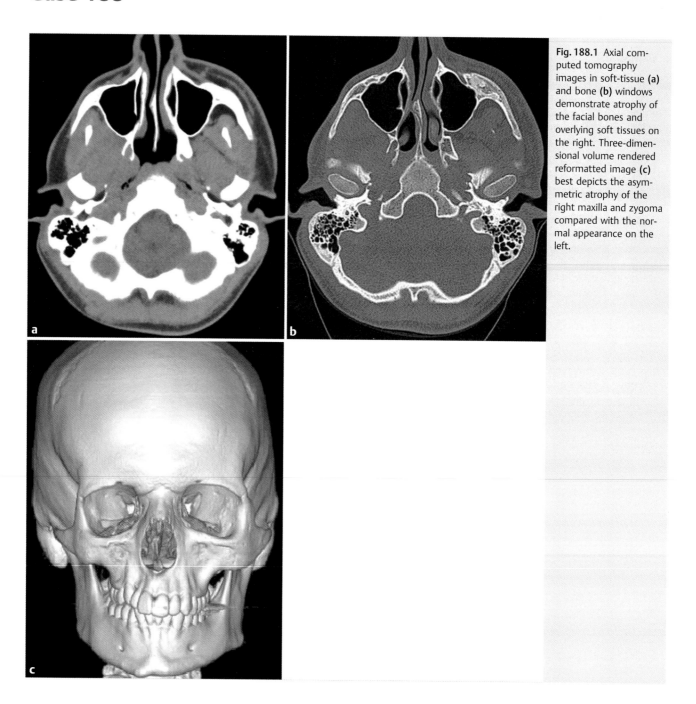

Fig. 188.1 Axial computed tomography images in soft-tissue (a) and bone (b) windows demonstrate atrophy of the facial bones and overlying soft tissues on the right. Three-dimensional volume rendered reformatted image (c) best depicts the asymmetric atrophy of the right maxilla and zygoma compared with the normal appearance on the left.

■ Clinical Presentation

A young adult man with progressive facial asymmetry (► Fig. 188.1)

■ Key Imaging Finding

Hemifacial atrophy

■ Diagnosis

Parry-Romberg syndrome (PRS). PRS, also referred to as progressive hemifacial atrophy, is a rare disorder that most often presents in adolescents and young adults. Although the exact etiology remains unknown, PRS has some morphological features that are similar to localized forms of scleroderma. Clinically, patients present with progressive unilateral facial asymmetry due to atrophy of the skin, subcutaneous soft tissues, musculature, and osseous structures, including the facial bones and orbits in some cases. Ocular involvement may result in enophthalmos secondary to atrophy of intraorbital fat with resultant decrease in orbital volume. A subset of patients also demonstrates neurological abnormalities with headaches being the most common clinical complaint, followed by trigeminal neuritis, facial paresthesias, and, occasionally, seizures; underlying parenchymal abnormalities are not uncommon.

Imaging of the head and neck reveals unilateral atrophy of the facial bones and soft tissues. The atrophy is limited to the affected side and does not cross midline. There is often a sharp demarcation between tissues that are involved and those that are spared; the demarcation has been termed *en coup de sabre*. Computed tomography is most useful for evaluating the extent of involvement, as well for reconstructive surgical planning in some patients.

Intracranial findings are not uncommon and may be ipsilateral, bilateral, or contralateral compared with the hemifacial involvement. Reported findings include parenchymal atrophy, nonspecific white matter lesions, intracranial calcifications, cortical dysplasia, leptomeningeal enhancement, and vascular abnormalities.

✓ Pearls

- PRS is a rare cause of progressive hemifacial atrophy; it most often presents in adolescents and young adults.
- Atrophy is unilateral and involves the skin, subcutaneous soft tissues, musculature, and osseous structures.

- Neurological symptoms and underlying parenchymal abnormalities are not uncommon in patients with PRS.

Suggested Reading

Sharma M, Bharatha A, Antonyshyn OM, Aviv RI, Symons SP. Case 178: Parry-Romberg syndrome. Radiology 2012; 262: 721–725

Case 189

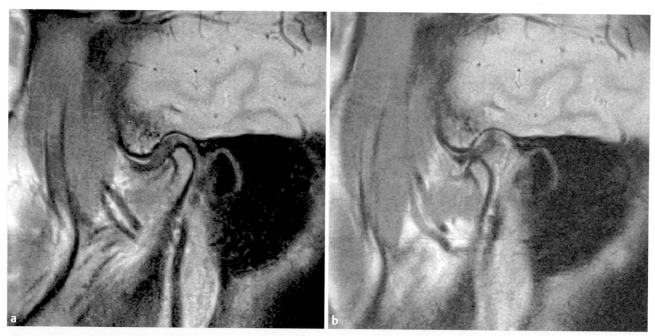

Fig. 189.1 Sagittal gradient echo image with the mouth closed **(a)** demonstrates anterior displacement of the hypointense meniscus with respect to the mandibular condyle. On the open-mouth view **(b)**, there is normal anterior translation of the mandibular condyle beneath the articular eminence with recapturing of the meniscus into normal position with respect to the mandibular condyle.

■ Clinical Presentation

A young adult woman with chronic jaw pain and "clicking" (▶ Fig. 189.1)

Key Imaging Finding

Displacement and recapturing of the temporomandibular joint (TMJ) meniscus

Diagnosis

Temporomandibular joint (TMJ) dysfunction. TMJ dysfunction is common in clinical practice and most often affects young to middle-aged patients with a female predominance. Common causes of TMJ dysfunction include meniscal displacement, joint effusions, and inflammatory or degenerative changes. It is important to correlate imaging findings clinically because findings of derangement may be seen in otherwise asymptomatic patients.

Articular disc or meniscal displacement is the most common cause of TMJ dysfunction. The meniscus is thinner at the center compared with the ends, which gives it a biconcave or "bow-tie" configuration on magnetic resonance imaging. A normal disc has homogeneous hypointensity within the anterior and intermediate bands and slightly hyperintense signal within the posterior band on T2, proton density, and gradient echo sequences. With meniscal degeneration, there is often increased T2 signal intensity within the meniscus, as well as meniscal thinning that is more pronounced anteriorly.

Under normal circumstances, the meniscus articulates with the mandibular condyle within the condylar fossa when the mouth is closed and translates anteriorly with the mandibular condyle beneath the articular eminence of the temporal bone when the mouth is opened. Meniscal displacement refers to an abnormal relationship between mandibular condyle and the overlying meniscus. Displacement may occur in any direction but is most common anteriorly. Sagittal closed-mouth views demonstrate anterior displacement or positioning of the meniscus with respect to the mandibular condyle. On open-mouth views, the meniscus can either remain displaced anteriorly or return to its normal position with respect to the mandibular condyle, which is referred to as reduction or recapturing.

The TMJ is a synovial joint and may also be affected by inflammatory and degenerative processes. Joint effusions are typically symptomatic and present with abnormal fluid within the joint space. They may occur with or independent of inflammatory or degenerative processes. Osteoarthritis occurs more frequently in the elderly population and results in meniscal degeneration with joint space narrowing, sclerosis, and osteophyte formation. Inflammatory arthropathies such as rheumatoid arthritis may cause bony erosions with demineralization. Synovial proliferation or synovitis are commonly associated with inflammatory arthropathies and are best evaluated on postcontrast studies that show abnormal synovial enhancement. Treatment of inflammatory or degenerative processes is geared toward the underlying etiology.

✓ Pearls

- Articular disc or meniscal displacement is the most common cause of TMJ dysfunction; most occur anteriorly.
- On open-mouth views, the meniscus can remain displaced or undergo reduction/recapturing.
- Osteoarthritis results in meniscal degeneration with joint space narrowing, sclerosis, and osteophyte formation.
- Inflammatory arthropathies such as rheumatoid arthritis may cause bony erosions with demineralization.

Suggested Reading

Tomas X, Pomes J, Berenguer J et al. MR imaging of temporomandibular joint dysfunction: a pictorial review. Radiographics 2006; 26: 765–781

Case 190

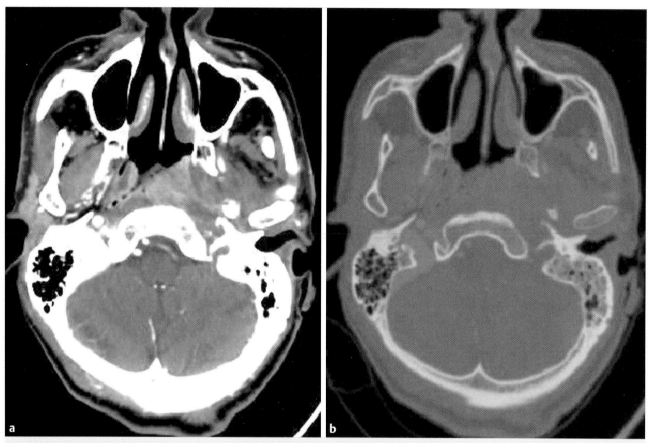

Fig. 190.1 Axial computed tomography (CT) image in soft-tissue windows **(a)** reveals a heterogeneous nasopharyngeal mass centered in the fossa of Rosenmüller on the left with mass effect on the nasopharyngeal airway. Corresponding axial CT image in bone window **(b)** demonstrates fluid within the left mastoid air cells as a result of eustachian tube obstruction.

▨ Clinical Presentation

A 58-year-old man with progressive nasal fullness and chronic ear "infections" (▶ Fig. 190.1)

■ Key Imaging Finding

Pharyngeal mucosal mass

■ Top 3 Differential Diagnoses

- **Squamous cell carcinoma (SCC).** SCC is the most common primary malignancy of the head and neck. It commonly originates in the nasopharynx or oropharynx. The lesions are clinically occult until late in the disease process. Nasopharyngeal carcinoma arises from the fossa of Rosenmüller. Patients may be asymptomatic or present with nasal obstruction or hearing deficits due to obstruction of the eustachian tube and subsequent accumulation of fluid within the middle ear and mastoid air cells. Oropharyngeal SCC commonly extends laterally to involve the parapharyngeal space. The imaging appearance is that of an ill-defined heterogeneously enhancing mass. There may be local spread and lymphatic spread to cervical lymph nodes, which characteristically demonstrate central necrosis. Treatment of nasopharyngeal and oropharyngeal carcinoma depends upon staging, which is determined by the local extent of the primary tumor, size and location of regional lymph node spread, and presence or absence of distant metastases.
- **Infection/Abscess.** Pharyngeal mucosal infections/abscesses most often result from adenoidal/tonsillar infections. Patients often present with fever and sore throat. Tonsillitis often demonstrates striated enhancement in a "tigroid" pattern without focal fluid collection. As the infection progresses and organizes, a rim-enhancing abscess may develop. With phlegmon, imaging often demonstrates ill-defined or partially organized inflammatory changes without complete rim enhancement. It is important to realize that the presence of complete rim enhancement is not 100% specific for an abscess because failed aspiration/drainage may occur in ~25% of cases of suspected abscesses on computed tomography. Prompt treatment is necessary to prevent retropharyngeal spread, which may allow for further spread to the mediastinum.
- **Lymphoma.** Non-Hodgkin lymphoma may involve the pharyngeal mucosa and appear similar to SCC. Patients with systemic lymphoma commonly have constitutional symptoms, along with abdominal lymphadenopathy, which are helpful discriminators. In the absence of constitutional symptoms or widespread disease, the presence of multiple, enlarged cervical lymph nodes without necrosis is also suggestive of lymphoma. In some cases biopsy may ultimately be necessary to establish the diagnosis.

■ Additional Differential Diagnoses

- **Thornwaldt cyst.** Thornwaldt cysts are benign developmental notochord remnants within the nasopharynx. They are cystic and midline, situated between the longus coli muscles. The amount of proteinaceous material determines the imaging appearances. Typically, they are hyperintense on T2 and variable but often hyperintense on T1 sequences. Although usually incidental findings, they may be associated with halitosis and may become superinfected. These can usually be differentiated from mucous retention cysts, which are typically off-midline and located within adenoidal tissue or pharyngeal mucosa.
- **Minor salivary gland tumor.** Benign (e.g., pleomorphic adenoma) and malignant (e.g., mucoepidermoid) minor salivary gland tumors may rarely involve the pharyngeal mucosal space. Imaging appearance is determined by the histology of the lesion. In general, benign lesions tend to be well-circumscribed, whereas more aggressive lesions are ill defined and heterogeneous with an imaging appearance that mimics SSC. Metastases and associated lymphadenopathy are uncommon.

■ Diagnosis

Nasopharyngeal squamous cell carcinoma

✓ Pearls

- Nasopharyngeal SCC arises at the fossa of Rosenmüller and may obstruct the eustachian tube.
- Striated tonsillar enhancement is seen with tonsillitis; abscesses show rim enhancement.
- The presence of constitutional symptoms or lymphadenopathy without necrosis suggests lymphoma.
- Thornwaldt cysts are midline notochord remnants and are often hyperintense on both T1 and T2 sequences.

Suggested Reading

Shin JH, Lee HK, Kim SY, Choi CG, Suh DC. Imaging of parapharyngeal space lesions: focus on the prestyloid compartment. Am J Roentgenol 2001; 177: 1465–1470

Case 191

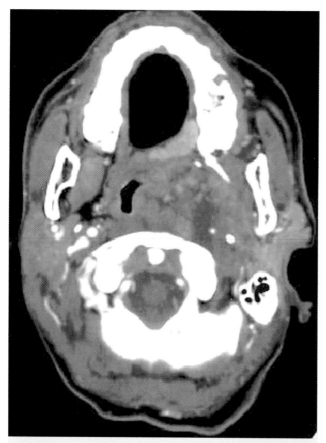

Fig. 191.1 Contrast-enhanced axial computed tomography image through the suprahyoid neck demonstrates heterogeneous hypodense attenuation centered within the left retropharyngeal space with irregular peripheral enhancement and mass effect on the aerodigestive tract. The hypoattenuation extends into the carotid space.

▨ Clinical Presentation

A 56-year-old man with sore throat (▶ Fig. 191.1)

■ Key Imaging Finding

Retropharyngeal mass

■ Top 3 Differential Diagnoses

• **Infection/abscess.** Patients with a retropharyngeal infection or abscess commonly present with fever, sore throat, and elevated white blood cell count. Involvement of the retropharyngeal space most often occurs secondary to spread of infection from tonsillar tissue. Lateral radiographs will show prevertebral soft-tissue swelling, prompting cross-section imaging. Contrast-enhanced computed tomography demonstrates soft-tissue swelling within the retropharyngeal space with associated inflammatory changes. Adenitis refers to inflammatory changes within retropharyngeal lymph nodes, which typically demonstrate enlargement and abnormal central hypoattenuation. Suppurative retropharyngeal adenitis may appear identical to an extralymphatic retropharyngeal abscess. If left untreated, suppurative adenitis may extend beyond the nodal capsule and result in a true retropharyngeal abscess. Phlegmon presents with ill-defined hypodensity and variable enhancement. As the infectious process becomes more organized, an abscess develops, demonstrating central fluid density with complete, peripheral rim enhancement. Prompt treatment is necessary because the retropharyngeal space allows for contiguous spread of infection into the mediastinum or within the danger space.

• **Nodal metastases.** The vast majority of nodal metastases within the retropharyngeal space result from spread of squamous cell carcinoma (SCC), which is the most common neoplasm of the pharyngeal mucosa. Involvement of the lateral retropharyngeal node of Rouviere is characteristic, and central necrosis is common. Extracapsular spread appears as disruption of the peripheral lymph node margin with ill-defined hypoattenuation extending into the surrounding soft tissues and portends a worse prognosis. Thyroid carcinoma (papillary variant) may also metastasize to the retropharyngeal lymph nodes, commonly resulting in central necrosis. Imaging of the remainder of the head and neck will help identify the primary lesion as originating from the pharyngeal mucosa (SCC) or thyroid gland.

• **Lymphoma.** Non-Hodgkin lymphoma commonly presents with lymphadenopathy within the neck. Patients with systemic lymphoma often have constitutional symptoms, along with abdominal lymphadenopathy, which are helpful discriminators. In the absence of constitutional symptoms or widespread disease, the presence of multiple, enlarged cervical lymph nodes without necrosis is suggestive of lymphoma. Unlike other nodal chains within the neck, however, isolated retropharyngeal lymph node enlargement may rarely be the initial presentation of lymphoma.

■ Additional Differential Diagnoses

• **Venolymphatic malformation.** Venolymphatic malformations represent a spectrum of venous and lymphatic developmental abnormalities. Pure venous malformations avidly enhance and may contain flow voids on T2 magnetic resonance imaging; the presence of phleboliths is pathognomonic. Pure lymphatic malformations may be unilocular or multilocular and demonstrate fluid attenuation and signal intensity. Fluid-fluid levels, most often due to hemorrhage, are characteristic. Many cases demonstrate characteristics of both. Venolymphatic malformations often cross fascial planes to involve multiple spaces of the neck.

■ Diagnosis

Nodal metastases with extracapsular spread (SCC involving the lateral retropharyngeal node of Rouviere)

✓ Pearls

• Retropharyngeal infections cause soft-tissue swelling and inflammation; abscesses reveal rim enhancement.
• SCC is the most common cause of retropharyngeal nodal metastases, followed by papillary thyroid cancer.

• Non-Hodgkin lymphoma commonly presents with constitutional symptoms and diffuse lymphadenopathy.
• Venolymphatic malformations have varying degrees of cystic/vascular components and cross fascial planes.

Suggested Reading

Shin JH, Lee HK, Kim SY, Choi CG, Suh DC. Imaging of parapharyngeal space lesions: focus on the prestyloid compartment. Am J Roentgenol 2001; 177: 1465–1470

Case 192

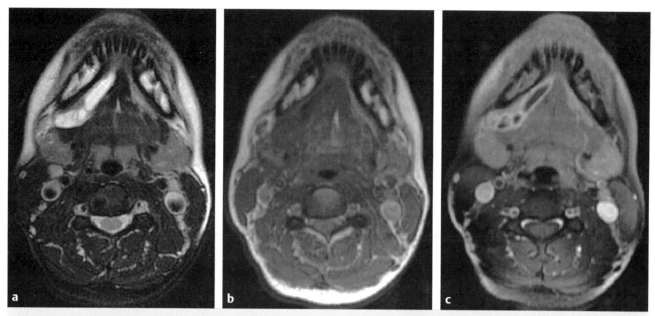

Fig. 192.1 Axial MR images through the floor of the mouth demonstrate a T2 hyperintense **(a)** and T1 hypointense **(b)** multiloculated cystic mass along the inner aspect of the mandible on the right with extension lateral to the mylohyoid muscle. Postcontrast axial T1 image with fat suppression **(c)** reveals intense peripheral and rim enhancement.

▧ Clinical Presentation

A 29-year-old man with jaw pain (▶ Fig. 192.1)

▩ Key Imaging Finding

Floor-of-the-mouth mass

▩ Top 3 Differential Diagnoses

- **Squamous cell carcinoma (SCC).** SCC is the most common neoplasm of the aerodigestive tract and is highly associated with tobacco usage. Common locations include the base of tongue, palate, and floor of the mouth. Patients are often asymptomatic until late in the disease process. The mylohyoid muscle divides floor-of-the-mouth carcinomas into sublingual (above) and submandibular (below) compartments. SCC often presents as an ill-defined enhancing mass. Lymphadenopathy, which may be centrally necrotic, is commonly seen.
- **Infection/abscess.** Cellulitis and abscesses within the floor of the mouth are commonly due to dental infections or procedures. Cellulitis presents with inflammatory changes that are typically ill defined, whereas abscesses are organized fluid collections with rim enhancement. The term *Ludwig angina* refers to a severe, potentially life-threatening infection with abscess formation involving the sublingual, submental, and submandibular spaces. The life-threatening nature of the infection results from airway compression.
- **Ranula.** Ranulas are mucous retention cysts of the salivary glands in the floor of the mouth. When confined to the sublingual space, they are referred to as simple ranulas; when they extend below the mylohyoid muscle into the submandibular space, they are referred to as diving or plunging ranulas. The plunging ranulas lack true cyst walls. Ranulas typically follow fluid attenuation and signal intensity and are most often unilocular. Peripheral enhancement may be seen, especially with superimposed infection.

▩ Additional Differential Diagnoses

- **Venolymphatic malformation.** Venolymphatic malformations represent a spectrum of venous and lymphatic developmental abnormalities. Pure venous malformations avidly enhance and may contain flow voids on T2 magnetic resonance imaging (MRI); the presence of phleboliths is pathognomonic. Pure lymphatic malformations may be unilocular or multilocular and demonstrate fluid attenuation and signal intensity. Fluid-fluid levels, most often due to hemorrhage, are characteristic. Many cases demonstrate characteristics of both. Venolymphatic malformations often cross fascial planes to involve multiple compartments and spaces of the neck.
- **Epidermoid/dermoid cyst.** Epidermoid and dermoid cysts are developmental abnormalities that may involve the oral cavity, oropharynx, or floor of mouth. Epidermoids contain epithelial elements, whereas dermoids contain epithelial elements along with dermal elements. Both appear cystic on imaging with low attenuation on computed tomography (CT) and T2 hyperintensity on MRI. There may be thin peripheral enhancement, if any. Dermoids may contain macroscopic fat, which is a key discriminator when present. Epidermoids demonstrate restricted diffusion.
- **Hemangioma.** Hemangiomas are benign vascular tumors that may involve the oral cavity or oropharynx; rarely, they may present as a submucosal floor-of-mouth mass. Capillary hemangiomas are common in infancy but naturally regress following a proliferative phase. CT and MRI demonstrate a well-circumscribed, lobulated, hyperdense and T2 hyperintense mass with avid enhancement.

▩ Diagnosis

Ranula (diving)

✓ Pearls

- SCC is the most common malignancy of the aerodigestive tract and may have associated necrotic adenopathy.
- Cellulitis and abscesses are typically of dental origin; Ludwig angina is severe and potentially life-threatening.
- Ranulas are mucous retention cysts and are characterized based upon their relation to the mylohyoid muscle.
- Venolymphatic malformations, epidermoid/dermoid cysts, and hemangiomas may involve the floor of the mouth.

Suggested Reading

Coit WE, Harnsberger HR, Osborn AG, Smoker WR, Stevens MH, Lufkin RB. Ranulas and their mimics: CT evaluation. Radiology 1987; 163: 211–216

Case 193

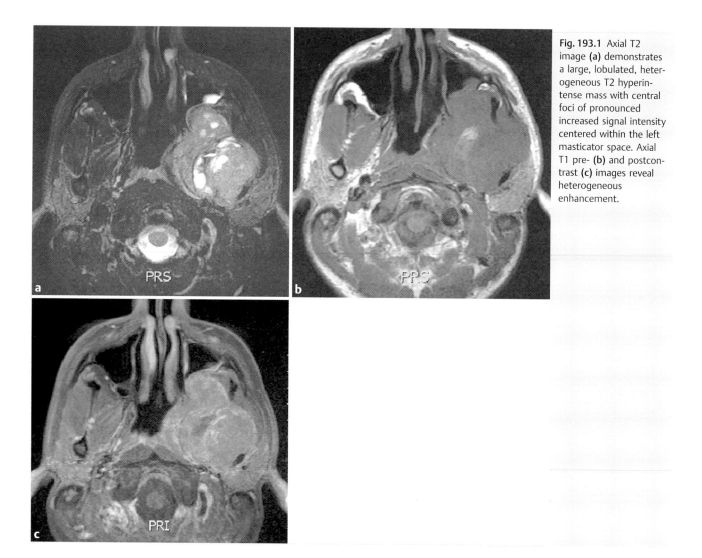

Fig. 193.1 Axial T2 image (a) demonstrates a large, lobulated, heterogeneous T2 hyperintense mass with central foci of pronounced increased signal intensity centered within the left masticator space. Axial T1 pre- (b) and postcontrast (c) images reveal heterogeneous enhancement.

■ Clinical Presentation

A young adult man with an enlarging facial mass and trismus (▶ Fig. 193.1)

■ Key Imaging Finding

Masticator space mass

■ Top 3 Differential Diagnoses

- **Infection/abscess.** Most infections of the masticator space evolve from a dental origin. Infections may present as osteomyelitis, cellulitis, or an organized abscess. Osteomyelitis has variable imaging appearances, including lucent, sclerotic, or mixed, and often mimics an aggressive, infiltrative process. Periosteal reaction may be seen. Care should be taken to evaluate the full extent of the infection because spread to other spaces and even the intracranial compartment can occur along nerve roots and fascial planes. Bony erosion and marrow infiltration are important findings, as are drainable fluid collections because these may alter clinical management.
- **Sarcoma.** Sarcomas within the masticator space most often arise from bone (chondrosarcoma, osteosarcoma, or Ewing sarcoma) or muscle (rhabdomyosarcoma). Occasionally, squamous cell carcinoma from a head and neck primary can secondarily involve the masticator space. Chondrosarcomas arise near the temporomandibular joint. There is typically a soft-tissue mass; the presence of a chondroid matrix is a helpful distinguishing characteristic. Osteosarcoma occurs anywhere in the mandible and is an aggressive lesion with bone formation and periosteal reaction. Ewing sarcoma typically presents within the first two decades of life with permeative bone destruction and a soft-tissue mass. The degree of periosteal reaction is variable. Rhabdomyosarcoma arises from the muscles of mastication and typically occurs in children. On magnetic resonance imaging (MRI), it may be difficult to distinguish between the types of sarcomas of the masticator space, as they all can be intermediate on T1 and variably hyperintense on T2 sequences and demonstrate heterogeneous enhancement.
- **Venolymphatic malformation.** Venolymphatic malformations represent a spectrum of venous and lymphatic developmental abnormalities. Pure venous malformations avidly enhance and may contain flow voids on T2 MRI; the presence of phleboliths is pathognomonic. Pure lymphatic malformations may be unilocular or multilocular and demonstrate fluid attenuation and signal intensity. Fluid-fluid levels, most often due to hemorrhage, are characteristic. Many cases demonstrate characteristics of both. Venolymphatic malformations often cross fascial planes to involve multiple spaces of the neck.

■ Additional Differential Diagnoses

- **Nerve sheath tumor.** Both schwannomas and neurofibromas may occur within the masticator space, typically involving the mandibular division of the trigeminal nerve (V₃). Schwannomas are usually more heterogeneous in appearance and may have regions of cystic degeneration. They are often intermediate on T1 and hyperintense on T2 sequences with heterogeneous but avid enhancement. Neurofibromas are generally more homogeneous and occur in the setting of neurofibromatosis type 1; they are commonly multiple and bilateral. MRI reveals intermediate T1 and hyperintense T2 signal intensity with heterogeneous enhancement. The target sign, characterized by central decreased and peripheral increased T2 signal intensity, is more frequently seen with neurofibromas.
- **Hemangioma.** Hemangiomas are unencapsulated, proliferative vascular neoplasms and represent the most common benign tumors of infancy. The proliferative growth phase typically occurs in the first year of life; infantile and RICH (rapidly involuting congenital hemangioma) variants then undergo involution with fatty replacement; NICH (noninvoluting congenital hemangioma) variants do not regress. Treatment is conservative unless there is mass effect on adjacent vital structures. Clinically, patients present with a superficial mass that is bluish or scarlet in color. MRI reveals a lobulated hyperintense T2 and slightly hyperintense T1 mass with avid enhancement.

■ Diagnosis

Sarcoma (chondrosarcoma)

✓ Pearls

- Most masticator space infections arise from a dental origin; look for signs of osteomyelitis or abscess.
- Masticator space sarcomas typically arise from bone or muscle; imaging findings often overlap.
- Venolymphatic malformations occur within the masticator space and may involve multiple compartments.
- Nerve sheath tumors (neurofibromas and schwannomas) occur along the mandibular division of cranial nerve V.

Suggested Reading

Shin JH, Lee HK, Kim SY, Choi CG, Suh DC. Imaging of parapharyngeal space lesions: focus on the prestyloid compartment. Am J Roentgenol 2001; 177: 1465–1470

Case 194

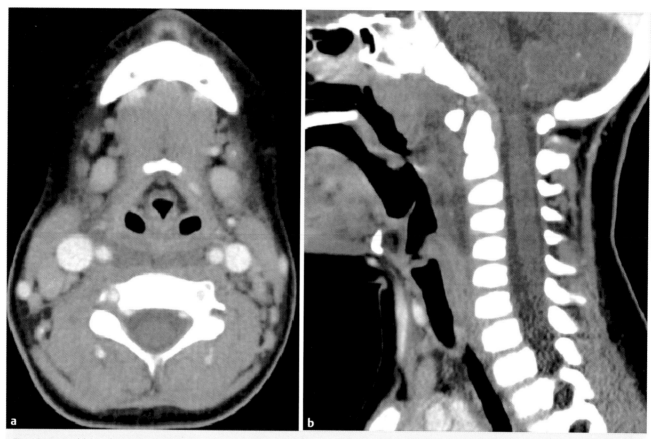

Fig. 194.1 Axial **(a)** and sagittal reformatted **(b)** postcontrast CT images of the neck demonstrate an ill-defined, hypodense fluid collection uniformly filling the retropharyngeal space and extending from the skull base to the C5–C6 level with tapering at the cranial and caudal ends. Associated lymphadenopathy is seen on the axial image **(a)**.

▓ Clinical Presentation

A young boy with neck pain (▸ Fig. 194.1)

■ Key Imaging Finding

Retropharyngeal fluid collection

■ Top 3 Differential Diagnoses

- **Abscess/phlegmon.** The retropharyngeal space lies posterior to the aerodigestive tract and anterior to the prevertebral musculature. It extends from the skull base to the mediastinum. Retropharyngeal infectious processes typically begin with suppurative lymphadenopathy that then extends into the retropharyngeal space. Tonsillitis and pharyngitis are the most common inciting events. Prior to abscess formation, retropharyngeal cellulitis or phlegmon presents as an ill-defined fluid collection often with inflammatory changes. This may mimic retropharyngeal edema. As the process becomes more organized, a focal collection forms with local mass effect and peripheral enhancement. An abscess is suggested when there is complete rim enhancement. It is important to describe the extent of the infectious process, as well as evaluate its effect on the airway and adjacent vasculature. Phlegmon is treated conservatively with antibiotics, whereas abscesses are surgically drained.
- **Retropharyngeal edema.** Retropharyngeal edema refers to noninfectious fluid within the retropharyngeal space. It is thought to represent lymphatic or inflammatory fluid, depending upon the etiology. Common causes include reactive edema secondary to infectious processes within the neck, radiation therapy, internal jugular venous occlusion, and calcific tendin-opathy of the longus colli tendons. Unlike phlegmon or abscesses, retropharyngeal edema uniformly spreads throughout and fills the retropharyngeal space. It has a characteristic "bow-tie" appearance on axial sequences and extends longitudinally throughout the retropharyngeal space with tapering at the cranial and caudal ends. There is no well-defined collection or enhancement. Calcific tendinopathy also demonstrates characteristic calcification of the longus colli tendons.
- **Retropharyngeal hemorrhage.** Retropharyngeal hematomas most often result from trauma or in the setting of an underlying coagulopathy. Spontaneous retropharyngeal hemorrhage or vascular rupture are less common etiologies. Retropharyngeal space hemorrhage can be significant due to the lack of anatomic constraints to tamponade the source of bleeding; therefore, prompt diagnosis and treatment is important. Retropharyngeal hemorrhage often mimics infectious processes on computed tomography (CT), demonstrating a fluid collection with mass effect and variable enhancement. Magnetic resonance imaging (MRI) is more sensitive and specific for identifying blood products. Characteristic findings include T1 hyperintensity and susceptibility on gradient echo or susceptibility-weighted imaging. Treatment is geared toward the underlying source of hemorrhage.

■ Diagnosis

Retropharyngeal edema secondary to pharyngitis

✓ Pearls

- Retropharyngeal infectious processes typically begin with suppurative lymphadenopathy.
- An abscess is suggested when there is a focal fluid collection with mass effect and rim enhancement.
- Retropharyngeal edema is noninfectious fluid that uniformly fills the retropharyngeal space.
- Retropharyngeal hemorrhage often mimics infectious processes on CT; MRI better identifies blood products.

Suggested Readings

Hoang JK, Branstetter BF, IV, Eastwood JD, Glastonbury CM. Multiplanar CT and MRI of collections in the retropharyngeal space: is it an abscess? Am J Roentgenol 2011; 196: W426–32

Muñoz A, Fischbein NJ, de Vergas J, Crespo J, Alvarez-Vincent J. Spontaneous retropharyngeal hematoma: diagnosis by mr imaging. Am J Neuroradiol 2001; 22: 1209–1211

Case 195

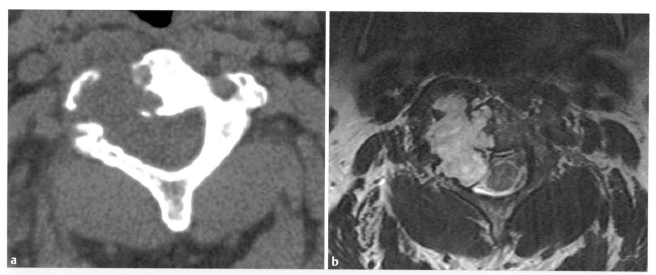

Fig. 195.1 Axial CT image through the upper cervical spine **(a)** shows bony destruction along the right side of the vertebral body with a prevertebral soft-tissue mass elevating the prevertebral musculature. Corresponding axial T2 MR image **(b)** demonstrates diffuse hyperintense signal intensity extending into the anterior prevertebral space with uplifting of the prevertebral musculature, as well as posterior extension into the epidural space of the spinal canal with leftward displacement of the cervical cord.

■ Clinical Presentation

A young adult man with globus sensation and vague neuropathy (▶ Fig. 195.1)

■ Key Imaging Finding

Prevertebral space mass

■ Top 3 Differential Diagnoses

• **Bony/epidural tumor.** Metastatic disease commonly involves the spine and prevertebral space. Breast and lung carcinoma are most often lytic, along with renal and thyroid carcinomas. Prostate (and occasionally breast) carcinoma produces sclerotic metastases. Metastases are typically hypointense on T1 and hyperintense on T2 sequences with avid enhancement; multiple lesions are common. Multiple myeloma is the most common primary bony malignancy in adults; plasmacytoma is the solitary variant. Patients are often > 40 years of age. Computed tomography (CT) demonstrates a poorly marginated, expansile lytic lesion. On magnetic resonance imaging (MRI), the lesions are typically isointense to cord on T1 and T2 sequences with homogeneous enhancement. Chordoma is an aggressive tumor that arises from notochordal remnants and is most common in young to middle-aged adults. It most often occurs within the sacrum and craniocervical junction. Patients with craniocervical involvement present with headache and ophthalmoplegia or neck pain and neuropathy. CT reveals a midline or slightly off-midline, expansile lesion with hyperdense foci centrally. Chordomas are classically hyperintense on T2 and often hypointense on T1 sequences with heterogeneous but avid

enhancement. Intratumoral hemorrhage is common. Lymphoma may involve the vertebral bodies and/or epidural space and is often homogeneous in signal and enhancement.

• **Disc-osteomyelitis.** Disc-osteomyelitis most often results from hematogenous spread of a distant bacterial infection; *Staphylococcus aureus* is the most common organism. MRI shows fluid signal intensity and enhancement centered at the disc space with adjacent endplate destruction and bony edema. Paraspinal phlegmon and abscess formation is typically seen. Tuberculous (TB) spondylitis is less common and typically occurs in immunocompromised patients. TB spondylitis characteristically affects the vertebral bodies with relative sparing of the disc space and is prone to subligamentous spread.

• **Nerve sheath tumor (NST).** NSTs include schwannomas (most common) and neurofibromas; neurofibromas may be sporadic or associated with neurofibromatosis type 1. Both are often circumscribed, T1 iso- to hypointense and T2 hyperintense with avid enhancement. Schwannomas may demonstrate cystic change and hemorrhage. Neurofibromas are more likely to demonstrate the "target" sign with centrally decreased and peripherally increased T2 signal intensity.

■ Additional Differential Diagnoses

• **Vascular abnormality.** Common vascular abnormalities within the prevertebral space include vertebral artery ectasia, aneurysms, and pseudoaneurysms. Although they may present a clinical dilemma on direct visualization, their vascular origin is typically readily identified on cross-sectional imaging studies, especially contrast-enhanced CT. Partially thrombosed aneurysms or pseudoaneurysms, however, may have a more complicated imaging appearance due to variant attenuation or signal intensity compared with the patent parent vessel.

• **Degenerative discogenic disease.** Degenerative changes of the cervical spine are common and progress with advancing

age. Anteriorly directed osteophytes project into the prevertebral space and often elevate the prevertebral musculature. The bony origin is readily identified on cross-sectional imaging. Anterior disc herniations are a less common discogenic cause of a prevertebral space mass and are often seen in the setting of trauma. MRI best depicts the disc herniation, which is often contiguous and follows similar signal intensity compared with the parent disc. Additional findings associated with trauma include bony fractures, ligamentous and soft-tissue injuries, as well as possible cord injury.

■ Diagnosis

Bony tumor (chordoma)

✓ Pearls

• Common prevertebral space tumors include metastases, multiple myeloma, chordoma, lymphoma, and NSTs.
• Disc-osteomyelitis involves the disc space and adjacent endplates with surrounding phlegmon or abscess.

• Discogenic disease (osteophytes and disc herniations) is a common cause of prevertebral space masses.

Suggested Reading

Harnsberger HR, Osborn AG. Differential diagnosis of head and neck lesions based on their space of origin. 1. The suprahyoid part of the neck. Am J Roentgenol 1991; 157: 147–154

Case 196

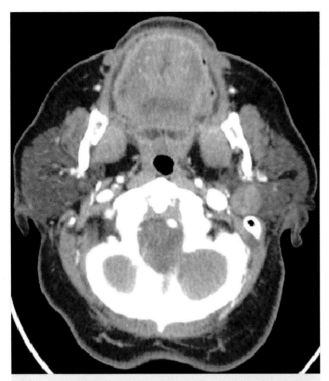

Fig. 196.1 Contrast-enhanced axial CT image demonstrates a well-circumscribed, round, hyperdense mass within the deep lobe of the left parotid gland.

■ Clinical Presentation

A 43-year-old man with vague jaw pain (▶ Fig. 196.1)

■ **Key Imaging Finding**

Unilateral parotid space mass

■ **Top 3 Differential Diagnoses**

• **Pleomorphic adenoma.** Benign parotid neoplasms are far more common (80%) than malignant primary neoplasms. Of all benign parotid neoplasms, pleomorphic adenoma is the most common (80%). Patients are often middle-aged and may be asymptomatic or present with nonspecific symptoms or a palpable mass. On computed tomography (CT), pleomorphic adenomas appear as well-circumscribed heterogeneous round, oval, or lobulated masses. They may be located within the superficial and/or deep parotid lobe, an important distinction for surgical planning; the facial nerve/retromandibular vein is the demarcation between the superficial and deep parotid lobes. On magnetic resonance imaging (MRI), the lesions are iso- to hypointense on T1 and characteristically hyperintense on T2 sequences. Delayed enhancement is typical.

• **Warthin tumor.** Warthin tumors, also known as papillary cystadenoma lyphomatosum, are the second most common benign parotid neoplasm and most commonly occur in middle-aged men. The may be both multifocal and bilateral. On imaging, the lesions are well-circumscribed with mixed cystic and solid components. CT findings include a slightly heterogeneous mass with enhancement of solid components. On MRI, the enhancing solid portions are generally hypointense on T1 and intermediate in signal on T2 sequences, whereas the cystic components typically follow fluid signal intensity (T1 hypo- and T2 hyperintense).

• **Parotid carcinoma.** Malignant neoplasms are more common in salivary glands other than the parotid gland (e.g., sublingual and submandibular). Of the malignant subtypes, mucoepidermoid is the most common in the parotid gland. Imaging appearance and clinical presentation vary based upon the aggressiveness of the lesion. In general, a well-circumscribed lesion is more characteristic of a low-grade neoplasm, whereas an ill-defined infiltrative appearance with intermediate density and T1/T2 signal intensity suggests a more aggressive lesion. Adenoid cystic carcinoma (ACC) is the second most common parotid malignancy and is typically an aggressive, infiltrative mass. Perineural spread is common, which leads to neuropathy involving the facial nerve, especially when located within the deep parotid lobe.

■ **Additional Differential Diagnoses**

• **Lymphadenopathy.** Lymphadenopathy may occur within the parotid gland from inflammatory, infectious, or neoplastic processes. Infectious or inflammatory etiologies typically resolve with follow-up imaging. Lymphoma may involve intraparotid lymph nodes and present as solitary, multiple, or bilateral masses. Lymphoma may also involve the parotid parenchyma in a diffuse, infiltrative pattern. Metastases from head and neck cancer (SCC) or skin cancer (SCC or melanoma) may also involve intraparotid lymph nodes, as intraparotid lymph nodes provide primary regional lymphatic drainage for portions of the scalp.

• **Branchial cleft cyst.** A developmental defect of the first branchial cleft may result in a type 1 branchial cleft cyst occurring anywhere from the external auditory canal to the angle of the mandible, including within the parotid gland parenchyma. The lesions are typically asymptomatic unless superinfected. Patients commonly present in adulthood with inflammation and/or a palpable mass. CT and MRI reveal a well-circumscribed cystic mass with varying degrees of peripheral enhancement.

■ **Diagnosis**

Pleomorphic adenoma

✓ **Pearls**

• Pleomorphic adenomas are benign, represent the most common parotid masses, and are bright on T2-weighted images.

• Warthin tumors are typically mixed cystic and solid, occur in middle-aged men, and may be bilateral.

• Malignant parotid tumors include mucoepidermoid and ACC (prone to perineural spread).

• Lymphadenopathy may result from inflammatory, infectious, or neoplastic processes.

Suggested Reading

Kinoshita T, Ishii K, Naganuma H, Okitsu T. MR imaging findings of parotid tumors with pathologic diagnostic clues: a pictorial essay. Clin Imaging 2004; 28: 93–101

Case 197

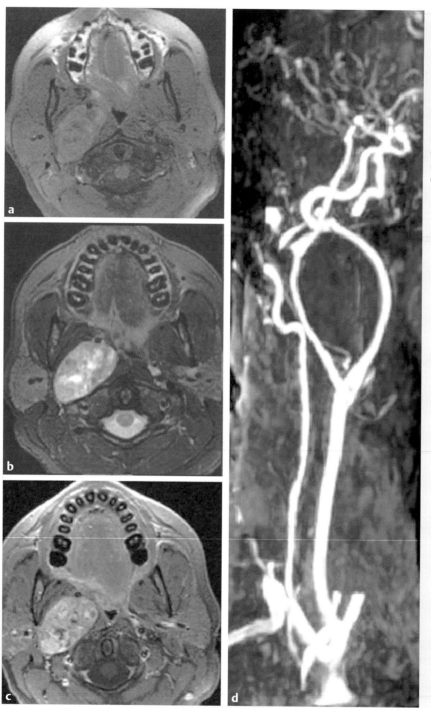

Fig. 197.1 Axial T1 precontrast with fat suppression (a), T2 (b), and T1 postcontrast with fat suppression (c) images through the neck demonstrate a heterogeneous, well-circumscribed T1 intermediate to hyperintense and T2 hyperintense mass that avidly enhances. There are small cystic foci internally. An oblique sagittal reformatted MR angiography image of the neck (d) reveals that the mass results in splaying of the right internal and external carotid arteries without significant internal hypervascularity. (Courtesy of Rebecca Cornelius, MD, University of Cincinnati.)

■ **Clinical Presentation**

A 48-year-old woman with "fullness in throat" (▶ Fig. 197.1)

◼ Key Imaging Finding

Carotid space mass

◼ Top 3 Differential Diagnoses

- **Paraganglioma.** Paragangliomas arise from neural crest cells and are most common in middle-aged women. Up to 10% are malignant and 10% may be bilateral. The two most common to present as carotid space masses are the carotid body tumor, which is the most common and occurs at the carotid bifurcation, and the glomus vagale, which occurs more superiorly along the course of the vagus nerve. The carotid body tumor splays the internal and external carotid arteries, which is characteristic but not pathognomonic, as other lesions may also occasionally splay the carotid arteries, including glomus vagale and nerve sheath tumors. Glomus vagale typically displaces the internal carotid artery anteriorly. Paragangliomas are highly vascular and commonly contain calcifications and flow voids, resulting in a "salt and pepper" appearance on magnetic resonance imaging (MRI). They are associated with multiple endocrine neoplasia syndromes but are typically hormonally inactive.
- **Nerve sheath tumor.** Both schwannomas and neurofibromas may occur within the carotid space, most often involving the vagus nerve or cervical nerve roots. When located more superiorly within the carotid space near the skull base, cranial nerves IX, XI, and XII may also be involved. Schwannomas are usually more heterogeneous with cystic and solid components when large. They are often intermediate in signal intensity on T1 and hyperintense on T2 sequences. Avid but heterogeneous enhancement of the solid components is typically seen. Neurofibromas are generally more homogeneous and occur in the setting of neurofibromatosis type 1, in which case they are most often multiple and bilateral. On computed tomography, the lesions are hypodense. MRI reveals intermediate signal intensity on T1 and heterogeneous signal on T2 sequences; enhancement is typical. Compared with schwannomas, neurofibromas more commonly demonstrate a target sign on T2 sequences with central decreased and peripheral increased signal intensity.
- **Vascular abnormality.** Vascular abnormalities and asymmetries are common causes of palpable abnormalities. The most important role of the radiologist is to identify the vascular origin of the abnormality so that inadvertent biopsy is avoided. Normal variants, such as a dominant jugular vein, are commonly seen. In the setting of hypertension or trauma, aneurysms and pseudoaneurysms can present as carotid space masses. Venous thrombosis as a result of recent line placement, surrounding inflammation or neoplasm, or hypercoagulable state can present a diagnostic dilemma; often, the wall and surrounding soft tissues enhance, mimicking a mass. The key is to identify the vascular origin of the abnormality.

◼ Additional Differential Diagnoses

- **Lymphadenopathy.** Lymph node enlargement may be reactive, inflammatory, or neoplastic in nature. Reactive and inflammatory etiologies typically demonstrate nonspecific lymph node enlargement that is often self-limiting. Squamous cell carcinoma from a head and neck origin is the most common cause of nodal metastases and often demonstrates lymphadenopathy with abnormal nodal architecture and central necrosis. Papillary thyroid carcinoma and atypical infections (e.g., *Myco-* *bacterium* and *Bartonella* subspecies) are additional causes of centrally necrotic cervical lymph nodes. Lymphoma commonly presents with prominent lymph node enlargement and may be of the Hodgkin or non-Hodgkin variant. Hodgkin lymphoma spreads in a contiguous fashion from the mediastinum and is most often unilateral. Non-Hodgkin lymphoma is typically bilateral with associated abdominal lymphadenopathy.

◼ Diagnosis

Nerve sheath tumor (vagal schwannoma)

✓ Pearls

- Paragangliomas arise from neural crest cells, may have a "salt and pepper" appearance, and avidly enhance.
- Schwannomas and neurofibromas may occur along the course of the vagus nerve within the carotid space.
- Vascular abnormalities and asymmetries may present as or mimic other carotid space masses.
- Lymphadenopathy within the neck may be reactive, inflammatory, or neoplastic in nature.

Suggested Reading

Fruin ME, Smoker WR, Harnsberger HR. The carotid space in the suprahyoid neck. Semin Ultrasound CT MR 1990; 11: 504–519

Case 198

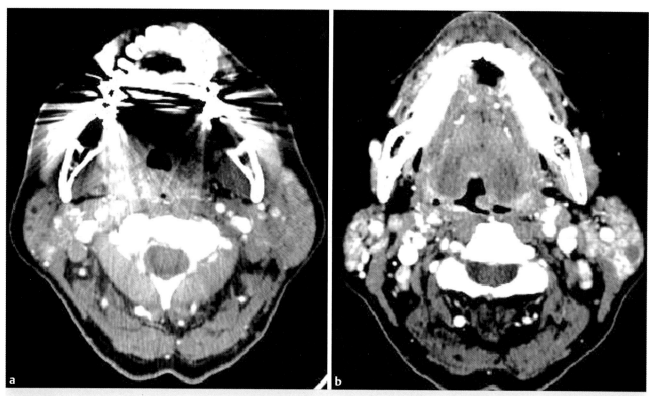

Fig. 198.1 Axial CT images through the neck **(a,b)** demonstrate multiple, bilateral hypodense masses and enhancing nodules within the parotid glands. (Courtesy of Rebecca Cornelius, MD, University of Cincinnati.)

■ Clinical Presentation

A 43-year-old woman with facial "swelling" (▶ Fig. 198.1)

■ Key Imaging Finding

Bilateral parotid space masses

■ Top 3 Differential Diagnoses

- **Lymphoepithelial lesions.** Benign lymphoepithelial lesions most often occur in patients with acquired immune deficiency syndrome (AIDS) who present with painless bilateral parotid gland enlargement. Pathologically, there is lymphocytic infiltration of the gland (similar to Sjögren syndrome) with lymphoepithelial cyst formation. Computed tomography (CT) and magnetic resonance imaging (MRI) reveal bilateral cystic and solid parotid lesions with diffuse gland enlargement. Associated cervical lymphadenopathy and tonsillar hypertrophy is commonly seen.
- **Sjögren syndrome.** Sjögren syndrome is an autoimmune disease that most commonly occurs in middle-aged to elderly women and results in lymphocytic infiltration of glandular tissue. The classic triad consists of parotid gland enlargement with keratoconjunctivitis sicca (dry eyes) and xerostomia (dry mouth). On CT and MRI, Sjögren syndrome presents as heterogeneous glandular enlargement with scattered enhancing nodules and fluid pockets. The appearance can mimic benign lymphoepithelial lesions or lymphoma. Patients with long-standing Sjögren syndrome are at increased risk for developing lymphoma.
- **Lymphadenopathy.** Lymphadenopathy may occur within the parotid gland from inflammatory, infectious, or neoplastic processes. Infectious or inflammatory etiologies typically resolve with follow-up imaging. Lymphoma may involve intraparotid lymph nodes and present as solitary, multiple, or bilateral masses. Lymphoma may also involve the parotid parenchyma in a diffuse, infiltrative pattern. Metastases from head and neck cancer (squamous cell carcinoma, SCC) or skin cancer (SCC or melanoma) may also involve intraparotid lymph nodes, as intraparotid lymph nodes provide primary regional lymphatic drainage for portions of the scalp.

■ Additional Differential Diagnoses

- **Warthin tumors.** Warthin tumors, also known as papillary cystadenoma lyphomatosum, are the second most common benign parotid neoplasm and most commonly occur in middle-aged men. The may be both multifocal and bilateral. On imaging, the lesions are well-circumscribed with mixed cystic and solid components. CT findings include a slightly heterogeneous mass with enhancement of solid components. On MRI, the enhancing solid portions are generally hypointense on T1 and intermediate in signal on T2 sequences, whereas the cystic components typically follow fluid signal intensity (T1 hypo- and T2 hyperintense).
- **Sarcoidosis.** Sarcoidosis is a multisystem granulomatous disorder that most commonly occurs in adult African Americans. Diffuse sarcoidosis can lead to granulomatous infiltration of glandular tissue, including the parotid and lacrimal glands. Patients typically have elevated angiotensin-converting enzyme levels and may also present with uveitis and cranial nerve deficits. On imaging, there is heterogeneous glandular enlargement that is usually bilateral and symmetric. Gallium 67 (Ga 67) scan will reveal the classic "panda sign" with increased uptake in the parotid and lacrimal glands.

■ Diagnosis

Sjögren syndrome

✓ Pearls

- Lymphoepithelial lesions occur in patients with AIDS and present with bilateral cystic and solid parotid lesions.
- Sjögren syndrome is characterized by parotid enlargement/ lesions, dry eyes, and dry mouth.
- Warthin tumors are typically mixed cystic and solid, occur in middle-aged men, and may be bilateral.
- Sarcoidosis results in bilateral heterogeneous parotid enlargement; the "panda sign" is seen on Ga 67 scans.

Suggested Reading

Kinoshita T, Ishii K, Naganuma H, Okitsu T. MR imaging findings of parotid tumors with pathologic diagnostic clues: a pictorial essay. Clin Imaging 2004; 28: 93–101

Case 199

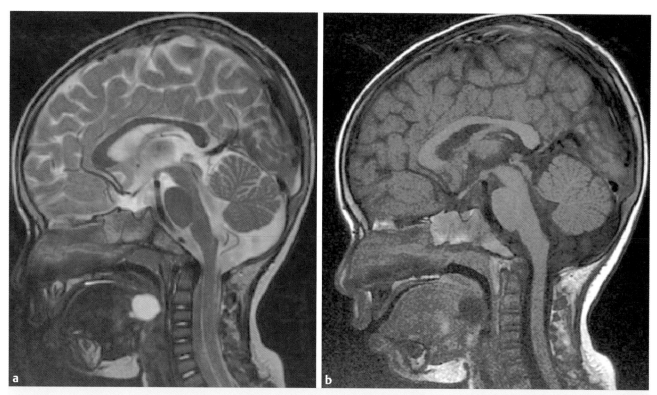

Fig. 199.1 Sagittal T2 **(a)** and T1 **(b)** MR images reveal a circumscribed cystic mass involving the root and base of the tongue. There is incidental note of a mega cisterna magna with hyperdynamic cerebrospinal fluid flow both intracranially and within the cervical spinal canal **(a).** The sphenoid sinus has yet to pneumatize in this child (open synchondroses).

■ Clinical Presentation

A young child with globus sensation (▶ Fig. 199.1)

■ Key Imaging Finding

Base of tongue mass in a child

■ Top 3 Differential Diagnoses

- **Thyroglossal duct cyst.** Thyroglossal duct cysts represent the most common congenital neck lesions. The vast majority (~85%) are midline. Approximately 25% are suprahyoid in location with the remaining 75% being infrahyoid. Suprahyoid lesions occur anywhere from the foramen cecum at the tongue base to the hyoid bone; infrahyoid lesions may be midline or paramedian and are characteristically embedded within the strap muscles. Thyroglossal duct cysts are most often well-circumscribed and may have lobulations or septations. They typically follow fluid attenuation (computed tomography, CT) or signal intensity (magnetic resonance imaging, MRI). Increased protein content may result in increased attenuation and T1 signal intensity. Superimposed infection or hemorrhage results in a heterogeneous imaging appearance, which may include peripheral enhancement.
- **Lingual thyroid.** Lingual thyroid refers to ectopic thyroid tissue located at the foramen cecum, involving the base and root of the tongue; 90% of ectopic thyroid cases occur in this location. It is important to evaluate the thyroid bed in the lower neck for the presence of additional thyroid tissue; in approximately 75% of cases, the lingual thyroid represents the only functioning thyroid tissue. Most patients are hypothyroid with the remainder of patients being euthyroid. On cross-sectional imaging, ectopic thyroid tissue follows thyroid attenuation and signal intensity. It is hyperdense on CT with moderate enhancement. On MRI, it is hyperintense on T1 and T2 sequences and demonstrates avid enhancement. Nuclear medicine thyroid imaging is also a useful adjunct in identifying functioning thyroid tissue. Rarely, thyroid cancer may occur in approximately 1 to 3% of cases; concerning imaging characteristics include soft-tissue nodular components or calcification.
- **Epidermoid/dermoid cyst.** Epidermoid and dermoid cysts are developmental abnormalities that may involve the oral cavity, oropharynx, or floor of the mouth. Epidermoids contain epithelial elements, whereas dermoids contain epithelial elements along with dermal elements. Both appear cystic on imaging with low attenuation on CT and T2 hyperintensity on MRI. There may be thin peripheral enhancement, if any. Dermoids may contain macroscopic fat, which is a key discriminator when present. Epidermoids demonstrate restricted diffusion.

■ Additional Differential Diagnoses

- **Hemangioma.** Hemangiomas are benign vascular tumors that may involve the oral cavity or oropharynx. Capillary hemangiomas are common in infancy but naturally regress after a proliferative phase. CT and MRI demonstrate a well-circumscribed, lobulated, hyperdense and T2 hyperintense mass with avid enhancement.
- **Tonsillar hypertrophy.** The lingual tonsils are a component of the Waldeyer ring and are located within the oropharynx along the base of the tongue. Tonsillar hypertrophy refers to enlargement of the tonsils that may occur in isolation or secondary to a local infectious or inflammatory process. It is most often symmetric; if asymmetric, it may mimic a mass. Contrast-enhanced CT demonstrates homogeneous hyperattenuation of tonsillar tissue. On MRI, tonsillar tissue is T2 hyperintense with enhancement similar to mucosal tissue.
- **Venolymphatic malformation.** Venolymphatic malformations represent a spectrum of venous and lymphatic developmental abnormalities. Pure venous malformations avidly enhance and contain flow voids on T2 MRI; the presence of phleboliths is pathognomonic. Pure lymphatic malformations may be unilocular or multilocular and demonstrate fluid attenuation and signal intensity. Fluid-fluid levels, most often due to hemorrhage, are characteristic. Venolymphatic malformations often cross fascial planes to involve multiple spaces of the neck.

■ Diagnosis

Thyroglossal duct cyst

✓ Pearls

- Thyroglossal duct cysts are common congenital lesions that present as circumscribed, midline cystic masses.
- Lingual thyroid is the most common form of ectopic thyroid; it is typically the only functioning thyroid tissue.
- Dermoid cysts contain epithelial and dermal elements; the presence of macroscopic fat is a key discriminator.
- Epidermoid cysts contain dermal elements; the presence of restricted diffusion is a key discriminator.

Suggested Reading

Fang WS, Wiggins RH, III, Illner A et al. Primary lesions of the root of the tongue. Radiographics 2011; 31: 1907–1922

Case 200

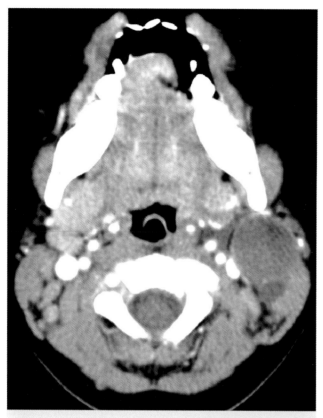

Fig. 200.1 Contrast-enhanced axial computed tomography image demonstrates a multicystic, nonenhancing mass at the angle of the mandible on the left, anterior and medial to the SCM muscle. Medially, a portion of the mass extends into the parapharyngeal space.

■ Clinical Presentation

An adolescent boy with neck swelling (▶ Fig. 200.1)

■ Key Imaging Finding

Cystic neck mass

■ Top 3 Differential Diagnoses

• **Congenital cyst.** *Thyroglossal duct cysts* (TDCs) represent the most common congenital cystic neck masses. They are typically midline (85%) or slightly off-midline and ~75% are infrahyoid in location. *Branchial cleft cysts* result from developmental abnormalities of the branchial apparatus. There are four types with the second being the most common, followed by the first. Type 1 branchial cleft cysts may occur anywhere from the external auditory canal to the angle of the mandible, including within the parotid gland. Type 2 branchial cleft cysts most commonly occur near the angle of the mandible anterior and medial to the sternocleidomastoid (SCM) muscle. Third and fourth branchial cleft cysts are rare and frequently result in sinus formation. Type 3 branchial cleft cysts occur deep to the SCM muscle or posteriorly, whereas type 4 branchial cleft cysts occur near the larynx or thyroid gland. *Thymic cysts* are the least common congenital cystic neck masses. They may occur anywhere along the tract of thymus descent from the angle of the mandible into the mediastinum. They are lateral in location, either deep or superficial to the SCM muscle, and may be unilocular or multilocular. All congenital cysts demonstrate fluid attenuation (computed tomography) or signal intensity (magnetic resonance imaging); internal debris and peripheral enhancement may be appreciated with superimposed infection or hemorrhage.

• **Abscess.** Abscesses may occur anywhere in the neck but are typically found within the peritonsillar, retropharyngeal, or perioral regions. Less common etiologies include penetrating trauma or postoperative complications. Clinical signs and symptoms include pain, fever, and elevated white blood cell count. Imaging characteristics include a rim-enhancing fluid collection with variable wall thickness and surrounding inflammatory changes. Percutaneous or surgical drainage with antibiotic therapy is commonly warranted.

• **Lymphatic malformation.** Lymphatic malformations are common in the neck and may occur in nearly any location. They may be unilocular or multilocular and demonstrate fluid attenuation and signal intensity. Fluid-fluid levels, most often due to hemorrhage, are characteristic. Peripheral enhancement may be seen in the setting of superimposed inflammation or infection; internal regions of enhancement, when present, correspond to venous components associated with a venolymphatic malformation. Lesions may grow quite large and insinuate between and cross fascial plains. Lymphatic malformations previously characterized as "cystic hygromas" are a common subtype that typically occur posteriorly and may be associated with chromosomal abnormalities, such as Turner or Down syndrome.

■ Additional Differential Diagnoses

• **Cystic lymph node.** Cystic lymph nodes may result from local or regional spread of infectious or malignant processes. Squamous cell carcinoma (SCC) and papillary thyroid cancer are the two most common primary neoplasms that demonstrate cystic metastases within cervical lymph nodes. Atypical infections, such as *Mycobacterium* and *Bartonella* subspecies, are the common infectious etiologies for cystic lymph nodes.

• **Cystic nerve sheath tumor.** Cystic nerve sheath tumors, such as a schwannomas, may occur within the neck and are typically oriented along the course of the traversing nerve; communication with the neural foramina may be seen with more central lesions and is characteristic. The presence of enhancing soft-tissue components is a useful discriminator to exclude a congenital cyst or pure lymphatic malformation.

■ Diagnosis

Lymphatic malformation

✓ Pearls

• The most common congenital cystic neck masses are TDCs (midline) and branchial cleft cysts (lateral).
• Abscesses commonly occur within the neck, are rim enhancing, and typically require drainage.

• Lymphatic malformations may be unilocular or multilocular, have fluid-fluid levels, and cross fascial planes.
• Cystic lymphadenopathy may occur from infectious or neoplastic (SCC and papillary thyroid) processes.

Suggested Reading

Lev S, Lev MH. Imaging of cystic lesions. Radiol Clin North Am 2000; 38: 1013–1027

Case 201

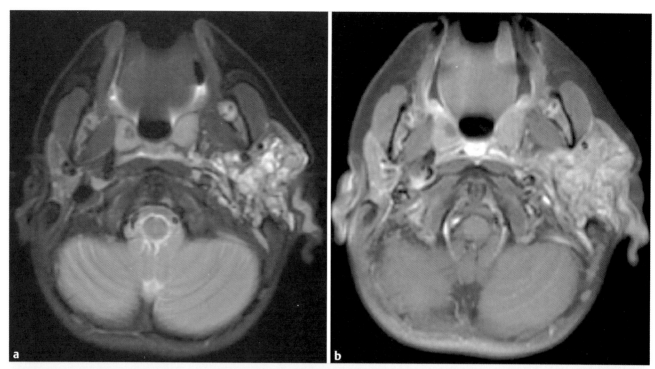

Fig. 201.1 Axial T2 image **(a)** reveals an ill-defined mass with mixed but predominantly hyperintense signal intensity extending from the superficial soft tissues overlying the left parotid gland to the deep parapharyngeal space. Avid enhancement is seen on the T1 postcontrast image with fat suppression **(b).**

■ Clinical Presentation

An adolescent boy with increased neck swelling (▸ Fig. 201.1)

Key Imaging Finding

Enhancing, infiltrating neck mass in an adolescent

Top 3 Differential Diagnoses

- **Venolymphatic malformation.** Venolymphatic malformations represent a spectrum of venous and lymphatic developmental abnormalities. Pure venous malformations avidly enhance and contain flow voids on T2 magnetic resonance imaging (MRI); the presence of phleboliths is pathognomonic. Pure lymphatic malformations may be unilocular or multilocular and demonstrate fluid attenuation and signal intensity. Fluid-fluid levels, most often due to hemorrhage, are characteristic. Peripheral and septal enhancement, which may extend into surrounding soft tissues, is more pronounced with superimposed infection. Many cases demonstrate characteristics of both. Venolymphatic malformations often cross fascial planes to involve multiple spaces of the neck.
- **Plexiform neurofibroma.** Plexiform neurofibromas are benign tumors that occur in ~5 to 15% of patients with neurofibromatosis type 1 (NF1). They may involve central or peripheral nerves and may be located anywhere in the body. They are often infiltrative with involvement of multiple spaces and compartments. Common locations in the head and neck region include the facial soft tissues, orbits, skull base, superficial and deep soft tissues of the neck, and within the cervical spine. The tumors are composed of multiple nerve fascicles and thickened

fibers with cellular proteinaceous matrix. Imaging reveals an ill-defined mass with heterogeneous, mixed T2 signal intensity and heterogeneous enhancement. The "target" sign, referred to as central regions of decreased and peripheral regions of increased T2 signal intensity, is often seen in association with neurofibromas. Approximately 5 to 10% of plexiform neurofibromas may undergo malignant degeneration.
- **Rhabdomyosarcoma.** Rhabdomyosarcoma is the most common soft-tissue sarcoma in children and adolescents. It arises from skeletal musculature within the head and neck. Common locations include the orbits, sinonasal cavities, and superficial and deep soft tissues of the neck. Lesions near the skull base may extend intracranially through skull-base foramina. Computed tomography and MRI are the preferred modalities to evaluate the size and extent of the tumor. Both may show an ill-defined and often infiltrative solid mass that may cross fascial planes. Enhancement of solid components is typically heterogeneous. Central necrosis or hemorrhage is common and results in a more heterogeneous appearance. When adjacent to bony structures, osseous erosion and destruction is often seen.

Additional Differential Diagnoses

- **Infection/inflammatory process.** Infections of the head and neck are common and may be localized or involve multiple spaces and compartments. Common etiologies include tonsillitis, pharyngitis, cellulitis, and lymphadenitis; infection as a sequela of trauma or surgery is less common. Patients often present with localized pain and swelling, fever, and elevated white blood cell count. Reactive lymphadenopathy is typically seen and may demonstrate central necrosis in the presence of atypical infections (*Mycobacterium* and *Bartonella* subspecies). Early in the infectious process, imaging reveals edematous inflammatory changes with fatty infiltration.

Superficial processes demonstrate overlying skin and fascial thickening. Enhancement, when present, is ill defined. As the infectious process becomes more organized, phlegmon develops with ill-defined regions of enhancement that may be peripheral but do not demonstrate complete rim enhancement around the central infectious process. With subsequent abscess formation, there is central fluid attenuation or signal intensity with complete rim enhancement. The presence of complete rim enhancement on imaging, however, is not entirely specific, as approximately 25% of cases will not have a drainable fluid collection at the time of intervention.

Diagnosis

Venolymphatic malformation

✓ Pearls

- Venolymphatic malformations often contain vascular and cystic components; phleboliths are pathognomonic.
- Plexiform neurofibromas are benign tumors which occur in ~5 to 15% of patients with NF1.
- Rhabdomyosarcoma arises from skeletal musculature and is the most common soft-tissue sarcoma in children.
- Infections of the neck are common and may be localized or involve multiple spaces and compartments.

Suggested Reading

Meuwly JY, Lepori D, Theumann N et al. Multimodality imaging evaluation of the pediatric neck: techniques and spectrum of findings. Radiographics 2005; 25: 931–948

Case 202

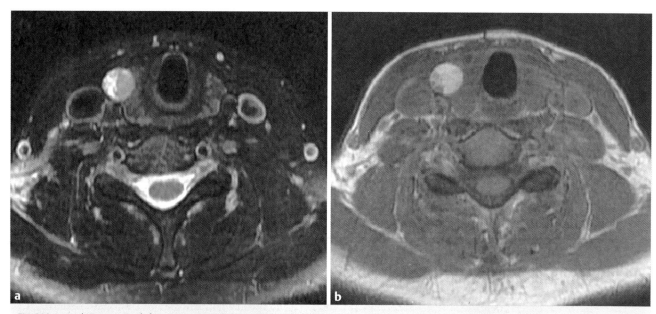

Fig. 202.1 Axial T2 image with fat suppression **(a)** demonstrates a circumscribed mass with heterogeneous increased signal intensity along the lateral aspect of the right thyroid lobe. The medial portion of the mass is hyperintense on unenhanced T1 sequences **(b)**, whereas the lateral aspect is hypointense.

■ Clinical Presentation

A middle-aged woman with chronic neck pain (► Fig. 202.1)

▨ Key Imaging Finding

Thyroid lesion

■ Top 3 Differential Diagnoses

- **Thyroid adenoma.** Benign thyroid adenomas are exceedingly common, representing roughly 75% of all thyroid nodules. They are often multiple and bilateral. The classic appearance on ultrasound (US) consists of a peripheral hypoechoic halo surrounding a circumscribed nodule. The nodule itself may have internal coarse calcifications or cystic changes. Lesions are hypodense on computed tomography (CT); on magnetic resonance imaging (MRI), they are typically T1 hypointense and T2 hyperintense. Thyroid adenomas may be hot or cold on technetium 99 m or iodine I 123 scans; malignant lesions are typically cold.
- **Differentiated thyroid carcinoma.** Differentiated thyroid carcinoma consists of papillary and follicular. Papillary carcinoma is the most common thyroid cancer, representing ~80% of cases. Its classic appearance on US consists of a thyroid lesion with numerous microcalcifications and/or cystic changes. Regional lymph node spread is often seen and commonly demonstrates cystic/necrotic lymph node enlargement with or without calcifications. Follicular carcinoma is less common but carries a worse prognosis due to the propensity for distant metastases. Its imaging appearance is less characteristic and often non-specific. In the absence of cystic change, microcalcifications, extracapsular spread, or regional lymph node spread, differentiated carcinoma may be indistinguishable from thyroid adenomas on imaging. Treatment includes thyroidectomy with I 131 ablation.
- **Colloid cyst.** Colloid cysts are benign thyroid lesions that are thought to result from cystic degeneration of adenomas. The presence of gelatinous colloid results in a characteristic US appearance, consisting of a cystic thyroid mass with internal hyperechoic foci and "comet tail" artifact. Its appearance on CT and MRI varies based upon its protein concentration. Most lesions are hypodense on CT and hyperintense on T2 MRI sequences. As the protein concentration increases, its density on CT and signal intensity on T1 MRI sequences also increases.

■ Additional Differential Diagnoses

- **Undifferentiated thyroid carcinoma.** Undifferentiated thyroid carcinomas are aggressive tumors and include medullary and anaplastic carcinomas. Medullary carcinoma is a neuroendocrine tumor that most commonly occurs in middle-aged patients. It may occur sporadically or in association with multiple endocrine neoplasia type 2. The primary lesion on US is hypervascular and may demonstrate microcalcifications. The majority of patients have metastatic lymphadenopathy at the time of diagnosis. Positron emission tomography and octreoscan imaging are useful for characterization of the tumor and post-treatment surveillance. Anaplastic thyroid carcinoma is an extremely aggressive tumor that is most common in elderly women. In many cases, patients have underlying multinodular goiter. Its imaging appearance is often aggressive, demonstrating a large, ill-defined mass with or without calcifications or central necrosis. Heterogeneous enhancement is noted on CT and MRI. The mass typically metastasizes to local lymph nodes and invades adjacent structures. Prognosis is dismal.
- **Parathyroid adenoma.** Parathyroid adenomas represent benign functioning tumors and are the most common cause of primary hyperparathyroidism. Although they may occur anywhere along the tract of developmental parathyroid descent and occasionally within the mediastinum, they are most commonly located along the posteroinferior margin of the thyroid gland. Preoperative localization is performed to identify the lesions and rule out the presence of multiple adenomas. On US, lesions are typically circumscribed, hypoechoic, and vascular. MRI reveals characteristic T2 hyperintensity. Heterogeneous enhancement is seen on both CT and MRI. Nuclear medicine sestamibi scans are useful in identifying parathyroid adenomas as foci of increased activity on delayed imaging. Treatment includes surgical resection.

■ Diagnosis

Colloid cyst

✓ Pearls

- Benign thyroid adenomas are exceedingly common; they are often multiple and bilateral.
- Differentiated thyroid carcinoma includes papillary (most common, cystic, microcalcifications) and follicular.
- Undifferentiated thyroid carcinomas are aggressive tumors and include medullary and anaplastic.
- Colloid cysts have a characteristic US appearance with internal hyperechoic foci and "comet tail" artifact.

Suggested Reading

Hoang JK, Lee WK, Lee M, Johnson D, Farrell S. US Features of thyroid malignancy: pearls and pitfalls. Radiographics 2007; 27: 847–860, discussion 861–865

Case 203

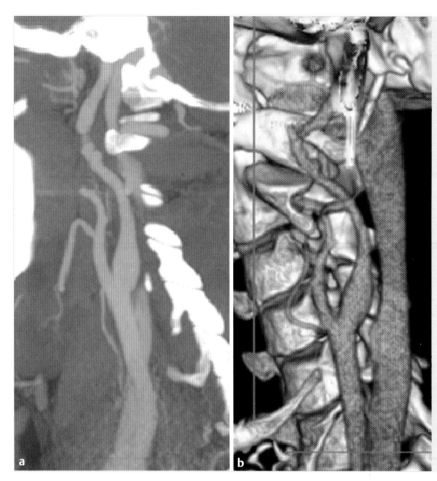

Fig. 203.1 Oblique sagittal maximum intensity projection **(a)** and three-dimensional volume rendered **(b)** images from a CTA demonstrate alternating regions of stenosis and dilatation involving the right ICA with a "string of beads" appearance, as well as a focal region of high-grade stenosis. (Courtesy of Richard Latchaw, MD.)

▓ Clinical Presentation

A 42-year-old woman with a history of transient ischemic attacks (▶ Fig. 203.1)

▨ Key Imaging Finding

Carotid artery stenosis

■ Top 3 Differential Diagnoses

- **Atherosclerosis.** Atherosclerosis is the most common cause of carotid artery stenosis. It typically occurs in older individuals and is more advanced in patients with a smoking history, hypertension, hyperlipidemia, and diabetes. The carotid bifurcation and proximal internal carotid artery (ICA) are the most common sites involved, followed by the parasellar ICAs. Doppler ultrasound is the initial screening study for the cervical carotid arteries. Typical findings include visualization of plaque with vessel stenosis, elevated velocities, and turbulent flow with aliasing. Magnetic resonance angiography (MRA) and computed tomography angiography (CTA) are used as confirmatory studies. Carotid endarterectomy (CEA) remains the treatment of choice in low-risk surgical candidates. Current guidelines recommend CEA for symptomatic lesions with > 50% stenosis (data from the NASCET trial) or asymptomatic lesions with > 60% stenosis (data from the ACAS trial). Although many recent trials have shown a benefit of endovascular carotid stent placement with distal embolic protection devices in many patient populations, current guidelines recommend this treatment only for high-risk surgical patients with symptomatic lesions of ≥ 70% stenosis. High-risk surgical patients are defined as follows: clinically significant cardiac disease, severe pulmonary disease (if general anesthesia will be used), recurrent stenosis after prior CEA, prior neck surgery or irradiation, contralateral recurrent laryngeal nerve paralysis,

contralateral carotid artery occlusion, and surgically inaccessible lesions.
- **Fibromuscular dysplasia (FMD).** FMD is a dysplastic vascular disease that primarily affects young women. The renal arteries are most commonly involved, followed by the carotid arteries. The medial fibroplasia variant is the most common subtype and presents with the classic "string of beads" appearance on imaging (CTA, MRA, digital subtraction angiography [DSA]) due to alternating regions of stenosis and dilatation. The disease results in vascular stenosis and subsequent hypertension (renal artery involvement) or stroke (ICA involvement). Patients are at increased risk for aneurysm formation and dissections. Symptomatic lesions are treated with angioplasty.
- **Dissection.** Carotid artery dissection may result from trauma, hypertension, iatrogenia, or vasculopathies such as FMD. Common imaging findings include an intramural hematoma and intimal flap. On unenhanced CT, acute dissections present with crescent-shaped increased density within the arterial wall. Unenhanced T1 sequences with fat suppression show a peripheral hyperintense intramural hematoma. DSA findings include luminal irregularity, tapered stenosis or occlusion, a double lumen, or an intimal flap. Some dissections may be managed medically with anticoagulation therapy and follow-up imaging to ensure stability or resolution. Symptomatic lesions or lesions that progress despite medical management often require intervention, including stent placement.

▨ Additional Differential Diagnoses

- **Iatrogenic.** The most common iatrogenic causes of carotid stenosis include clamp injury during surgical procedures or vasculitis secondary to radiation therapy for head and neck

cancer. Treatment depends upon symptoms and morphology of the lesions with endovascular therapy (angioplasty or stent placement) favored over surgical intervention.

■ Diagnosis

Fibromuscular dysplasia

✓ Pearls

- Atherosclerosis is the most common cause of carotid artery stenosis; it typically occurs in older individuals.
- Carotid stents are indicated for symptomatic lesions of ≥ 70% stenosis in high-risk surgical patients.

- FMD primarily affects young women; angioplasty is the primary treatment option for symptomatic lesions.
- Most dissections are due to hypertension or trauma; treatment depends upon morphology and symptoms.

Suggested Readings

Executive committee for the asymptomatic carotid atherosclerosis study (ACAS). Endarterectomy for asymptomatic carotid artery stenosis. JAMA 1995; 273: 1421–1428

Gurm HS, Yadav JS, Fayad P et al. SAPPHIRE Investigators. Long-term results of carotid stenting versus endarterectomy in high-risk patients. N Engl J Med 2008; 358: 1572–1579

North American Symptomatic Carotid Endarterectomy Trial Collaborators. Beneficial effect of carotid endarterectomy in symptomatic patients with high-grade carotid stenosis. N Engl J Med 1991; 325: 445–453

Roffi M, Yadav JS. Carotid stenting. Circulation 2006; 114: e1–e4

Case 204

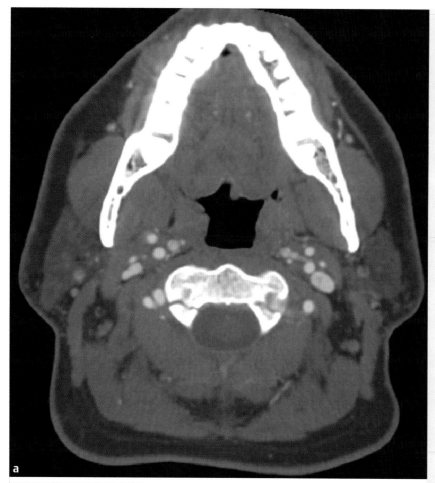

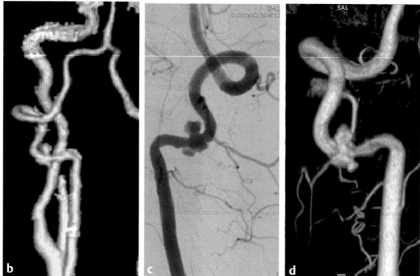

Fig. 204.1 Contrast-enhanced axial CT image from a neck CTA at the skull base **(a)** demonstrates a vertebral fracture through the left foramen transversarium with an ovoid area of opacification adjacent to the right vertebral artery. Reformatted three-dimensional (3-D) CTA **(b)**, conventional angiographic **(c)**, and 3-D volume rendered angiographic **(d)** images depict a multilobular outpouching along the distal cervical right vertebral artery. (Case courtesy of Adam J. Zuckerman, DO.)

■ Clinical Presentation

A 36-year-old cyclist with neck pain following a collision (▶ Fig. 204.1)

■ Key Imaging Finding

Vascular neck injury

■ Top 3 Differential Diagnoses

- **Dissection.** Arterial dissections are the result of intimal injury. They most commonly involve the cervical internal carotid and vertebral arteries; vertebral injury is most common in the V_3 segment near the skull base where the vessel is most mobile. Early dissection can often present with complete occlusion of the vessel lumen preceded by a segment of tapered narrowing. Classic angiographic findings include the presence of an intimal flap or irregular segmental luminal narrowing. Computed tomography (CT) angiography reveals eccentric luminal narrowing with relative enlargement of the cross-sectional area of the affected artery compared with contralateral side secondary to thickening from mural hematoma. Axial fat-suppressed T1 magnetic resonance imaging (MRI) demonstrates an eccentric, crescentic periarterial rim of signal abnormality along the margin of a flow void. Dissections can be complicated by pseudoaneurysm, thromboembolic, or occlusive phenomena. First-line treatment involves anticoagulation with refractory cases necessitating endovascular or surgical intervention.
- **Pseudoaneurysm.** Pseudoaneurysms are typically due to penetrating or blunt trauma and are frequently associated with arterial dissection. They can also be due to infectious or iatrogenic causes. Pseudoaneurysms are commonly ovoid in appearance and located at the distal aspect of a stenotic segment. Doppler ultrasound of a pseudoaneurysm may demonstrate the classic "to and fro" appearance. Management is dependent upon size, location, and etiology. Patients are at risk for expansion of the lesion with compression of adjacent structures and possible rupture. They are also prone to thrombus formation with distant emboli. Treatment options include surgical resection/reconstruction or endovascular stent placement with or without coil embolization of the pseudoaneurysm.
- **Vascular occlusion.** Complete or partial vascular occlusion commonly occurs in association with blunt or penetrating neck injuries. Vascular imaging with CT or conventional angiography demonstrates decreased or absent opacification of the involved vascular structures with or without other associated vascular injuries, including an underlying dissection or intramural hematoma.

■ Additional Differential Diagnoses

- **Arteriovenous fistula (AVF).** AVFs are usually the result of a penetrating neck injury with partial transection of an artery and adjacent vein. AVFs may also occur spontaneously or be the result of blunt trauma with cervical spine fracture, infection, or iatrogenia. Patients often present with a neck bruit or ischemic symptoms; however, up to 30% of cases may be asymptomatic. AVFs can be diagnosed angiographically with early venous filling during the arterial phase. CT and MRI provide additional detail on the relationship of an AVF to surrounding structures. Endovascular treatment aims to close the fistula while preserving flow in the parent artery.

■ Diagnosis

Pseudoaneurysm of the right vertebral artery

✓ Pearls

- Dissections result from intimal injury; common findings include an intramural hematoma and intimal flap.
- Pseudoaneurysms commonly result from traumatic injuries; they are at risk of expansion and rupture.
- Complete or partial vascular occlusion commonly occurs in association with blunt or penetrating neck injuries.
- AVFs are direct communications between an artery and vein, typically due to penetrating injuries.

Suggested Reading

Núñez DB, Jr, Torres-León M, Múnera F. Vascular injuries of the neck and thoracic inlet: helical CT-angiographic correlation. Radiographics 2004; 24: 1087–1098, discussion 1099–1100

Case 205

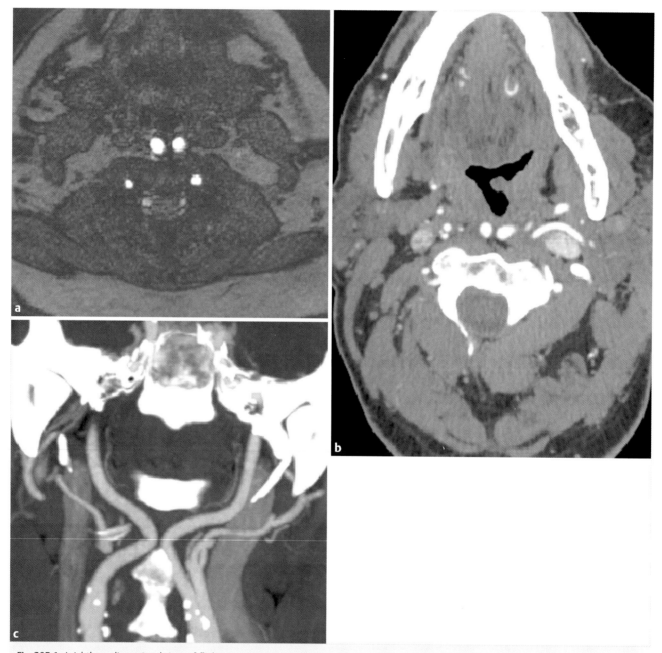

Fig. 205.1 Axial three-dimensional time-of-flight magnetic resonance **(a)**, axial computed tomography angiography (CTA) **(b)**, and coronal reformatted maximum intensity projection CTA **(c)** images demonstrate medial deviation of the cervical internal carotid arteries, which closely approximate at the midline and indent the posterolateral aerodigestive tract. Eccentric calcifications are seen within the carotid vasculature **(c)**, consistent with atherosclerotic disease. (Courtesy of Michael Zapadka, DO.)

■ Clinical Presentation

A 64-year-old woman referred for a vascular workup (▶ Fig. 205.1)

■ Key Imaging Finding

Medial deviation of the carotid arteries along the posterior aspect of the aerodigestive tract

■ Diagnosis

Medialization/"kissing" carotid arteries. The cervical portions of the carotid arteries are commonly tortuous, especially in older adults with hypertension and atherosclerotic disease. This tortuosity can result in medial deviation of the carotid artery into the retropharyngeal space along the posterior aspect of the aerodigestive tract, simulating a pathological, pulsatile, submucosal mass. When this occurs below the hyoid bone, it involves the common carotid artery; when this occurs above the hyoid bone, it involves the internal carotid artery. Deviation is most often unilateral or bilateral but asymmetric. Bilateral medial deviation with close approximation of the carotid

arteries in the midline retropharyngeal space is referred to as "kissing" carotid arteries.

Medial deviation of the carotid arteries is often asymptomatic and found incidentally. Occasionally, however, patients may experience a globus sensation or possibly symptoms related to airway narrowing. Indentation of the aerodigestive tract may mimic a submucosal mass on clinical inspection. Cross-sectional imaging easily identifies and classifies the abnormality as carotid in origin, preventing inadvertent biopsy, which would be catastrophic.

✓ Pearls

- Tortuosity of the carotid arteries can result in medial deviation into the retropharyngeal space.
- Bilateral medial deviation is referred to as "kissing" carotid arteries due to their close approximation.

- Indentation of the aerodigestive tract may mimic a submucosal mass on clinical inspection.
- Cross-sectional imaging easily identifies the carotid origin, preventing inadvertent and catastrophic biopsy.

Suggested Reading

Muñoz A, De Vergas J, Crespo J. Imaging and clinical findings in patients with aberrant course of the cervical internal carotid arteries. Open Neuroimaging J 2010; 4: 174–181

Case 206

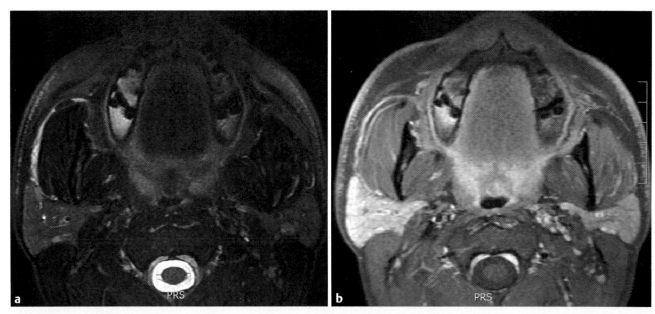

Fig. 206.1 Axial high-resolution T2 image with fat suppression **(a)** reveals asymmetric enlargement of the right parotid gland with mild increased signal intensity compared with the left. There is also dilatation and increased signal within Stenson duct on the right with an ovoid hypointense filling defect distally. Axial postcontrast T1 image with fat suppression **(b)** demonstrates asymmetric enlargement and increased enhancement of the right parotid gland, as well as dilatation of Stenson duct with surrounding inflammatory enhancement.

■ Clinical Presentation

A young adult woman with facial pain that is exasperated by eating (► Fig. 206.1)

■ Key Imaging Finding

Parotid gland enlargement with increased signal intensity and enhancement

■ Diagnosis

Parotitis (due to ductal obstruction by stone). Parotitis refers to inflammation of the parotid gland; it may be unilateral or bilateral depending upon the underlying etiology. Common causes include infection, ductal obstruction, and autoimmune or granulomatous processes. Rarely, parotitis may be a chronic or recurrent process with an unknown etiology.

Infectious etiologies may be bacterial or viral (e.g., mumps) and are more often bilateral. Human immunodeficiency virus parotitis results in characteristic bilateral lymphoepithelial lesions. Ductal obstruction is most often the result of sialolithiasis (stones); less common sources of obstruction include traumatic injury to Stenson duct or an obstructing neoplasm. Obstructive processes are typically unilateral. Autoimmune etiologies include Sjögren syndrome, which results in bilateral solid nodules and fluid pockets. Sarcoidosis is a granulomatous disease that commonly involves the parotid and lacrimal glands.

Clinically, patients with parotitis present with localized swelling overlying the parotid gland(s). In the case of an obstructing process, there is typically pain that is exasperated by eating. Treatment is directed toward the underlying etiology.

On imaging, parotitis presents with diffuse gland enlargement and avid enhancement. On computed tomography (CT), the gland is hypodense due to edema; on magnetic resonance imaging, there is associated increased T2 signal intensity. With an obstructing process, Stenson duct will be dilated proximal to the level of obstruction with surrounding inflammation and enhancement. Sialolithiasis is best evaluated on CT because the vast majority are calcified. Occasionally, sialography may be needed to evaluate the duct. Chronic parotitis, in contrast, typically demonstrates an atrophic gland with intraglandular calcifications.

✓ Pearls

- Parotitis refers to inflammation of the parotid gland; it may be unilateral or bilateral depending upon the cause.
- Acute parotitis presents with diffuse gland enlargement, abnormal density/signal, and enhancement.

- Chronic parotitis typically demonstrates an atrophic gland with intraglandular calcifications.
- With obstructing processes, Stenson duct will be dilated with surrounding inflammation and enhancement.

Suggested Reading

Yousem DM, Kraut MA, Chalian AA. Major salivary gland imaging. Radiology 2000; 216: 19–29

Case 207

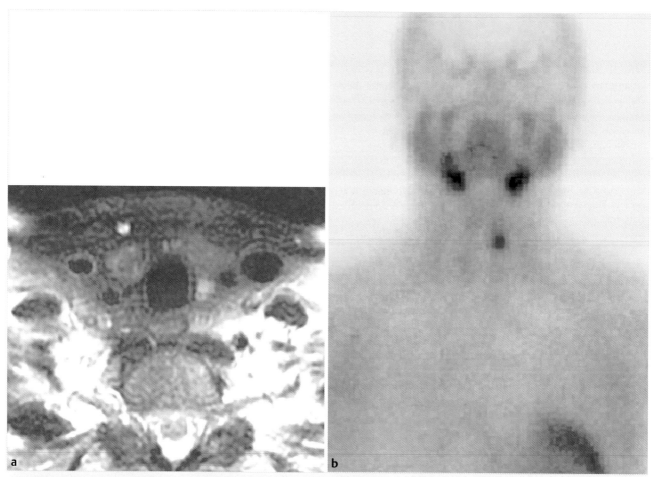

Fig. 207.1 Axial T2 image with fat suppression **(a)** reveals a hyperintense lesion along the posterior aspect of the left thyroid lobe. Delayed image from a Tc99 m sestamibi scan **(b)** in a different patient with the same diagnosis reveals a region of increased activity on the left with clearance of radiotracer from the surrounding thyroid gland. (Image B courtesy of Kamal Singh, MD.)

■ Clinical Presentation

An adult woman with abnormal laboratory result (▶ Fig. 207.1)

■ Key Imaging Finding

Lesion with increased activity along the posterior aspect of the thyroid gland

■ Diagnosis

Parathyroid adenoma. The parathyroid glands regulate serum calcium concentrations through the production of parathormone (PTH). Parathormone causes increased serum calcium by reabsorbing calcium from bones via osteoclasts, increasing renal calcium resorption, and decreasing renal phosphate resorption. PTH also increases vitamin D production, which in turn increases gastrointestinal tract calcium absorption. Hyperparathyroidism (HPT) is caused by inappropriate elevation of PTH and subsequent increased serum calcium concentrations. It is most often due to a primary hyperfunctioning adenoma; parathyroid hyperplasia and carcinoma are less common causes. Common presenting symptoms include fatigue, psychosis, and depression ("moans"); abdominal pains ("groans"); renal calculi ("stones"); and bony pain or pathological fractures ("bones").

Most individuals have paired superior and inferior parathyroid glands that are situated along the posterior margin of the thyroid gland. They commonly measure 5 mm in maximal dimension; adenomas are typically larger. Ectopic parathyroid glands may occur anywhere from a location just superior to the thyroid gland to the mediastinum. Identifying the site of a parathyroid adenoma and excluding an ectopic location are important factors in preoperative imaging.

Parathyroid imaging often consists of a combination of ultrasound (US), magnetic resonance imaging (MRI), and technetium 99 m (Tc99m) sestamibi scintigraphy. Using multiple modalities increases the overall sensitivity and specificity in detecting and localizing parathyroid adenomas. On US, parathyroid adenomas appear as circumscribed, homogeneously hypoechoic masses deep to the thyroid gland. There is internal flow that is more pronounced along its periphery, which is fairly characteristic. Evaluation for an ectopic adenoma is limited. On MRI, parathyroid adenomas are most often iso- to hypointense on T1 and hyperintense on T2 sequences. The enhancement pattern is variable, although most adenomas will show some enhancement. As with US, evaluation for an ectopic adenoma is limited because cervical lymph nodes may mimic the appearance of an adenoma on MRI.

Tc99 m sestamibi scintigraphy is the most common modality for identifying parathyroid adenomas. Both thyroid and parathyroid glands demonstrate normal physiological uptake of sestamibi; however, adenomas demonstrate increased and prolonged uptake of the radiopharmaceutical, allowing for their detection, especially on delayed imaging. The addition of single-photon emission computed tomography imaging on delayed sequences further increases the sensitivity and specificity. Scintigraphy is superior in the detection of ectopic adenomas, especially when located in the mediastinum.

✓ Pearls

- HPT causes increased serum calcium concentrations; patients present with "moans, groans, stones, and bones."
- Multimodality preoperative imaging increases sensitivity and specificity for parathyroid adenoma detection.

- Adenomas are homogeneously hypoechoic with peripheral vascular flow on US and T2 hyperintense on MRI.
- On Tc99 m sestamibi scintigraphy parathyroid adenomas demonstrate increased and prolonged tracer uptake.

Suggested Reading

Johnson NA, Tublin ME, Ogilvie JB. Parathyroid imaging: technique and role in the preoperative evaluation of primary hyperparathyroidism. Am J Roentgenol 2007; 188: 1706–1715

Case 208

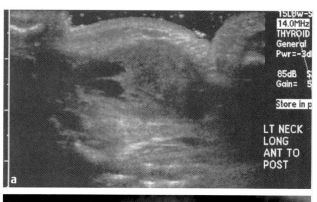

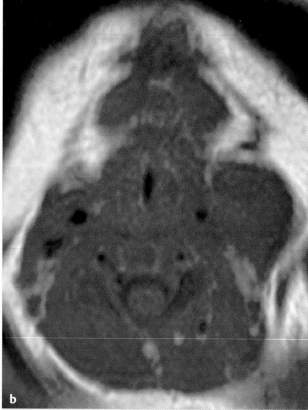

Fig. 208.1 Longitudinal gray-scale US image **(a)** of the left neck reveals a well-marginated mass that is isointense to musculature but slightly heterogeneous. Axial T1 MR image **(b)** demonstrates fusiform enlargement of the left SCM muscle, corresponding to the US abnormality.

■ **Clinical Presentation**

A 2-month-old boy with a difficult delivery and progressive torticollis (▶ Fig. 208.1)

■ Key Imaging Finding

Enlargement of the sternocleidomastoid (SCM) muscle in a child with torticollis

■ Diagnosis

Fibromatosis colli. Fibromatosis colli is a rare disorder characterized by isolated fibromatosis involving the SCM muscle. It is typically undetectable at birth but progresses over the first few weeks or months of life. Although the exact etiology remains unclear, a history of birth trauma or a difficult delivery is found in > 90% of cases. Most patients are asymptomatic and may present with a localized neck mass; ~20% of patients present with torticollis involving the affected side.

Ultrasound (US) is the initial modality of choice and is often diagnostic. Most cases reveal a homogeneously enlarged SCM muscle. Less common findings include a focal, well-defined or ill-defined hypoechoic mass within the SCM muscle. The typical computed tomography appearance consists of homogeneous enlargement of the SCM muscle without a focal mass or attenuation abnormality. Magnetic resonance imaging (MRI) demonstrates similar findings with iso- to hypointense T1 and iso- to slightly hyperintense T2 signal intensity within the SCM.

✓ Pearls

- Fibromatosis colli is a rare disorder characterized by isolated fibromatosis involving the SCM muscle.
- Most cases are asymptomatic with or without a localized neck mass; approximately 20% of patients present with torticollis.

- US is the modality of choice and is often diagnostic; most cases show a homogeneously enlarged SCM muscle.
- MRI demonstrates similar SCM enlargement with iso- to slightly hyperintense T2 signal intensity.

Suggested Reading

Robbin MR, Murphey MD, Temple HT, Kransdorf MJ, Choi JJ. Imaging of musculo-skeletal fibromatosis. Radiographics 2001; 21: 585–600

Case 209

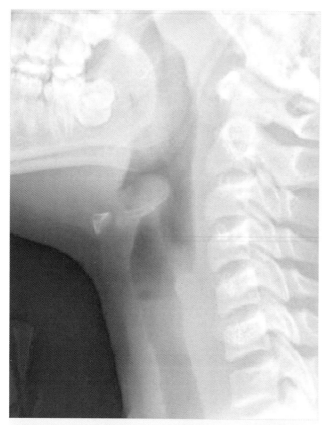

Fig. 209.1 Lateral plain film view of the soft tissues of the neck demonstrates enlargement of the epiglottis with a "thumbprint" appearance. Prevertebral soft tissues are normal in thickness.

▨ Clinical Presentation

A 12-year-old girl with a sore throat and difficulty swallowing (▶ Fig. 209.1)

■ Key Imaging Finding

Epiglottic enlargement

■ Diagnosis

Epiglottitis. Epiglottitis is an acute-onset, progressive supraglottic infection that may lead to life-threatening airway obstruction. It is more common in children than adults and its incidence has drastically decreased secondary to widespread administration of the *Haemophilus influenza* type b vaccine.

Epiglottitis is usually suspected clinically and may be confirmed with direct visualization under monitored conditions and with personnel trained in airway management. Lateral radiographs of the soft tissues of the neck show characteristic enlargement of the epiglottis with a classic "thumbprint" appearance. Clinical mimics include peritonsillar or retropharyngeal abscesses, which may be distinguished on plain films or computed tomography. It is important to remember that a negative radiograph does not entirely exclude the diagnosis of epiglottitis if there is a high clinical suspicion because findings may be subtle, especially when imaged early.

Treatment consists of broad-spectrum antibiotics and airway monitoring and management.

✓ Pearls

- Epiglottitis is a rapidly progressive supraglottic infection that may lead to life-threatening airway obstruction.
- Lateral radiographs of the neck show characteristic "thumbprint" enlargement of the epiglottis.
- Clinical mimics include peritonsillar or retropharyngeal abscesses, which may be differentiated on imaging.

Suggested Reading

O'Brien WT, Sr, Lattin GE, Jr. "My airway is closing". J Fam Pract 2005; 54: 423–425

Case 210

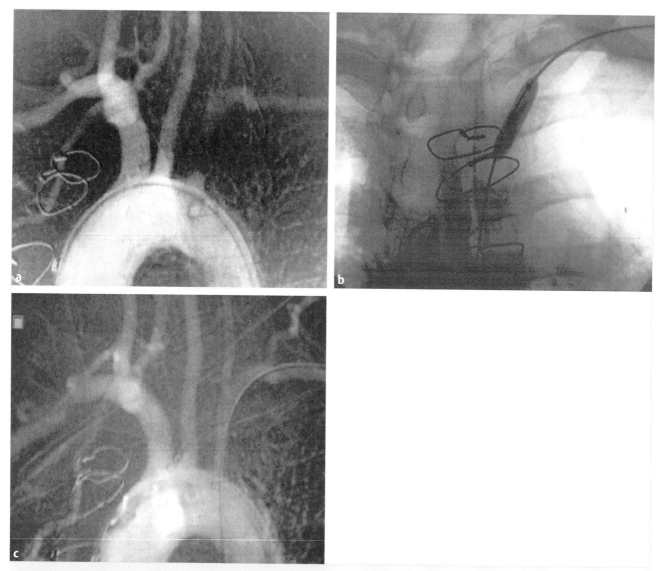

Fig. 210.1 Aortic arch digital subtraction angiogram **(a)** demonstrates cutoff of the proximal left subclavian artery with delayed filling of the distal left subclavian artery via retrograde flow through the vertebral artery. Balloon angioplasty of the left subclavian artery occlusion was performed **(b)** with satisfactory angiographic result **(c).** (Courtesy of David D. Gover, MD.)

■ Clinical Presentation

A 60-year-old man experiencing dizziness and ataxia with exercise (▶ Fig. 210.1)

■ Key Imaging Finding

Subclavian artery occlusion with retrograde filling distally via the ipsilateral vertebral artery

■ Diagnosis

Subclavian steal. Subclavian steal is a phenomenon that occurs secondary to subclavian artery stenosis or occlusion proximal to the origin of the vertebral artery. The distal subclavian arterial supply comes from retrograde filling via the ipsilateral vertebral artery. Subclavian steal most commonly occurs secondary to atherosclerotic disease in elderly men, although congenital and additional acquired etiologies exist. The clinical presentation is variable; patients may be asymptomatic, have decreased blood pressure or a weak pulse in the affected arm, or experience vertebrobasilar insufficiency, often associated with exercise of the upper extremity.

Conventional angiography shows cutoff or stenosis of the subclavian artery with lack of antegrade opacification within the ipsilateral vertebral artery in the early arterial phase, followed by delayed retrograde filling of the distal subclavian artery via the vertebral artery. Computed tomography angiography (CTA), two-dimensional time-of-flight magnetic resonance angiography (MRA), and contrast-enhanced MRA will demonstrate the region of stenosis or occlusion, but will not identify flow reversal in the vertebral artery, as they are not sensitive to direction of flow. Phase-contrast MRA, however, is sensitive to flow direction and will demonstrate flow reversal in the ipsilateral vertebral artery. Duplex ultrasound of the ipsilateral vertebral artery may show complete reversal of flow, although diminished peak systolic velocities are an early sign. Additionally, markedly increased contralateral vertebral artery peak systolic flow or a parvus-tardus waveform in the peripheral ipsilateral subclavian artery are secondary findings, especially if identified or exacerbated following exercise of the upper extremity.

Treatment options include endovascular balloon angioplasty with possible stent placement and surgery. Surgical options include a common carotid or innominate artery to subclavian artery bypass, depending upon the anatomic location of the lesion.

✓ Pearls

- Subclavian steal is characterized by proximal stenosis/occlusion and distal filling via the vertebral artery.
- Patients commonly present with vertebrobasilar insufficiency when exercising the affected arm.
- Phase-contrast MR imaging will show flow reversal within the ipsilateral vertebral arterial.
- Treatment options include angioplasty with possible stent placement versus surgical bypass procedures.

Suggested Readings

Henry M, Amor M, Henry I, Ethevenot G, Tzvetanov K, Chati Z. Percutaneous transluminal angioplasty of the subclavian arteries. J Endovasc Surg 1999; 6: 33–41

Kliewer MA, Hertzberg BS, Kim DH, Bowie JD, Courneya DL, Carroll BA. Vertebral artery Doppler waveform changes indicating subclavian steal physiology. Am J Roentgenol 2000; 174: 815–819

Sueoka BL. Percutaneous transluminal stent placement to treat subclavian steal syndrome. J Vasc Interv Radiol 1996; 7: 351–356

Case 211

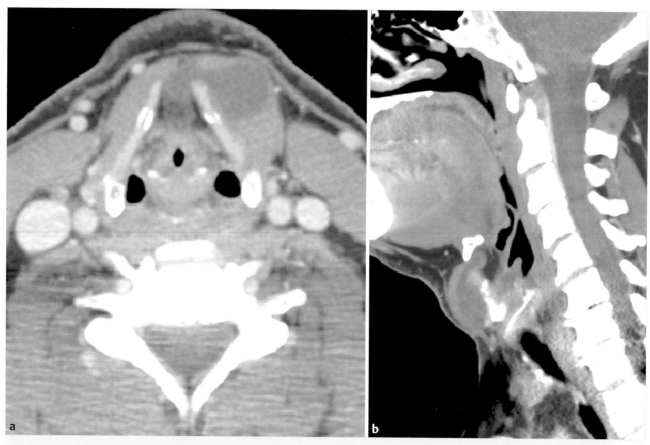

Fig. 211.1 Axial **(a)** and reformatted sagittal **(b)** contrast-enhanced computed tomography images reveal a nonenhancing fluid attenuation mass along the undersurface of the hyoid bone and embedded within the strap muscles on the left. Portions of the mass are midline **(b)** and off-midline to the left **(a)**.

■ Clinical Presentation

A 49-year-old man with a slowly growing neck mass (▶ Fig. 211.1)

■ Key Imaging Finding

Cystic neck mass embedded within strap muscles

■ Diagnosis

Thyroglossal duct cyst (TGDC). The thyroid gland originally develops at the level of the foramen cecum along the floor of the primitive pharynx and descends to its normal position in the lower neck. Its migration path extends from the foramen cecum and passes anterior to and through the hyoid bone and strap muscles, as well as anterior to the laryngeal cartilage and thyroid membrane. The thyroglossal duct exists as a normal structure during thyroid descent, maintaining a connection between the gland and the foramen cecum. It typically involutes toward the end of the first trimester of development. Should any portion of the duct persist, it may result in development of a TGDC.

TGDCs represent the most common congenital neck masses and most often present in children and young adults. Approximately 75% of cases occur at or below the hyoid bone with the remainder being suprahyoid in location. Eighty-five percent are midline in location, whereas 15% of cases are slightly off-midline. They may be discovered incidentally or present as an enlarging neck mass. Oftentimes, superimposed infection results in growth and inflammation of the cyst with subsequent clinical presentation.

On imaging, TGDCs present as midline or slightly off-midline cystic masses. The majority occur at or below the hyoid bone and are often characteristically embedded in the strap muscles. Suprahyoid TGDCs occur anywhere from the foramen cecum/base or root of tongue to the hyoid bone. On ultrasound, the cysts are anechoic or hypoechoic with increased through-transmission. Heterogeneity, including internal debris, is noted with superimposed infection. Computed tomography demonstrates a well-circumscribed hypodense cystic mass extending along the path of craniocaudad descent. Enhancement, when present, is peripheral and increased with superimposed infection. Magnetic resonance imaging demonstrates similar findings with internal fluid signal intensity (decreased T1 and increased T2) and occasional peripheral enhancement. Increased proteinaceous content may result in increased T1 signal intensity.

Treatment includes surgical resection using the Sistrunk procedure. When using this technique, recurrence rates are low. Rarely (< 1% of cases), thyroid carcinoma may occur within a TGDC due to ectopic foci of thyroid tissue. The carcinoma is typically of the papillary subtype and is usually only discovered on pathological specimens. The presence of prospective imaging findings to suspect carcinoma within a TGDC is uncommon.

✓ Pearls

- TGDCs are the most common congenital neck masses; they most often present in children and young adults.
- Approximately 75% of TGDCs occur at or below the hyoid bone; 85% are midline with the remainder slightly off-midline.
- Cross-sectional imaging reveals a well-circumscribed cystic mass along the path of thyroid decent.
- Appearance is heterogeneous with superimposed infection, including internal debris and peripheral enhancement.

Suggested Reading

Koeller KK, Alamo L, Adair CF, Smirniotopoulos JG. Congenital cystic masses of the neck: radiologic-pathologic correlation. Radiographics 1999; 19: 121–146, quiz 152–153

Case 212

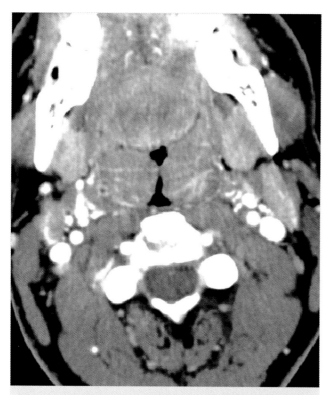

Fig. 212.1 Axial contrast-enhanced computed tomography image through the oropharynx reveals marked enlargement and apposition of the palatine tonsils with a striated or "tigroid" enhancement pattern. There is no focal fluid collection to suggest abscess.

▓ Clinical Presentation

A 26-year-old man with a sore throat and globus sensation (▶ Fig. 212.1)

■ Key Imaging Finding

Tonsillar enlargement with striated, "tigroid" enhancement

■ Diagnosis

Tonsillitis. Tonsillitis represents the most common infection of the deep neck structures among children, adolescents, and young adults. Patients often present with fever, sore throat, odynophagia, dysphagia, and otalgia. Early on, there is tonsillar enlargement with or without exudates. As the infection progresses, it may spread to the peritonsillar region with ensuing phlegmon and potential abscess formation. A peritonsillar abscess is far more common than an intratonsillar abscess. The most common inciting organisms are *Steptococcus* subspecies, *Staphylococcus aureus*, and *Haemophilus influenza*; polymicrobial etiology is common.

On imaging, tonsillitis demonstrates tonsillar enlargement and apposition, referred to as the "kissing tonsils." There is characteristic linear, striated, or "tigroid" enhancement. As the process spreads to the peritonsillar region, phlegmon may develop and present as relatively ill-defined regions of inflammatory changes with fat-stranding and variable degrees of enhancement. A peritonsillar abscess is suggested when there is complete rim enhancement; the presence of rim enhancement, however, is not pathognomonic for abscess formation because it has a specificity of ~75%.

Tonsillitis is treated with antibiotics and supportive care; abscesses require aspiration or surgical drainage.

✓ Pearls

- Tonsillitis is the most common infection of the deep neck structures in children, adolescents, and young adults.
- Tonsillitis reveals tonsillar enlargement, apposition ("kissing tonsils"), and striated or "tigroid" enhancement.

- Peritonsillar abscess is suggested with complete, rim enhancement, which has a specificity of 75%.
- Tonsillitis is treated with antibiotics and supportive care; abscesses require aspiration or surgical drainage.

Suggested Reading

Capps EF, Kinsella JJ, Gupta M, Bhatki AM, Opatowsky MJ. Emergency imaging assessment of acute, nontraumatic conditions of the head and neck. Radiographics 2010; 30: 1335–1352

Case 213

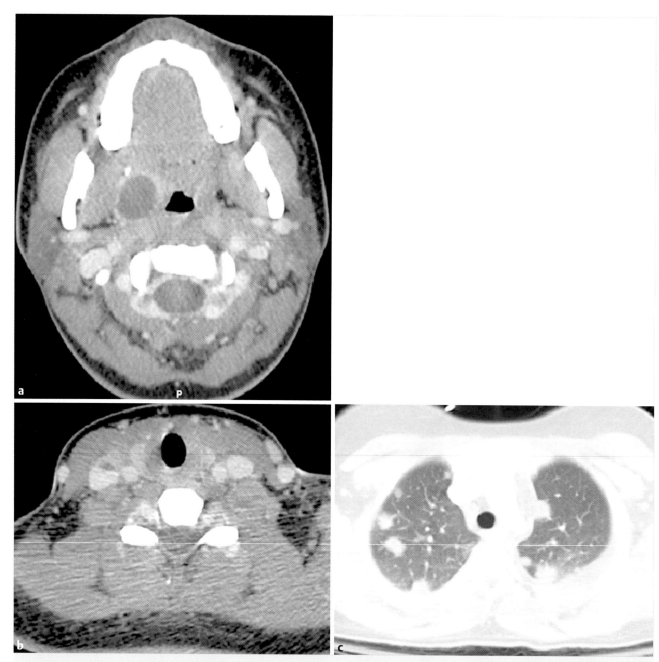

Fig. 213.1 Contrast-enhanced CT image through the oropharynx **(a)** reveals a rim-enhancing right peritonsillar abscess. Image through the lower neck **(b)** demonstrates a hypodense thrombus along the anterior aspect of the right internal jugular vein. Image through the chest in lung windows **(c)** reveals multiple peripheral pulmonary nodules. (Reprinted with permission: O'Brien WT, Cohen RA. Appl Radiol 2011;40[1]:37–38.)

■ Clinical Presentation

A 16-year-old girl with worsening sore throat and new onset cough and chest pain (▶ Fig. 213.1)

■ Key Imaging Finding

Peritonsillar abscess, jugular vein thrombus, and pulmonary septic emboli

■ Diagnosis

Lemierre syndrome. Lemierre syndrome is a rare entity characterized by an oropharyngeal infection with subsequent development of internal jugular venous (IJV) thrombosis and distant septic emboli. The lungs are the most common site of septic emboli; however, nearly any organ system may be involved.

Lemierre syndrome classically occurs in otherwise healthy adolescents and young adults. Patients present with sepsis following an antecedent oropharyngeal infection. Diagnosis is frequently delayed due to the indolent nature of the infection, as well as the rarity of the syndrome. Diagnosis is made based upon a combination of characteristic imaging findings and confirmatory blood cultures. *Fusobacterium necrophorum* is the most common causative organism; however, most cases are polymicrobial. Treatment includes antibiotic therapy tailored to

susceptibility analyses and drainage of any organized fluid collections. The use of anticoagulation therapy is controversial because it may propagate the infection but is often used with success.

The primary oropharyngeal infection is best evaluated by computed tomography (CT). Peritonsillar or retropharyngeal abscesses present with rim-enhancing fluid collections that exert mass effect on the aerodigestive tract. IJV thrombosis may be evaluated with CT or ultrasound; both modalities reveal filling defects within the internal jugular vein. Distant septic emboli are most often evaluated with CT, especially with pulmonary involvement. Pulmonary septic emboli present as multiple, peripheral pulmonary nodules that may demonstrate a feeding vessel extending into the nodules, as well as cavitation.

✓ Pearls

- Lemierre syndrome is characterized by an oropharyngeal infection, IJV thrombosis, and distant septic emboli.
- The lungs are the most common site of septic emboli; however, nearly any organ system may be involved.

- Diagnosis is made based upon characteristic imaging findings and confirmatory blood cultures.
- Treatment includes antibiotic therapy and drainage of any organized fluid collections.

Suggested Reading

O'Brien WT, Cohen RA. Lemierre's syndrome. Appl Radiol 2011; 40: 37–38

Case 214

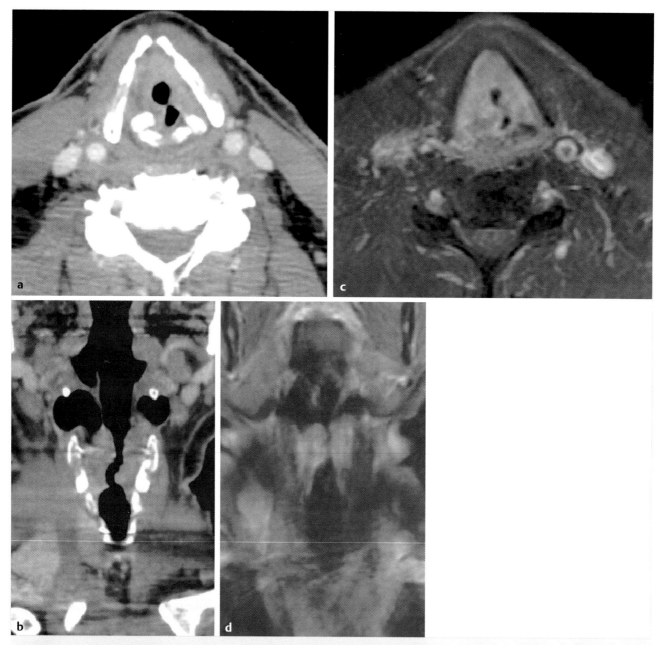

Fig. 214.1 Axial contrast-enhanced CT image **(a)** demonstrates a glottic mass involving the left greater than right true vocal cords and anterior commissure. There is extension into the paraglottic space and medialization of the right vocal cord and arytenoid. Coronal reformatted image **(b)** shows superior extension into the supraglottic space with replacement of fat within the false vocal cords. Axial **(c)** and coronal **(d)** postcontrast T1 MR images with fat suppression better demonstrate the glottic mass with supraglottic extension.

■ Clinical Presentation

A 72-year-old man with hoarseness (▶ Fig. 214.1)

■ Key Imaging Finding

Glottic mass

■ Diagnosis

Glottic carcinoma. Glottic carcinoma involves intrinsic structures of the larynx, including the true vocal cords and the anterior and posterior commissures. Squamous cell carcinoma (SCC) is by far the most common histological subtype (>90%), is more common in men, and is associated with tobacco and alcohol use. Lymphoma, chondrosarcoma, minor salivary gland tumors, and neurogenic tumors are less common tumors that may involve the glottis. Patients typically present with hoarseness; hemoptysis is a less common presentation. The superficial portions of the lesions are identified by direct visualization. Imaging (most often computed tomography, CT) is used to evaluate the underlying extent of disease and help with staging and management.

Understanding the pertinent laryngeal anatomy is a critical component in the evaluation of glottic carcinoma. The glottis consists of the true vocal cords, anterior commissure, and posterior commissure. The supraglottic larynx includes the epiglottis, aryepiglottic folds, laryngeal ventricle, false vocal cords, and the superficial mucosa of the arytenoids. The subglottic larynx includes portions of the larynx below the true vocal cords to the level of the first tracheal ring. Thyroid cartilage partially encases the larynx anteriorly. The paraglottic space refers to the space between the glottis and inner margin of the thyroid cartilage, as well as the space between the glottis and hypopharyngeal structures posteriorly.

Glottic carcinoma often originates along the true vocal cords and is prone to spread into adjacent structures; this also can include lymphatic spread to level II and III lymph nodes. It initially presents as a bulky mass with variable enhancement on CT. Key imaging components to staging include unilateral or bilateral true vocal cord involvement; extension into or across the anterior or posterior commissures; supraglottic or subglottic spread; extension into the paraglottic space; cartilaginous erosion or invasion (arytenoids, thyroid, cricoid); cord mobility (paralysis on imaging); presence of lymphadenopathy (may be necrotic with SCC); and involvement of critical vascular, neurological, or aerodigestive structures of the neck.

The determination of tumor involvement centers on the presence of abnormal soft-tissue attenuation or replacement of normal fat. Cartilaginous invasion is more problematic because imaging findings may represent inflammatory or reactive changes as opposed to true tumor involvement. Imaging findings that suggest cartilaginous invasion include extralaryngeal spread through the cartilage, lysis or irregular borders, sclerosis, and cartilage expansion. Sclerosis is the most sensitive finding, and extralaryngeal spread through the cartilage is the most specific finding. On magnetic resonance imaging (MRI), increased T2 signal on fat-suppressed sequences or enhancement within cartilage are the most helpful findings; however, these changes may also be reactive or inflammatory. Overall, CT is less sensitive for cartilage invasion and MRI is less specific; therefore, a combination of both may be useful.

Early-stage disease may be treated primarily with radiation therapy. More advanced disease typically involves both surgical and radiation therapy with or without adjuvant chemotherapy. Voice-sparring surgeries (partial laryngectomies) are preferred when appropriate. Options include a vertical hemilaryngectomy for cases with bilateral cord and anterior commissure involvement that includes less than one-third of the contralateral cord; and supracricoid or supraglottic laryngectomies for more extensive tumor with involvement of the ipsilateral arytenoid, paraglottic space, or supraglottic larynx. Total laryngectomy (with or without pharyngectomy) is indicated in cases with hyoid invasion, cricoid involvement, interarytenoid disease, bilateral arytenoid disease, or subglottic extension > 1 cm.

Post-treatment surveillance is important to evaluate for recurrent or residual disease. Postradiation changes within the neck, such as edema, fatty infiltration, and mucositis, may complicate imaging findings.

✓ Pearls

- Glottic carcinoma involves intrinsic structures of the larynx; SCC is the most common histological subtype.
- Understanding the pertinent laryngeal anatomy is a critical component in the evaluation of glottic carcinoma.
- Determination of tumor involvement includes abnormal soft tissue, replacement of fat, and cartilage invasion.
- Voice sparring surgeries (partial laryngectomies) are preferred over total laryngectomy when appropriate.

Suggested Reading

Yousem DM, Tufano RP. Laryngeal imaging. Magn Reson Imaging Clin N Am 2002;
10: 451–465

Case 215

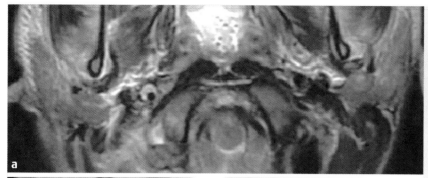

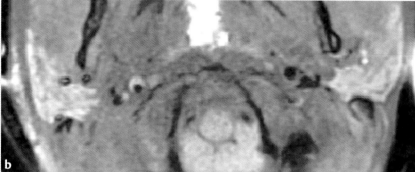

Fig. 215.1 Axial T2 MR image **(a)** demonstrates a crescent of hyperintense signal along the margin the right ICA with narrowing of the adjacent patent flow void. The cross-sectional diameter of the right ICA is enlarged compared with the left. Axial T1 MR image with FS **(b)** reveals persistent eccentric hyperintensity along the margin of the right ICA lumen. Both images show fluid within the nasopharynx and sinus cavities secondary to support tubing (not imaged).

▨ Clinical Presentation

An adolescent boy involved in a motor vehicle crash (▶ Fig. 215.1)

▤ Key Imaging Finding

Eccentric arterial wall hyperintensity with vessel enlargement and luminal narrowing

▤ Diagnosis

Arterial dissection. Arterial dissections within the neck most often occur in the setting of trauma. Spontaneous dissections are more common in patients with underlying predispositions, such as those with hypertension, fibromuscular dysplasia, polycystic kidney disease, vasculitis, or connective tissue disorders. Dissections of the carotid artery typically involve the cervical portion of the internal carotid artery (ICA) up to the level of the pertrous segment. Extension further into the intracranial ICA is uncommon. Vertebral artery dissections most often involve the V_3 segment near the craniocervical junction where the vessel is most mobile or the V_2 segment, which is located within the transverse foramina of the cervical spine, in the setting of vertebral fractures.

Arterial injury may result in an intramural hematoma or an intimal tear, which allows for blood to enter the media portion of the arterial wall. Extension to the adventitia layer may result in pseudoaneurysm formation. Intramural hematomas and diversion of blood flow into a false lumen may result in narrowing of the primary vascular channel. Possible clinical manifestations include arterial stenosis, primary occlusion, or thromboembolic disease. Some patients may present with Horner syndrome with involvement of the sympathetic chain along the course of the carotid artery. Headache and localized neck pain are seen in most patients.

On unenhanced computed tomography (CT), acute dissections commonly present as crescent-shaped regions of increased density within the wall of the involved artery. Although the lumen of the vessel is often narrowed, the overall cross-sectional diameter of the artery is increased due to the presence of an intramural hematoma. Contrast-enhanced CT angiography may show

luminal irregularity, narrowing, or a dissection flap. Occasionally, longitudinal extension of a dissection flap may result in tapered narrowing or even occlusion of the vessel.

Conventional magnetic resonance imaging (MRI) sequences are helpful in evaluating the size and signal intensity of the artery and its wall. As with CT, the involved vessel typically has an increased diameter due to the presence of an intramural hematoma. The signal intensity of the hematoma varies based upon the stage of blood products and resultant paramagnetic effects. In the acute and chronic stages, the intramural hematoma is typically isointense compared with surrounding tissues, making it less conspicuous. In the subacute phase (roughly 7 to 60 days); however, intrinsic T1 hyperintensity readily identifies the intramural hematoma and is best seen on unenhanced axial T1 sequences with fat suppression (FS). Time-of-flight imaging and contrast-enhanced MR angiography will demonstrate regions of luminal irregularity, narrowing, or occlusion but are limited in evaluating the vessel wall.

Digital subtraction angiography (DSA) similarly evaluates the vessel lumen but cannot evaluate the vessel wall. Findings of dissection on DSA include luminal irregularity, tapered eccentric stenosis or occlusion ("string" sign), a double lumen, or an intimal flap.

Patients with extracranial dissections of the neck and clinical and hemodynamic stability are typically treated initially with anticoagulation therapy. Endovascular or surgical treatment of dissections may be required in patients who are unstable due to the dissection, fail medical management, have persistent thromboemboli, or have a dissecting pseudoaneurysm.

✓ Pearls

- Dissections result from intimal injury; common findings include an intramural hematoma and intimal flap.
- On unenhanced CT, acute dissections present with crescent-shaped increased density within the arterial wall.
- In the subacute phase, unenhanced T1 sequences with FS show a peripheral hyperintense intramural hematoma.
- DSA findings include luminal irregularity, tapered stenosis or occlusion, a double lumen, or an intimal flap.

Suggested Reading

Rodallec MH, Marteau V, Gerber S, Desmottes L, Zins M. Craniocervical arterial dissection: spectrum of imaging findings and differential diagnosis. Radiographics 2008; 28: 1711–1728

Case 216

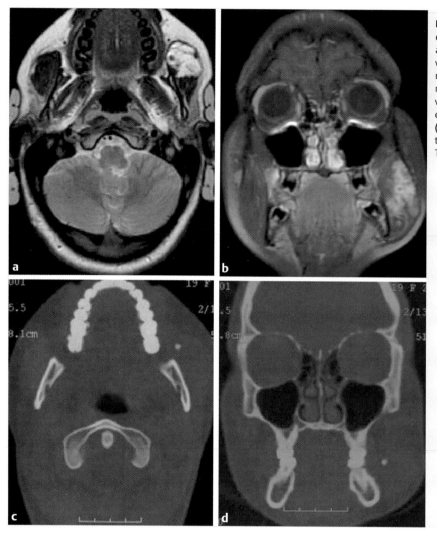

Fig. 216.1 Axial T2 image **(a)** demonstrates a circumscribed, lobulated hyperintense mass along the anterior margin of the masseter muscle within the left masticator space. There is a small region of decreased T2 signal intensity within the mass medially. Coronal T1 postcontrast image with fat suppression **(b)** shows prominent enhancement. Axial **(c)** and coronal reformatted **(d)** CT images reveal a round phlebolith within the mass, corresponding to the focal region of T2 hypointensity.

▧ Clinical Presentation

A young adult man with mild facial asymmetry and focal skin discoloration (▶ Fig. 216.1)

■ Key Imaging Finding

Enhancing mass with phlebolith

■ Diagnosis

Venous malformation. Vascular malformations are classified as slow-flow or high-flow lesions and are common in the head and neck region. It is important to distinguish vascular malformations from vascular tumors with endothelial hyperplasia, such as hemangiomas. Although it occasionally may be impossible to distinguish between a low-flow vascular malformation and a hemangioma on imaging, the terms should not be used interchangeably because they are different lesions altogether.

Slow-flow vascular malformations encompass a spectrum of anomalies that include capillary, lymphatic, and/or venous components. High-flow vascular malformations include arteriovenous malformations and arteriovenous fistulas.

Venous malformations (VMs) are the most common low-flow vascular malformation overall and especially in adults. Most are solitary, but multiple lesions are not uncommon, especially when familial. On pathological examination, the lesions have thin-walled, dilated capillary and cavernous vascular channels. Clinically, they are soft and compressible and often increase in size with Valsalva maneuvers. They demonstrate growth proportional to somatic growth. Superficial lesions commonly have overlying discoloration of the skin that is typically bluish in color.

On computed tomography (CT), VMs present as lobulated hypodense or heterogeneous lesions that demonstrate delayed enhancement, which progresses from the periphery to the central portions of the mass. Phleboliths are characteristic; fatty components may also be seen. Magnetic resonance imaging (MRI) is the preferred modality for characterizing VMs in terms of their extent and effect on adjacent structures. As with CT, lesions are usually lobulated and often demonstrate internal septations. Abnormal venous structures may be noted in the region of the underlying lesion. VMs are typically hypo- to iso-intense on T1 and hyperintense on T2 sequences. Signal characteristics are more heterogeneous in the setting of hemorrhage or thrombosis. Phleboliths typically appear hypointense on all sequences. Postcontrast sequences demonstrate avid enhancement.

Asymptomatic VMs may be left alone. Symptomatic lesions or those that result in a cosmetic deformity may be treated with sclerotherapy, laser therapy, or surgical resection.

✓ Pearls

- Slow-flow vascular malformations are composed of capillary, lymphatic, and/or venous elements.
- VMs are the most common slow-flow vascular malformations and are often seen in the head and neck.
- CT demonstrates a lobulated lesion with delayed enhancement; phleboliths are characteristic.
- MRI is preferred for evaluating the extent of the lesion and its effect on adjacent structures.

Suggested Reading

Dubois J, Soulez G, Oliva VL, Berthiaume MJ, Lapierre C, Therasse E. Soft-tissue venous malformations in adult patients: imaging and therapeutic issues. Radiographics 2001; 21: 1519–1531

Case 217

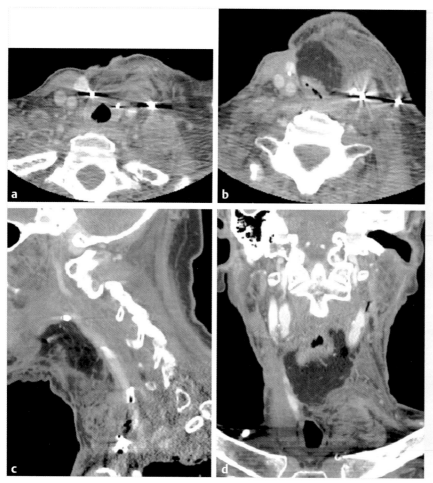

Fig. 217.1 Axial (**a,b**), sagittal formatted (**c**), and coronal reformatted (**d**) contrast-enhanced computed tomography images show post-operative changes consistent with a left modified radical neck dissection and placement of a myocutaneous flap. There is atrophy of the musculature within the flap, as well as regions of fatty infiltration from radiation therapy. No masslike enhancement is seen within the surgical bed or along the surgical margins. (Courtesy of Michael Zapadka, DO.)

▪ Clinical Presentation

A 61-year-old man post laryngectomy and modified left radical neck dissection with reconstruction (▶ Fig. 217.1)

■ Key Imaging Finding

Postoperative and post-treatment changes within the neck.

■ Diagnosis

Postoperative neck. Radiologists play an important role in the follow-up of patients who have undergone various forms of neck dissection and reconstruction. To evaluate for postoperative complications or tumor recurrence, a basic knowledge of the various surgical procedures and imaging appearances is necessary.

The nodal groups of the neck are categorized as levels I through VI. Level I lymph nodes are divided into submental and submandibular. Level II lymph nodes are located along the upper third of the jugular vein above the level of the hyoid bone and include the jugulodigastric nodes. Level III lymph nodes are located along the middle third of the jugular vein from the hyoid bone superiorly to the cricothyroid notch inferiorly. Level IV lymph nodes are located along the lower third of the jugular vein from the cricothyroid notch superiorly to the clavicle inferiorly. Level V lymph nodes are located within the posterior triangle along the course of the spinal accessory nerve, including the supraclavicular lymph nodes. Level VI lymph nodes are located within the anterior midline neck from the hyoid bone to the suprasternal notch.

Various types of neck dissections are performed for the treatment of head and neck cancer. Radical neck dissection includes removal of all ipsilateral lymph node groups and the spinal accessory nerve, submandibular gland, internal jugular vein (IJV), and sternocleidomastoid muscle. A modified radical neck dissection, which is more commonly performed, consists of removal of ipsilateral lymph node groups with preservation of some of the extralymphatic structures that are removed in a radical neck dissection. A selective neck dissection refers to removal of certain ipsilateral lymph node groups with preservation of the remaining lymph node groups and extralymphatic structures. As the name implies, an extended neck dissection is the most extensive and consists of removal of ipsilateral lymph node groups, extralymphatic structures, and additional structures, which may include the strap and trapezius musculature,

platysma, thyroid gland, cranial nerves, carotid artery, and overlying skin. Extended neck dissections commonly involve a myocutaneous flap.

Surgical flaps allow for more extensive primary dissections with relative preservation of function and aesthetics. Local flaps reposition adjacent tissues into or over the surgical defect. Pedicle flaps involve rotation of flap components to cover a surgical defect with preservation of the native vascular supply. Examples include pectoralis and trapezius flaps. Free flaps consist of tissues removed from a remote donor site with microvascular anatamoses at the surgical site. Examples include rectus abdominus free flaps and radial forearm flaps for intraoral reconstruction with use of portions of the fibula, ilium, or scapula for mandibular reconstruction. Simple flaps contain one tissue type, whereas complex flaps contain two or more tissue types (e.g., myocutaneous flaps). Because the native nerve innervation within myocutaneous flaps is sacrificed, the involved musculature within the flaps undergoes atrophy with fatty replacement over time.

On postoperative imaging, there is typically a sharp demarcation between surgical flaps and native tissues. Adjuvant radiation therapy may alter the imaging appearance, however, because early radiation changes include skin thickening, fatty stranding, and edema. Late radiation changes include thickening of the musculature with atrophy of glandular tissues. Tumor recurrence typically occurs within the first 2 years following treatment and most often occurs either within the tumor bed or at the surgical margins. It is often isodense or isointense to musculature with variable enhancement. It may be difficult to distinguish recurrence from early enhancing fibrosis. Follow-up imaging is helpful because recurrence will continue to progress, whereas fibrosis will often retract. Lymph node spread is difficult to evaluate in the post-treatment neck because fat planes are often obliterated; interval enlargement and increased enhancement suggest metastatic infiltration.

✓ Pearls

- Surgical flaps allow for more extensive primary dissections and are classified as local, pedicle, or free flaps.
- The musculature within myocutaneous flaps undergoes progressive fatty atrophy due to denervation.

- Recurrence often occurs within the first 2 years of treatment within the tumor bed or at the surgical margins.

Suggested Reading

Saito N, Nadgir RN, Nakahira M et al. Posttreatment CT and MR imaging in head and neck cancer: what the radiologist needs to know. Radiographics 2012; 32: 1261–1282, discussion 1282–1284

Case 218

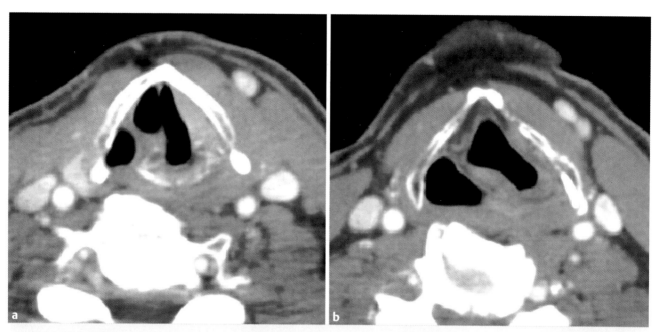

Fig. 218.1 Axial contrast-enhanced CT image at the level of the larynx **(a)** demonstrates medial deviation of the right true vocal cord with ipsilateral dilatation of the laryngeal ventricle, resulting in a "sail" sign. A dilated piriform sinus is partially seen on the right. Axial CT image superior to the level of the larynx **(b)** shows dilatation of the right piriform sinus and medial deviation and thickening of the aryepiglottic fold.

■ **Clinical Presentation**

A 50-year-old man with hoarseness (▶ Fig. 218.1)

■ Key Imaging Finding

Medial deviation of vocal cord and aryepiglottic fold with dilated laryngeal ventricle and piriform sinus

■ Diagnosis

Vocal cord paralysis (VCP). VCP results from dysfunction of the recurrent laryngeal nerve (RLN), which provides motor innervation to the true vocal cords. Pathology affecting RLN function may occur anywhere along its path from the brain stem, through the cervical neck, and into portions of the mediastinum. Peripheral nerve dysfunction is more common than central etiologies. The inferior course of the RLN is longer on the left, making the left side more prone to injury or pathology. Common causes of RLN dysfunction include iatrogenia (thyroidectomy), infectious or inflammatory neuropathy, compressive neoplasms along the course of the vagus and RLNs, and vascular injuries or aneurysms within the carotid sheath or mediastinum. The most common presenting symptom is hoarseness; however, many patients are asymptomatic.

To evaluate for pathological causes of RLN dysfunction, it is important to first understand the course of the vagus and recurrent laryngeal nerves. The vagus nerve exists from the medulla and courses through the pars vascularis of the jugular foramen. It descends through the cervical neck within the carotid sheath posterolateral to the carotid arteries and posteromedial to the jugular veins. On the right side of the neck, the RLN branches at the level of the subclavian artery, courses posteriorly beneath the brachiocephalic artery, and ascends in the tracheoesophageal groove to the larynx. On the left side, the RLN branches at the level of the aortic arch, passes anteriorly and below the aortic arch and ligamentum arteriosum through the aorticopulmonary window, and ascends in the tracheoesophageal groove to the larynx. The RLNs enter the larynx along the posterior aspect of the cricoarytenoid joints and innervate the intrinsic muscles of the larynx with the exception of the cricothyroid muscle, which receives its motor innervation from the superior laryngeal nerve.

Contrast-enhanced computed tomography (CT) is the imaging modality of choice in evaluating for vocal cord dysfunction. Imaging is ideally performed with the patient undergoing quiet respiration, which optimizes evaluation of the larynx. Common findings of VCP include medial displacement of the ipsilateral true vocal cord, anteromedial displacement and rotation of the ipsilateral arytenoid cartilage, and dilatation of the ipsilateral laryngeal ventricle, the combination of which leads to a characteristic "sail" sign on axial images. Additional findings include ipsilateral dilatation of the piriform sinus and medial rotation and thickening of the aryepiglottic fold. In the setting of a more central lesion involving the vagus nerve and pharyngeal plexus, secondary findings include dilatation of the ipsilateral oropharynx, atrophy of the ipsilateral pharyngeal constrictor musculature, and contralateral deviation of the uvula.

Treatment options are geared toward the underlying cause of vocal cord dysfunction. Unfortunately, a causative etiology is not identified on CT in the majority of cases. Being able to distinguish between a central or peripheral cause, however, is helpful in guiding further workup and management.

✓ Pearls

- VCP results from dysfunction of the RLN; pathology or injury may occur anywhere along its course.
- Axial CT images commonly show the "sail" sign ipsilateral to the side of VCP.
- Additional findings include ipsilateral piriform sinus dilatation and aryepiglottic fold rotation/thickening.
- Central lesions show oropharynx dilatation, pharyngeal constrictor atrophy, and contralateral uvula deviation.

Suggested Readings

Chin SC, Edelstein S, Chen CY, Som PM. Using CT to localize side and level of vocal cord paralysis. Am J Roentgenol 2003; 180: 1165–1170

Paquette CM, Manos DC, Psooy BJ. Unilateral vocal cord paralysis: a review of CT findings, mediastinal causes, and the course of the recurrent laryngeal nerves. Radiographics 2012; 32: 721–740

Case 219

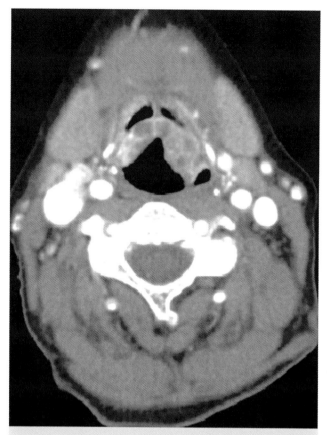

Fig. 219.1 Contrast-enhanced axial CT image demonstrates a bulky epiglottic mass, eccentric to the left, with heterogeneous enhancement. Subsequent images (not shown) revealed extension into the aryepiglottic folds.

■ Clinical Presentation

A 51-year-old man with globus sensation and dysphagia (▶ Fig. 219.1)

■ Key Imaging Finding

Supraglottic mass

■ Diagnosis

Supraglottic carcinoma. Supraglottic carcinoma involves the structures of the larynx above the glottis, including the epiglottis, aryepiglottic folds, laryngeal ventricle, false vocal cords, and superficial mucosa of the arytenoids. Squamous cell carcinoma (SCC) is by far the most common histological subtype; minor salivary gland neoplasms and infectious or granulomatous processes are far less common. Patients are most often middle-aged to elderly men who present with dysphagia or pain. There is an increased incidence with tobacco and alcohol usage. The superficial portions of the lesions are identified by direct visualization. Imaging (most often computed tomography [CT]) is used to evaluate the underlying extent of disease and help with staging and management.

The larynx is divided into the glottic, supraglottic, and subglottic spaces. The glottis consists of the true vocal cords, anterior commissure, and posterior commissure. The supraglottic larynx includes the epiglottis, aryepiglottic folds, laryngeal ventricle, false vocal cords, and superficial mucosa of the arytenoids. The subglottic larynx includes portions of the larynx below the true vocal cords to the level of the first tracheal ring. Thyroid cartilage partially encases the larynx anteriorly. The paraglottic space refers to the space between the glottis and inner margin of the thyroid cartilage, as well as the space between the glottis and hypopharyngeal structures posteriorly; it predominantly contains fat. The preepiglottic space is a wedge-shaped region that is also composed primarily of fat and is located anterior to the epiglottis and posterior to the hyoid bone and thyrohyoid ligament. The preepiglottic space is contiguous with the paraglottic space laterally.

Supraglottic SCC may involve any portion of the supraglottic space. Epiglottic SCC may present as a midline symmetric or off-midline asymmetric mass; aryepiglottic SCC is asymmetric in appearance. Supraglottic SCC spreads to level II lymph nodes; regional lymphatic spread is often bilateral with epiglottic SCC. Epiglottic SCC may spread into the preepiglottic and paraglottic spaces, which allows for further spread into the glottic space. Aryepiglottic SCC has a propensity for spread into the adjacent hypopharynx (piriform sinus). Supraglottic SCC initially presents as a bulky mass with variable enhancement on CT. Key imaging components to staging include the number of supraglottic structures involved; spread into the preepiglottic or paraglottic spaces; spread to adjacent laryngeal or extralaryngeal spaces of the neck, including the glottic space, oropharynx/tongue base, and hypopharynx; cartilaginous invasion; cord mobility; presence of lymphadenopathy (may be necrotic with SCC); and involvement of critical vascular, neurological, or aerodigestive structures of the neck.

The determination of tumor involvement centers on the presence of abnormal soft-tissue attenuation or replacement of normal fat. Cartilaginous invasion is more problematic because imaging findings may represent inflammatory or reactive changes as opposed to true tumor involvement. Imaging findings that suggest cartilaginous invasion include extralaryngeal spread through the cartilage, lysis or irregular borders, sclerosis, and cartilage expansion. Sclerosis is the most sensitive finding, and extralaryngeal spread through the cartilage is the most specific finding. On magnetic resonance imaging (MRI), increased T2 signal on fat-suppressed sequences or enhancement within cartilage are the most helpful findings; however, these changes may also be reactive or inflammatory. Overall, CT is less sensitive for cartilage invasion and MRI is less specific; therefore, a combination of both may be useful.

Early-stage disease may be treated primarily with radiation therapy. More advanced disease typically involves both surgical and radiation therapy with or without adjuvant chemotherapy. Tumors limited to the supraglottic space are often amenable to supraglottic laryngectomy (usually horizontal) with voice preservation. Transglottic extension, involvement of the paraglottic space, or cartilaginous invasion are contraindications to this approach.

Post-treatment surveillance is important to evaluate for recurrent or residual disease. Postradiation changes within the neck, such as edema, fatty infiltration, and mucositis, may complicate imaging findings.

✓ Pearls

- Supraglottic SCC often involves the epiglottis, aryepiglottic folds, laryngeal ventricle, and/or false cords.
- Supraglottic SCC spreads to level II lymph nodes; regional spread is often bilateral with epiglottic tumors.

- Determination of tumor involvement includes abnormal soft tissue, replacement of fat, and cartilage invasion.

Suggested Reading

Yousem DM, Tufano RP. Laryngeal imaging. Magn Reson Imaging Clin N Am 2002; 10: 451–465

Case 220

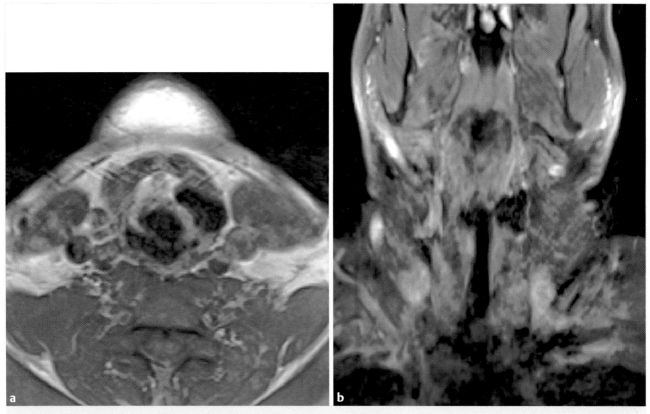

Fig. 220.1 Axial unenhanced T1 magnetic resonance image through the neck **(a)** demonstrates a lobulated focal air-filled sac on the left centered within the supraglottic fat and extending beyond the thyrohyoid membrane. Coronal T1 postcontrast image with fat suppression **(b)** shows communication of the air-filled sac with the laryngeal ventricle.

■ Clinical Presentation

A 51-year-old man with intermittent neck pain (▶ Fig. 220.1)

▨ Key Imaging Finding

Air-filled sac centered within the supraglottic fat

▨ Diagnosis

Laryngocele. The laryngeal appendix or saccule refers to a small air-filled recess that extends cephalad from the laryngeal ventricle within the supraglottic fat. In the setting of appendiceal obstruction or increased laryngeal pressure (e.g., wind/horn instrument players), an air and/or fluid-filled laryngocele may develop due to dilatation of the laryngeal appendix/saccule. Some clinicians will refer to a fluid-filled laryngocele as a saccular cyst, whereas others reserve the term *saccular cyst* for a mucous-containing cyst that does not communicate with the laryngeal ventricle.

Laryngoceles are categorized as internal, which remain within the paraglottic space and are bound by the thyrohyoid membrane, or mixed, which include components of an internal laryngocele with extension beyond the thyrohyoid membrane. A purely external laryngocele is rare and occurs with decompression of the internal component and persistence of the external component of a mixed laryngocele. Laryngoceles are most often incidental and asymptomatic. When symptomatic, common clinical presentations include a globus sensation and hoarseness. Large internal laryngoceles may cause cough and, rarely, airway compromise. Large mixed or purely external laryngoceles may present as a palpable mass.

On computed tomography, laryngoceles most often present as blind-ending air-filled pockets located within the supraglottic fat at the expected location of the laryngeal appendix. When fluid-filled, the attenuation may be consistent with simple fluid or demonstrate increased attenuation, if proteinaceous. On magnetic resonance imaging, air-filled lesions are hypointense on all pulse sequences. Fluid-filled lesions are typically hypointense on T1 and hyperintense on T2 sequences. As the internal protein content increases, there is increased T1 and decreased T2 signal intensity. Mild peripheral enhancement may be seen. Solid enhancement is indicative of an underlying mass, whereas prominent rim enhancement with surrounding inflammatory changes suggests superimposed infection, termed a *laryngopyocele*.

When presented with a suspected laryngocele, it is important to look closely for an underlying mass as the cause of laryngeal appendiceal obstruction. It is also important to describe the size and full extent of the lesion, especially in terms or internal, mixed, or external, to help guide surgical planning.

✓ Pearls

- A laryngocele results from obstruction of the laryngeal appendix or increased laryngeal pressures.
- Laryngoceles may be internal, mixed, or external based upon their relationship to the thyrohyoid membrane.

- It is important to look closely for an underlying mass as the cause of laryngeal appendiceal obstruction.
- A laryngopyocele refers to an infected laryngocele; rim enhancement and inflammatory changes are seen.

Suggested Reading

Catena JR, Moonis G, Glastonbury CM et al. MDCT and MR imaging evaluation of the laryngeal appendix and laryngoceles. Neurographics. 2011; 1: 74–83

Case 221

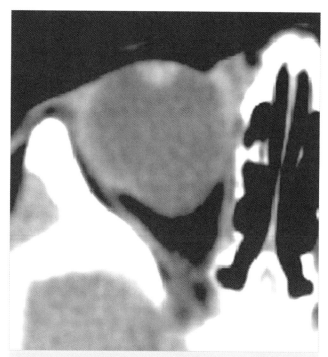

Fig. 221.1 Magnified axial computed tomography image through the right orbit reveals a focal contour abnormality along the posterior aspect of the globe.

■ Clinical Presentation

History withheld (▶ Fig. 221.1)

■ Key Imaging Finding

Globe contour abnormality

■ Top 3 Differential Diagnoses

- **Globe trauma.** Injury to the globe is an important finding in a trauma patient because it may result in temporary or permanent loss of vision, depending on the type and extent of injury. Globe rupture (open globe injury) is a severe form of injury that may result from blunt or penetrating trauma. Globe rupture is suspected when there is a focal globe contour abnormality, scleral deformity, foreign body or gas within the globe, and/or when there is loss of orbital volume, which may lead to the "flat tire" sign. Additional findings include vitreous hemorrhage, dislocation of the lens, and retinal or choroidal detachments.
- **Coloboma.** The globe has three layers posteriorly with the sclera representing the outermost layer, the choroid representing the middle layer, and the retina representing the innermost layer. The posterior segment contains the vitreous humor. Coloboma refers to a congenital scleral defect that results in a focal globe abnormality at or near the optic nerve insertion onto the globe. It is present at birth, although most

often presents in childhood. It may be sporadic and unilateral or associated with syndromes, in which case it is more often bilateral. Associated syndromes include morning glory, CHARGE (*c*oloboma of the eye, *h*eart anomaly, choanal *a*tresia, growth and developmental *r*etardation, and *g*enital and *e*ar anomalies), and Aicardi syndromes. Imaging reveals an enlarged globe with a focal protrusion of the vitreous in the region of the optic nerve head.

- **Staphyloma.** Staphyloma is an acquired sclera defect that commonly results from severe degenerative myopia. Less common etiologies include glaucoma, infection, and trauma. Imaging reveals an enlarged globe that is elongated in the anterior-posterior dimension, as well as a focal region of sclera thinning and protrusion of the vitreous. The focal globe abnormality is typically posterior in location and often along the lateral aspect of the optic nerve insertion onto the globe. An anterior version with a corneal defect may be associated with inflammatory conditions.

■ Additional Differential Diagnoses

- **Axial myopia.** Axial myopia refers to unilateral or bilateral elongation of the globe in the anterior-posterior dimension, resulting in an ovoid configuration. It is commonly idiopathic and chronic but may be associated with orbital infections and

thyroid orbitopathy. The abnormal globe configuration often results in proptosis. A focal acquired sclera defect, staphyloma, may coexist. Imaging reveals characteristic anteroposterior elongation of the globe without a focal mass.

■ Diagnosis

Coloboma

✓ Pearls

- Globe rupture is suspected with a focal contour abnormality, foreign body, and/or loss of intraocular volume.
- Coloboma refers to a congenital scleral defect at or near the optic nerve insertion onto the globe.

- Staphyloma is an acquired sclera defect that commonly results from severe degenerative myopia.
- Axial myopia refers to elongation of the globe in the anterior-posterior dimension, resulting in an ovoid configuration.

Suggested Readings

Kubal WS. Imaging of orbital trauma. Radiographics 2008; 28: 1729–1739

Osborne DR, Foulks GN. Computed tomographic analysis of deformity and dimensional changes in the eyeball. Radiology 1984; 153: 669–674

Smith M, Castillo M. Imaging and differential diagnosis of the large eye. Radiographics 1994; 14: 721–728

Betts AM, O'Brien WT, Davies BW, Youssef OH. A systemic approach to CT evaluation of orbital trauma. Emerg Radiol 2014; 21(5): 511–531

Case 222

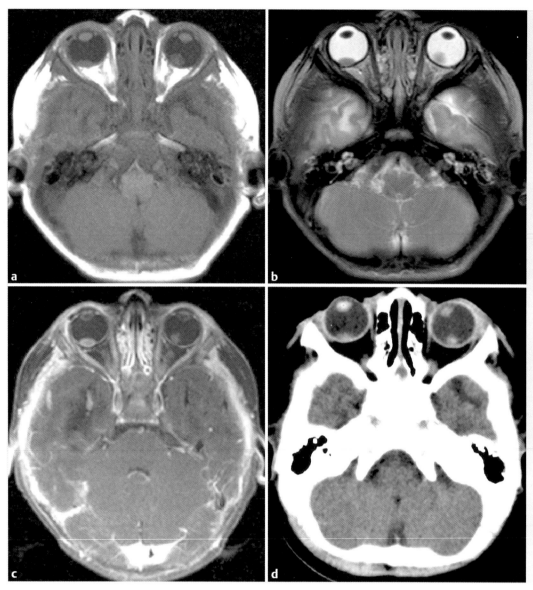

Fig. 222.1 Axial MR images **(a–c)** demonstrate bilateral T1 iso- to hyperintense **(a)** and T2 hypointense **(b)** globe masses with enhancement **(c)**. The lesions are hyperdense on CT **(d)**. Globe size is normal and there is no extension beyond the globe margin. Decreased T1 and increased T2 signal intensity in the anterior temporal lobes represent regions of unmyelinated white matter.

■ **Clinical Presentation**

A 3-month-old boy with leukocoria (▶ Fig. 222.1)

▨ Key Imaging Finding

Globe mass/lesion in a child

▨ Top 3 Differential Diagnoses

- **Retinoblastoma.** Retinoblastoma is a malignant neoplasm of the retina and represents the most common globe tumor in children. Nearly all cases present prior to 5 years of age with leukocoria (white pupillary reflex) being the most common presenting sign. Approximately 75% are unilateral, whereas the remainder are bilateral. Trilateral (bilateral globe plus pineal gland involvement) and quadrilateral (trilateral plus suprasellar involvement) disease is seen in familial cases. Unenhanced computed tomography (CT) demonstrates a hyperdense globe mass with calcifications (95%). Globe size is normal to slightly enlarged. The mass is hyperintense on T1 and hypointense on T2 sequences with avid enhancement. Treatment options include chemotherapy, radiation, and enucleation. Distinguishing features include a normal globe size and presence of calcification.
- **Persistent hyperplastic primary vitreous (PHPV).** PHPV results from persistence of the embryonic vascularity within the vitreous, which may result in vitreous hemorrhage, cataracts, and retinal detachment. In severe disease, phthisis bulbi may occur with globe deformity. Characteristic imaging findings include microphthalmia and increased density in the vitreous. The density may change location with repositioning of the patient. Magnetic resonance imaging (MRI) findings consist of increased T1 and T2 signal within the vitreous. Calcifications are not a feature of PHPV. This may be difficult to distinguish from other entities, especially noncalcified retinoblastoma. Key distinguishing features are microphthalmia in a full-term infant.
- **Coats disease.** Coats disease occurs primarily in young boys and is characterized by subretinal exudates, retinal detachment, and vascular anomalies of the retina. The primary imaging findings are exudates in the region of the retina and retinal detachment. CT reveals increased density within the affected globe without calcification. Subretinal exudates are better visualized on MRI as regions of increased T1 and T2 signal. Distinguishing features include normal globe size and lack of calcification.

▨ Additional Differential Diagnoses

- **Retinopathy of prematurity (ROP).** ROP, also referred to as retrolental fibroplasia, occurs as a sequela of prolonged oxygen therapy in premature infants, resulting in abnormal vascular development and hemorrhage. Imaging features include bilateral (usually) microphthalmia. Resultant hemorrhage leads to increased density within the globe and retinal detachment. Calcification may occur in advanced cases. Bilateral involvement and a history of prematurity help distinguish this entity from other differential considerations.
- **Toxocariasis.** Ocular toxocariasis results from a hypersensitivity reaction to the larval form of *Toxocara*. The infection is transmitted through contact with dogs and cats. Patients present with unilateral visual disturbances. On CT, imaging findings include hyperdensity within the globe, often without a focal mass. The lesion is isointense on T1- and hyperintense on T2-weighted sequences. Distinguishing features include normal globe size, lack of calcification, and history of contact with dogs or cats.

▨ Diagnosis

Retinoblastoma (bilateral)

✓ Pearls

- Retinoblastoma is the most common globe tumor in children and presents with leukocoria and calcification.
- PHPV is due to persistent embryonic vascularity and presents as microphthalmia in a full-term infant.
- Coats disease is characterized by retinal detachment and lack of calcification with a normal globe size.
- ROP is caused by prolonged oxygenation; bilateral microphthalmia without calcification is characteristic.

Suggested Reading

Chung EM, Specht CS, Schroeder JW. From the archives of the AFIP: pediatric orbit tumors and tumorlike lesions: neuroepithelial lesions of the ocular globe and optic nerve. Radiographics 2007; 27: 1159–1186

Case 223

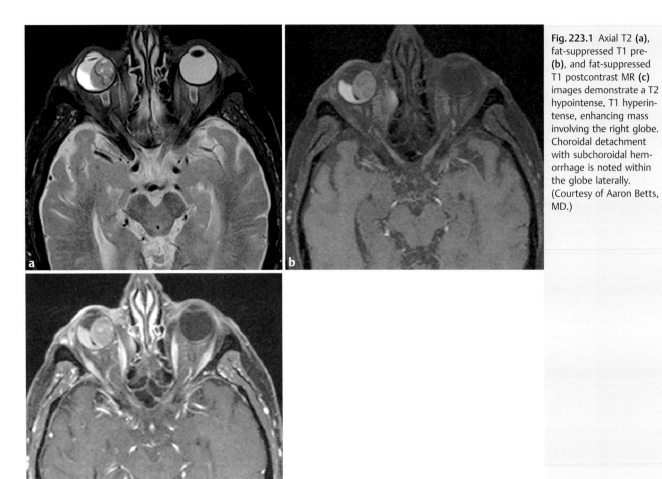

Fig. 223.1 Axial T2 (**a**), fat-suppressed T1 pre- (**b**), and fat-suppressed T1 postcontrast MR (**c**) images demonstrate a T2 hypointense, T1 hyperintense, enhancing mass involving the right globe. Choroidal detachment with subchoroidal hemorrhage is noted within the globe laterally. (Courtesy of Aaron Betts, MD.)

■ Clinical Presentation

An adult man with visual disturbances (▶ Fig. 223.1)

▓ Key Imaging Finding

Globe mass in adult

▓ Top 3 Differential Diagnoses

- **Hematoma/hemorrhage.** Intraocular hemorrhage occurs secondary to trauma, including iatrogenia, in the vast majority of cases. Hemorrhage related to an underlying coagulopathy or neoplasm is less common. On computed tomography (CT), hemorrhage or hematoma presents as a hyperdense mass that may be well-defined or ill-defined. If subretinal or subchoroidal in location, a characteristic "V" or biconvex configuration may be seen, respectively, and is consistent with detachment. The appearance of hemorrhage on magnetic resonance imaging (MRI) is variable based upon the stage of blood products. Blooming may be seen on gradient echo or susceptibility-weighted imaging.
- **Melanoma.** Ocular melanoma is a primary malignancy of melanocytes within the globe and represents the most common ocular tumor in adults. Secondary, metastatic involvement from nonocular melanoma is much less common. The vast majority of lesions occur in the choroid with the remainder occurring in the cilia or iris. Patients are typically middle-aged to older adults who present with painless visual loss.

Both CT and MRI demonstrate a dome- or mushroom-shaped mass with a broad attachment to the choroid and avid enhancement. Superimposed choroidal or retinal detachments are commonly seen. Lesions are hyperdense on CT and characteristically hyperintense on T1 and hypointense on T2 sequences due to the presence of melanin. Treatment and prognosis is based upon the size, depth, and extraocular extension of the lesions.
- **Metastases.** Metastases to the globe typically occur in adults with advanced disease. Breast and lung cancer are the most common primary tumors, followed by hypervascular tumors, such as renal cell and thyroid carcinoma. Due to hematogenous spread, the lesions are commonly posterior in location and involve the uvea and choroid. Superimposed choroidal or retinal detachments may be seen. Metastatic foci are hyperdense on CT, more so with superimposed hemorrhage, and avidly enhance. Lesions are variable in MRI signal intensity but often intermediate to hypointense on T2 sequences with enhancement.

▓ Additional Differential Diagnoses

- **Orbital pseudotumor.** Orbital pseudotumor is an idiopathic inflammatory process that is most-often ill-defined and may involve any portion of the orbit. More common forms involve the extraocular muscles (EOMs) and diffuse involvement of the intra- and extraconal spaces. Globe involvement is typically ill defined with enhancement. Its MRI appearance varies, but most lesions are hypointense on T1 and isointense on T2 sequences compared with the EOMs. Chronic, sclerosing lesions have decreased signal intensity.
- **Choroidal hemangioma.** Choroidal hemangioma is a hamartoma that may occur sporadically or in association with Sturge-Weber syndrome (SWS). On CT and MRI, the lesions

may be solitary and focal or lentiform and diffuse with avid enhancement. They are hyperdense on CT and typically hyperintense on both T1 and T2 sequences.
- **Choroidal osteoma.** Choroidal osteomas are uncommon, benign tumors that calcify/ossify. The vast majority are solitary and unilateral, and they are more common in young adult women. CT reveals a focal or lentiform calcified mass along the posterior aspect of the globe at the choroidal-retinal junction. On MRI, the lesions are typically hypointense on T2 and variable in signal on T1 sequences due to calcification/ossification. Avid enhancement is often seen.

▓ Diagnosis

Ocular melanoma (with choroidal detachment)

✓ Pearls

- Melanoma is characteristically hyperdense on CT with T1 hyperintense and T2 hypointense signal intensity.
- Orbital pseudotumor is an idiopathic inflammatory process; most lesions are ill defined with enhancement.

- Choroidal hemangioma is a vascular hamartoma that may occur sporadically or in association with SWS.
- Choroidal osteomas are uncommon, benign tumors that calcify/ossify and demonstrate avid enhancement.

Suggested Reading

Smoker WRK, Gentry LR, Yee NK, Reede DL, Nerad JA. Vascular lesions of the orbit: more than meets the eye. Radiographics 2008; 28: 185–204, quiz 325

Case 224

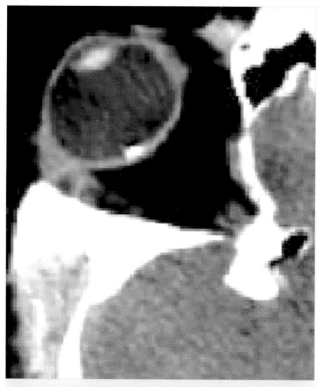

Fig. 224.1 Magnified axial CT image through the right orbit shows a focal region of calcification along the posterior aspect of the globe.

■ Clinical Presentation

A patient with decreased visual acuity (▶ Fig. 224.1)

■ Key Imaging Finding

Globe calcification

■ Top 3 Differential Diagnoses

- **Scleral plaque.** Scleral plaques are commonly seen in middle-aged and elderly adults and are thought to be degenerative in nature and incidental. They occur at the site of extraocular muscle (EOM) insertion onto the globe, are commonly bilateral, and most often involve the medial (most common) and lateral rectus muscles. Their appearance and location are characteristic.
- **Optic nerve head drusen (ONHD).** ONHD refers to a process of acellular deposition and calcification associated with degenerating nerve fibers at the optic nerve head. It is typically asymptomatic, although mild visual field deficits may occur. Its main clinical significance is that it may mimic papilledema (normally associated with increased intracranial pressure) on fundoscopic

examination. Computed tomography (CT) is useful in identifying calcified optic nerve head drusen, as well as ruling out retroorbital causes of true papilledema. Drusen characteristically presents as small calcifications (<3 mm) at the optic nerve insertion onto the globe.
- **Retinal hamartoma.** Tuberous sclerosis (TS) results in hamartomas involving various anatomic sites. Retinal hamartomas frequently occur in the setting of TS and are often asymptomatic; when present, they represent a major diagnostic criterion for TS. The majority of lesions calcify and have the appearance of a giant drusen. Additional findings of TS, including subependymal nodules and cortical tubers, are useful discriminators.

■ Additional Differential Diagnoses

- **Neoplasm.** Retinoblastoma is a malignant neoplasm of the retina and represents the most common globe tumor in children. Nearly all cases present prior to 5 years of age with leukocoria (white pupillary reflex) being the most common presenting sign. Approximately 75% are unilateral; the remainder are bilateral. Trilateral (bilateral globe plus pineal gland involvement) and quadrilateral (trilateral plus suprasellar involvement) disease is seen in familial cases. Unenhanced CT demonstrates a hyperdense globe mass with calcifications (95%). Globe size is normal to mildly increased. The mass is hyperintense on T1 and hypointense on T2 sequences with avid enhancement. Treatment options include chemotherapy, radiation, and enucleation. Choroidal osteomas are uncommon, benign tumors that calcify/ossify. The vast majority are solitary and unilateral, and they are more common in young adult women. CT reveals a focal or lentiform calcified mass along the posterior aspect of the globe at the choroidal-retinal junction. On magnetic resonance imaging, the lesions are typically hypointense on T2 and variable in signal on T1

sequences due to calcification/ossification. Avid enhancement is typically seen.
- **Foreign body.** Foreign bodies (FBs) occur in the setting of penetrating trauma or in patients with occupational exposures. Metallic FBs demonstrate increased density and streak artifact. They may be identified on plain radiography or CT. Nonmetallic FBs are less characteristic and most often demonstrate soft-tissue attenuation; wood may mimic air density. Associated findings of trauma should raise suspicion for a possible FB.
- **Phthisis bulbi.** Phthisis bulbi refers to end-stage ocular degeneration due to an underlying insult. Common causes include ocular trauma and myriad long-standing, infectious or inflammatory processes. Imaging demonstrates an irregular, shrunken globe with coarse calcifications. The calcifications may mimic an underlying mass; however, the combination of calcifications with a shrunken globe is characteristic of phthisis bulbi. Atrophy of the optic nerve is a helpful secondary finding that may be seen in chronic cases.

■ Diagnosis

Retinal hamartoma

✓ Pearls

- Scleral plaques occur in older patients, are degenerative, and are located at the EOM insertions onto the globe.
- ONHD occurs at the optic nerve insertion onto the globe and may mimic papilledema on fundoscopic exam.

- Retinal hamartomas frequently occur in the setting of TS and have the appearance of a giant drusen.
- Common neoplasms with calcification include retinoblastoma (malignancy in children) and choroidal osteoma.

Suggested Reading

LeBedis CA, Sakai O. Nontraumatic orbital conditions: diagnosis with CT and MR imaging in the emergent setting. Radiographics 2008; 28: 1741–1753

Case 225

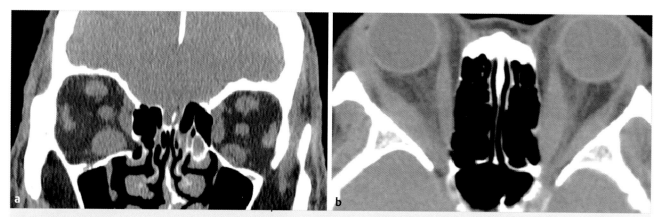

Fig. 225.1 Coronal CT image **(a)** demonstrates bilateral enlargement of the extraocular muscles, right greater than left, with more pronounced involvement of the inferior recti muscles. Axial CT in a different patient with the same diagnosis **(b)** reveals bilateral enlargement of the bellies of the recti musculature with sparing of the myotendinous junctions, as well as radiological proptosis.

■ Clinical Presentation

Middle-aged women with proptosis and the same underlying diagnosis (► Fig. 225.1)

■ Key Imaging Finding

Enlarged extraocular muscles

■ Top 3 Differential Diagnoses

- **Thyroid associated orbitopathy (TAO).** TAO, also known as Graves ophthalmopathy, is the most common cause of proptosis in adults. TAO is an autoimmune inflammatory condition characterized by enlargement of multiple extraocular muscle bellies with typical sparing of the myotendinous junctions. It is most commonly bilateral and preferentially affects the inferior > medial > superior > lateral > superior oblique muscles ("I'M SLOW" mnemonic). Increased orbital fat and lacrimal gland enlargement can also be seen. Look for stretching or compression of the optic nerve. TAO tends to affect young and middle-aged adults, women more so than men. Corticosteroid treatment is effective, but some will require surgical therapy for uncontrolled mass effect.
- **Orbital pseudotumor.** Orbital pseudotumor, the most common cause of a painful orbital mass in adults, is an idiopathic inflammatory disease, causing infiltrative or masslike soft-tissue enhancement involving any part of the orbit. Extra-ocular muscle (EOM) involvement, including the myotendinous junction, is the most common pattern. There may be involvement of multiple EOMs, but the findings are most commonly unilateral. When isolated lateral rectus muscle enlargement is seen, it is most likely due to orbital pseudotumor and essentially never due to thyroid orbitopathy. Other presentations include enlargement of the lacrimal gland and involvement of retro bulbar fat. Intracranial extension of pseudotumor into the cavernous sinus is known as Tolosa-Hunt syndrome.
- **Infectious myositis.** Infectious cellulitis-myositis may be a complication of sinonasal infection, most often involving the ethmoids. The most common finding is enlargement of the medial rectus muscle with associated ethmoid sinus disease. Secondary findings, in addition to adjacent sinus opacification, include subperiosteal abscess formation, osseous erosion or osteitis, and inflammatory intraorbital fat stranding.

■ Additional Differential Diagnoses

- **Neoplasm.** Neoplasms that may involve the EOMs include lymphoma, leukemia, rhabdomyosarcoma, and metastases. Lymphoma has many imaging manifestations but most commonly presents as a homogenously enhancing, painless, orbital mass in an elderly patient (> 60 years of age). It may also involve the lacrimal glands or occasionally the EOMs, simulating thyroid orbitopathy. Rhabdomyosarcoma is the most common soft-tissue sarcoma in childhood. The vast majority occur within orbital soft tissues, rather than within the EOMs. Lesions are isodense to muscle on computed tomography (CT), hypointense on T1, and hyperintense on T2 with moderately avid enhancement.
- **Sarcoidosis.** Approximately 25% of sarcoid patients have associated ophthalmic disease. The most common imaging findings include masslike lacrimal gland enlargement with enhance-ment, EOM enlargement, optic nerve thickening and enhancement, and orbital pseudotumor-like intraorbital masses. The most common presenting signs/symptoms include acute uveitis, chronic dacroadenitis, and lacrimal gland enlargement.
- **Vascular congestion.** High-flow arteriovenous shunting may result in increased intraorbital pressure and vascular congestion. Carotid-cavernous fistulas are the most common cause and consist of abnormal communications between the carotid artery and cavernous sinus. The vast majority are direct fistulas that result from trauma. Chemosis, pulsatile exophthalmos, and an orbital bruit are commonly found clinically. Magnetic resonance imaging demonstrates a convex lateral border of the cavernous sinus, increased cavernous sinus flow voids, enlarged ipsilateral superior ophthalmic vein and extraocular muscles, and proptosis.

■ Diagnosis

Thyroid-associated orbitopathy

✓ Pearls

- Thyroid orbitopathy is the most common cause of EOM enlargement; it is most often bilateral.
- Pseudotumor presents as a painful orbital mass; myotendinous junction involvement is characteristic.
- Infectious myositis is most commonly secondary to intraorbital extension from ethmoid sinus disease.
- Orbital lymphoma most commonly presents as an indolent painless mass in an elderly patient.

Suggested Reading

LeBedis CA, Sakai O. Nontraumatic orbital conditions: diagnosis with CT and MR imaging in the emergent setting. Radiographics 2008; 28: 1741–1753

Case 226

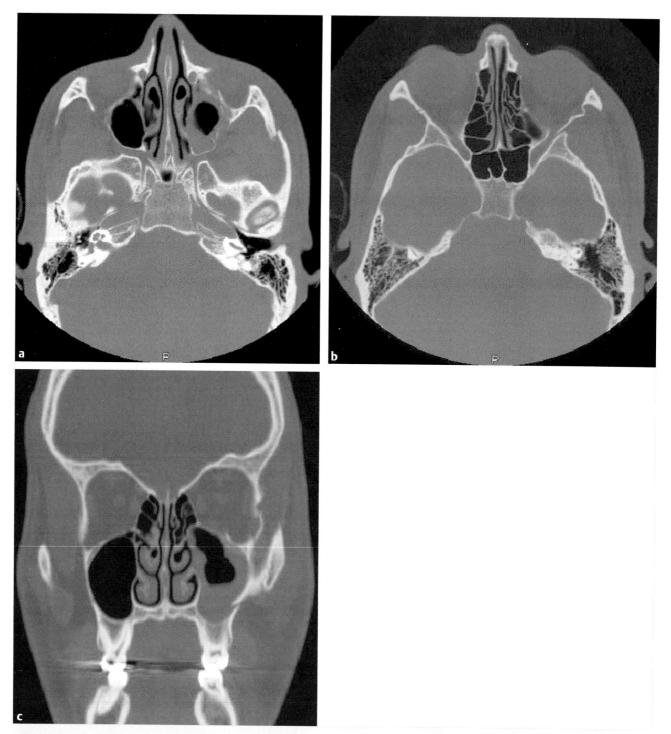

Fig. 226.1 Axial computed tomography image through the facial bones **(a)** demonstrates a fracture of the left lateral maxillary sinus wall that extends into the inferior orbital wall, as well as a displaced fracture of the zygomatic arch. An axial image more superior **(b)** reveals a fracture of the left lateral orbital wall. Coronal image **(c)** depicts fractures of the left inferior and lateral orbital walls, as well as the lateral maxillary sinus wall. Maxillary sinus opacification is seen **(a–c)**.

■ Clinical Presentation

An adult man with facial and orbital pain after trauma (▶ Fig. 226.1)

■ Key Imaging Finding

Orbital fracture

■ Top 3 Differential Diagnoses

- **Orbital wall blowout fracture.** An orbital wall blowout fracture results from a direct blow to the globe. Increased intraorbital pressure is transmitted to the thin orbital floor, resulting in a characteristic fracture pattern. A fracture fragment may protrude inferiorly into the maxillary sinus with a "trap door" appearance; a "Bombay door" configuration occurs with two fragments along the orbital floor. Intraorbital fat is usually displaced inferiorly into the maxillary sinus, and there is often a hyperdense air-fluid level within the sinus due to hemorrhage. The inferior rectus muscle may extend into or through the site of fracture, resulting in muscle entrapment. Imaging findings suggestive of clinical entrapment include a focal change in course or contour of the rectus musculature in the region of fracture. It is important to evaluate for globe injury, as well as additional orbital and facial fractures. A fracture through the medial orbital wall (lamina papyracea) results in herniation of orbital fat into the ethmoid sinus with associated hemorrhage; entrapment of the medial rectus muscle may be seen.
- **Zygomaticomaxillary complex fracture.** A zygomaticomaxillary complex fracture (also referred to as a tripod fracture) is a common facial fracture that is caused by a direct blow to the zygomatic bone. The fractures involve the zygomatic arch and inferior and lateral orbital walls, resulting in disassociation of the anterior zygoma from the remainder of the facial bones. Patients commonly present with facial swelling, a localized deformity, and, occasionally, the inability to open the jaw due to impingement upon the mandibular coronoid process from the fracture fragment.
- **Le Fort fracture.** Le Fort fractures are characterized by some form of facial disassociation as a result of bilateral fractures and are categorized into three major subtypes. All subtypes involve fractures of the pterygoid plates. Le Fort I fractures occur through the maxillary bone below the orbital floor. There may be extension into one or both maxillary sinuses. The inferior portion of the maxilla below the fracture site is disassociated from the remainder of the facial bones. In Le Fort II fractures, the fracture is pyramidal in shape, involving the bilateral maxilla and converging superiorly and medially through the inferior and medial orbital walls and nasal bridge. The nasal bridge and maxilla below the fracture is disassociated from the remainder of the facial bones. The Le Fort III fracture is the most severe and is characterized by complete craniofacial disassociation. This complex set of fractures involves the bilateral zygomaticofrontal sutures, the nasofrontal suture, and the lateral, medial, and inferior orbital walls. Pure Le Fort-type fractures as described are unusual; most fractures are complex with components of different subtypes.

■ Diagnosis

Zygomaticomaxillary complex (tripod) fracture

✓ Pearls

- Orbital wall blowout fractures are due to a direct blow to the globe; muscle entrapment may be seen.
- Zygomaticomaxillary complex fractures involve the zygoma, inferior orbital wall, and lateral orbital wall.
- Le Fort fractures are characterized by varying degrees of facial disassociation; type III is the most severe.

Suggested Reading

Dolan KD, Jacoby CG, Smoker WR. The radiology of facial fractures. Radiographics 1984; 4: 575–663

Betts AM, O'Brien WT, Davies BW, Youssef OH. A systemic approach to CT evaluation of orbital trauma. Emerg Radiol 2014; 21(5): 511–531

Case 227

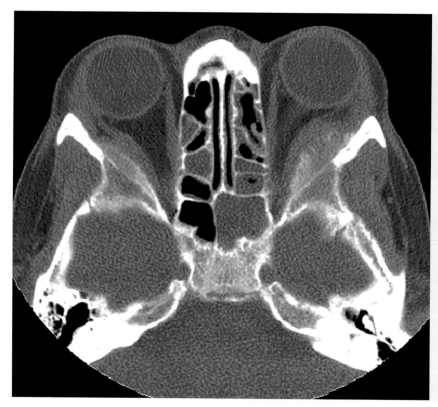

Fig. 227.1 Axial CT image demonstrates abnormal spiculated sclerosis along the left lateral orbital wall with periosteal reaction in a "sunburst" pattern. There is inward displacement of the lateral rectus muscle and mild proptosis. Less pronounced periosteal reaction is noted along the inner margin of the right lateral orbital wall with inward displacement of the lateral rectus muscle. There is paranasal sinus opacification involving the left sphenoid and bilateral ethmoid sinuses. (Courtesy of Rocky Saenz, DO.)

▓ Clinical Presentation

A patient with progressive diplopia (▶ Fig. 227.1)

▧ Key Imaging Finding

Sclerotic orbital wall mass

▧ Top 3 Differential Diagnoses

- **Intraosseous meningioma.** Although meningiomas represent the most common intracranial extraaxial masses, intraosseous meningiomas are quite rare. As with dural-based meningiomas, the intraosseous variant occurs most often in adult women. The orbits, paranasal sinuses, and facial bones are commonly involved locations in the head and neck. Computed tomography (CT) reveals focal bony expansion with sclerosis, mixed sclerosis and lucency, or "ground glass" attenuation. Cortical thickening may also be seen. The margin of the inner table is typically irregular, which is a distinguishing feature from fibrous dysplasia (FD) but may mimic an underlying malignant lesion. This entity differs from the benign, smooth, bony reactive changes or hyperostosis associated with an underlying extraaxial meningioma that is far more common.
- **Fibrous dysplasia.** FD occurs most often in young adults and is more common in women. The calvarium, skull base, and facial bones are most often affected in the head and neck. The classic appearance on CT is focal bony expansion with ground glass attenuation of the diploic space; sclerotic and cystic or lytic variants are less common. The inner margin is smooth (in contrast to meningioma and malignant lesions) and typically does not demonstrate significant cortical thickening (in contrast to Paget disease). On magnetic resonance imaging (MRI), FD is typically hypointense on both T1 and T2 sequences and demonstrates avid enhancement; regions of cystic involvement, however, are T2 hyperintense. The MRI appearance can mimic aggressive lesions; therefore, CT is preferred in suspected cases of FD.
- **Malignancy.** Metastatic disease commonly involves the calvarium. Typically, lesions present as soft-tissue infiltration or soft-tissue masses with bony destruction; focal sclerosis is less common. Malignancies prone to sclerotic metastases include neuroblastoma in children, prostate and breast carcinoma in adults, and lymphoma at any age. Neuroblastoma has a predilection for the sphenoid bone/lateral orbital wall. Primary bone tumors are less common and include Ewing sarcoma in children and osteosarcoma in young adults or the elderly with a history of Paget disease or prior radiation therapy. Both Ewing and osteosarcoma present as focal, aggressive bone-forming tumors with periosteal reaction on CT; lytic lesions are less common. MRI most often reveals intermediate T1 and T2 signal intensity with avid but heterogeneous enhancement; calcified portions are hypointense.

▧ Additional Differential Diagnoses

- **Paget disease.** Paget disease occurs in elderly patients and consists of three stages: lytic, sclerotic, and mixed. Calvarial involvement during the lytic phase results in a characteristic large lytic lesion with erosion of the outer table, referred to as osteoporosis circumscripta. During the sclerotic phase, there is expansion and sclerosis of the cortex and diploic spaces, which may be diffuse or focal. In the mixed phase, a combination of lytic and sclerotic lesions results in the characteristic "cotton wool" appearance of the skull.

▧ Diagnosis

Malignancy (neuroblastoma metastases)

✓ Pearls

- Intraosseous meningioma presents with bony expansion, increased density, and irregularity of the inner table.
- FD occurs in young adults; the classic appearance is focal bony expansion with "ground glass" attenuation.
- Primary and metastatic malignancies may involve the orbital wall, especially neuroblastoma in children.
- Paget disease occurs in elderly patients with bony/cortical expansion and lytic, sclerotic, or mixed attenuation.

Suggested Readings

Daffner RH, Yakulis R, Maroon JC. Intraosseous meningioma. Skeletal Radiol 1998; 27: 108–111

D'Ambrosio N, Lyo JK, Young RJ, Haque SS, Karimi S. Imaging of metastatic CNS neuroblastoma. Am J Roentgenol 2010; 194: 1223–1229

Case 228

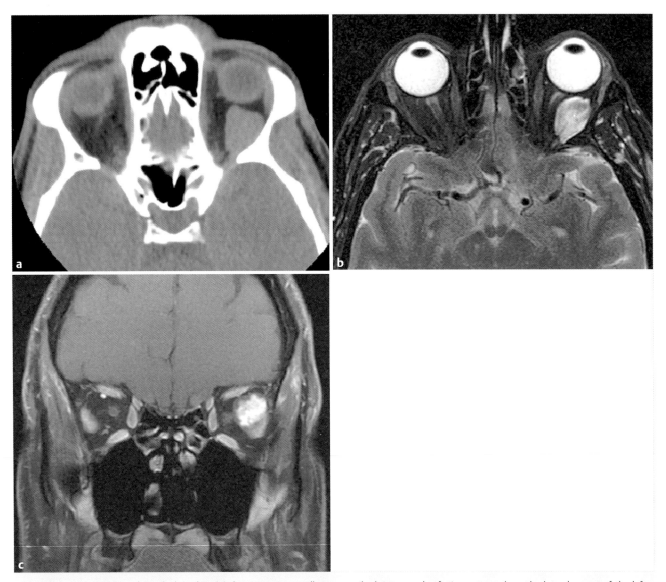

Fig. 228.1 Axial CT image through the orbits **(a)** demonstrates a well-circumscribed, intraconal soft-tissue mass along the lateral aspect of the left orbit. Axial T2 MR image with fat suppression **(b)** shows diffuse heterogeneous but predominantly increased signal intensity. Coronal T1 postcontrast image **(c)** with fat suppression reveals avid enhancement of the mass, as well as its intraconal location and medial displacement of the optic nerve sheath complex.

■ Clinical Presentation

A 52-year-old man with noncontrast head computed tomography (CT) performed for headaches (▶ Fig. 228.1)

▨ Key Imaging Finding

Circumscribed, enhancing orbital mass

▣ Top 3 Differential Diagnoses

- **Cavernous hemangioma.** Orbital cavernous hemangiomas are truly non-neoplastic, encapsulated vascular malformations (VMs). They represent the most common intraorbital masses and often present with proptosis or pain. Lesions are well-circumscribed a with round, oval, or lobulated configuration. Most commonly, they are intraconal and retrobulbar in location, although they may occur anywhere within the orbit. They are typically hyperdense on CT, hypointense on T1, and hyperintense on T2 magnetic resonance imaging (MRI) sequences. Intense enhancement is the rule. Calcifications are occasionally seen and are characteristic. Larger lesions may remodel adjacent bony structures.
- **Lymphatic malformation.** Orbital lymphatic malformations are benign hamartomatous lesions that occur in children and young adults. Patients typically present with proptosis as the lesion enlarges. Although they most commonly involve the extraconal compartment, orbital lymphatic malformations may involve any and multiple compartments. They are typically multilocular, cystic, and prone to hemorrhage. Fluid-fluid levels are common and characteristic after episodes of hemorrhage. Enhancement of septations is typically seen.
- **Meningioma.** Orbital meningiomas most often occur in middle-aged women; they may also occasionally occur in children with neurofibromatosis type 2 (NF2). Extraconal involvement is typically due to intraorbital spread from a sphenoid wing or cavernous sinus meningioma. Optic nerve sheath meningiomas, on the other hand, are true intraconal lesions that typically do not extend intracranially, a differentiating feature from an optic nerve glioma. Meningiomas enhance avidly and may have calcifications. The enhancement pattern is characterized as a "tram track" configuration on axial images (bright nerve sheath/meningioma enhancement peripherally and hypodense [CT] or hypointense [T1 MRI] optic nerve centrally). Meningiomas commonly are associated with hyperostosis.

▨ Additional Differential Diagnoses

- **Metastases.** Metastases may involve any portion of the orbit, including the bony orbit, globe, intraconal, and extraconal spaces. Breast and lung cancer are the most common primary tumors in adults, followed by prostate, gastrointestinal, genitourinary, and soft-tissue sarcomas. In children, neuroblastoma, leukemia, Wilms tumor, and Ewing sarcoma are most common. Larger lesions may result in proptosis and loss of visual acuity.
- **Lymphoma.** Lymphoma usually involves the orbit secondarily and is of the non-Hodgkin variant. Patients are often elderly and present with proptosis or painless swelling. Lymphomatous infiltrates are commonly well-circumscribed and may be bilateral, a helpful distinguishing feature. CT may show increased density with enhancement. Lesions are low to intermediate in signal intensity on T1 and variable in signal intensity on T2 sequences. Common areas of involvement include the lacrimal gland and superior aspect of the orbit.
- **Nerve sheath tumor.** Both schwannomas and neurofibromas may occur within the orbit. Schwannomas are usually more heterogeneous and prone to cystic degeneration. They are often intermediate in signal intensity on T1 and hyperintense on T2 sequences with heterogeneous but avid enhancement. Neurofibromas are generally more homogeneous but less well defined and typically occur in the setting of NF1; they are commonly multiple and bilateral. MRI reveals an intermediate T1 and hyperintense T2 signal intensity mass with heterogeneous enhancement. The "target" sign, characterized by central decreased and peripheral increased T2 signal intensity, is more frequently seen with neurofibromas than schwannomas.

▨ Diagnosis

Cavernous hemangioma

✓ Pearls

- Cavernous hemangiomas/VMs are the most common orbital masses, intensely enhance, and may have calcifications.
- Lymphatic malformations are often multilocular cystic lesions; hemorrhagic fluid-fluid levels are characteristic.
- Extraconal meningiomas involve the orbit secondarily; intraconal meningiomas occur along the optic nerve.
- Metastases and lymphoma involve the orbit secondarily and may involve multiple orbital structures.

Suggested Reading

Tanak A, Mihara F, Yoshiura T. et al. Differentiation of cavernous hemangioma from schwannoma of the orbit. Am J Roentgenol 2004; 183: 1799–1804

Case 229

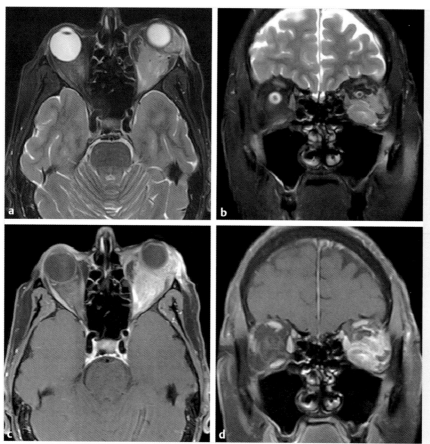

Fig. 229.1 Axial **(a)** and coronal **(b)** T2 images with fat suppression reveal an ill-defined left orbital mass that is intermediate in signal intensity and involves intraconal structures, the inferior and lateral rectus muscles, and portions of the extraconal space inferiorly and laterally. There is visible proptosis **(a–c)**, as well as displacement and asymmetric cerebrospinal fluid effacement of the optic nerve sheath complex on the left **(b)**. Axial **(c)** and coronal **(d)** postcontrast T1 images with fat suppression demonstrate diffuse, avid enhancement of the infiltrative mass.

■ Clinical Presentation

An adult woman with proptosis (▶ Fig. 229.1)

■ Key Imaging Finding

Infiltrative orbital lesion in an adult

■ Top 3 Differential Diagnoses

- **Orbital pseudotumor.** Orbital pseudotumor, also referred to as idiopathic orbital inflammatory disease, is the most common cause of a painful orbital mass in adults. It commonly presents with infiltrative or masslike soft-tissue enhancement involving any part of the orbit or with extraocular muscle enlargement that includes the myotendinous junction; when isolated lateral rectus muscle enlargement is seen, it is most likely due to orbital pseudotumor and essentially never due to thyroid orbitopathy. Other presentations include enlargement of the lacrimal gland and involvement of retro bulbar fat. Intracranial extension of pseudotumor into the cavernous sinus is known as Tolosa-Hunt syndrome.
- **Leukemia/lymphoma.** Orbital involvement of leukemia and lymphoma has a variety of presentations, which include ill-defined infiltration of the intra- and/or extraconal spaces or a well-defined enhancing mass that is typically extraconal in location. Lacrimal gland involvement is also common. Because lymphoproliferative disorders are systemic processes,

lesions may be unilateral or bilateral. Lesions enhance fairly avidly. T2 magnetic resonance imaging (MRI) signal varies, ranging from hypo- to hyperintense depending upon the cellularity of the lesion.

- **Granulomatous process.** Sarcoidosis and Wegener granulomatosis commonly involve orbital structures. Sarcoidosis is a systemic disease characterized by noncaseating granulomas; Wegener granulomatosis is a systemic vasculitis that primarily affects the kidneys and respiratory tract. Both processes often present with ill-defined and infiltrative enhancing orbital masses; scleral involvement is also commonly seen. Additional findings of sarcoid include optic nerve involvement and abnormal intracranial meningeal enhancement. Secondary findings for Wegener granulomatosis include adjacent sinus involvement with bony erosions. Soft-tissue lesions on MRI are variable but commonly demonstrate intermediate to hypointense T1 and T2 signal intensity with enhancement.

■ Additional Differential Diagnoses

- **Infectious process.** Orbital infections may result from adjacent sinonasal infections, hematogenous spread of a distant infection, direct spread from an overlying cellulitis, or in cases of trauma or iatrogenia. Fungal infections are more common in immunocompromised patients. Periorbital cellulitis refers to infection involving the preseptal soft tissues; orbital cellulitis refers to postseptal extension of the infectious process. The orbital septum consists of fibrous tissue that extends from the anterior bony periosteum of the orbit to the palprebal soft tissues. It is a barrier to the spread of infection from superficial preseptal soft tissues into the orbital compartment. Patients with postseptal orbital cellulitis commonly present with proptosis, ophthalmoplegia, altered visual acuity, and chemosis. Imaging reveals inflammatory changes with fatty infiltration and ill-defined regions of enhancement. Focal abscesses demonstrate central fluid attenuation or

signal intensity with rim enhancement. Complications include vision loss, thrombosis of the superior ophthalmic vein, and intracranial spread of the infectious process, all of which should be interrogated on cross-sectional imaging.

- **Metastases.** Metastases may involve any portion of the orbit, including the bony orbit, globe, intraconal, and extraconal spaces. Breast and lung cancer are most common in adults, followed by prostate, gastrointestinal, genitourinary, and soft-tissue sarcomas. Schirrhous breast metastases may result in progressive enophthalmos. In children, neuroblastoma, leukemia, Wilms tumor, and Ewing sarcoma represent the most common primary neoplasms with orbital involvement. Intraorbital lesions may be well defined or ill defined with infiltrative enhancement. Larger lesions may result in proptosis and loss of visual acuity.

■ Diagnosis

Orbital lymphoma

✓ Pearls

- Orbital pseudotumor commonly presents with infiltrative or masslike soft-tissue enhancement.
- Lymphoproliferative processes have a variety of presentations, including ill- or well-defined orbital masses.

- Sarcoidosis and Wegener granulomatosis are systemic processes that often have helpful secondary findings.
- Patients with orbital cellulitis often present with fatty infiltration and ill-defined regions of enhancement.

Suggested Reading

Müller-Forell W, Pitz S. Orbital pathology. Eur J Radiol 2004; 49: 105–142

Case 230

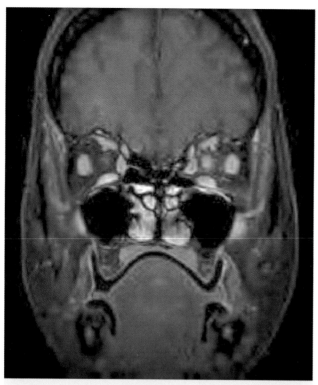

Fig. 230.1 Coronal T1 postcontrast image with fat suppression demonstrates diffuse enlargement and abnormal enhancement involving the left optic nerve with some mild adjacent inflammatory changes. There is normal enhancement of the extraocular muscles.

■ Clinical Presentation

A young adult woman with visual changes (► Fig. 230.1)

▨ Key Imaging Finding

Optic nerve enlargement and enhancement

▨ Top 3 Differential Diagnoses

- **Optic neuritis.** Optic neuritis is most often due to demyelination secondary to an autoimmune or viral process. Other etiologies include ocular infection, toxic or metabolic degeneration, ischemia, or meningitis/encephalitis. Multiple sclerosis (MS) involves the optic nerve in roughly one-third of cases. Approximately one-half to three-fourths of patients who present with their first episode of optic neuritis will develop MS within 15 years. Patients present with ipsilateral orbital pain with eye movement and vision loss that occurs over hours to days. Magnetic resonance imaging (MRI) demonstrates abnormal increased T2/fluid-attenuated inversion recovery signal intensity within the affected optic nerve, best visualized on coronal sequences. Postcontrast studies may reveal abnormal optic nerve enlargement and enhancement. In chronic stages, the optic nerve may become atrophic.
- **Optic nerve glioma.** Optic nerve gliomas are low-grade neoplasms (typically juvenile pilocytic astrocytomas) that most often occur between 5 and 15 years of age; they are a common cause of optic nerve enlargement in children. Patients present with vision loss with or without proptosis. Optic nerve gliomas may occur sporadically or be associated with neurofibromatosis type 1 (NF1); bilateral optic nerve involvement is pathognomonic for NF1. Tumors cause enlargement, elongation and "buckling" of the optic nerve, resulting in the

"dotted i" sign on axial images. Enlargement and benign bony remodeling of the optic canal may also be seen. The enhancement pattern is variable. Optic nerve gliomas may extend along the optic pathways (optic chiasm, tracts, and radiations). NF1 predominantly involves the optic nerve with preservation of nerve morphology. Non-NF1 cases most often involve the optic chiasm or hypothalamus, are larger and more masslike, commonly have cystic degeneration, and may extend beyond the optic pathways.
- **Optic nerve sheath meningioma.** Meningiomas arise from arachnoid rests in the meninges covering the optic nerve. Eighty percent occur in women and typically present in the fourth decade of life with progressive loss of vision (optic nerve atrophy). They may occur as tubular (most common), fusiform, or eccentric masses associated with the optic nerve. The lesions may be hyperdense on computed tomography; calcification is common (20 to 25%). On MRI, they are typically isointense to gray matter on T1 and variable in signal on T2 sequences. Enhancement is intense and relatively homogeneous. The "tram track" sign on postcontrast imaging represents linear bands of enhancement surrounding the central nonenhancing optic nerve. Sphenoid bone and/or optic canal hyperostosis may be seen.

▨ Additional Differential Diagnoses

- **Leukemia/lymphoma.** Leukemia and non-Hodgkin lymphoma may involve the orbit in a variety of presentations. Involvement of the optic nerve sheath complex with regions of enhancement is the least common manifestation. When present, lesions are often (but not exclusively) bilateral.
- **Sarcoidosis.** Sarcoidosis is a systemic process characterized by noncaseating granulomas. Symptomatic central nervous

system involvement (neurosarcoidosis) occurs in approximately 5% of sarcoidosis patients. Isolated optic nerve involvement is rare but should be considered in the differential diagnosis of an optic nerve lesion. Varying degrees and patterns of enhancement are seen, but nodular enhancement is most common.

▨ Diagnosis

Optic neuritis

✓ Pearls

- Optic neuritis is commonly due to demyelination; the majority of patients will develop MS within 15 years.
- Optic nerve gliomas are common causes of nerve enlargement in children; they are often associated with NF1.

- Optic nerve sheath meningiomas occur most often in women and demonstrate "tram track" enhancement.

Suggested Readings

LeBedis CA, Sakai O. Nontraumatic orbital conditions: diagnosis with CT and MR imaging in the emergent setting. Radiographics 2008; 28: 1741–1753

Kornreich L, Blaser S, Schwarz M et al. Optic pathway glioma: correlation of imaging findings with the presence of neurofibromatosis. Am J Neuroradiol 2001; 22: 1963–1969

Case 231

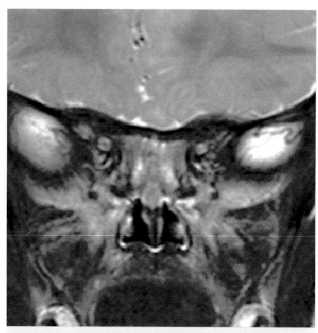

Fig. 231.1 Coronal T2 MR image through the orbits reveals decreased caliber of the optic nerves, significantly more so on the left, without appreciable abnormal signal intensity.

■ Clinical Presentation

A young boy with decreased visual acuity, more pronounced on the left (▶ Fig. 231.1)

■ **Key Imaging Finding**

Small-caliber optic nerve(s)

■ **Top 2 Differential Diagnoses**

• **Optic nerve atrophy.** Optic nerve atrophy is often the end result of chronic optic nerve injury, typically associated with long-standing optic neuritis. In children and young adults, demyelinating processes are the most common etiology, whereas ischemic neuropathy is the most common cause in middle-aged and older adults and is more pronounced in the setting of diabetes mellitus, hypertension, and hyperlipidemia. Acutely, optic neuritis typically presents with optic nerve edema, abnormal signal intensity, and mild nerve enlargement on magnetic resonance imaging (MRI). Enhancement is commonly seen, especially during periods of active injury or inflammation. Chronically, there is optic nerve volume loss; the presence of abnormal signal or enhancement is variable in late-stage disease. Perineural inflammation or neuritis may be seen with both acute and chronic disease.

• **Optic nerve hypoplasia.** Optic nerve hypoplasia (ONH) refers to congenital underdevelopment of the optic nerve. It is more often bilateral and is commonly associated with additional central nervous system malformations or syndromes, including septooptic dysplasia (SOD). Optic symptoms present in early childhood and include loss of visual acuity, nystagmus, and strabismus. Nonorbital symptoms are dependent upon additional underlying malformations but commonly include developmental delay and endocrinopathies because hypothalamic-pituitary anomalies are commonly associated with optic nerve hypoplasia and SOD. MRI is the imaging modality of choice and demonstrates decreased caliber of one or both optic nerves and the optic chiasm. In the setting of SOD, the septum pellucidum is partially or completely absent; schizencephaly, pituitary hypoplasia, and an ectopic posterior pituitary are often coexistent. Cortical malformations, heterotopias, and complete or partial agenesis of the corpus callosum may be seen.

■ **Diagnosis**

Optic nerve hypoplasia (SOD)

✓ **Pearls**

• Optic nerve atrophy is often the end result of chronic optic nerve injury, typically long-standing optic neuritis.

• Demyelinating disease occurs more often in younger patients; ischemic neuropathy occurs in older adults.

• ONH refers to underdevelopment of the optic nerve, is most often bilateral, and is associated with SOD.

Suggested Reading

Barkovich AJ, Fram EK, Norman D. Septo-optic dysplasia: MR imaging. Radiology 1989; 171: 189–192

Case 232

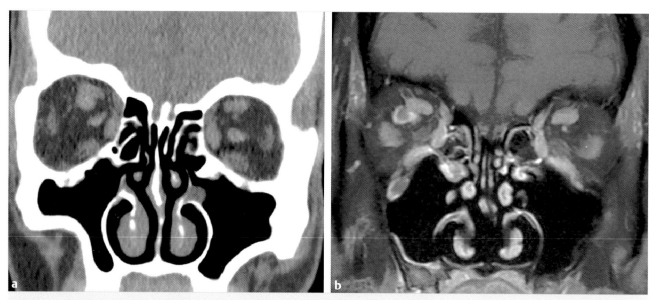

Fig. 232.1 Coronal unenhanced CT image **(a)** demonstrates significant enlargement of the right superior ophthalmic vein compared with the left. Coronal postcontrast T1 weighted MR image with fat suppression **(b)** reveals central decreased signal intensity within the right superior ophthalmic vein with peripheral enhancement.

■ Clinical Presentation

A 70-year-old man with eye pain, headache, and loss of visual acuity (▶ Fig. 232.1)

▧ Key Imaging Finding

Superior ophthalmic vein enlargement

■ Top 3 Differential Diagnoses

- **Venous/cavernous sinus thrombosis.** Cavernous sinus thrombosis most often results from extension of an adjacent infectious or inflammatory process, typically involving the orbits or sinonasal cavities. Contrast-enhanced computed tomography (CT) or magnetic resonance imaging (MRI) reveals enlargement and decreased enhancement within the thrombosed cavernous sinus. Peripheral enhancement is commonly seen. In the subacute phase, thrombus is typically hyperintense on T1 and T2 MRI sequences. Increased venous and orbital pressures result in exophthalmos and enlargement of the superior ophthalmic vein (SOV). SOV thrombosis may result from extension of cavernous sinus thrombosis, secondary occlusion from mass effect or an infectious/inflammatory process, or a hypercoagulable state. Contrast-enhanced studies typically reveal enlargement and lack of enhancement within the SOV.
- **Carotid-cavernous fistula (CCF).** CCFs refer to abnormal communications between the carotid artery and cavernous sinus. They are classified as direct (more common) or indirect. Direct CCFs are high-flow arteriovenous shunts with rapid presentation of symptoms, including pulsatile exophthalmos, orbital bruit, chemosis, and, occasionally, intracranial hemorrhage. The vast majority result from trauma; rupture of a cavernous carotid aneurysm is a much less common cause. Indirect CCFs are slow-flow shunts between dural branches of the internal or external carotid artery and the cavernous sinus. They most often occur spontaneously and have a more insidious onset of symptoms. Increased venous pressure associated with CCFs results in enlargement of the cavernous sinus and the ipsilateral SOV. MRI demonstrates a convex lateral border of the cavernous sinus, increased cavernous sinus flow voids, enlarged ipsilateral SOV and extraocular muscles (EOMs), and proptosis. Cavernous sinus enlargement may be bilateral because there are venous communications with the contralateral side. Angiography demonstrates early venous filling in the arterial phase. Endovascular treatment options are favored and include glue or coil embolization.
- **Venous varix.** Varices represent congenital malformations with enlargement of venous structures. In the orbit, the superior ophthalmic vein is most commonly involved. Patients may be asymptomatic or present with proptosis that is worsened by Valsalva maneuver. Contrast-enhanced CT or MRI reveals focal or diffuse enlargement and enhancement of the involved venous structures; prominent flow voids are seen on T2 sequences. Identifying vascular continuity is the key to distinguishing varices from other nonvascular, enhancing orbital masses. Occasionally, phleboliths may be present and are best depicted on CT. Complications include venous thrombosis and variceal hemorrhage.

■ Additional Differential Diagnoses

- **Normal variant.** Occasionally, SOVs may be asymmetrically prominent, making the distinction between a normal variant and pathological enlargement difficult. However, normal variation is asymptomatic. Careful evaluation should be made to exclude abnormalities of the orbit and cavernous sinus that may lead to SOV enlargement prior to a presumptive diagnosis of a normal variant; follow-up imaging may be beneficial.
- **Increased intracranial or intraorbital pressure.** Elevated intracranial or intraorbital pressures may lead to SOV enlargement. Secondary findings of increased intracranial pressure include diffuse sulcal and cisternal effacement. Increased intraorbital pressure may be due to underlying orbital or cavernous sinus masses or infiltrative or inflammatory processes or the orbit, such as Grave's orbitopathy and orbital pseudotumor.

■ Diagnosis

Venous thrombosis

✓ Pearls

- Cavernous sinus thrombosis presents with enlargement and decreased enhancement within the cavernous sinus.
- CCFs present with cavernous sinus enlargement, flow voids, enlarged SOV and EOMs, and proptosis.
- Varices refer to congenital venous enlargement that is worsened by Valsalva maneuver.

Suggested Readings

Poon CS, Sze G, Johnson MH. Orbital lesions: differentiating vascular and non-vascular etiologic factors. Am J Roentgenol 2008; 190: 956–965

Razek AA, Castillo M. Imaging lesions of the cavernous sinus. Am J Neuroradiol 2009; 30: 444–452

Case 233

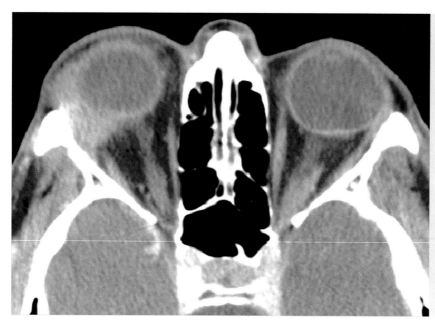

Fig. 233.1 Axial contrast-enhanced CT image through the orbits demonstrates diffuse enlargement of the right lacrimal gland, including the orbital and palpebral lobes, with enhancement.

■ **Clinical Presentation**

A 55-year-old woman with proptosis (▶ Fig. 233.1)

■ Key Imaging Finding

Lacrimal gland enlargement and enhancement

■ Top 3 Differential Diagnoses

- **Infectious dacryoadenitis.** The lacrimal gland is responsible for tear production and sits in the anterior superolateral aspect of the orbit along the margin of the superior and lateral rectus muscles. It is composed of an orbital lobe posteriorly and a palpebral lobe anteriorly. Infectious dacryoadenitis is an inflammatory process of the lacrimal gland that most often affects children and young adults; it is typically a unilateral process. Cross-sectional imaging demonstrates diffuse enlargement of the gland with increased enhancement. There are often surrounding inflammatory changes involving the orbital fat. Bony structures are typically normal.
- **Epithelial neoplasm.** Pleomorphic adenoma is the most common primary epithelial tumor of the lacrimal gland and typically involves the orbital lobe. It results in unilateral gland enlargement with proptosis. Computed tomography (CT) reveals a well-circumscribed enhancing mass, often with benign bony remodeling. Magnetic resonance imaging (MRI) reveals a hypo- to isointense T1 and intermediate to hyperintense T2 mass (compared with rectus musculature) with

moderate enhancement. Treatment requires complete surgical resection; recurrences are common. Adenoid cystic carcinoma (ACC) and mucoepidermoid carcinoma are malignant epithelial tumors and are less common. They tend to be infiltrative, grow rapidly, diffusely enhance, and result in overlying bony erosion. ACC is prone to perineural spread.
- **Lymphoproliferative lesion.** Lymphoid hyperplasia refers to a benign lymphoproliferative process that may affect the lacrimal glands. It is typically bilateral and symmetric with involvement of both orbital and palpebral lobes. Although it may be indistinguishable from lymphoma on imaging, it tends to be more heterogeneous in signal intensity and enhancement, whereas lymphoma is more homogeneous. Lymphoma may be unilateral or bilateral (more common) and is isodense compared with musculature on CT, with mild, homogeneous enhancement. On MRI, lymphoma is T1 isointense and variable in T2 signal intensity; restricted diffusion may be seen due to increased cellularity. Leukemia may appear similar and often involves overlying bony structures.

■ Additional Differential Diagnoses

- **Sarcoid.** Sarcoid is a systemic disease characterized by noncaseating granulomas. It represents the most common noninfectious inflammatory process of the lacrimal glands. Common orbital findings include uveitis and bilateral, symmetric lacrimal gland enlargement, typically involving both orbital and palpebral lobes, with increased enhancement. Lacrimal glands are isointense on T1 and hyperintense on T2 sequences compared with musculature. Look for interstitial lung disease with or without lymphadenopathy on chest X-ray or CT.
- **Sjögren syndrome.** Sjögren syndrome is an autoimmune disease that most commonly occurs in middle-aged to elderly women and results in lymphocytic infiltration of lacrimal and salivary glands. Patients classically present with keratoconjunctivitis sicca (dry eyes) and xerostomia (dry mouth). Early lacrimal gland involvement demonstrates bilateral, symmet-

ric gland enlargement involving both orbital and palpebral lobes with heterogeneous enhancement. Chronically, there is gland atrophy with regions of fatty replacement. Parotid glands may also be enlarged with scattered enhancing nodules and fluid pockets.
- **Orbital pseudotumor.** Orbital pseudotumor, the most common cause of a painful orbital mass in adults, is an idiopathic inflammatory disease that may involve any part of the orbit. Extraocular muscle involvement, including the myotendinous junction, is the most common pattern. Lacrimal gland involvement is less common and may be unilateral (most common) or bilateral. Imaging reveals gland enlargement involving orbital and palpebral lobes with variable enhancement. Lesions are typically iso- to hypointense on T1 and T2 sequences.

■ Diagnosis

Lymphoma

✓ Pearls

- Infectious dacryoadenitis, epithelial neoplasms, and orbital pseudotumor tend to be unilateral processes.
- Lymphoproliferative lesions, sarcoid, and Sjögren syndrome more often occur in a bilateral, symmetric fashion.

- Lymphoma may be unilateral or bilateral; pleomorphic adenoma is the most common primary epithelial tumor.

Suggested Reading

Gao Y, Moonis G, Cunnane ME, Eisenberg RL. Lacrimal gland masses. Am J Roentgenol 2013; 201: W371–81

Case 234

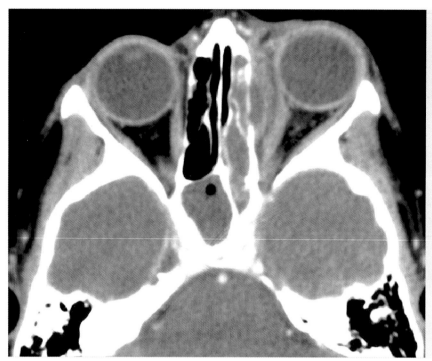

Fig. 234.1 Contrast-enhanced axial computed tomography image demonstrates opacification of the sphenoid and left ethmoid sinuses with a hypodense collection along the medial aspect of the left orbit/lamina papyracea. There is lateral deviation of the left medial rectus muscle and mild propotosis.

■ Clinical Presentation

A young boy with facial pain and visual difficulties (▶ Fig. 234.1)

▦ Key Imaging Finding

Hypodense collection along the medial orbit/lamina papyracea

▦ Diagnosis

Subperiosteal abscess. Imaging, particularly contrast-enhanced computed tomography, plays a key role in the evaluation of orbital infections because the clinical distinction between periorbital and orbital cellulitis is difficult. Periorbital cellulitis refers to infection involving the preseptal soft tissues; orbital cellulitis refers to postseptal extension of the infectious process. The orbital septum consists of fibrous tissue that extends from the anterior bony periosteum of the orbit to the palprebal soft tissues. It serves as a barrier to the spread of infection from superficial preseptal soft tissues into the orbital compartment.

The distinction between preseptal and postseptal infections is important, as preseptal cellulitis may be treated on an outpatient basis with oral antibiotics, whereas postseptal infections often require intravenous antibiotic therapy and occasional drainage of the infectious collections. Both groups of patients commonly present with periorbital soft-tissue swelling and erythema. Patients with orbital cellulitis may also have proptosis, ophthalmoplegia, altered visual acuity, and chemosis.

Orbital cellulitis most often results from the spread of ethmoid sinusitis into the orbit; trauma or postoperative causes of orbital cellulitis are less common. Subperiosteal abscesses from ethmoid sinusitis typically present as hypodense collections along the medial aspect of the orbit/lamina papyracea in the extraconal space. Surrounding inflammatory changes may be seen within the orbital fat. Bony destruction is not generally seen because the infection spreads via perivascular routes. Associated mass effect and increased intraorbital pressure commonly results in proptosis. Complications include vision loss, thrombosis of the superior ophthalmic vein, and intracranial spread of the infectious process, all of which should be interrogated on cross-sectional imaging.

✓ Pearls

- Imaging plays a key role in the distinction between periorbital (preseptal) and orbital (postseptal) cellulitis.
- Preseptal cellulitis is treated in an outpatient setting; postseptal infections require intravenous antibiotics and possible drainage.

- Subperiosteal abscesses (most often from ethmoid sinusitis) present as collections along the medial orbit.
- Complications include vision loss, venous thrombosis, and intracranial spread of the infectious process.

Suggested Reading

LeBedis CA, Sakai O. Nontraumatic orbital conditions: diagnosis with CT and MR imaging in the emergent setting. Radiographics 2008; 28: 1741–1753

Case 235

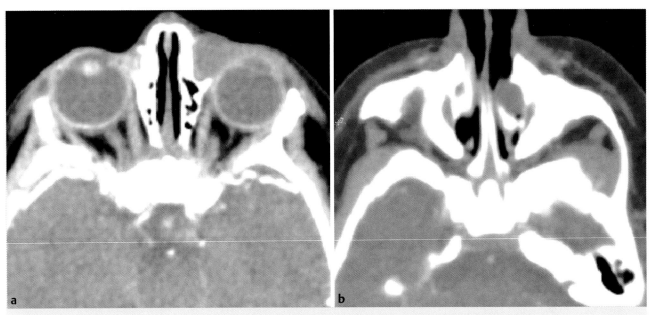

Fig. 235.1 Contrast-enhanced axial CT images **(a,b)** demonstrate a fluid attenuation lesion expanding the NLD in the region of the medial canthus **(a)** and extending into the nasal cavity **(b)**. The lesion causes mass effect on the left globe with associated asymmetry in orientation of the lens.

■ Clinical Presentation

An infant with facial swelling (▶ Fig. 235.1)

Key Imaging Finding

Fluid attenuation mass along the course of the nasolacrimal duct (NLD)

Diagnosis

Dacryocystocele. An NLD dacryocystocele, also referred to as a NLD mucocele, is the next most common congenital cause of nasal obstruction in infants following choanal atresia. They result from both proximal and distal obstruction of the nasolacrimal apparatus and subsequent buildup of fluid. Lesions may be unilateral or bilateral. Clinically, patients present with a bluish mass in the medial canthus region and/or within the nasal cavity, depending upon the size and extent of the lesion. Dacryocystoceles must be treated promptly, either conservatively through ductal massage or with invasive procedures because infants are obligate nasal breathers and the lesions are prone to superimposed infection, referred to as dacryocystitis.

Computed tomography (CT) is the imaging modality of choice and demonstrates a well-defined, fluid attenuation mass in the region of the medial canthus and/or nasal cavity and in direct continuity with the NLD. The mass often results in adjacent benign bony remodeling or displacement involving the nasolacrimal cavity, nasal septum, or inferior turbinate. Prominent peripheral or adjacent soft-tissue enhancement is indicative of dacryocystitis. Magnetic resonance imaging reveals similar findings with internal fluid signal intensity (T1 hypointense/T2 hyperintense).

✓ Pearls

- Dacryocystoceles result from proximal and distal obstruction of the NLD with buildup of fluid.
- Dacryocystoceles are the next most common congenital cause of nasal obstruction following choanal atresia.

- CT demonstrates a fluid density in the medial canthus and/or nasal cavity mass in continuity with the NLD.
- Prominent peripheral or adjacent soft-tissue enhancement is indicative of dacryocystitis.

Suggested Reading

Lowe LH, Booth TN, Joglar JM, Rollins NK. Midface anomalies in children. Radiographics 2000; 20: 907–922, quiz 1106–1107, 1112

Case 236

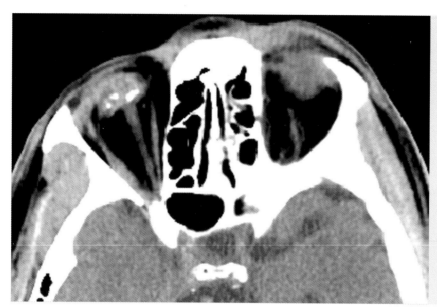

Fig. 236.1 Axial computed tomography image shows a shrunken, deformed right globe with dystrophic calcifications. There is secondary volume loss/atrophy affect of the ipsilateral optic nerve. (Courtesy of Aaron Betts, MD.)

▤ Clinical Presentation

A young child with a history of perinatal infection and long-standing unilateral visual loss (▶ Fig. 236.1)

▨ Key Imaging Finding

Shrunken, deformed globe with dystrophic calcifications

▨ Diagnosis

Phthisis bulbi. Phthisis bulbi refers to end-stage ocular degeneration due to an underlying insult. Common causes include ocular trauma and a myriad of long-standing, infectious, inflammatory, or autoimmune processes. Rarely, phthisis bulbi may occur in the setting of underlying tumor necrosis associated with retinoblastoma and melanoma. Patients present with blindness in the affected eye; treatment options include enucleation with prosthesis placement.

Imaging demonstrates an irregular, disorganized, shrunken globe with coarse calcifications. Atrophy of the optic nerve is a helpful secondary finding that may be seen in chronic cases. The associated volume loss often results in enophthalmos.

✓ Pearls

- Phthisis bulbi refers to end-stage ocular degeneration often due to trauma or an infectious/inflammatory insult.
- Computed tomography demonstrates an irregular, disorganized, shrunken globe with coarse calcifications.

- Atrophy of the optic nerve and enophthalmos associated with volume loss are helpful secondary findings.

Suggested Reading

LeBedis CA, Sakai O. Nontraumatic orbital conditions: diagnosis with CT and MR imaging in the emergent setting. Radiographics 2008; 28: 1741–1753

Case 237

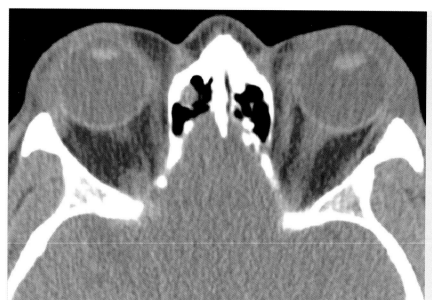

Fig. 237.1 Axial computed tomography image through the orbits demonstrates posterior displacement/dislocation of the lens on the left; the right side is normal.

■ Clinical Presentation

A 54-year-old man with facial/orbital trauma (▶ Fig. 237.1)

■ Key Imaging Finding

Displacement/dislocation of the lens

■ Diagnosis

Lens dislocation. The lens represents the demarcation between the anterior and posterior segments of the globe. It is attached to the overlying sclera via zonular fibers. Lens dislocation results from tearing of the zonular fibers, which may result from trauma (most common) or underlying connective tissue disorders, such as Ehlers-Danlos syndrome and homocystinuria. The dislocation may be partial or complete depending on the presence or absence of intact zonular fibers.

Post-traumatic lens dislocations are typically posterior. Computed tomography shows malpositioning/ dislocation of the hyperdense lens. It is important to look for additional globe or orbital injuries. Spontaneous lens dislocations associated with Marfan syndrome are commonly bilateral and superotemporal in location. Those associated with homocystinuria are also bilateral but typically inferonasal in location. Treatment is ultimately surgical in most cases.

✓ Pearls

- Lens dislocations may result from trauma or connective tissue disorders (Ehlers-Danlos syndrome and homocystinuria).
- Post-traumatic lens dislocations are typically posterior; anterior is less common.

- Lens dislocations associated with Marfan syndrome are commonly bilateral and superotemporal in location.
- Lens dislocations associated with homocystinuria are typically bilateral and inferonasal in location.

Suggested Readings

Kubal WS. Imaging of orbital trauma. Radiographics 2008; 28: 1729–1739

Betts AM, O'Brien WT, Davies BW, Youssef OH. A systemic approach to CT evaluation of orbital trauma. Emerg Radiol 2014; 21(5): 511–531

Case 238

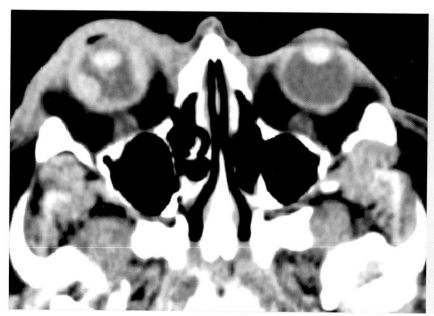

Fig. 238.1 Axial computed tomography image shows soft-tissue swelling overlying the right orbit with lenticular/biconvex hemorrhages along the lateral aspects of the right globe. The asymmetric orientation of the right lens compared with the left was projectional.

■ Clinical Presentation

A 68-year-old man post fall (▶ Fig. 238.1)

■ Key Imaging Finding

Lenticular/biconvex hemorrhages along the lateral aspects of the globe

■ Diagnosis

Choroidal detachment. The globe has three layers posteriorly with the sclera representing the outermost layer, the choroid representing the middle layer, and the retina representing the innermost layer. The choroid extends from the ora serrata anteriorly to the optic nerve head posteriorly. Vascular structures allow for its attachment to the overlying sclera. With choroidal detachment, fluid (proteinaceous or hemorrhagic) accumulates between and results in separation of the choroid and sclera. Common causes include inflammatory processes, trauma, and iatrogenia, all of which result in decreased intraocular pressure.

On imaging, choroidal detachments present as lenticular or biconvex fluid collections along the lateral margins of the globe. The collections are hyperdense compared with the vitreous on computed tomography. Unlike retinal detachments, a V-shaped configuration and extension to the optic disc are typically not seen, although choroidal detachments may occasionally mimic the appearance of a retinal detachment in the absence of the characteristic biconvex configuration.

✓ Pearls

- With choroidal detachment, fluid (proteinaceous or hemorrhagic) accumulates between the choroid and sclera.
- On imaging, choroidal detachments present as biconvex fluid collections along the lateral margins of the globe.

- Unlike retinal detachments, a V-shaped configuration and extension to the optic disc are typically not seen.

Suggested Readings

Kubal WS. Imaging of orbital trauma. Radiographics 2008; 28: 1729–1739

Betts AM, O'Brien WT, Davies BW, Youssef OH. A systemic approach to CT evaluation of orbital trauma. Emerg Radiol 2014; 21(5): 511–531

Case 239

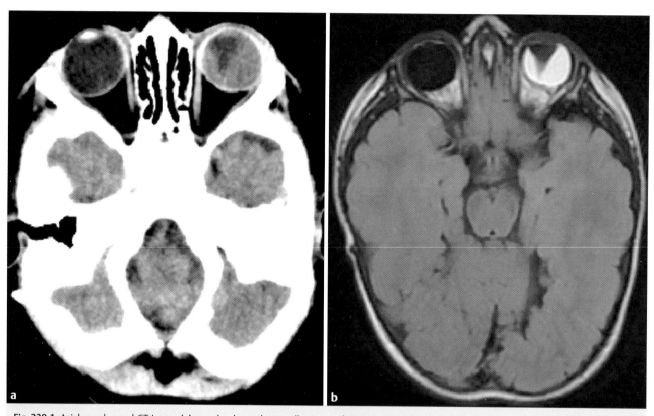

Fig. 239.1 Axial unenhanced CT image **(a)** reveals a hyperdense collection in the posterior segment of the left globe with a V-shaped configuration; the apex is located at the optic disc. Axial fluid-attenuated inversion recovery MR image **(b)** demonstrates the collection to be hyperintense compared with the adjacent vitreous.

■ Clinical Presentation

A young girl with progressive visual impairment (► Fig. 239.1)

▦ Key Imaging Finding

Ocular detachment with a V-shaped configuration

▦ Diagnosis

Retinal detachment. The globe has three layers posteriorly with the sclera representing the outermost layer, the choroid representing the middle layer, and the retina representing the innermost layer. The retina is the sensory layer of the globe, and when damaged, significant visual impairment may result. It has firm attachments anteriorly at the ora serrata and posteriorly at the optic disc. When fluid, typically hemorrhage, accumulates beneath the retina, there is uplifting of the more loosely attached portions of the retina between the ora serrata and optic disc, which often gives rise to the characteristic V-shaped configuration of a retinal detachment with its apex located at the optic disc. Small, large, or long-standing retinal hemorrhages may have a less characteristic imaging appearance without the classic V-shaped configuration.

Common causes of retinal detachment include inflammatory processes, neoplastic processes, and trauma. If noted in a young child with a questionable history, nonaccidental trauma should be a consideration. On computed tomography (CT), subretinal hemorrhage is typically hyperdense compared with the adjacent vitreous. Its appearance on magnetic resonance imaging (MRI) is variable depending upon the stage of breakdown of blood products. Most cases demonstrate increased signal on T1 and fluid-attenuated inversion recovery sequences with iso- to hyperintense T2 signal intensity. Treatment options include scleral buckling or banding, placement of a silicone sponge, and intraocular gas or silicone oil tamponade.

✓ Pearls

- The retina is the sensory layer of the globe, and when damaged, significant visual impairment may result.
- Retinal detachment often results in a characteristic V-shaped configuration with its apex at the optic disc.

- Retinal hemorrhage is hyperdense on CT; its MRI appearance is variable due to the stage of blood products.

Suggested Readings

Kubal WS. Imaging of orbital trauma. Radiographics 2008; 28: 1729–1739

Betts AM, O'Brien WT, Davies BW, Youssef OH. A systemic approach to CT evaluation of orbital trauma. Emerg Radiol 2014; 21(5): 511–531

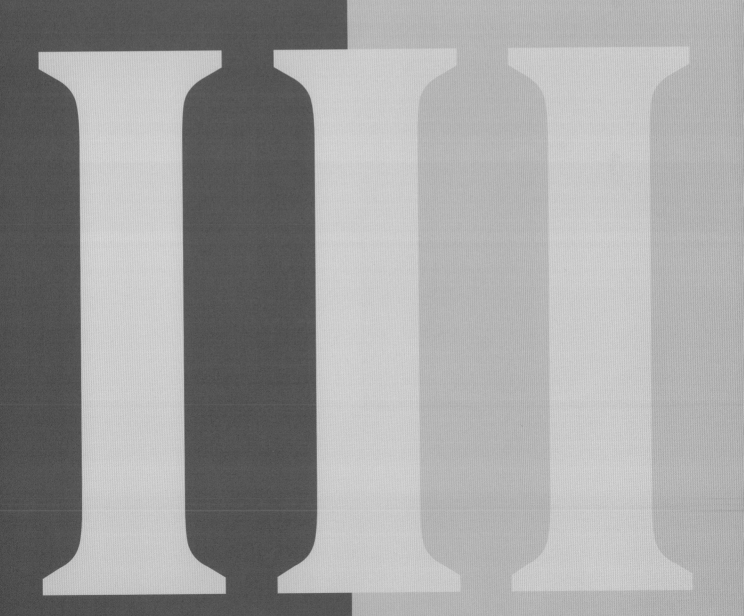

Section III

Spine

Case 240

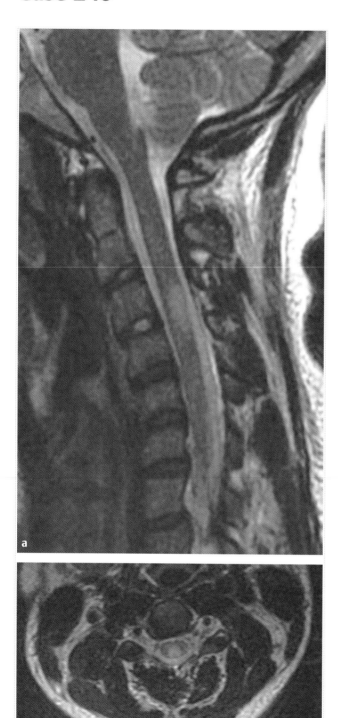

Fig. 240.1 Sagittal **(a)** and axial **(b)** T2-weighted images through the cervical spine demonstrate a hyperintense cord lesion involving the midposterior aspect of the cord at the C3–4 level; there is no cord expansion.

■ **Clinical Presentation**

A young adult with myelopathy (▶ Fig. 240.1)

■ Key Imaging Finding

Cord signal abnormality

■ Top 3 Differential Diagnoses

- **Demyelinating disease.** Demyelinating processes, such as multiple sclerosis (MS) and acute disseminated encephalomyelitis (ADEM), may affect the spinal cord in addition to the brain. Isolated cord disease is seen in ~10 to 20% of cases. The lesions are hyperintense on T2 sequences and most commonly located along the posterolateral aspect of the cord. There is little edema, if any; enhancement may be seen during periods of active demyelination. The plaques are typically small, usually spanning < 2 vertebral bodies in length. Patients commonly present with neurological deficits. MS demonstrates relapsing and remitting symptoms, whereas ADEM is characteristically monophasic after an antecedent viral infection or vaccination. Devic disease (neuromyelitis optica) affects the optic nerves and spinal cord with sparing of the brain parenchyma; Devic disease is now considered a separate entity from MS because it responds differently to therapy.
- **Transverse myelitis (TM).** TM refers to abnormalities involving both the ventral and dorsal cord at a particular level. Transverse myelitis may be caused by a variety of factors, including infectious, ischemic, autoimmune (collagen vascular diseases), demyelinating, and paraneoplastic processes. When no causative factor is identified, it is termed *idiopathic TM*. Patients with TM present with pain and sensorimotor deficits corresponding to the affected level. Imaging findings include abnormal cord signal, which may affect the whole cord at that level; enhancement is variable.
- **Intramedullary neoplasm.** The most common intramedullary neoplasms include ependymomas, which are most common in adults, and astrocytomas, which are more common in children. Ependymomas may be either myxopapillary at the caudal end of the cord or cellular within the central portion of the cord. Both neoplasms may extend up to 4 vertebral bodies in length, although astrocytomas may rarely be holocord. In general, ependymomas are more circumscribed and heterogeneous; intratumoral cysts and cord edema are commonly seen. Astrocytomas are typically more ill defined and diffuse, causing fusiform cord expansion.

■ Additional Differential Diagnoses

- **Cord contusion.** Cord contusions occur in the setting of trauma and often present with acute onset neurological deficits. There is increased T2 signal intensity and edema within the involved segment(s) of the cord. Foci of hemorrhage and cord expansion may also be seen. Secondary findings to suggest contusion include spinal fractures, marrow edema, ligamentous injury, and soft-tissue injuries. The cervical spine is the most common portion of the spine involved.
- **Cord ischemia.** The spinal cord arterial supply consists of a single anterior spinal artery and paired posterior spinal arteries. Cord infarcts are multifactorial and may be caused by arterial occlusion, usually the anterior spinal artery, or venous hypertension. Imaging findings of arterial infarcts include central increased T2 signal intensity involving the cord gray matter, as well as cord edema and swelling. Venous edema and infarcts are less specific in their imaging pattern and are often due to spinal dural arteriovenous fistulas or underlying causes of impaired venous drainage.
- **Subacute combined degeneration.** Subacute combined degeneration results from a vitamin B12 deficiency and is often due to pernicious anemia or malabsorption (e.g., Crohn disease). Patients present with weakness, spasticity, ataxia, and loss of proprioception. Imaging demonstrates signal abnormality involving the posterior columns with a characteristic "inverted V" appearance on axial sequences. Treatment consists of B12 replacement therapy.

■ Diagnosis

Demyelinating disease (ADEM)

✓ Pearls

- Demyelinating disease commonly affects the posterolateral aspect of the cord; active lesions may enhance.
- The most common intramedullary neoplasms include ependymomas (adults) and astrocytomas (children).
- Cord contusions occur in the setting of trauma; hemorrhage, edema, and cord expansion may be seen.
- Cord ischemia is usually due to arterial occlusion; signal abnormality preferentially affects central gray matter.

Suggested Reading

Bourgouin PM, Lesage J, Fontaine S et al. A pattern approach to the differential diagnosis of intramedullary spinal cord lesions on MR imaging. Am J Roentgenol 1998; 170: 1645–1649

Case 241

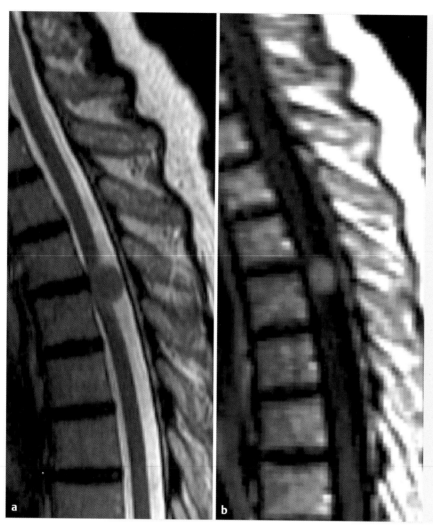

Fig. 241.1 Sagittal T2 magnetic resonance (MR) image **(a)** demonstrates a circumscribed intradural extramedullary isointense mass displacing and compressing the cord anteriorly. A subtle CSF cleft and acute angles between the lesion and cord confirms an extramedullary location. Sagittal T1 postcontrast MR image **(b)** reveals homogeneous, solid enhancement. (Courtesy of Paul M. Sherman, MD.)

■ Clinical Presentation

A young adult man with chronic back pain and neuropathy (▶ Fig. 241.1)

■ Key Imaging Finding

Enhancing intradural extramedullary spinal mass

■ Top 3 Differential Diagnoses

- **Nerve sheath tumor.** Schwannomas represent the most common intradural extramedullary masses. They may be purely intradural (most common), intra- and extradural with a classic "dumbbell" configuration, or, rarely, extradural. They may cause bony remodeling with foraminal enlargement or posterior vertebral body scalloping. Schwannomas are typically well-circumscribed, iso- to hypointense to cord on T1, variably hyperintense on T2, and enhance intensely. Cystic change and hemorrhage may be seen with larger lesions. Most cases are solitary and sporadic; they may be multiple in the setting of neurofibromatosis type 2 (NF2). Neurofibromas (NFs) are often indistinguishable from schwannomas on imaging, especially when solitary and sporadic (90%). However, they are more likely to demonstrate the "target" sign with central decreased and peripherally increased T2 signal intensity. Multiple NFs are seen in patients with NF1. Plexiform NFs are a specific subtype that demonstrate T2 hypointense septations and may undergo malignant degeneration in 5% of cases (suggested by rapid growth). Additional spinal stigmata of NF1 include thoracic scoliosis/kyphosis, vertebral anomalies, meningocele, and dural ectasia.
- **Meningioma.** Meningiomas are the second most common intradural extramedullary masses and are more common in women and patients with NF2. The vast majority (90%) are intradural; the remainder present as intra- and extradural, extradural, or, rarely, paraspinal or intraosseous. They are most common in the thoracic spine (80%), followed by the cervical and lumbar spine. They are typically round and may have a broad dural base. Meningiomas are isointense to cord on T1 and iso- to hyperintense on T2 images. Up to 5% may calcify. Flow voids may occasionally be present. The lesions intensely enhance; the presence of a dural tail is a useful discriminator but is less common than with intracranial meningiomas.
- **Metastatic disease.** Cerebrospinal fluid (CSF) metastases may result from hematogenous spread of a distant primary tumor or dissemination from a primary central nervous system (CNS) tumor. Common extra-CNS tumors with a propensity for hematogenous spread to the spine include lung, breast, and melanoma; CNS tumors prone to CSF dissemination include high-grade astrocytomas, medulloblastomas, germ cell tumors, choroid plexus neoplasm, and ependymomas. CSF metastases may present in one of several patterns, including a solitary intradural extramedullary mass, multiple enhancing masses, smooth or nodular leptomeningeal infiltration with "sugar coating" of the cord/ nerve roots, and thickening of the cauda equina. Extensive disease may fill the thecal sac, resulting in slightly increased precontrast T1 signal of the CSF ("dirty" or "ground glass" appearance of the CSF). Rarely, metastases may present as an intramedullary mass. Bony lesions of the spine may be seen in association with hematogenous metastases.

■ Additional Differential Diagnoses

- **Lymphoma/leukemia.** Lymphoma and leukemia have a variety of imaging appearances within the spine, including leptomeningeal infiltration, intradural extramedullary spinal masses, epidural masses, and vertebral masses; leptomeningeal involvement is most common and presents with smooth or nodular enhancement. Intradural extramedullary masses typically occur in the setting of diffuse CSF involvement; a focal, solitary mass is rare. Intradural extramedullary lesions are often well-circumscribed with homogeneous enhancement.
- **Paraganglioma.** Paragangliomas are neural crest tumors that most often occur in the adrenal gland, followed by the head and neck region; occasionally, they may present in the spine as intradural, extramedullary masses. They typically occur in the lumbar spine along the filum and cauda equina. Magnetic resonance imaging reveals a well-circumscribed T2 hyperintense avidly enhancing mass. A hemosiderin cap and vascular flow voids may be seen. There is characteristic increased activity on nuclear medicine metaiodobenzylguanidine (MIBG) scans.

■ Diagnosis

Meningioma

✓ Pearls

- Nerve sheath tumors (specifically schwannoma) are the most common intradural extramedullary spinal masses.
- Meningiomas are more common in women and patients with NF2; they may have a broad dural base.
- CSF malignancies may result from hematogenous spread, drop metastases, or lymphoma/leukemic infiltration.

Suggested Reading

Carra BJ, Sherman PM. Intradural spinal neoplasms: a case based review. J Am Osteopath Coll Radiol. 2013; 2: 13–21

Case 242

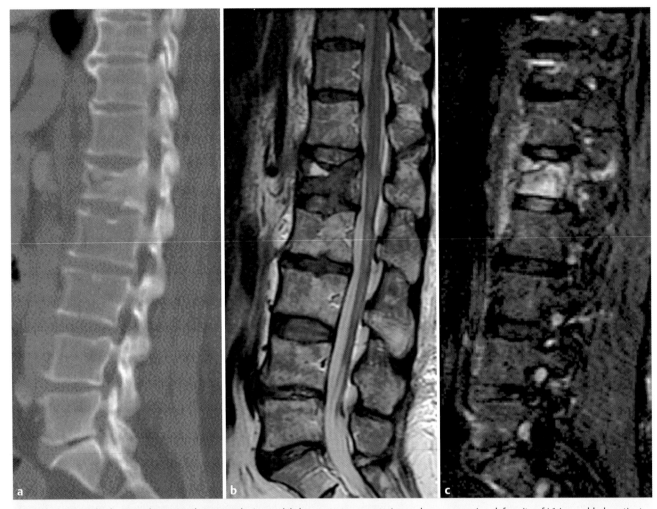

Fig. 242.1 Sagittal reformatted computed tomography image **(a)** demonstrates an anterior wedge compression deformity of L1 in an elderly patient. There is sclerosis of the posterior vertebral body. Sagittal T2-weighted MR image **(b)** shows the L1 compression fracture with focal edema/fluid signal anteriorly and decreased signal intensity within the remainder of the vertebral body. Sagittal short tau inversion recovery image **(c)** paramidline extending through the pedicle demonstrates extension of abnormal signal/marrow edema into the vertebral body pedicle with normal pedicle signal at other levels. (Case courtesy of Sonia Kaur Ghei, MD.)

■ Clinical Presentation

A 72-year-old woman with acute back pain (▶ Fig. 242.1)

■ Key Imaging Finding

Vertebral body wedge compression deformity

■ Top 3 Differential Diagnoses

- **Traumatic fracture.** Traumatic vertebral fractures tend to occur in the lower thoracic and upper lumbar spine; a history of fall or significant trauma is usually present. These most often involve the superior end plate of the vertebral body with surrounding marrow edema. If the fracture extends into the posterior elements, abnormal marrow signal intensity will typically be seen in these regions as well. Surrounding paravertebral soft-tissue swelling or hematoma is often present. This soft-tissue edema or hematoma should be smooth and rim shaped, rather than irregular or nodular.
- **Insufficiency fracture.** Insufficiency fractures of the spine tend to occur in older osteoporotic patients. These have a similar imaging characteristics compared to traumatic fractures but can occur at any level. In an older patient, the images should be carefully examined for signs of underlying malignancy because the spine is a common site of metastatic disease and a fracture may be the presenting abnormality. Marrow edema in insufficiency fractures is limited to the vertebral body; extension of abnormal signal into the pedicles suggests an underlying lesion or trauma. In addition, any soft-tissue edema or hematoma should be relatively smooth and rim shaped. Acute fractures with bone marrow edema may be amenable to symptomatic relief with vertebroplasty; post-treatment images show decreased signal intensity on all magnetic resonance imaging (MRI) sequences. Occasionally, vertebral osteonecrosis, referred to as Kummel disease, may occur in the setting of insufficiency fractures (less frequently with traumatic fractures) with interposition of an intravertebral gas or fluid cleft between collapsed bony components.
- **Pathological fracture.** A pathological fracture may occur anywhere in the spine where there is an underlying lesion. There are four MRI features that suggest an underlying malignant etiology: (1) abnormal marrow signal with ill-defined margins (all fractures will demonstrate increased T2 and short tau inversion recovery [STIR] signal secondary to marrow edema and hemorrhage, but it is typically well defined if benign); (2) abnormal marrow signal extending into the pedicles; (3) associated soft-tissue lesion with irregular or nodular borders (smooth paravertebral soft-tissue swelling is normally seen surrounding a fracture); and (4) marked enhancement (mild enhancement can normally be seen with benign fractures). Also, because traumatic fractures tend to occur in the upper lumbar spine, an underlying lesion should be considered in a younger patient with a lower lumbar spine fracture, particularly if there is no history of significant antecedent trauma.

■ Diagnosis

Pathological fracture (metastatic disease)

✓ Pearls

- Traumatic fractures often involve the superior end plates within the lower thoracic and upper lumbar spine.
- Insufficiency fractures tend to occur in older, osteoporotic patients and spare the posterior elements.

- Nontraumatic edema involving the pedicles or marked enhancement is concerning for a pathological fracture.
- Pathological fracture should be considered in a younger patient with an atraumatic lower lumbar spine fracture.

Suggested Readings

Haba H, Taneichi H, Kotani Y et al. Diagnostic accuracy of magnetic resonance imaging for detecting posterior ligamentous complex injury associated with thoracic and lumbar fractures. J Neurosurg 2003; 99 Suppl: 20–26

Shih TT, Huang KM, Li YW. Solitary vertebral collapse: distinction between benign and malignant causes using MR patterns. J Magn Reson Imaging 1999; 9: 635–642

Wintermark M, Mouhsine E, Theumann N et al. Thoracolumbar spine fractures in patients who have sustained severe trauma: depiction with multi-detector row CT. Radiology 2003; 227: 681–689

Case 243

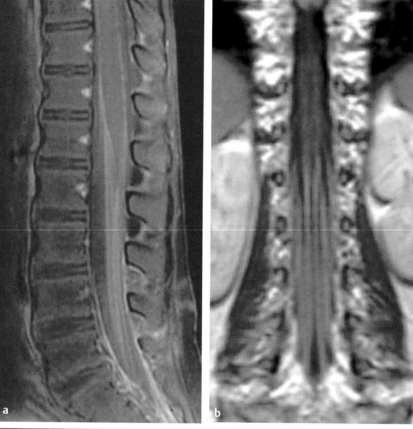

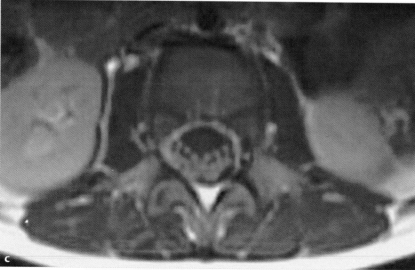

Fig. 243.1 Sagittal **(a)**, coronal **(b)**, and axial **(c)** T1 postcontrast images with **(a)** and without **(b,c)** fat suppression demonstrate diffuse, smooth avid enhancement of the distal cord/conus and nerves roots of the cauda equina. (Reprinted with permission: Zapadka M. J Am Osteopath Coll Radiol 2012;1(1):29–32.)

▇ Clinical Presentation

A young girl with progressive bilateral lower extremity weakness over the past week (▶ Fig. 243.1)

■ Key Imaging Finding

Smooth enhancement of the cauda equina

■ Top 3 Differential Diagnoses

- **Leptomeningitis.** Leptomeningitis may result from hematogenous spread (most common), direct spread from a spinal infection, or inoculation from iatrogenic or surgical complications. Patients commonly present with fever, headache, and stiff neck. Symptoms are more severe with bacterial meningitis as opposed to viral meningitis; atypical infections, such as *Cryptococcus* and *Tuberculosis*, may be seen in immunocompromised patients. Meningitis is typically diagnosed clinically with confirmatory cerebrospinal fluid (CSF) analysis. Imaging is usually reserved for refractory cases or to evaluate for complications of meningitis. Imaging may be normal, especially early in the disease course. The most common magnetic resonance imaging (MRI) findings include smooth or nodular leptomeningeal enhancement along the surface of the cord, conus, and cauda equina. The CSF may also appear "dirty" on unenhanced sequences due to the presence of inflammatory cells. Treatment for viral meningitis is supportive; bacterial infections require intravenous (IV) antibiotic therapy.
- **Leptomeningeal carcinomatosis.** Leptomeningeal carcinomatosis most often results from hematogenous spread of a distant primary malignancy or CSF dissemination of a primary central nervous system (CNS) malignancy. CNS tumors prone to CSF dissemination include high-grade gliomas, germ cell tumors, medulloblastoma, choroid plexus tumors, and ependymoma. Systemic tumors include lung and breast carcinoma, as well as hematologic malignancies such as leukemia and lymphoma. MRI demonstrates variable enhancement patterns, including focal masslike enhancement; smooth leptomeningeal enhancement along the surface of the cord, conus, and cauda equina; and nodular leptomeningeal enhancement (most common). Prognosis is typically poor.
- **Guillain-Barré syndrome (GBS).** GBS represents an acute, monophasic inflammatory demyelinating polyneuropathy that is thought to result from an autoimmune response to an antecedent infection or vaccination. Patients typically present initially with progressive, ascending weakness involving the lower extremities; there is often no sensory involvement. Later in the disease course, the upper extremities and brain stem may become involved. CSF analysis shows increased protein without pleocytosis and nerve conduction studies show signs of demyelination. MRI classically reveals smooth enhancement of the nerve roots of the cauda equina with early preferential involvement of the ventral motor nerve roots. Enhancement is also commonly seen along the distal cord and conus. Treatment includes plasmapheresis and/or IV immunoglobulin.

■ Additional Differential Diagnoses

- **Neurosarcoidosis.** Sarcoidosis is a systemic, inflammatory, granulomatous (noncaseating) disease with a peak onset in the third and fourth decades. Symptomatic CNS involvement is relatively uncommon and most often presents with smooth or nodular (most common) dural and/or leptomeningeal enhancement, preferentially involving the basal cisterns. Within the spine, the enhancement commonly involves the cord, conus, and cauda equina. If not already obtained, look for lymphadenopathy with or without interstitial lung disease on chest X-ray or computed tomography.
- **Chronic inflammatory demyelinating polyneuropathy (CIDP).** CIDP represents a chronic, acquired, mixed motor and sensory polyneuropathy. Patients present with ascending motor weakness involving the lower and upper extremities with additional sensory disturbances; symptoms are often present for months to years. In contrast with GBS, an antecedent infection or vaccination is seen in less than one-third of cases. MRI reveals focal or diffuse enlargement, T2 hyperintensity, and enhancement involving the nerve roots of the cauda equina that often extends into the extraspinal peripheral nerves. Symptoms generally improve with corticosteroid therapy.

■ Diagnosis

Guillain-Barré syndrome

✓ Pearls

- Meningitis, carcinomatosis, and sarcoidosis often present with smooth or nodular leptomeningeal enhancement.
- GBS results from an antecedent infection or vaccination and presents with ascending motor weakness.
- CIDP is a chronic demyelinating polyneuropathy with motor and sensory involvement; nerve roots are enlarged.

Suggested Reading

Zapadka M. Diffuse cauda equina nerve root enhancement. JAOCR J Am Osteopath Coll Radiol. 2012; 1: 29–32

Case 244

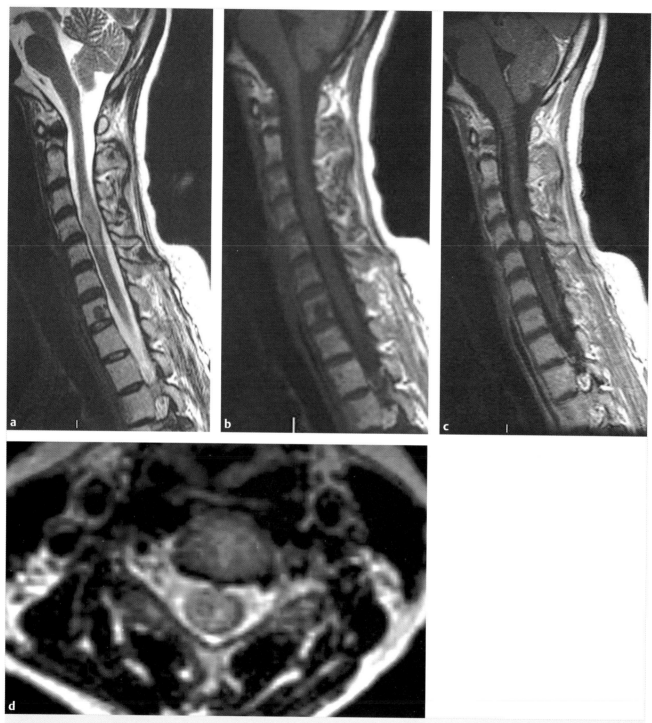

Fig. 244.1 Sagittal T2 (**a**), T1 pre- (**b**), and T1 postgadolinium (**c**) images demonstrate an ill-defined T2 hyperintense, T1 isointense expansile intramedullary mass within the cervical cord with a homogeneously enhancing nodular component and surrounding cord edema. Axial T2 image (**d**) confirms that the mass is intramedullary. Additional findings include an enhancing lesion within the C7 vertebral body and subtle leptomeningeal enhancement along the surface of the cord (**c**).

Clinical Presentation

A young adult woman with neck pain and paresthesias (▶ Fig. 244.1)

◼ Key Imaging Finding

Enhancing intramedullary spinal mass

◼ Top 3 Differential Diagnoses

- **Ependymoma.** Ependymoma is the most common spinal cord tumor in adults. They may occur at any age but have a peak incidence in the fourth and fifth decades of life. The cellular variant originates from the ependymal lining of the central canal and most commonly occurs within the cervical followed by thoracic spine. It is a circumscribed, central lesion that typically has symmetric cord expansion but may have exophytic components. It usually spans 3 to 4 vertebral segments with surrounding cord edema. Intratumoral cysts are present in the majority of cases, and adjacent cord syrinx is common. Enhancement may be intense and homogenous or nodular and heterogeneous. Hemorrhage is seen more often than with astrocytoma and presents as a T2 hypointense hemosiderin cap along the cranial and/or caudal end of the tumor. The myxopapillary variant occurs in the conus medullaris, filum terminale, or cauda equina. When located along the filum or cauda equina, it may mimic an extramedullary mass. It is a circumscribed ovoid or lobular mass, which commonly spans 2 to 4 vertebral segments. Mucin may cause T1 hyperintensity. The solid components intensely enhance. Both subtypes may cause widening of the interpediculate distance and scalloping of the vertebral bodies. The cellular variant may also cause scoliosis, whereas the myxopapillary variant may extend through neural foramina.

- **Astrocytoma.** Astrocytomas are the most common intramedullary spinal cord tumor in children and young adults. They are most common in the cervical followed by thoracic spine but may also be holocord. Common imaging presentation includes an infiltrating, expansile mass spanning up to 4 vertebral segments. Fusiform but eccentric expansion of cord is typical with occasional exophytic components. Syrinx and cystic components are less common compared with ependymoma. Solid components are T1 hypo- or isointense and T2 hyperintense with heterogeneous enhancement. They are typically low grade with an 80% 5-year survival.
- **Demyelinating disease.** Demyelinating disease may affect any portion of the cord but preferentially involves the posterolateral cervical cord. The lesions are often "flame shaped" and T2 hyperintense with little cord swelling or edema. Enhancement may be seen during periods of active demyelination. Concomitant brain lesions are usually present, although isolated cord disease is seen in 10 to 20% of cases. Lesions typically span < 2 vertebral segments and involve less than half the cross-sectional area of the cord. Acute disseminated encephalomyelitis, however, may be more extensive, involving multiple segments and a larger cross-sectional area of the cord.

◼ Additional Differential Diagnoses

- **Hemangioblastoma.** Hemangioblastomas are low-grade neoplasms of the cord and cerebellum. In the cord, 75% are sporadic and 25% are associated with von Hippel-Lindau (VHL) syndrome, in which case they are often multiple. They are subpial and most often dorsal in location. Hemangioblastomas are typically isointense on T1 and hyperintense on T2 sequences with surrounding cord edema. Signal is more heterogeneous with hemorrhage. Smaller lesions demonstrate solid enhancement, whereas larger lesions demonstrate the characteristic cystic mass with enhancing mural nodule. Prominent flow voids may be seen. The brain and entire spine should be imaged if VHL is suspected.
- **Metastatic disease.** Intramedullary metastases are relatively uncommon. The most common primary neoplasms include lung carcinoma (especially small cell), breast carcinoma, melanoma, lymphoma, and renal cell carcinoma. There is typically a nidus of enhancement and extensive edema. Pial metastatic lesions can mimic hemangioblastomas.

◼ Diagnosis

Metastatic disease (breast cancer)

✓ Pearls

- Ependymomas are the most common cord tumor in adults; a characteristic hemosiderin cap may be seen.
- Astrocytomas are the most common cord tumors in children and present as infiltrating, expansile masses.

- Demyelinating disease preferentially involves the posterolateral cord; enhancement suggests active disease.
- Hemangioblastomas are highly vascular lesions that may be sporadic or associated with VHL syndrome.

Suggested Reading

Carra BJ, Sherman PM. Intradural spinal neoplasms: a case based review. J Am Osteopath Coll Radiol. 2013; 2: 13–21

Case 245

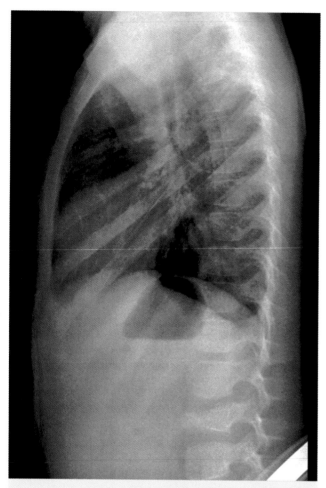

Fig. 245.1 Lateral radiograph of the chest shows marked flattening of the L3 vertebral body with preservation of the disc spaces and alignment, consistent with vertebra plana. (Case courtesy of Eva Escobedo, MD.)

■ Clinical Presentation

A 12-year-old boy with a cough (▶ Fig. 245.1)

■ Key Imaging Finding

Vertebra plana in a child

■ Top 3 Differential Diagnoses

- **Langerhans cell histiocytosis (LCH).** LCH is a group of idiopathic disorders characterized by the proliferation of Langerhans cells and mature eosinophils. It is by far the most common cause of vertebra plana in children. It most commonly occurs at a single site, but it can also occur at multiple levels. Compression may be progressive and rapid. More often, Langerhans cell histiocytosis manifests as a lytic lesion rather than vertebra plana. Bone lesions, especially with the eosinophilic granuloma form of LCH, may be asymptomatic.
- **Leukemia/lymphoma.** Leukemia is the most common pediatric primary malignancy. Loss of vertebral height and/or increased sclerosis are common findings in the vertebral body. Secondary lymphoma is much more common than primary lymphoma in the pediatric spine and presents in a similar manner. Constitutional symptoms and involvement of multiple levels are seen more commonly with these diseases, as opposed to LCH, which more commonly involves a single level.
- **Osteomyelitis.** Both bacterial and granulomatous (*Mycobacterium tuberculosis* [TB]) infection can present as vertebra plana. It has also been reported with chronic recurrent multifocal osteomyelitis, which is more likely inflammatory in nature rather than a true infection. Bacterial infection commonly involves the intervertebral disc with disc destruction and vertebral body end plate erosions. TB spondylitis, on the other hand, more commonly results in predominant bony destruction with relative disc preservation, which can manifest as vertebra plana. However, some form of vertebral end plate irregularity, sclerosis, or destruction is usually present.

■ Additional Differential Diagnoses

- **Trauma.** Traumatic vertebral body fractures may result in vertebral body collapse, particularly wedge compression fractures, burst fractures, and Chance fractures. Patients present acutely with a history of significant trauma. Computed tomography is ideal for identifying and characterizing the pattern of fracture. Magnetic resonance imaging is useful in evaluating for marrow edema, ligamentous stability/injury, and cord injury. A Chance or seatbelt fracture refers to a horizontal fracture of the neural arch due to flexion injury associated with rapid motor vehicle deceleration in patients wearing lap belts. The thoracolumbar junction is most commonly involved. A burst fracture refers to a complex, comminuted compression fracture of the vertebral body with disbursement of fracture fragments. It occurs in the setting of significant trauma and is most common at the thoracolumbar junction. Involvement of the posterior cortical margin of the vertebral body differentiates a burst fracture from a simple wedge compression fracture.
- **Metastases.** Neuroblastoma is the third most common primary malignancy in children and can metastasize to any bone. Peak age incidence for neuroblastoma is 2 to 3 years of age. Radiographic presentation of neuroblastoma metastases to the spine has a variety of appearances, including focal lucent lesions, regions of sclerosis, and loss of vertebral body height. Involvement of multiple levels is often seen.

■ Diagnosis

Langerhans cell histiocytosis

✓ Pearls

- Langerhans cell histiocytosis is the most common cause of vertebra plana in children.
- The most common osseous manifestation of Langerhans cell histiocytosis is a focal lytic lesion.
- Leukemia or lymphoma may present with multiple levels of vertebral body collapse and sclerosis.
- TB may demonstrate predominantly bony destruction with relative preservation of the disc space.

Suggested Readings

Chang MC, Wu HT, Lee CH, Liu CL, Chen TH. Tuberculous spondylitis and pyogenic spondylitis: comparative magnetic resonance imaging features. Spine 2006; 31: 782–788

Kilborn TN, Teh J, Goodman TR. Paediatric manifestations of Langerhans cell histiocytosis: a review of the clinical and radiological findings. Clin Radiol 2003; 58: 269–278

Kriss VM. My aching back: a serious complaint in children. Curr Probl Diagn Radiol 2001; 30: 23–30

Case 246

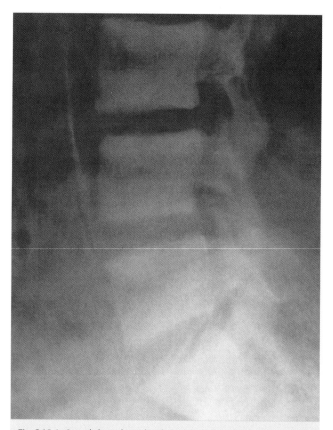

Fig. 246.1 Coned-down lateral radiograph of the lumbar spine shows superior and inferior end plate sclerosis at all levels. There is relative lucency within the central vertebral bodies between the areas of end plate sclerosis with an indistinct transition between the areas of sclerosis and the central areas of lucency. (Case courtesy of M. Jason Akers, MD.)

■ Clinical Presentation

An adult man with back pain (▶ Fig. 246.1)

Key Imaging Finding

"Rugger jersey" appearance of the spine

Top 3 Differential Diagnoses

- **Renal osteodystrophy.** Renal osteodystrophy represents a constellation of musculoskeletal abnormalities that occur in chronic renal failure, including osteomalacia, secondary hyperparathyroidism, and osteosclerosis. Osteosclerosis is common and results from an increased amount of abnormal osteoid. A classic site for osteosclerosis is the vertebral body end plates. The "rugger jersey" appearance of the spine is created by the relative lucency of the central aspect of the vertebral bodies between the sclerotic end plates. The margins between the sclerotic and lucent portions of the vertebral body are smudgy, rather than sharp. Look for extraskeletal evidence of chronic renal failure, including surgical clips in the abdomen from nephrectomy or renal transplant and dialysis catheters in the chest.

- **Osteopetrosis.** Osteopetrosis represents a group of hereditary disorders characterized by abnormal osteoclastic activity, resulting in dense bones. The "sandwich" appearance of the vertebral bodies is classic for osteopetrosis. The appearance is similar to the "rugger jersey" spine of renal osteodystrophy with the difference being a sharp margin between the sclerotic end plates and more lucent bone centrally. The classic "bone-in-bone" appearance occurs within the pelvis and long bones.

- **Paget disease.** Paget disease occurs in middle-aged and elderly patients and is characterized by excessive and abnormal bony remodeling. Most cases are polyostotic and the majority of cases involve the pelvis, spine, skull, femur, or tibia. The more common appearance of Paget disease in the spine is the "picture frame" vertebral body caused by overall increased density with sclerosis most marked at the periphery and a relatively lucent center. As in other bones, the classic features of Paget disease in the spine are bony (vertebral) enlargement, coarsened trabeculae, and overall increased bone density.

Additional Differential Diagnoses

- **Metastatic disease.** Classic primary tumors that cause sclerotic bone metastases include prostate, breast, lymphoma, carcinoid, bladder, and medulloblastoma. Tumor cells most often spread to the vertebral body hematogenously. Metastatic deposits may occur as discrete or ill-defined lesions or involve the marrow diffusely. Magnetic resonance imaging shows solitary or multiple, low T1 and variable T2 signal intensity lesions with heterogeneous enhancement. Diffuse involvement of the vertebral bodies causes diffusely low vertebral body signal as the metastases replace normal fatty marrow.

- **Myelofibrosis.** Myelofibrosis is bone marrow fibrosis that is most commonly secondary to leukemia, lymphoma, or metastatic disease. The disease initially involves primary sites of active hematopoiesis, including the vertebrae, ribs, and pelvis and later secondary sites in the proximal and distal aspects of long bones. Myelofibrosis manifests as very low marrow signal intensity on all sequences. Radiographs may be normal, but when abnormal, will show diffuse marrow sclerosis.

Diagnosis

Renal osteodystrophy

✓ Pearls

- The "rugger jersey" appearance of the vertebral bodies in renal osteodystrophy has smudgy margins.
- The "sandwich" vertebrae in osteopetrosis have sharp interfaces between sclerotic and lucent bone.

- Paget disease is characterized by bony enlargement, coarsened trabeculae, and increased bone density.
- With diffuse spine metastases, there is decreased marrow signal due to replacement of normal fatty marrow.

Suggested Readings

Graham TS. The ivory vertebra sign. Radiology 2005; 235: 614–615

Wittenberg A. The rugger jersey spine sign. Radiology 2004; 230: 491–492

Case 247

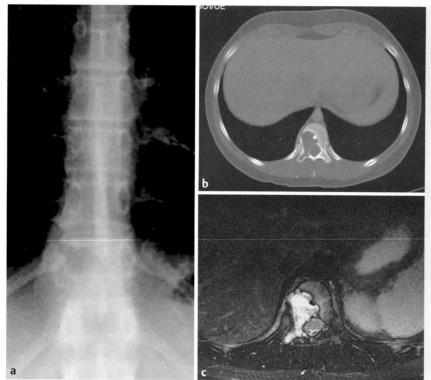

Fig. 247.1 Frontal radiograph of the thoracic spine **(a)** shows lucent expansion/absence of the right T11 pedicle. Corresponding axial CT image **(b)** shows an expansile lytic lesion involving the right posterior T11 body and pedicle. There is cortical thinning and regions of bony dehiscence. Axial T2 magnetic resonance image **(c)** shows fluid-fluid levels within the lesion and slight epidural extension. (Case courtesy of M. Jason Akers, MD.)

■ Clinical Presentation

An adult man with back pain (▶ Fig. 247.1)

■ Key Imaging Finding

Posterior element lytic lesion

▦ Top 3 Differential Diagnoses

- **Aneurysmal bone cyst (ABC).** ABCs are benign expansile lesions containing thin-walled, blood-filled cavities and are thought to occur as a result of trauma. They can be isolated or associated with other tumors. ABCs are usually seen in children and young adults and commonly occur in long-bone metaphyses and the posterior elements of the spine. In the spine, ABCs are classically centered in the pedicle and extend into the vertebral body. The pedicle appears expanded or absent on anteroposterior radiographs of the spine. Cortical thinning and focal cortical destruction are common. There may also be extension into the epidural space causing canal stenosis. Fluid-fluid levels result from hemorrhage within the lesion and are characteristic.
- **Osteoblastoma.** Osteoblastomas are benign osteoid-forming tumors thought to be a larger version (> 1.5 cm) of osteoid osteoma. Forty percent occur in the spine and originate in the posterior elements, often extending into the vertebral body. They present as expansile lesions with narrow zones of transition and variable mineralization. The matrix is better visualized on computed tomography than radiographs. There may be an aneurysmal bone cyst component with fluid-fluid levels. Tumors can incite an inflammatory response with associated peritumoral edema that extends beyond the margins of the lesion.
- **Infection (tuberculosis).** TB causes granulomatous infection of the spine and adjacent soft tissues. Isolated posterior element involvement can occur, particularly in the thoracic spine. Patients usually have prominent epidural and paraspinal disease with large paraspinal abscesses dissecting over multiple levels. TB spondyltitis is more likely to spare intervertebral discs while causing prominent bony destruction.

■ Additional Differential Diagnoses

- **Metastases.** Metastases usually occur in older patients and involve the posterior vertebral body initially with extension into the posterior elements. Metastases most commonly spread to the spine hematogenously. Lytic metastases tend to be less expansile and more permeative in appearance, occurring as a destructive lesion with an associated soft-tissue mass. Multiple vertebral levels may be involved.
- **Langerhans cell histiocytosis (LCH).** LCH is a disease occurring in children that is characterized by abnormal histiocyte proliferation producing granulomatous skeletal lesions. The classic presentation in the spine is vertebra plana with preservation of the disc space. LCH can also present as an aggressive lytic lesion with soft-tissue mass and extension into the spinal canal. Other sites of involvement include the skull with a "beveled" edge appearance, mandible, long bones, ribs, and pelvis.

■ Diagnosis

Aneurysmal bone cyst

✓ Pearls

- ABCs are benign, expansile, lytic lesions that contain fluid-fluid levels due to internal hemorrhage.
- Osteoblastoma has an osteoid matrix and typically has peritumoral edema that extends beyond the lesion.
- Posterior element involvement of the thoracic spine with paraspinal abscesses suggests TB spondylitis.
- Lytic metastases typically occur in older patients, appear permeative/destructive, and affect multiple levels.

Suggested Readings

DiCaprio MR, Murphy MJ, Camp RL. Aneurysmal bone cyst of the spine with familial incidence. Spine 2000; 25: 1589–1592

Shaikh MI, Saifuddin A, Pringle J, Natali C, Sherazi Z. Spinal osteoblastoma: CT and MR imaging with pathological correlation. Skeletal Radiol 1999; 28: 33–40

Case 248

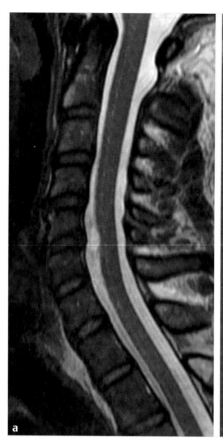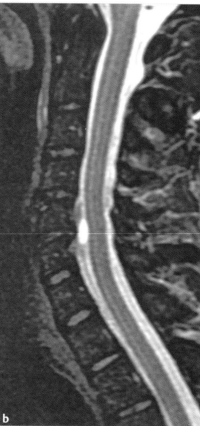

Fig. 248.1 Sagittal T2 **(a)** and short tau inversion recovery **(b)** images demonstrate a small, circumscribed intradural extramedullary cyst along the ventral aspect of the cord at the C5–6 level. The cyst is slightly hyperintense relative to surrounding CSF.

■ **Clinical Presentation**

A patient with chronic neck pain (▶ Fig. 248.1)

■ Key Imaging Finding

Intradural extramedullary cyst

■ Top 3 Differential Diagnoses

- **Meningeal cyst.** Meningeal cysts are classified according to their location and the presence or absence of neural tissue within the cyst. Type 1 cysts include extradural arachnoid cysts without neural elements (type 1A) and sacral meningoceles (type 1B). Extradural arachnoid cysts result from congenital or acquired dural defects and are most commonly located posteriorly within the mid to lower thoracic spine; they may extend into the neural foramina. Type 2 meningeal cysts are extradural cysts that contain neural elements and are commonly referred to as perineural or Tarlov cysts. They are very common and most often seen in the spine and sacrum in the region of the neural foramina. Type 3 meningeal cysts are intradural arachnoid cysts and may be congenital or acquired. They occur most frequently in the thoracic spine and may cause symptomatic cord compression. The signal intensity of meningeal cysts on magnetic resonance imaging (MRI) is often slightly hyperintense compared with cerebrospinal fluid (CSF) due to decreased CSF pulsations and, occasionally, increased protein content within the cysts. With computed tomographic myelography, there is often delayed contrast filling of meningeal cysts.
- **Epidermoid or dermoid cyst.** Epidermoid and dermoid cysts are benign lesions that may be congenital or acquired, especially in the setting of instrumentation during surgery or lumbar puncture. Epidermoid cysts are composed of desquamatized epithelium; dermoids also contain keratin debris and skin appendages. Congenital lesions result from inclusion of cutaneous ectodermal elements within the neuroectoderm during development and are most common in the lumbosacral region. An overlying tract or sinus may be identified in the superficial soft tissues. Patients may be asymptomatic or present with symptoms related to mass effect on the cord or nerve roots or with symptoms related to local infection or meningitis. MRI is the modality of choice and demonstrates a circumscribed mass with signal characteristics similar to but slightly hyperintense compared with CSF. Peripheral inflammatory enhancement may be seen with superimposed infection. Dermoid elements may contain macroscopic fat; epidermoid elements typically show restricted diffusion. An intrathecal ruptured dermoid or epidermoid often results in a chemical meningitis. The cord and conus should be closely evaluated to look for a low-lying cord or imaging findings suggestive of cord tethering.
- **Neuroenteric cyst.** Neuroenteric cysts are rare developmental anomalies that represent persistent elements of the primitive neuroenteric canal. Approximately half of patients have associated vertebral anomalies with possible communication between the spinal canal and the alimentary tract. Additional associations include spina bifida, diastematomyelia, and Klippel-Feil syndrome. The imaging appearance of a neuroenteric cyst depends upon its location. Common locations include the posterior mediastinum, abdomen, retroperitoneum, and within the spinal canal. Intraspinal cysts present as anterior intradural extramedullary cystic masses that may be unilocular or multilocular. When associated spinal anomalies are present, neuroenteric cyst should be a leading differential consideration, despite its overall rarity. The cysts typically follow CSF signal intensity, although the signal may vary slightly due to a lack of CSF pulsations or the presence of proteinaceous content.

■ Diagnosis

Meningeal cyst (type 3)

✓ Pearls

- Meningeal cysts are classified based upon their location and presence or absence of neural tissue in the cyst.
- Type 2 meningeal cysts (perineural or Tarlov cysts) are common, extradural, and contain neural elements.
- Dermoid cysts may contain macroscopic fat; epidermoid cysts typically show restricted diffusion.
- When spinal anomalies are present, neuroenteric cyst should be a leading consideration for an intradural cyst.

Suggested Reading

Khosla A, Wippold FJ, II. CT myelography and MR imaging of extramedullary cysts of the spinal canal in adult and pediatric patients. Am J Roentgenol 2002; 178: 201–207

Case 249

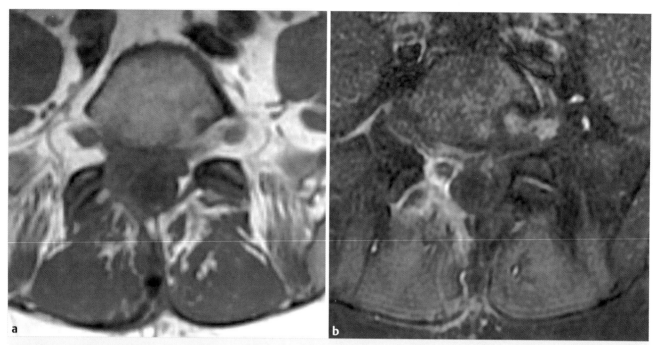

Fig. 249.1 Axial unenhanced T1 image at the level of prior discectomy **(a)** demonstrates hypointense tissue surrounding the right lateral recess. Axial postcontrast T1 image **(b)** with fat suppression shows diffuse enhancement of the tissue around the cerebrospinal fluid–filled lateral recess.

■ Clinical Presentation

A 41-year-old man with L4–5 prior discectomy and recurrent symptoms (▶ Fig. 249.1)

◼ Key Imaging Finding

Postoperative enhancement

◼ Top 3 Differential Diagnoses

- **Granulation tissue.** Granulation tissue or scar commonly forms following spinal surgery. It is most pronounced in the region of discectomy, which presents a diagnostic challenge when attempting to distinguish granulation tissue from a recurrent disc herniation because both entities appear similar on unenhanced magnetic resonance imaging sequences. Classically, granulation or scar tissue enhances homogeneously, allowing for differentiation from a recurrent disc. However, within the first 3 to 6 months following surgery, granulation tissue may demonstrate peripheral rather than homogeneous enhancement, making the distinction between scar tissue and a recurrent disc impossible on imaging. A follow-up examination will often reveal the more characteristic homogeneous enhancement pattern associated with scarring.
- **Recurrent disc.** Recurrent disc herniation is a not uncommon cause of recurrent back pain following surgical discectomy. The herniation often occurs in the region of prior surgery. On unenhanced sequences, a recurrent disc typically follows similar signal intensity compared with the parent disc; this

finding is not specific, however, because granulation tissue may have a similar appearance. Therefore, postcontrast imaging is key to distinguishing between a recurrent disc and granulation or scar tissue. On postcontrast T1 sequences, disc material characteristically demonstrates peripheral rather than homogeneous enhancement. The specificity of this finding increases with time from the original surgery.
- **Infection.** Infection is a dreaded complication of spinal surgery, especially in the presence of hardware instrumentation. Patients often present clinically with back pain, fever, and elevated white blood cell count and erythrocyte sedimentation rate. Imaging findings depend upon the stage of infection. Initially, the infectious process results in ill-defined, inflammatory, or phlegmonous enhancement. As the infection becomes more organized, an abscess forms, demonstrating central fluid signal intensity with a rim-enhancing capsule. In the early stages, medical management with antibiotics may be adequate. Once an abscess forms, however, surgical drainage is often necessary.

◼ Diagnosis

Granulation tissue

✓ Pearls

- Classically, granulation or scar enhances homogeneously, allowing for differentiation from a recurrent disc.
- A recurrent disc herniation characteristically demonstrates peripheral rather than homogeneous enhancement.

- Early infection results in ill-defined, inflammatory enhancement; an abscess demonstrates rim enhancement.

Suggested Reading

Hancock CR, Quencer RM, Falcone S. Challenges and pitfalls in postoperative spine imaging. Appl Radiol 2008; 37: 23–34

Case 250

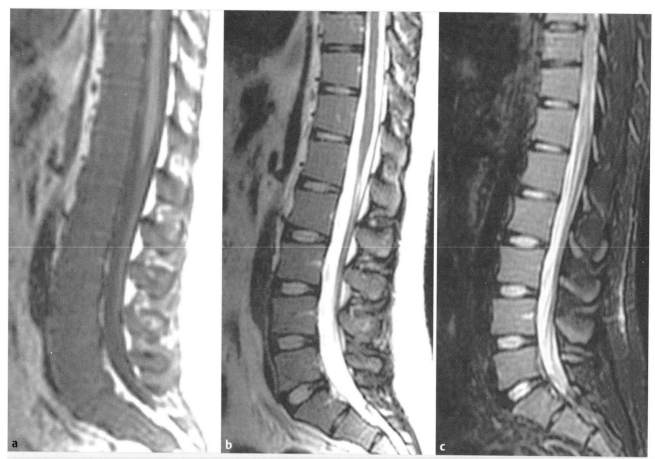

Fig. 250.1 SagittalT1-weighted MR image **(a)** demonstrates diffuse decreased marrow signal intensity, which is hypointense compared with paraspinal musculature and intervertebral discs. No focal abnormality is seen on T1- or T2-weighted **(b)** sequences. Sagittal short tau inversion recovery image **(c)** shows diffuse abnormal increased marrow signal intensity within the visualized portions of the spine and sacrum.

▓ Clinical Presentation

A 24-year-old man with increasing fatigue (▶ Fig. 250.1)

▨ Key Imaging Finding

Diffuse abnormal marrow signal intensity

▨ Top 3 Differential Diagnoses

- **Hematopoietic marrow.** In children and young adults, bone marrow progresses from predominantly hematopoietic at birth to predominantly fatty marrow in adulthood. In adults, residual hematopoietic marrow persists in the axial skeleton (spine and flat bones) and proximal shafts of the femur and humerus. T1-weighted magnetic resonance imaging (MRI) sequences are ideal in evaluating for marrow abnormalities. Normal T1 bone marrow signal intensity in adults is brighter than adjacent paraspinal musculature. In the setting of chronic illness or anemia, however, marrow reconversion occurs with replacement of fatty marrow with hematopoietic marrow. Increased concentrations of hematopoietic marrow results in decreased T1 signal intensity that may be iso- to hypointense compared with paraspinal musculature. Fluid-sensitive fat-suppressed (FS) T2 and postcontrast FS T1 sequences are helpful in distinguishing hematopoietic marrow from more aggressive marrow infiltrative processes, both of which may demonstrate decreased T1 signal intensity. On these sequences, hematopoietic marrow is typically hypointense, whereas infiltrative processes are most often hyperintense.
- **Myeloproliferative disorder.** Myeloproliferative disorders refer to abnormal proliferation of marrow elements. Common diffuse infiltrative processes include multiple myeloma (plasma cells), leukemia (white blood cells), and myelofibrosis (supporting collagen and fibrous tissue). These proliferative disorders replace normal fatty marrow, resulting in diffuse decreased T1 signal intensity compared with paraspinal musculature. Multiple myeloma is the most common primary bone malignancy and occurs in middle-aged and older adults. It results in bony resorption due to increased osteoclastic activity and inflammatory response. Any bone may be involved, but the most common locations include the spine and calvarium. Bony involvement may be focal or diffuse. Focal involvement results in "punched out" lucencies on plain radiographs. Diffuse involvement leads to marrow infiltration with decreased T1 and increased FS T2 signal intensity with enhancement. Leukemia may occur in patients of any age but is commonly seen in adolescents and young adults. Diffuse involvement results in decreased T1 and increased FS T2 signal intensity with enhancement. Signal intensity must be evaluated closely because the diffuse nature of marrow infiltration may inadvertently be overlooked. Myelofibrosis is unique in that proliferation of fibrous elements results in decreased signal intensity on all MRI sequences.
- **Lymphoma.** Lymphomatous involvement of the spine may be primary or secondary (far more common). Lesions may be solitary, multiple, or diffuse. Diffuse involvement most often demonstrates imaging features similar to leukemia with diffuse decreased T1 and increased FS T2 signal intensity with enhancement. A characteristic feature of lymphoma is extraspinous spread into adjacent soft tissues and compartments without cortical disruption.

▨ Additional Differential Diagnoses

- **Metastases.** Metastatic disease represents the most common malignancy to involve bone. Bones with increased hematopoietic marrow, including the axial skeleton, are preferentially involved due to relatively increased blood flow. Common primary malignancies include breast, lung, and prostate carcinomas, as well as gastrointestinal and genitourinary neoplasms. Diffuse marrow infiltration in the setting of metastatic disease is uncommon; more common patterns of involvement include discreet lesions that may be solitary or multiple. The majority of metastatic foci are hypointense on T1 and hyperintense on FS T2 sequences with enhancement. Sclerotic lesions from breast or prostate primaries may be hypointense on all sequences.
- **Treatment-related marrow changes.** Radiation, chemotherapy, and granulocyte-colony stimulating factor (G-CSF) are commonly used in the treatment of malignancies. In the acute setting (4-6 weeks), radiation therapy results in marrow edema with increased signal intensity on fat-suppressed T2 sequences. In the chronic setting, radiation induces fatty marrow replacement confined to the treatment field. Chemotherapy results in similar changes with less pronounced chronic fatty marrow. G-CSF causes stimulation of marrow, resulting in diffuse increased signal on fat-suppressed T2 sequences, which may mimic residual or recurrent disease.

▨ Diagnosis

Myeloproliferative disorder (leukemia)

✓ Pearls

- Hematopoietic marrow occurs in the setting of chronic illness/anemia and is hypointense to musculature on T1.
- Cellular marrow infiltrative processes result in decreased T1 and increased FS T2 signal with enhancement.
- Myelofibrosis results in proliferation of marrow support elements with decreased signal on all sequences.
- Metastatic foci typically present with discreet masses; diffuse marrow infiltration is uncommon.

Suggested Reading

Long SS, Yablon CM, Eisenberg RL. Bone marrow signal alteration in the spine and sacrum. Am J Roentgenol 2010; 195: W178–200

Case 251

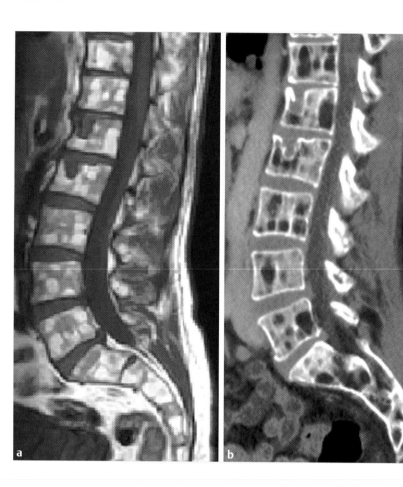

Fig. 251.1 Sagittal T1 MR image **(a)** demonstrates multifocal regions of increased signal intensity throughout the visualized portions of the spine; the relatively hypointense regions are normal. Prominent superior end plate Schmorl nodes are visualized at the L1 and L2 levels. Sagittal reformatted postcontrast CT image **(b)** shows corresponding regions of hypoattenuation within the spine; the degree of hypoattenuation approximates that of the superficial fat. (Courtesy of Sheri Albers, DO.)

▣ Clinical Presentation

An adult patient with back pain (▶ Fig. 251.1)

■ **Key Imaging Finding**

Multifocal regions of increased T1 marrow signal intensity

■ **Top 3 Differential Diagnoses**

- **Focal fatty marrow.** Bone marrow consists of a mixture of hematopoietic and fatty marrow, as well as the underlying supporting structures. As patients age, hematopoetic marrow is replaced by predominantly fatty marrow. This process may be diffuse or focal and presents as regions of increased T1 and T2 signal with loss of signal on short tau inversion recovery (STIR) or other fat-suppressed sequences. In contrast to hemangiomas, the characteristic vertical striations and "polka dot" appearance (axial images) are not typically seen with focal fatty marrow.

- **Multiple hemangiomas.** Vertebral body hemangiomas are endothelial-lined vascular structures interspersed between the bony trabeculae of the spine. They may be solitary or multiple and are most commonly seen in the thoracic and lumbar spine. The vast majority of lesions are incidental and asymptomatic. Plain radiographs and computed tomography (CT) demonstrate focal fat attenuation with prominence of vertical striations within the trabeculae, leading to the characteristic "honeycomb" (sagittal, coronal) and polka dot (axial images) appearances. Magnetic resonance imaging (MRI) signal intensity may be variable depending upon the fatty and vascular components within the lesion. Predominantly fatty lesions are hyperintense on T1- and T2-weighted sequences with loss of signal on fat-suppressed sequences. In the absence of characteristic vertical striations or polka dot appearance on axial sequences, hemangiomas may appear identical to focal fatty marrow. With increased vascularity, the signal characteristics are more variable and atypical. Aggressive or compressive hemangiomas are rare, tend to be less well defined, have intermediate T1 signal intensity, and may demonstrate internal flow voids.

- **Osteoporosis.** Osteoporosis refers to demineralization of bony structures with decreased cellular and increased fatty marrow components. It may be diffuse or focal and presents as regions of increased T1 and variable but typically increased T2 signal intensity, similar to fatty marrow. Occasionally, hyperintense signal on STIR sequences may be seen in the setting of increased vascular as opposed to fatty components within the region of demineralization. The vast majority of patients are elderly; children with osteoporosis typically have underlying congenital or acquired causes of bony demineralization.

■ **Additional Differential Diagnoses**

- **Melanoma or hemorrhagic metastases.** Melanoma or hemorrhagic metastases are the rare exceptions to the rule that most T1 hyperintense lesions in the spine are benign. Patients with metastatic melanoma may presents with solitary or multiple bony lesions. Lesions are typically well-circumscribed and hyperintense on T1 sequences due to the propensity for hemorrhage, as well as inherent T1 shortening associated with melanin. They are often heterogeneously hypointense on T2 and demonstrate abnormal enhancement. By the time of widespread metastases, the diagnosis is usually known.

- **Intraosseous lipoma/lipomatosis.** Solitary intraosseous lipomas of the vertebral bodies are in and of themselves rare lesions; spinal lipomatosis, which is characterized by multifocal intraosseous lipomas, is exceedingly rare. Lipomatous lesions typically follow fat attenuation (CT) and signal intensity (MRI), although lesions with calcification or reactive surrounding bony changes may have a more heterogeneous appearance, especially on MRI. The key distinguishing features of these benign lesions include fat attenuation/signal intensity and a lack of enhancement.

■ **Diagnosis**

Intraosseous lipomatosis

✓ **Pearls**

- As patients age, hematopoetic marrow is replaced by fatty marrow, which may appear diffuse or multifocal.
- Vertebral body hemangiomas often demonstrate a characteristic "honeycomb" or "polka dot" (axial) appearance.

- Osteoporosis refers to bony demineralization with decreased cellular and increased fatty marrow components.
- Melanoma is a rare exception to the rule that the vast majority of T1 hyperintense spinal lesions are benign.

Suggested Reading

Hanrahan CJ, Shah LM. MRI of spinal bone marrow: part 2, T1-weighted imaging-based differential diagnosis. Am J Roentgenol 2011; 197: 1309–1321

Case 252

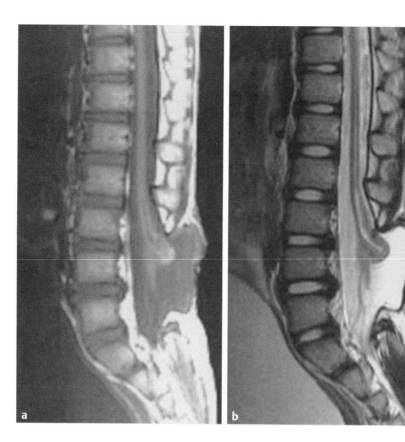

Fig. 252.1 Sagittal T1 **(a)** and T2 **(b)** images demonstrate fetal elongation of the cord with herniation of cerebrospinal fluid–filled meninges and the neural placode through a posterior lumbosacral bony defect. The sac extends beyond the level of the skin surface. The T1 image best depicts a defect in the overlying skin and subcutaneous fat. There is also marked distension of an atonic, neurogenic bladder.

Clinical Presentation

A young girl with long-standing neurological and orthopedic deficits (▶ Fig. 252.1)

■ Key Imaging Finding

Open lumbosacral spinal dysraphism

■ Top 3 Differential Diagnoses

- **Myelomeningocele (MMC).** MMC is a congenital defect caused by improper closure of the primary neural tube, resulting in herniation of meninges and neural elements through a midline osseous defect with no overlying skin covering. MMCs represent roughly 98% of all open spinal dysraphisms, and nearly all cases occur in the setting of a Chiari II malformation. The herniated elements extend beyond or above the level of the skin surface, which helps distinguish MMC from myelocele. The abnormality is commonly seen during fetal ultrasound screening; fetal magnetic resonance imaging better characterizes the lumbosacral and craniocervical junction defects. Imaging shows herniation of cerebrospinal fluid–filled meninges and the neural placode through a posterior osseous defect. Findings at the craniocervical junction include cerebellar tonsillar herniation through the foramen magnum, cervicomedullary kinking, tectal beaking, and

a small posterior fossa. In cases where prenatal imaging was not performed, the first imaging study may be postoperative because the diagnosis is clinically apparent at birth.
- **Myelocele.** Myeloceles are similar to MMCs in that they are also caused by improper closure of the primary neural tube. Both entities result in herniation of meninges and neural elements through a midline osseous defect with no overlying skin covering. In contrast to MMCs, which protrude beyond the skin surface, however, myeloceles remain flush with the skin surface. Myeloceles are rare in comparison with MMCs.
- **Hemimyelomeningocele/hemimyelocele.** Hemimyelomeningoceles and hemimyeloceles are extremely rare. They are characterized by the findings associated with an underlying MMC or myelocele with the addition of diastematomyelia or splitting of the neural placode/cord. One of the two hemicords fails to undergo proper neurulation.

■ Diagnosis

Myelomeningocele (with prior surgery)

✓ Pearls

- MMC refers to herniation of meninges and neural elements through an osseous defect with no skin covering.
- MMCs represent 98% of open dysraphisms; nearly all cases occur in the setting of Chiari II malformation.

- The key distinction between myeloceles and MMCs is that myeloceles remain flush with the skin surface.
- Hemimyelomeningoceles and hemimyeloceles are extremely rare and have underlying diastematomyelia.

Suggested Reading

Rufener SL, Ibrahim M, Raybaud CA, Parmar HA. Congenital spine and spinal cord malformations—pictorial review. Am J Roentgenol 2010; 194 Suppl: S26–S37

Case 253

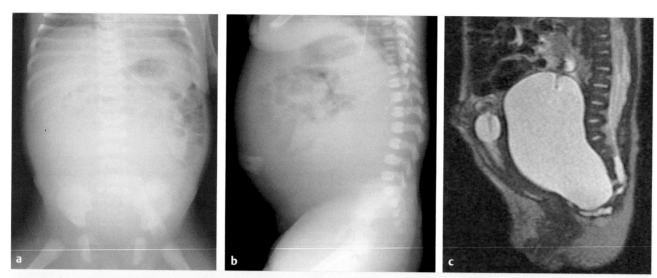

Fig. 253.1 Frontal **(a)** and lateral **(b)** radiographs of the abdomen demonstrate a large noncalcified presacral mass displacing the bowel superiorly and anteriorly. The lower sacrum and coccyx are not identified. Sagittal T2-weighted MR image **(c)** defines the large, presacral cystic mass that extends posterior to the spine but is separate from the spinal canal. The bladder (containing a Foley catheter) is compressed anteriorly. (Case courtesy of Sandra L. Wootton-Gorges, MD.)

■ **Clinical Presentation**

A full-term infant girl with a distended abdomen (▶ Fig. 253.1)

■ Key Imaging Finding

Presacral mass in an infant

■ Top 3 Differential Diagnoses

- **Sacrococcygeal teratoma (SCT).** SCTs are rare tumors that arise from multipotential cells and contain all three germ layers. SCTs are the most common tumors of the caudal region in infants. They may be extrapelvic, intrapelvic, or both. Most are benign at birth, but beyond the neonatal period the risk of malignancy increases. Cystic lesions are more often benign. Radiographs show the soft-tissue mass. Calcifications are seen in 60%, and vary in their appearance. The sonographic, computed tomography (CT), and magnetic resonance imaging (MRI) appearance is typically heterogeneous and varies based upon the tumor composition (solid versus cystic, fatty or calcified components, etc.). MRI demonstrates the extent of the lesions, as well as intraspinal extension.
- **Anterior meningocele.** Anterior sacral meningoceles (ASMs) are rare herniations of cerebrospinal fluid (CSF)-distended meninges through a sacral foramen or defect. MRI is the modality of choice to define the lesion, but CT may be useful to demonstrate the bony defect. ASMs may be associated with genitourinary and/or anorectal malformations, as well as neurofibromatosis type 1. They may also occur as part of the Currarino triad (anorectal malformation, sacral osseous defect [scimitar sacrum], and presacral mass).
- **Rectal duplication cyst.** Rectal duplication cysts account for 5% of enteric duplication cysts. They are spherical, thin-walled, uni-or multilocular cystic lesions that may communicate with the rectal lumen. Pathologically, they contain smooth muscle in the wall and have a rectal mucosal lining. Radiographs may demonstrate widening of the retrorectal space. Ultrasound shows characteristic hypoechogenicity of the muscular wall. CT and MRI reveal a nonenhancing cystic mass; the presence of mucinous content may result in regions of increased T1 signal intensity. The imaging appearance is more complex with superimposed infection.

■ Additional Differential Diagnoses

- **Cystic lymphatic malformation.** Macrocystic lymphatic malformations are fluid-filled lymphatic spaces resulting from malconnection of lymphatic vessels with the central lymphatic system. They appear as a thin-walled uni- or multilocular cystic masses with enhancing walls and septa. Fluid-fluid levels may be seen and are characteristic of superimposed hemorrhage.
- **Dermoid cysts.** Dermoid cysts are developmental lesions that may rarely occur in the presacral region. They are cystic masses containing mucoid fluid, calcification (one-third of cases), and macroscopic fatty tissue (two-thirds to three-fourths of cases). Associated malformations include anorectal and osseous defects as part of the Currarino triad.
- **Adnexal mass.** Ovarian cysts are common in neonatal girls and can be very large. They result from maternal hormonal stimulation of the ovarian follicles and typically resolve. Ultrasound confirms the ovarian location of the cyst. Cysts > 6 cm are at risk of torsion.

■ Diagnosis

Sacrococcygeal teratoma

✓ Pearls

- SCTs are the most common caudal region tumor in infants; the appearance varies based upon composition.
- SCTs may be intrapelvic, extrapelvic, or both; they may also demonstrate intraspinal extension.
- ASMs are CSF herniations through neural foramina or bony defects; they may have associated anomalies.
- Ovarian cysts are relatively common in neonatal girls; larger lesions are at risk of ovarian torsion.

Suggested Reading

Kocaoglu M, Frush DP. Pediatric presacral masses. Radiographics 2006; 26: 833–857

Case 254

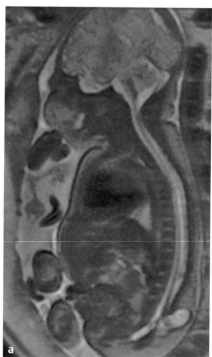 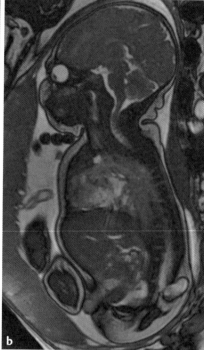

Fig. 254.1 Sagittal T2-weighted image through the fetal spine (a) demonstrates fetal elongation of the cord with herniation of CSF-filled meninges and the neural placode through a posterior bony defect at the lumbosacral junction. Sagittal high-resolution T2-weighted image (b) outlines an intact skin surface posteriorly, confirming a closed spinal dysraphism. The craniocervical junction appears normal.

■ Clinical Presentation

A fetal magnetic resonance image (MRI) after abnormal anatomic survey on ultrasound (▶ Fig. 254.1)

■ Key Imaging Finding

Closed lumbosacral spinal dysraphism with subcutaneous mass

■ Top 3 Differential Diagnoses

- **Lipomyelomeningocele/lipomyelocele.** Both lipomyelomeningoceles and lipomyeloceles result from a defect in primary neurulation, which allows for mesenchymal elements (lipomatous tissue) to enter the neural tube. The fatty tissue is in continuity with the subcutaneous fat and interfaces with the neural placode through a posterior bony defect. The overlying skin covering is intact. The key differentiating feature between a lipomyelomeningocele and a lipomyelocele is the location of the interface between the lipomatous tissue and neural placode. With a lipomyelocele, the interface is within the spinal canal; with a lipomyelomeningocele, the interface is outside of the spinal canal. MRI best depicts the fatty elements that are readily identified on fat-suppressed sequences; it also allows for optimal evaluation of the neural placode.
- **Meningocele.** A meningocele refers to herniation of cerebrospinal fluid (CSF)-filled meninges through a bony defect. They may occur anywhere in the spine, but are most common at the lumbosacral junction in association with a posterior bony defect and intact skin surface. Although the neural placode/cord is not present within the herniated sac, patients often present with clinical signs of cord tethering. Initial screening is typically performed with ultrasound; MRI is diagnostic and best evaluates the herniated contents and neural elements.
- **Terminal myelocystocele.** Terminal myelocystoceles refer to fetal elongation of the cord with herniation of CSF-filled meninges (meningocele) and a large terminal syrinx through a posterior osseous defect at the lumbosacral junction. This results in a CSF-filled subcutaneous mass of variable size that often appears as a cyst within a cyst, where the inner cyst is the syrinx and the outer cyst is the meningocele; neural elements surround the inner syrinx. In contrast to a myelomeningocele, terminal myelocystoceles have an intact skin covering and are not associated with Chiari II malformations.

■ Diagnosis

Terminal myelocystocele

✓ Pearls

- Lipomyelomeningoceles/lipomyeloceles refer to mesenchymal elements (fat) entering the neural tube.
- The key distinction between lipomyelomeningoceles/lipomyeloceles is the location of the fat-placode interface.
- Meningocele refers to herniation of CSF-filled meninges through a bony defect with an intact skin surface.
- Terminal myelocystocele refers to herniation of meninges and a large terminal syrinx through a bony defect.

Suggested Reading

Rufener SL, Ibrahim M, Raybaud CA, Parmar HA. Congenital spine and spinal cord malformations—pictorial review. Am J Roentgenol 2010; 194 Suppl: S26–S37

Case 255

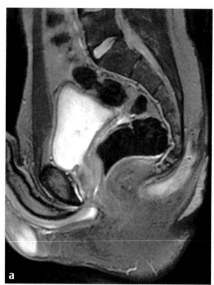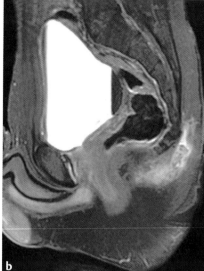

Fig. 255.1 Sagittal T2 MR image of the lumbo-sacral junction (a) demonstrates a T2 hyper-intense tract extending from the subcutaneous soft tissues to the region of the coccyx with surrounding inflammatory changes. Sagittal T1 postcontrast image with fat suppression (b) shows enhancement along the course of the tract, including the perirectal region.

Clinical Presentation

A 19-year-old man with perirectal pain (▶ Fig. 255.1)

■ Key Imaging Finding

Posterior lumbosacral tract

■ Top 3 Differential Diagnoses

- **Dermal sinus tract.** A dermal sinus tract results from inclusion of cutaneous ectodermal elements within the neuroectoderm during development. The tract is lined by squamous epithelium and may remain superficial or extend into deep paraspinal tissues or even into the spinal canal. It can be midline or paramedian and often includes dermoid or epidermoid elements; intradural dermoids commonly involve the conus medullaris or cauda equina. Patients often present incidentally with a dimple and/or hair patch noted over the lumbosacral junction on physical examination. Less commonly, patients may present with symptoms related to local infection or meningitis secondary to extension into the thecal sac. Ultrasound may be used for initial screening. The dermal sinus tract is typically hypoechoic compared with subcutaneous fat; intrathecal components are hyperechoic compared with surrounding cerebrospinal fluid (CSF). Magnetic resonance imaging (MRI) is the confirmatory modality of choice and demonstrates a fluid signal intensity tract (T1 hypointense/T2 hyperintense) extending various lengths within the subcutaneous tissues. Inflammatory enhancement is noted along the course of the tract. It is important to evaluate for intraspinal extension. Dermoid elements often demonstrate macroscopic fat; epidermoid elements follow CSF signal intensity but may show restricted diffusion. An intrathecal ruptured dermoid or epidermoid may cause chemical meningitis. The cord and conus should be closely evaluated to look for a low-lying cord or imaging findings suggestive of cord tethering, which may be associated with a dermal sinus tract.
- **Pilonidal sinus tract.** Pilonidal disease was initially thought to represent a developmental abnormality, but it is now generally accepted as an acquired process secondary to a superficial infection of hair follicle. The infected follicle causes a secondary inflammatory response, resulting in a sinus lined with epithelial cells and granulation tissue. It occurs most frequently in young adult men who either present with chronic irritation or discomfort overlying the sacrum superior to the anus or present acutely with abscess formation. The sinus tract is typically midline and extends deep and inferiorly towards the coccyx. If the sinus tract extends to the ischioanal fossa, it may be confused with a fistula-in-ano. MRI reveals abnormal increased T2 signal intensity within and along the sinus tract. Inflammatory enhancement is typically seen; abscesses demonstrate rim enhancement. A lateral location is less common but does occur. Surgical resection requires excision of the entire tract; recurrence rates may be as high as 30%.
- **Anal fistula (fistula-in-ano).** Fistula-in-ano is caused by an infection of the anal glands between the internal and external sphincters. Abscess formation causes a local inflammatory response, often with fistula formation extending to the perineum. Because there is direct communication of the tract with the anal lumen, the tract is referred to as a fistula rather than a sinus. Abscesses and tracts may be multiple, so preoperative MRI is vital to the initial workup and treatment planning. On MRI, a fistula-in-ano demonstrates increased T2 signal intensity and inflammatory T1 contrast enhancement along the course and surrounding the fistula. Focal abscesses demonstrate rim enhancement. Surgical resection is difficult and recurrence rates are high, especially when multiple.

■ Diagnosis

Pilonidal sinus tract

✓ Pearls

- Dermal sinus tracts result from inclusion of cutaneous ectodermal elements within the neural ectoderm.
- It is important to evaluate for coexistent (epi)dermoids and cord tethering in the setting of dermal sinus tracts.
- Pilonidal sinus tracts result from superficial inflammation and may extend inferiorly into paraspinal tissues.
- Fistula-in-ano refers to infection of the intersphincteric anal glands, often with extension to the perineum.

Suggested Readings

Rufener SL, Ibrahim M, Raybaud CA, Parmar HA. Congenital spine and spinal cord malformations—pictorial review. Am J Roentgenol 2010; 194 Suppl: S26–S37

Taylor SA, Halligan S, Bartram CI. Pilonidal sinus disease: MR imaging distinction from fistula in ano. Radiology 2003; 226: 662–667

Case 256

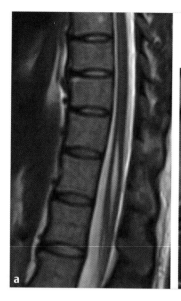

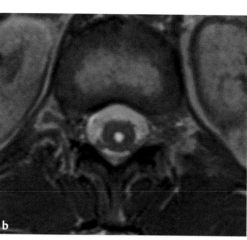

Fig. 256.1 Sagittal T2 magnetic resonance image **(a)** demonstrates a central region of increased fluid signal intensity within the distal cord/conus with tapering at the cranial and caudal ends. Axial T2 image **(b)** shows a central location and rounded configuration, which measured 3 mm in transverse dimension.

▨ Clinical Presentation

A young adult with nonspecific back pain (▶ Fig. 256.1)

■ Key Imaging Finding

Distal cord fluid collection

■ Top 3 Differential Diagnoses

- **Prominence of the central spinal canal.** Prominence of the central spinal cord canal is a common finding that is asymptomatic and incidental. It may occur transiently in the neonatal period or persist into adulthood. Magnetic resonance imaging reveals a round or ovoid region of cerebrospinal fluid (CSF) signal intensity in continuity with the central spinal canal measuring < 2 to 3 mm in maximal cross-sectional dimension.
- **Ventriculus terminalis.** Ventriculus terminalis refers to focal dilatation of the central spinal cord canal at the level of the conus. It is also referred to as a terminal or fifth ventricle. In the vast majority of cases, ventriculus terminalis is an incidental finding in an asymptomatic patient; occasionally, it may be present in the setting of fetal elongation of the cord or cord developmental anomalies. Large lesions may rarely cause neurological symptoms and require treatment. The classic imaging appearance includes a central round or ovoid region of CSF signal intensity in the distal cord/conus, measuring < 4 mm in cross-sectional dimension and extending a few centimeters or less in craniocaudal dimension. Larger variants, which may measure a few centimeters in cross-sectional dimension, are relatively uncommon but also characteristically located in the region of the conus.
- **Syrinx.** Hydromyelia is defined as dilatation of the central canal, whereas syringomyelia refers to a CSF cavity within the cord separate from the central canal. Because these entities are often indistinguishable on imaging, the terms *syrinx* or *syringomyelia* are commonly used for a region of abnormal CSF signal intensity within the cord. A cord syrinx may be an isolated finding or occur in the setting of underlying abnormalities such as Chiari I malformation or in association with a cord tumor, cord compression, or trauma. Depending upon the underlying etiology and chronicity, there may be underlying cord edema, as well as variable cord size, including a normal-sized cord, focal enlargement, or atrophy. The most common locations include the cervical followed by the thoracic cord. When a syrinx is found, it often requires further evaluation of the neuroaxis, including imaging of the craniocervical junction and at times contrast-enhanced imaging, to exclude an underlying cord tumor.

▨ Additional Differential Diagnoses

- **Cord myelomalacia.** Cord myelomalacia results from an underlying cord insult that is typically ischemic, post-traumatic, or hemorrhagic in nature. Similar to encephalomalacia in the brain parenchyma, there is focal volume loss with CSF signal intensity and surrounding gliosis. Focal cord volume loss is a helpful differentiating feature. Although the remaining differentials may occasionally demonstrate cord volume loss, they more characteristically present a normal-sized cord or focal cord enlargement.
- **Cystic cord tumor.** Ependymomas are the most common cord tumors in adults and commonly present with hemorrhage and cystic components within the tumor and/or a syrinx at its cranial or caudal end. The tumor itself causes cord enlargement and demonstrates enhancement of the solid components. Astrocytomas are the most common cord neoplasms in children and may also demonstrate cystic components and associated syrinx but less frequently than with ependymoma. Hemangioblastomas are highly vascular cord tumors that may occur sporadically or in association with von Hippel-Lindau disease. Smaller lesions demonstrate solid enhancement, whereas larger lesions present as a cystic mass with a subpial enhancing nodule.

■ Diagnosis

Ventriculus terminalis

✓ Pearls

- Prominence of the central spinal cord canal is a common incidental finding and is typically < 2 to 3 mm in size.
- Ventriculus terminalis (fifth ventricle) refers to focal dilatation of the central spinal cord canal at the conus.
- Syrinx represents abnormal CSF signal within the cord; underlying anomalies or cord injury may be seen.
- Cord tumors may have inherent cystic components or result in a cord syrinx, often at its cranial or caudal end.

Suggested Readings

Sherman JL, Barkovich AJ, Citrin CM. The MR appearance of syringomyelia: new observations. Am J Roentgenol 1987; 148: 381–391

Sigal R, Denys A, Halimi P, Shapeero L, Doyon D, Boudghène F. Ventriculus terminalis of the conus medullaris: MR imaging in four patients with congenital dilatation. Am J Neuroradiol 1991; 12: 733–737

Case 257

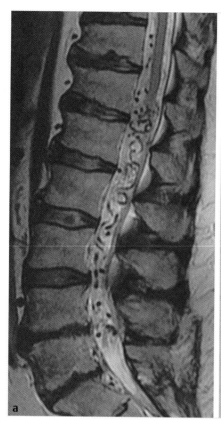 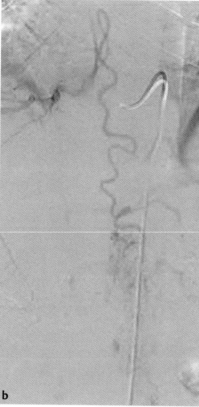

Fig. 257.1 Sagittal T2-weighted magnetic resonance image **(a)** demonstrates multiple, serpentine extramedullary, intradural vascular flow voids in the lumbar spine. Subsequent spinal digital subtraction angiogram image **(b)** during the arterial phase of a right T10 intercostal artery injection reveals an enlarged anterior spinal artery with early filling of a plexus of intradural veins from arteriovenous shunting. (Case courtesy of Matthew Moore, MD.)

▨ Clinical Presentation

A 55-year-old man with progressive lower extremity weakness (▶ Fig. 257.1)

■ Key Imaging Finding

Prominent paraspinal flow voids

■ Top 3 Differential Diagnoses

- **Dural arteriovenous fistula (AVF).** There are four types of spinal arteriovenous shunt lesions. The most common is the type I dural AVF, which accounts for 70 to 80% of cases and is a direct arteriovenous connection (no intervening nidus) within the spinal dura mater itself. The lesion drains into distended pial veins, which are seen as extramedullary, intradural serpentine flow voids on sagittal T2 sequences or multiple, enhancing serpentine vessels on enhanced sagittal T1 sequences. The arteriovenous shunting causes venous hypertension, leading to chronic cord ischemia. There cord ischemia presents as a "flame-shaped" region of cord edema with sparing of the periphery and is best seen on T2 sequences. Patients, typically men, present in the fifth or sixth decades with progressive lower extremity weakness, which is exacerbated by exercise. Spinal angiogram is the gold standard for diagnosis, localization, and treatment, which consists of endovascular coiling. Care must be taken to identify and avoid the spinal arteries and their feeders, including the artery of Adamkiewicz (typically found on the left between T8 and T12). The type IV AVF or "perimedullary fistula" is the other true AVF, which may be indistinguishable from the type I dural AVF on magnetic resonance imaging.

- **Spinal cord arteriovenous malformation (AVM).** The remaining two types of spinal arteriovenous shunt lesions (types II and III) represent true AVMs with an intervening nidus. Both of these lesions present with prominent extramedullary flow voids; however, unlike the type I and IV lesions, an intramedullary component is present, representing the nidus. The spinal type II AVM is similar to a brain AVM with an intramedullary nidus, enlarged feeding arteries, and enlarged draining veins. Patients commonly present with acute onset of symptoms due to intralesional or subarachnoid hemorrhage. Type III, or juvenile AVM, is a rare lesion that typically occurs in the first through third decades of life. The large AVM has both intramedullary and extramedullary components, often with significant involvement of paraspinal soft tissues.

- **Collateral venous flow from inferior vena cava (IVC) occlusion.** IVC occlusion may cause prominent collateral epidural and/or intradural veins. Common etiologies of IVC occlusion include trauma, extrinsic compression, tumor invasion, and hypercoagulable states. It is important to evaluate the IVC for evidence of thrombus, adjacent mass effect, or internal susceptibility artifact related to an IVC filter. Treatment is geared toward the underlying etiology.

■ Additional Differential Diagnoses

- **Spinal cord neoplasm with increased vascular flow.** Paraspinal flow voids may be seen with several intradural neoplasms, both intra- and extramedullary. Hemangioblastoma classically presents as an expansile intramedullary mass with serpentine flow voids. Smaller lesions demonstrate solid enhancement, whereas larger lesions present as a cystic mass with an enhancing mural nodule. On occasion, ependymomas and paragangliomas may also have associated flow voids related to increased vascular flow. An enhancing mass is the common and distinguishing feature associated with these lesions.

- **Cerebrospinal fluid (CSF) pulsations.** Normal CSF pulsations are seen dorsal to the cord on T2 sequences. They have ill-defined margins, which easily differentiate them from the well-defined vascular flow voids seen with spinal arteriovenous shunt lesions. The lack of corresponding abnormality on non-T2-weighted sequences allows for identification of this common artifact.

■ Diagnosis

Dural arteriovenous fistula (type I)

✓ Pearls

- Type I dural AVFs result in vascular shunting with chronic cord ischemia and progressive weakness.
- Spinal cord AVMs are similar to brain AVMs with a vascular nidus and arteriovenous shunting.
- Collateral epidural and intradural veins may be seen with IVC occlusion, simulating an AVF or AVM.
- Hemangioblastomas, ependymomas, and paragangliomas may have prominent paraspinal flow voids.

Suggested Readings

Krings T, Geibprasert S. Spinal dural arteriovenous fistulas. Am J Neuroradiol 2009; 30: 639–648

Rodesch G, Lasjaunias P. Spinal cord arteriovenous shunts: from imaging to management. Eur J Radiol 2003; 46: 221–232

Case 258

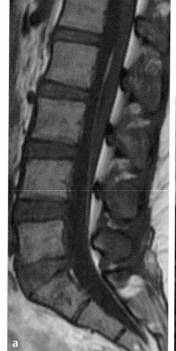

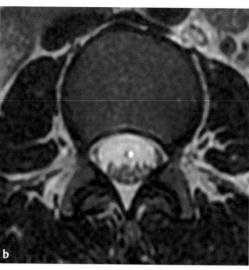

Fig. 258.1 Sagittal T1-weighted image **(a)** demonstrates a linear region of T1 hyperintensity along the filum/cauda equina beginning at the L1–2 level and extending inferiorly. Axial T2 image **(b)** shows a rounded region of hyperintense signal along the left lateral aspect of the filum, centered within the thecal sac.

▓ Clinical Presentation

A young adult man with chronic back pain (▶ Fig. 258.1)

■ Key Imaging Finding

Intrathecal fat

■ Top 3 Differential Diagnoses

- **Fatty infiltration of the filum.** Also known a fibrolipomatous thickening of the filum terminale or filar lipoma, fatty infiltration of the filum is a relatively common finding on lumbar spine magnetic resonance imaging (MRI). Patients are often asymptomatic, although the lesion may be associated with clinical signs of cord tethering in a minority of patients. A low-lying cord, when present, is most often seen in symptomatic patients. Imaging demonstrates characteristic linear fatty signal intensity (increased signal on T1/T2 and decreased signal on fat-suppressed sequences) along a normal-sized or mildly thickened filum. It typically extends from the conus to the termination of the thecal sac and measures < 2 to 3 mm in transverse dimension. Chemical shift artifact may be seen.
- **Subpial lipoma.** A subpial lipoma represents focal fatty infiltration isolated to the cord. It may occur at any level, is most common in the thoracic spine, and most often occurs dorsally. When located in the lumbar spine, it typically involves the distal cord or conus and does not extend along the filum terminale. The lipoma may vary significantly from a few millimeters to centimeters in size. Subpial lipomas may be incidental or associated with spinal dysraphism and neurological deficits corresponding to the involved spinal level.
- **Terminal lipoma.** A terminal lipoma refers to fatty infiltration along the distal cord and conus without an overlying spinal dysraphism. The cord is low lying, typically extending to the lumbosacral junction, and there is an indistinct junction between the cord and associated lipoma. Patients often present with clinical signs of cord tethering and progressive neurological symptoms.

■ Additional Differential Diagnoses

- **Lipomyelocele.** Both lipomyelomeningoceles and lipomyeloceles result from a defect in primary neurulation, which allows for mesenchymal elements (lipomatous tissue) to enter the neural tube. The fatty tissue is in continuity with the subcutaneous fat and interfaces with the neural placode through a posterior bony defect. The overlying skin covering is intact. The key differentiating feature between a lipomyelomeningocele and a lipomyelocele is the location of the interface between the lipomatous tissue and neural placode. With a lipomyelocele, the interface is within the spinal canal; with a lipomyelomeningocele, the interface is outside of the spinal canal. MRI best depicts the fatty elements, which are readily identified on fat-suppressed sequences; it also allows for optimal evaluation of the neural placode.
- **Teratoma.** A teratoma is a germ cell tumor that contains elements from all three germ layers. It most often occurs at the sacrum (sacrococcygeal teratoma) and is commonly diagnosed prenatally or in the early neonatal period. Intrathecal teratomas are exceedingly rare and have similar imaging characteristics to teratomas elsewhere. Lesions typically present with cystic and solid components, as well as characteristic macroscopic fat. Additional components include calcifications, teeth, and hair. Prognosis is dependent upon the classification in terms of internal or external location. MRI shows a large mass centered at the sacrum with variable extension into adjacent compartments and structures. Characteristic calcifications, macroscopic fat, and fat-fluid levels are useful discriminators. Solid components heterogeneously enhance.

■ Diagnosis

Fatty infiltration of the filum

✓ Pearls

- Fatty infiltration of the filum is linear, measures 2 to 3 mm in size, and is most often asymptomatic and incidental.
- Subpial lipoma represents focal fatty infiltration isolated to the cord; it does not extend along the filum.
- Terminal lipoma involves the distal aspect of a low-lying cord without an overlying spinal dysraphism.
- Lipomyelocele occurs in the setting of a spinal dysraphism; the placode–lipoma interface is in the thecal sac.

Suggested Reading

Rufener SL, Ibrahim M, Raybaud CA, Parmar HA. Congenital spine and spinal cord malformations—pictorial review. Am J Roentgenol 2010; 194 Suppl: S26–S37

Case 259

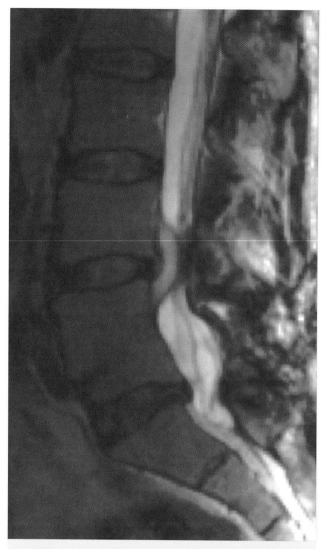

Fig. 259.1 Sagittal T2 magnetic resonance image demonstrates a hyperintense anterior epidural mass centered at the L3–4 level. There is a congenital segmentation anomaly with partial fusion of L4 and L5, as well as L5-S1 disc dessication with a disc bulge.

▇ Clinical Presentation

A middle-aged adult man with back pain; history otherwise withheld (▸ Fig. 259.1)

▓ Key Imaging Finding

Epidural spinal mass

▓ Top 3 Differential Diagnoses

- **Disc extrusion.** Disc extrusion refers to herniations with migration of the disc fragment within the anterior epidural space. There is often disc dessication and height loss with intact end plates. The extruded fragment is usually similar in signal intensity and in continuity with the parent disc, unless it becomes sequestered. There may be peripheral enhancement. Epidural hematomas may be seen in association with acute disc extrusions.
- **Epidural hematoma.** Epidural hematomas may occur spontaneously or result from trauma, transient venous hypertension (cough), iatrogenia, or coagulopathy. They are most often due to rupture of the epidural venous plexus. Most occur within the dorsal thoracolumbar spine in adults and cervicothoracic spine in children. They are generally biconvex and surrounded by epidural fat. Acute hemorrhage is T1 isointense, whereas subacute or chronic is most often T1 hyperintense. Hemorrhage is variable in T2 signal intensity depending upon the composition of blood products. On gradient echo imaging, hemorrhagic blood products are often hypointense. Peripheral enhancement is common; focal enhancement may represent extravasation.
- **Epidural abscess.** Epidural abscesses are commonly associated with disc-osteomyelitis. They most often occur anteriorly and are associated with paraspinal phlegmon or abscess formation. They may result from hematogenous dissemination of a distant infection or direct inoculation from surgical procedures or epidural anesthesia. The latter are less common and occur dorsally. *Staphylococcus aureus* (70 to 75%) is the most common organism; *Mycobacterium tuberculosis* infection most often occurs in immunocompromised patients. *Staphylococcus aureus* infections are centered at the disc space, whereas tuberculosis spondylitis results in relative sparing of the disc. Epidural abscesses follow fluid signal with peripheral rim and adjacent dural enhancement.

▓ Additional Differential Diagnoses

- **Metastatic disease.** Epidural foci from metastatic disease are often contiguous with a pedicle or posterior vertebral body lesion. A pathological compression fracture may be present. The masses are typically T1 hypointense and variable in T2 signal intensity with diffuse or heterogeneous enhancement depending upon the presence of necrosis or hemorrhage. Common primary tumors include breast, lung, and prostate carcinoma. Non-Hodgkin lymphoma may also present as an extradural mass. Lymphoma is typically iso- to hyperdense on computed tomography, isointense on T1, and variable on T2 sequences with intense homogeneous enhancement.
- **Epidural lipomatosis.** Lipomatosis refers to abnormal proliferation of epidural fat. It is most commonly seen in the thoracolumbar spine. Causative etiologies include excessive steroids (exogenous or endogenous) and obesity, although it may also be idiopathic. The lesions follow fat signal on all sequences and do not enhance. There may be compression of the spinal canal and neural structures.
- **Synovial cyst.** Synovial cysts result from degenerative facet disease and most commonly occur in the lumbar spine. They may extend into the posterolateral epidural space or through the neural foramen. The cyst follows fluid signal and has a T2 hypointense margin. Peripheral enhancement may be seen, as can hemorrhage or calcification. Patients commonly present with pain or radiculopathy.

▓ Diagnosis

Epidural abscess

✓ Pearls

- Disc extrusions occur anterior to the thecal sac and commonly follow the signal intensity of the parent disc.
- Epidural hematomas are most often dorsal and may occur spontaneously or due to an inciting event.
- Epidural abscesses have rim enhancement and most commonly are associated with disc-osteomyelitis.
- Synovial cysts result from degenerative facet disease and may compress the posterolateral thecal sac.

Suggested Reading

Chhabra A, Batra K, Satti S, et al. Spinal epidural space: anatomy, normal variations, and pathological lesions. Neurographics 2006; 5(1)

Case 260

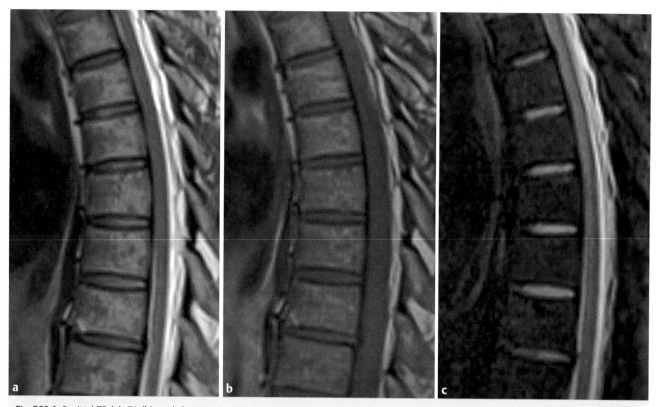

Fig. 260.1 Sagittal T2 **(a)**, T1 **(b)**, and short tau inversion recovery (STIR) **(c)** images demonstrate a long-segment posterior epidural fluid collection that is hyperintense on all pulse sequences, including the fat-suppressed STIR sequence. There is anterior displacement of the thecal sac and linear hypointensities traversing the epidural collection.

■ Clinical Presentation

A young adult man with back pain and headache (▶ Fig. 260.1)

■ Key Imaging Finding

Epidural fluid collection

■ Top 3 Differential Diagnoses

- **Epidural hematoma.** Epidural hematomas most often result from trauma or iatrogenia (e.g., lumbar puncture). Less often, they may be due an underlying coagulopathy or vascular malformation, occur spontaneously, or have an unknown cause. Patients present with pain with or without neurological deficits. Epidural hematomas may span several vertebral segments or occur focally. They are more common in the thoracolumbar region, followed by the cervical spine. Computed tomography (CT) reveals a hyperdense epidural collection. The magnetic resonance imaging (MRI) appearance varies based upon the timing of hemorrhage. Acute hemorrhage is typically isointense on T1 and becomes hyperintense in the subacute phase. T2 signal intensity is most often hyperintense but heterogeneous. "Capping" of the hematoma by epidural fat is often seen on sagittal sequences. Chronically, hypointensity on all sequences may be seen due to hemosiderin deposition. Gradient echo (GRE) sequences are helpful, demonstrating susceptibility artifact from blood products. Peripheral inflammatory enhancement may be seen. Treatment options include conservative management versus surgical decompression, depending upon the size and severity of the hematoma.
- **Epidural abscess.** Epidural abscesses are most often the result of disc-osteomyelitis and therefore typically occur in the anterior epidural space. Less common etiologies that occur in the posterior epidural space include postoperative complications, iatrogenia, and facet septic arthritis. Disc-osteomyelitis is most often pyogenic and caused by hematogenous dissemination of *Staphylococcus aureus*. Tuberculosis spondylitis is less common and most often involves the thoracic spine. Infectious processes occur locally and spread into adjacent soft tissues and compartments. Phlegmon presents as ill-defined regions of inflammatory signal and enhancement. As the infectious process becomes more organized, abscesses develop with rim-enhancing fluid collections, which may be focal or spread throughout the epidural space. Pyogenic abscesses commonly restrict diffusion. Treatment typically consists of intravenous antibiotic therapy and drainage of any fluid collections.
- **Cerebrospinal fluid (CSF) leak.** CSF leaks may result from iatrogenia (e.g., lumbar puncture), postoperative complication, trauma, or occur spontaneously. Patients often present with positional headaches that are worse when sitting or standing and improved when lying down. The majority will resolve spontaneously with conservative therapy consisting of bed rest, caffeine, and hydration. Blood patch or surgical repair may be necessary in refractory cases. Spinal fluid collections follow CSF attenuation (CT) and signal intensity (MRI) with compression of the thecal sac. Regions remote from the site of leakage may demonstrate retraction of the thecal sac due to a paucity of CSF and enlargement of epidural veins. The site of leakage may be interrogated with CT myelography or radionuclide cisternography. Intracranial findings of intracranial hypotension include a "sagging" brain, dural thickening with subdural collections, and diffuse pachymeningeal enhancement.

■ Additional Differential Diagnoses

- **Epidural lipomatosis.** Epidural lipomatosis refers to abnormal proliferation of epidural fat. It is most commonly seen in the thoracolumbar spine and is more common in men. Causative etiologies include excessive steroids (exogenous or endogenous) and obesity, although it may also be idiopathic. Patients may be asymptomatic or present with symptoms from compressive neuropathy. MRI demonstrates increased proliferation of fat signal intensity (increased signal on T1/T2 sequences and decreased signal on fat-suppressed sequences) within the epidural space with compression of the thecal sac. Axial images may demonstrate a characteristic Y-shaped or polygonal configuration due to the presence of meningovertebral ligaments that serve as anchors for the dural sac. Treatment is medical and geared toward the underlying cause.

■ Diagnosis

Epidural hematoma

✓ Pearls

- Hematomas often result from trauma or iatrogenia; they are typically T1 iso-bright, T2 bright, and GRE dark.
- Epidural abscesses most often result from disc-osteomyelitis and present as rim-enhancing fluid collections.
- CSF leaks may show CSF collections compressing the thecal sac or thecal sac retraction due to hypotension.

Suggested Reading

Koch BL, Moosbrugger EA, Egelhoff JC. Symptomatic spinal epidural collections after lumbar puncture in children. Am J Neuroradiol 2007; 28: 1811–1816

Case 261

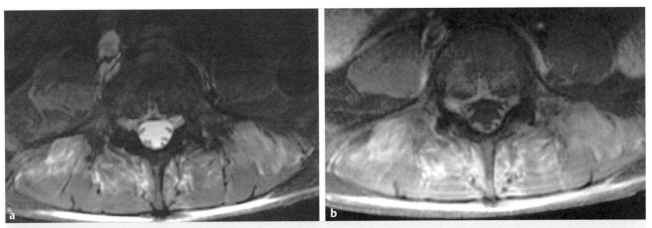

Fig. 261.1 Axial T2 **(a)** and T1 postcontrast **(b)** MR images with incomplete fat suppression reveal abnormal increased T2 signal intensity and enhancement throughout the paraspinal musculature of the lumbar spine. There is also abnormal enhancement of the descending nerve roots of the cauda equina.

■ Clinical Presentation

A 22-year-old man with chronic immunodeficiency and back pain (▶ Fig. 261.1)

■ Key Imaging Finding

Diffuse, symmetric paraspinal musculature signal and enhancement

■ Top 3 Differential Diagnoses

- **Myositis.** Myositis refers to inflammation of the musculature due to a variety of underlying causes, including infectious, inflammatory, postradiation, autoimmune, and idiopathic etiologies. Infectious myositis may be bacterial or viral and affect immunocompetent or immunocompromised hosts. Routes of spread include hematogenous spread of a distant infection or local spread from an adjacent infectious process, such as soft-tissue or bony infections. Early infection demonstrates muscle edema with ill-defined, diffuse increased T2 signal intensity with or without enhancement. Bacterial infections may progress to frank abscess formation with a rim-enhancing fluid collection that may mimic a soft-tissue mass. Radiation therapy results in vascular and soft-tissue injury that manifests as diffuse muscle edema confined to the treatment field; diffuse inflammatory enhancement may be seen. Autoimmune etiologies, such as polymyositis and dermatomyositis, commonly involve the extremities with eventual extension into the musculature of the neck. Magnetic resonance imaging (MRI) shows diffuse, symmetric muscle edema that progresses to atrophy in the chronic stages.
- **Trauma.** Injury to paraspinal musculature results in focal (more common) or diffuse edema with or without hemorrhage. The extent and degree of abnormal signal intensity on MRI depends upon the type and severity of injury. MRI demonstrates abnormal increased T2 signal intensity within the involved musculature and surrounding soft tissues. Foci of hemorrhage have variable signal intensity depending upon the stage of hemorrhage and may appear masslike in the setting of an intramuscular hematoma. Regions of inflammatory enhancement may be seen. In severe trauma, it is important to evaluate the spine, supporting ligamentous structures, and cord for associated injury.
- **Denervation.** Denervation injury may result from a variety of causes, including trauma, infection, and congenital or degenerative compression. MRI in the first few days of denervation is most often normal. In the subacute phase, muscle edema is seen as regions of diffuse increased T2 signal intensity; this may begin as early as 2 days after the initial denervation injury and peaks between 2 and 4 weeks. If the underlying cause is corrected, signal intensity and function are typically restored. Regions of enhancement may be seen. Should the condition persist into the chronic stage, however, muscle atrophy with fatty replacement ensues.

■ Additional Differential Diagnoses

- **Rhabdomyolysis.** Rhabdomyolysis refers to a severe muscular condition that results from loss of cell membrane integrity. Underlying etiologies include trauma, ischemia, excessive exercise, and autoimmune causes. The lack of cell membrane integrity results in migration of intracellular contents into the extracellular compartment with associated muscle edema. Complications in severe cases include renal failure and compartment syndrome. MRI reveals abnormal increased T2 signal intensity within the involved musculature. Regions of enhancement may be seen. In the setting of myonecrosis, a linear and dotted pattern of signal abnormality and enhancement is referred to as the "stipple sign."

■ Diagnosis

Myositis (infectious)

✓ Pearls

- Myositis refers to inflammation and edema of the musculature; imaging appearance varies based upon etiology.
- Injury to paraspinal musculature results in focal or diffuse edema with or without hemorrhage.
- Denervation presents with muscle edema in the subacute phase and fatty infiltration in the chronic phase.
- Rhabdomyolysis refers to severe muscle injury that may result in renal failure and compartment syndrome.

Suggested Reading

May DA, Disler DG, Jones EA, Balkissoon AA, Manaster BJ. Abnormal signal intensity in skeletal muscle at MR imaging: patterns, pearls, and pitfalls. Radiographics 2000; 20: S295–S315

Case 262

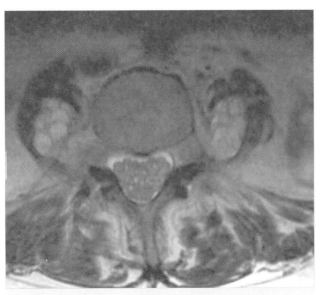

Fig. 262.1 Axial T2 image demonstrates diffuse enlargement and increased signal intensity involving the nerve roots of the cauda equina and extradural nerve roots along the psoas musculature. (Courtesy of Paul M. Sherman, MD.)

▨ Clinical Presentation

A young man with long-standing neurological deficits (▶ Fig. 262.1)

▨ Key Imaging Finding

Diffuse, multiple nerve root enlargement

▨ Top 3 Differential Diagnoses

- **Chronic inflammatory demyelinating polyneuropathy (CIDP).** CIDP represents a chronic, acquired, mixed motor and sensory polyneuropathy. Patients present with motor weakness involving the extremities with additional sensory disturbances; symptoms are often present for months to years and are slowly progressive. An antecedent infection or vaccination is seen in less than one-third of cases. Pathological evaluation demonstrates a characteristic "onion bulb" appearance due to episodes of demyelination with repair. Magnetic resonance imaging (MRI) reveals focal or diffuse enlargement, T2 hyperintensity, and enhancement involving the nerve roots of the cauda equina, which often extend into the extraspinal peripheral nerves. Symptoms generally improve with corticosteroid therapy.
- **Neurofibromatosis type 1 (NF1).** NF1, also known as von Recklinghausen disease, is the most common neurocutaneous syndrome. It may occur sporadically or be inherited in an autosomal dominant fashion. The genetic defect affects chromosome 17q12 and results in decreased production of neurofibromin, which acts as a tumor suppressor. The disease affects the brain, skull, orbits, spine, musculoskeletal system, and skin/integumentary system. Spinal manifestations of NF1 include multiple neurofibromas with extension through and expansion of the neuroforamina. Neurofibromas are more likely than schwannomas to demonstrate the "target sign," which refers to peripheral increased and central decreased T2 signal intensity. Large, retroperitoneal plexiform neurofibromas are prone to malignant degeneration, which is best characterized by interval growth. Additional spinal manifestations include kyphoscoliosis, dural ectasia with posterior vertebral body scalloping, and lateral thoracic meningoceles. Rarely, intramedullary lesions may occur in patients with NF1.
- **Hereditary motor-sensory neuropathy (HMSN).** HMSN refers to a group of inherited disorders that may result in diffuse nerve root enlargement and neurological symptoms affecting motor and sensory pathways. Two of the more common syndromes include Charcot-Marie-Tooth disease and Dejerine-Sottas disease. The clinical presentation varies depending upon the specific underlying syndrome; however, symptoms are generally chronic and progressive. Imaging often reveals diffuse, fusiform enlargement, abnormal signal intensity, and enhancement of the extraspinal peripheral nerves and/or nerve roots of the cauda equina. In some patients, nerve root enhancement without enlargement may be seen. The impaired neurological function associated with motor nerves results in denervation. In the acute setting, denervation produces edema within the involved musculature; chronically, there is muscle atrophy with volume loss and fatty replacement, which is a helpful distinguishing feature, when present. Confirmatory diagnosis is typically made by sural nerve biopsy.

▨ Additional Differential Diagnoses

- **Guillain-Barré syndrome (GBS).** GBS represents an acute, monophasic inflammatory demyelinating polyneuropathy that is thought to result from an autoimmune response to an antecedent infection or vaccination. Patients present with progressive ascending weakness of the lower extremities without sensory involvement. MRI classically reveals smooth enhancement of the nerve roots of the cauda equina with early preferential involvement of the ventral motor nerve roots. Enhancement is also commonly seen along the distal cord and conus. Mild nerve root enlargement may be seen. Treatment includes plasmapheresis and/or intravenous immunoglobulin.

▨ Diagnosis

Chronic inflammatory demyelinating polyneuropathy

✓ Pearls

- CIDP is a chronic, acquired, mixed motor and sensory polyneuropathy with ascending motor weakness.
- NF1 reveals neurofibromas, kyphoscoliosis, dural ectasia, vertebral body scalloping, and lateral meningoceles.
- HMSN results in diffuse nerve root enlargement, motor and sensory deficits, and muscle denervation.
- GBS represents an acute, monophasic demyelinating polyneuropathy with progressive ascending weakness.

Suggested Readings

Cellerini M, Salti S, Desideri V, Marconi G. MR imaging of the cauda equina in hereditary motor sensory neuropathies: correlations with sural nerve biopsy. Am J Neuroradiol 2000; 21: 1793–1798

Rodriguez D, Young Poussaint T. Neuroimaging findings in neurofibromatosis type 1 and 2. Neuroimaging Clin N Am 2004; 14: 149–170, vii

Zapadka M. Diffuse cauda equina nerve root enhancement. JAOCR J Am Osteopath Coll Radiol. 2012; 1: 29–32

Case 263

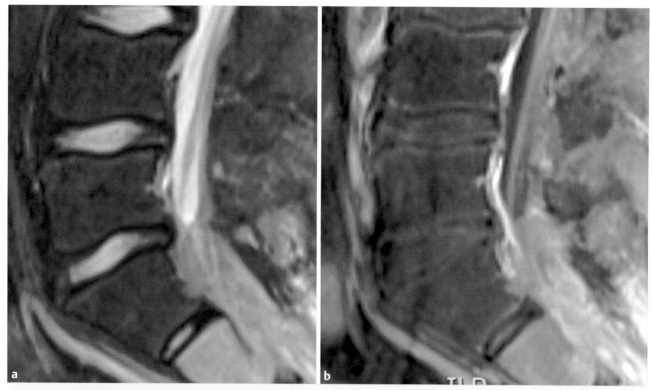

Fig. 263.1 Axial short tau inversion recovery image **(a)** through the lumbosacral junction demonstrates diffuse hyperintense marrow infiltration of the S2 vertebral body with cortical breakthrough posteriorly and extension into the epidural space. Sagittal T1 postcontrast image with fat suppression **(b)** reveals homogeneous enhancement.

■ Clinical Presentation

An adult man with low back pain (▶ Fig. 263.1)

■ Key Imaging Finding

Sacral mass in an adult

■ Top 3 Differential Diagnoses

- **Metastases.** Metastatic disease commonly involves the spine. The most common primary neoplasms include breast, lung, and prostate carcinoma. Breast and lung carcinoma are most often lytic, along with renal and thyroid carcinomas. Prostate (and occasionally breast) carcinoma produces sclerotic metastases. Computed tomography (CT) demonstrates bony involvement in better detail than magnetic resonance imaging (MRI), whereas MRI is superior in evaluating the soft-tissue component. Metastases are typically hypointense on T1 and hyperintense on T2 with avid enhancement.
- **Chordoma.** Chordoma is a malignant tumor that arises from notochordal remnants. It most commonly affects the sacrum, skull base, and spine in young to middle-aged adults and is more common in men. It represents the most common primary sacral tumor. Patients with sacral involvement often present with localized pain and neuropathy. CT reveals a midline, expansile, lytic mass with hyperdense foci centrally. Chordomas are classically hyperintense on T2 sequences with hypointense fibrous septations. They are typically hypo- to isointense on T1 sequences with heterogeneous but avid enhancement.
- **Giant cell tumor (GCT).** GCT is a neoplasm that is locally aggressive and composed of giant cells that lead to bony resorption. It represents the second most common primary bony neoplasm of the sacrum. Conventional radiographs and CT demonstrate a lytic, expansile lesion with no internal matrix; central necrosis or hemorrhage may be seen. The margins are often nonsclerotic, although some lesions demonstrate a thin sclerotic rim. On MRI, GCTs are often hypointense to intermediate in signal on T1 and iso- to hyperintense on T2 sequences. Internal bony septations are curvilinear and hypointense in T2 signal. Heterogeneous but avid enhancement is typically seen. The presence of multiple loculations with fluid-fluid levels suggests a superimposed aneurysmal bone cyst (ABC), which is commonly associated with GCTs.

■ Additional Differential Diagnoses

- **Lymphoma.** Lymphoma has a variety of manifestations within the spine, including osseous, epidural, and various forms of intradural involvement. It is more often secondary than primary. Bony involvement may appear lytic and permeative or sclerotic on CT. MRI demonstrates hypointense T1 and variable T2 marrow infiltration with homogeneous enhancement. Epidural extension is common. Lesions may be multiple or solitary.
- **Chondrosarcoma.** Chondrosarcoma is a malignant primary bone tumor that may involve the spine. It may occur at any age but is most common in middle-aged patients who present with localized pain and neuropathy. CT demonstrates an expansile lesion with internal chondroid matrix in an "arcs and swirls" pattern. The soft-tissue component is variable in attenuation. On MRI, the chondroid matrix is hyperintense on T2 sequences, whereas internal calcifications are hypointense. Heterogeneous enhancement is typically seen.
- **Plasmacytoma.** Plasmacytoma is the result of abnormal proliferation of plasma cells; it is the solitary form of multiple myeloma. Patients are typically ≥ 40 years of age. Presentation depends upon the location of the mass; pain and neuropathy are common. CT demonstrates a poorly defined, expansile, lytic lesion. On MRI, lesions are typically hypo- to isointense to cord on T1 and iso- to hyperintense on T2 sequences; curvilinear regions of hypointense T2 signal are commonly seen. The majority of lesions demonstrate homogeneous enhancement. Extension into the epidural space is common. Patients must be followed to exclude multiple myeloma.

■ Diagnosis

Lymphoma

✓ Pearls

- Metastases (most often breast, lung, and prostate) represent the most common neoplasms to affect the sacrum.
- Chordomas and chondrosarcomas are classically hyperintense in T2 signal with linear hypointense components.
- GCT presents as an expansile lytic lesion; there may be central necrosis, hemorrhage, or a co-existent ABC.
- Osseous lymphoma may appear lytic and permeative or sclerotic on CT; homogeneous enhancement is typical.

Suggested Reading

Diel J, Ortiz O, Losada RA, Price DB, Hayt MW, Katz DS. The sacrum: pathologic spectrum, multimodality imaging, and subspecialty approach. Radiographics 2001; 21: 83–104

Case 264

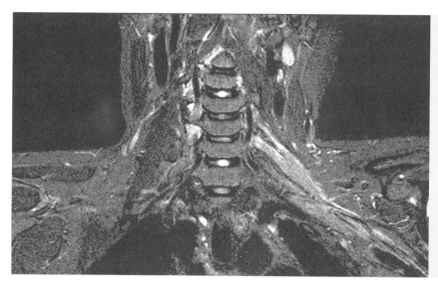

Fig. 264.1 Coronal short tau inversion recovery image shows abnormal enlargement and increased signal intensity within the visualized portions of the brachial plexus on the left.

■ Clinical Presentation

Unilateral upper arm loss of muscular tone and decreased reflexes (▶ Fig. 264.1)

▧ Key Imaging Finding

Enlarged brachial plexus nerve roots

▧ Top 3 Differential Diagnoses

- **Trauma.** The brachial plexus is composed of the C5-T1 nerve roots that extend into trunks, divisions, cords, and terminal branches as they progresses laterally. Brachial plexus injuries are most often seen in birth-related trauma and adolescents involved in motor vehicle accidents. Birth-related injuries commonly involve C5–7 (Erb-Duchenne palsy); C8-T1 involvement is less common (Klumpke palsy). Injuries range from stretching (most common) to avulsions and are classified as either preganglionic or postganglionic. Preganglionic injuries do not recover spontaneously, whereas postganglionic injuries often do. Stretching injuries result in nerve root enlargement, increased T2 signal intensity, and enhancement. Surrounding hematoma may be seen.

- **Brachial plexitis.** Brachial plexitis refers to inflammation involving the brachial plexus. The most common cause is radiation therapy, typically used in the treatment of breast or apical lung cancer. Less common causes include viral infections, immune-mediated neuropathy, and idiopathic. Compared with neoplastic processes, radiation brachial plexitis typically presents with diffuse thickening and indistinct signal abnormality that is often confined to the treatment field; fibrosis may be seen in the chronic setting. The viral, immune-mediated, and idiopathic forms of brachial plexitis have a variety of imaging appearances, ranging from normal to nerve root enlargement, abnormal signal intensity, and enhancement, depending upon the severity and underlying etiology. Chronic plexitis of motor nerves may result in denervation. In the acute setting, denervation produces edema within the innervated musculature; chronically, there is muscle atrophy with volume loss and fatty replacement.

- **Neoplasm.** Secondary neoplastic involvement of the brachial plexus is more common than primary nerve sheath tumors (NSTs). Common secondary causes include lymphatic spread of breast cancer (most common), direct spread from lung cancer (Pancoast tumor), lymphomatous involvement, and hematogenous spread from distant primary or hematologic malignancies. Magnetic resonance imaging (MRI) demonstrates focal or diffuse nerve root enlargement, increased T2 signal intensity, and abnormal enhancement, which may be masslike. Primary tumors include schwannomas and neurofibromas, as well as malignant peripheral NSTs in the setting of NF1. These primary lesions appear more focal compared with secondary involvement and present as T2 hyperintense, enhancing lesions. Schwannomas are more likely to undergo cystic degeneration. Neurofibromas tend to be more uniform in signal intensity and may demonstrate the "target sign," which refers to peripheral increased and central decreased T2 signal intensity. Central lesions may extend through and expand the neural formina.

▧ Additional Differential Diagnoses

- **Hypertrophic neuropathy.** Hypertrophic neuropathy refers to a variety of disorders that result in enlargement and degeneration of involved nerves. The condition may be acquired (e.g., chronic inflammatory demyelinating polyneuropathy [CIDP]) or genetic (e.g., hereditary motor-sensory neuropathy [HMSN]). Two of the more common congenital syndromes (HMSN) include Charcot-Marie-Tooth disease and Dejerine-Sottas disease. Symptoms depend upon the underlying etiology; however, most patients present with a chronic, progressive neuropathy with motor and sensory components. MRI often reveals diffuse fusiform enlargement, abnormal signal intensity, and enhancement of the extraspinal peripheral nerves. The impaired neurological function associated with motor nerves may result in denervation. In the acute setting, denervation produces edema within the involved musculature; chronically, there is muscle atrophy with volume loss and fatty replacement.

▧ Diagnosis

Brachial plexitis

✓ Pearls

- Stretching injury causes enlargement, abnormal signal, and enhancement; surrounding hematoma may be seen.
- Brachial plexitis refers to inflammation of the brachial plexus; radiation therapy is the most common cause.

- Neoplastic involvement of the brachial plexus may be secondary (more common) or primary NSTs.
- Patients with hypertrophic neuropathy (CIDP, HMSN) commonly present with chronic, progressive symptoms.

Suggested Reading

Aralasmak A, Karaali K, Cevikol C, Uysal H, Senol U. MR imaging findings in brachial plexopathy with thoracic outlet syndrome. Am J Neuroradiol 2010; 31: 410–417

Case 265

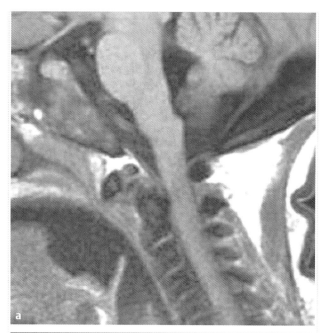

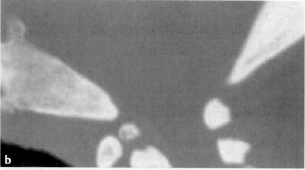

Fig. 265.1 Sagittal T1 magnetic resonance (MR) **(a)** and reformatted computed tomography **(b)** images demonstrate an ossific fragment along the superior margin of a truncated dens articulating with a hypertrophic anterior arch of C1. The MR image shows anterior subluxation of the atlantodental articulation with respect to the proximal portion of the dens, resulting in spinal canal stenosis. Bony structures are diffusely sclerotic due to underlying osteopetrosis.

■ **Clinical Presentation**

A 20-year-old man with neck pain and neurological deficits (▶ Fig. 265.1)

■ Key Imaging Finding

Dens abnormality

■ Top 3 Differential Diagnoses

• **Odontoid fracture.** Odontoid/dens fractures occur in the setting of significant trauma. They are categorized into three types: type I refers to an avulsion fracture of the tip of the dens at the insertion of the alar ligament; type II refers to a fracture through the base of the dens; and type III is a fracture of the base of the dens that extends into the body of C2. Types I and III are typically stable after treatment with spinal immobilization, whereas type II fractures are most common and have a relatively high incidence of nonunion and instability. Acutely, fractures present as a lucency through the dens with surrounding soft-tissue edema. The lack of corticated margins and normal developmental appearance of both C1 and C2 are useful findings to distinguish a fracture from congenital anomalies such as os odontoideum or persistent ossiculum terminal.

• **Os odontoideum.** An os odontoideum refers to an ossification along the superior margin of the body of C2. It is typically an unstable anomaly that may be confused with a type II

odontoid fracture. Flexion and extension views are helpful in characterizing the degree of instability. Secondary findings that help differentiate a congenital os odontoideum from an odontoid fracture include a well-corticated convex superior margin of the C2 vertebral body and a rounded, hypertrophic anterior arch of C1.

• **Persistent ossiculum terminale.** A persistent ossiculum terminale is a congenital fusion anomaly where the terminal ossicle along the superior margin does not fuse with the remainder of the dens. Normal fusion typically occurs within the late first or early part of the second decades of life. The bony fragment may be confused with a type I odontoid fracture; in fact, imaging may not be able to distinguish between the two. Sclerotic margins are useful in distinguishing it from a fracture in the acute trauma setting; however, remote fractures may appear identical. A persistent ossiculum terminale is typically an incidental finding that does not lead to spinal instability.

■ Additional Differential Diagnoses

• **Odontoid erosion.** Inflammatory arthropathies of the cervical spine, especially rheumatoid arthritis and juvenile chronic arthritis, may lead to bony erosions, pannus formation, ligamentous laxity with instability, and possible ankylosis. When severe, the erosions may cause bony fragments, simulating

fractures. Irregular margins of the bony fragments and secondary findings of inflammatory arthropathy are useful discriminators to distinguish from fractures. Ligamentous laxity may lead to instability at the atlantodental articulation.

■ Diagnosis

Os odontoideum (patient with osteopetrosis)

✓ Pearls

• Odontoid fractures occur with significant trauma and are categorized into three subtypes; type II is most common.
• Os odontoideum is an ossification superior to the body of C2, mimics a type II fracture, and may be unstable.

• Persistent ossiculum terminale is a fusion anomaly that is incidental and may mimic a type I dens fracture.
• Inflammatory arthropathies may result in bony erosions, pannus formation, and ligamentous laxity.

Suggested Readings

Lustrin ES, Karakas SP, Ortiz AO et al. Pediatric cervical spine: normal anatomy, variants, and trauma. Radiographics 2003; 23: 539–560

Munera F, Rivas LA, Nunez DB, Jr, Quencer RM. Imaging evaluation of adult spinal injuries: emphasis on multidetector CT in cervical spine trauma. Radiology 2012; 263: 645–660

Smoker WR. Craniovertebral junction: normal anatomy, craniometry, and congenital anomalies. Radiographics 1994; 14: 255–277

Case 266

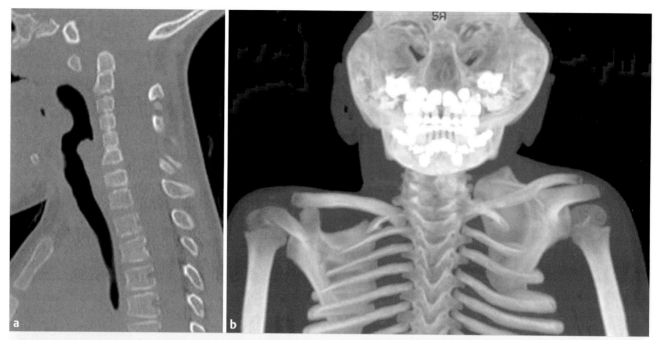

Fig. 266.1 Reformatted sagittal computed tomography image of the cervical spine **(a)** demonstrates decreased anteroposterior dimension and partial fusion of the C3–6 vertebral bodies. There is also an abnormal craniocervical junction with platybasia and a widened atlantodental articulation. Volume rendered coronal reformatted image **(b)** reveals an elevated scapula on the left with an abnormal bony articulation with the lower cervical spine.

■ **Clinical Presentation**

A 4-year-old girl with neck and back deformities (▶ Fig. 266.1)

■ Key Imaging Finding

Cervical spine segmentation anomaly in a young child

■ Top 3 Differential Diagnoses

- **Congenital spinal fusion/Klippel-Feil syndrome (KFS).** KFS refers to failed segmentation of two or more cervical vertebral segments with or without associated segmentation anomalies of the thoracic and lumbar spine. Congenital spinal fusion is more common in girls and may be sporadic, familial, or associated with multisystem syndromes such as VACTERL (vertebral defects, anal atresia, cardiac defects, tracheoesophageal fistula, renal anomalies, and limb abnormalities). The segmentation defect involves the vertebral bodies with or without involvement of the posterior elements and facets. Congenital causes of spinal fusion can often be distinguished from secondary causes based upon decreased size of the vertebral bodies. The C2–3 level is most often involved, followed by the lower cervical (C5–6) and upper thoracic spine. Clinical manifestations are varied and proportional to the degree and extent of segmentation anomalies. Patients often present with a shortened neck and limited range of motion. Anomalies of the craniocervical junction are commonly associated with KFS and may lead to instability. Additional associated anomalies include developmental cord anomalies, vascular developmental anomalies and variants, hearing loss, and Sprengel deformity (congenitally high scapula). KFS is characterized into three types. Type I is the most severe with multilevel segmentation anomalies of the cervical and upper thoracic spine, as well as neurological defects. Type II is most common and involves segmentation anomalies of one or more cervical levels. Type III consists of fusion anomalies of the cervical and lumbar or lower thoracic spine.
- **Juvenile chronic arthritis (JCA).** JCA is an inflammatory arthropathy that commonly involves the cervical spine and craniocervical junction. Chronic inflammation often leads to erosive changes, spinal fusion/ankylosis, and instability. Erosive changes are commonly seen at the altantodental articulation, as well as along the facets and uncovertebral joints. Fusion/ankylosis commonly involves the vertebral bodies and facet joints. Instability is associated with the inflammatory component of the arthropathy and is most common at the craniocervical junction but may also occur throughout the cervical spine. Computed tomography is ideal for evaluation of bony structures, including characterizing the fusion abnormalities and osseous erosions; magnetic resonance imaging provides superior soft-tissue evaluation, especially in identifying T2 hyperintense and enhancing inflammatory synovitis and pannus formation. JCA is classified into several groups based upon the distribution of the arthropathy and presence or absence of rheumatoid factor. Patients with cervical involvement often present with neck pain and limited range of motion. Juvenile rheumatoid arthritis may be monoarticular (most common), typically involving a large joint, or polyarticular. Those with Still disease present at a young age with systemic involvement, including fever, hepatosplenomegaly, and chronic anemia. Patients with juvenile ankylosing spondylitis are human leukocyte antigen (HLA)-B27 positive and have arthropathy of the sacroiliac joints, as well as enthesopathy.
- **Surgical spinal fusion.** Surgical spinal fusion in children is most often due to trauma or congenital or acquired causes of instability. Postoperative changes are often readily identified based upon the presence of surgical hardware and/or postoperative changes in the overlying soft tissues. Surgical fusion in the setting of prior trauma without hardware in place can often be distinguished from congenital segmentation anomalies based upon the relatively normal size of the vertebral bodies.

■ Diagnosis

Klippel-Feil syndrome

✓ Pearls

- KFS refers to failed segmentation of two or more cervical vertebral segments; it is more common in girls.
- KFS is associated with craniocervical, cord, and vascular anomalies, as well as Sprengel deformity.
- JCA is an inflammatory arthropathy that often leads to erosions, spinal fusion/ankylosis, and instability.
- Surgical spinal fusion in children is most often due to trauma or congenital or acquired causes of instability.

Suggested Readings

Resnick D. Inflammatory disorders of the vertebral column: seronegative spondyloarthropathies, adult-onset rheumatoid arthritis, and juvenile chronic arthritis. Clin Imaging 1989; 13: 253–268

Ulmer JL, Elster AD, Ginsberg LE, Williams DW, III. Klippel-Feil syndrome: CT and MR of acquired and congenital abnormalities of cervical spine and cord. J Comput Assist Tomogr 1993; 17: 215–224

Case 267

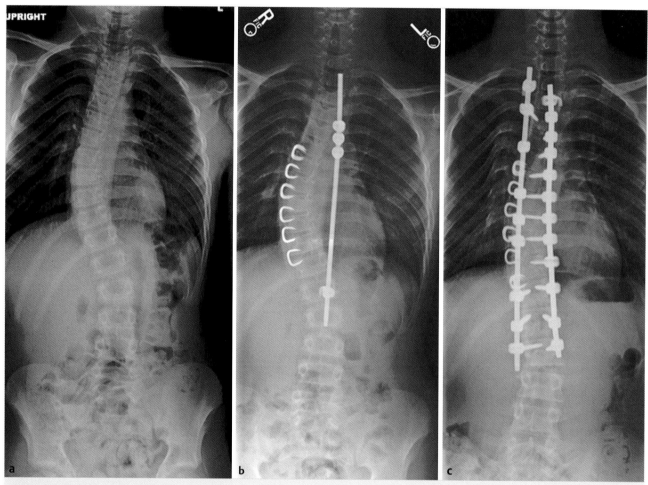

Fig. 267.1 Frontal view from a scoliosis survey in a 10-year-old boy **(a)** demonstrates convex right curvature of the thoracic spine with its apex at T9–10 and a Cobb angle of 42 degrees measured from the superior end plate of T4 to the inferior end plate of T12. There is a mild compensatory convex left curvature of the lumbar spine. Frontal view from a scoliosis survey at age 11 **(b)** reveals interval vertebral body stapling along the thoracic curvature convexity and placement of a growing hybrid rod along the concavity; the thoracic curve measures ~35 degrees. Frontal view form a scoliosis survey at age 14 **(c)** shows interval removal of the hybrid rod with spinal fusion from T2-L2. There is significant correction of the thoracic curvature, which now measures < 20 degrees. The iliac crest apophysis is not seen on images **(a)** or **(b)**, consistent with a Risser score of 0. On image **(c)**, the iliac crest apophysis is readily seen extending roughly three-fourths of the way across the iliac crest, consistent with a Risser score of 3.

▓ Clinical Presentation

An adolescent child with abnormal exam on school physical (▶ Fig. 267.1)

■ Key Imaging Finding

Lateral spinal curvature in a skeletally immature patient

■ Diagnosis

Scoliosis. Scoliosis refers to one or more lateral curvatures of the spine with a Cobb angle ≥ 10 degrees, often with a rotatory component. Approximately 80% of cases are idiopathic, whereas the remainder have an underlying developmental or acquired cause. Idiopathic scoliosis may also be classified based upon patient age as infantile (0 to 3 years), juvenile (4 to 10 years), adolescent (11 to 18 years), and adult. Juvenile and adolescent idiopathic scoliosis are far more common in girls and present with a convex right curve (dextroscoliosis).

Spinal curvature typically increases or progresses during periods of skeletal growth. Once skeletal maturity is achieved, curvatures < 30 degrees are often stable, whereas those > 30 degrees typically continue to progress, although at rates much less than those in skeletally immature patients. The Risser index (Risser sign) is used on scoliosis studies to determine the degree of skeletal maturity and is helpful in determining appropriate management and treatment options. It is based upon the degree of ossification of the iliac crest apophysis. The index ranges from 0 to 5, where 4 and 5 suggest skeletal maturity pre- and postapophyseal fusion, respectively. During the time of skeletal immaturity, follow-up imaging ranges from 4 to 12 months with an average of every 6 months; closer intervals are used for periods of rapid growth.

The apex of the curvature may be a vertebral body or intervertebral disc space and is defined by the portion of the spine that is furthest away from midline. The end vertebrae are those with the maximal tilt at the cranial and caudal ends of the curve and are used to measure the angle of curvature. When measuring the degree of curvature, the Cobb angle, the measurement is made along the superior end plate of the cephalad end vertebra and inferior end plate of the caudal vertebra. It is important to measure the curvature at the same levels on subsequent examinations to properly evaluate its progression. There is some degree of intraobserver variability, as well as intrinsic variability, in the measurement of Cobb angles; maintaining consistency between studies is most important. Secondary curves form as a compensatory mechanism for the primary curve and have a smaller angle of curvature.

Plain radiographs are the imaging modality of choice in diagnosing and following scoliosis, especially idiopathic cases. Computed tomography and magnetic resonance imaging are useful for atypical curvatures, such as those with an early onset, convex left curvature (levoscoliosis), or rapid progression, as well as to exclude or further evaluate underlying congenital or secondary causes of scoliosis, such as vertebral anomalies, tethered cord, masses, etc. In contrast to idiopathic cases, secondary causes may have accompanying neurological deficits or pain.

Treatment options for idiopathic scoliosis depend upon the age of onset, curvature severity, and curvature progression. External bracing is intended to stabilize the spinal curvature and is typically used for curves between 20 and 45 degrees. External bracing has varying degrees of success; an early age at presentation and rapid progression are less responsive to external bracing. Surgery is generally indicated for idiopathic scoliosis with a curvature > 45 degrees or in those with progressive curvature who cannot tolerate external bracing or when external bracing fails. The ultimate goal of surgery is fusion with correction of the curvature to the greatest degree possible. In skeletally immature patients, surgical options without fusion, including internal bracing (e.g., vertebral body stapling along the convexity) or "growing" or lengthening fusion rods, are preferred until definitive fusion can be performed when skeletal maturity is reached. To preserve mobility, surgeons attempt to avoid fusion within the cervical and lower lumbar spine when possible. In cases of congenital or acquired causes of scoliosis, the surgical option depends upon the underlying etiology.

✓ Pearls

- Scoliosis refers to lateral curvature of the spine with a Cobb angle ≥ 10 degrees, often with a rotatory component.
- Idiopathic scoliosis is more common in girls and has a convex right curvature (dextroscoliosis).
- A Risser index is used to determine the degree of skeletal maturity and is helpful in predicting progression.
- Treatment options depend on curve severity and progression and include external bracing and surgical correction.

Suggested Reading

Kim H, Kim HS, Moon ES et al. Scoliosis imaging: what radiologists should know. Radiographics 2010; 30: 1823–1842

Case 268

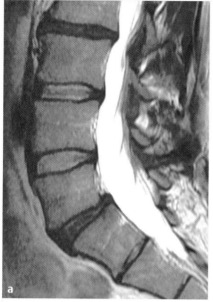
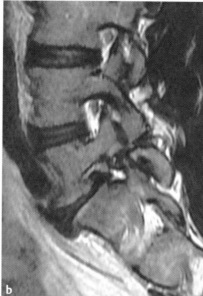

Fig. 268.1 Sagittal T2 image in the midline **(a)** demonstrates grade I anterolisthesis on L5 with respect to S1, as well as intervertebral disc dessication and height loss at L5-S1 and disc dessication at L2–3. Off-midline sagittal T2 image **(b)** reveals a pars defect at L5 with neuroforaminal narrowing and compression of the exiting L5 nerve root. Axial CT image **(c)** shows bilateral L5 pars defects at the vertebral body level with mild increased AP dimension of the spinal canal.

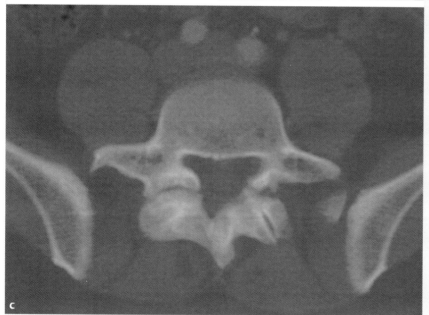

■ **Clinical Presentation**

A 34-year-old man with chronic low back pain (▶ Fig. 268.1)

■ Key Imaging Finding

Bilateral pars defects with listhesis

■ Diagnosis

Spondylolisthesis. Spondylolisthesis refers to abnormal displacement of a vertebral body with respect to another. It most often occurs at the L5-S1 level, followed by the L4–5 level. Causes of spondylolisthesis include isthmic (pars interarticularis defect), degenerative, dysplastic, traumatic, and pathological etiologies. Pars defects and degenerative changes are by far the most common causes of spondylolisthesis.

The pars interarticularis represents the portion of the neural arch between the lamina and the pedicle, facet, and transverse process. A fracture through this region is referred to as spondylolysis. When there is associated displacement at the region of the pars defect, spondylolisthesis occurs. Spondylolysis occurs at the L5 level in ~90% of cases; most of the remaining cases occur at the L4 level. Although the precise etiology of spondylolysis is not fully understood, it is widely accepted that repetitive injury during periods of development results in pars interarticularis stress fractures. The increased incidence in young athletes supports this theory.

Patients with spondylolisthesis typically present in adolescence or young adulthood with lower back pain and occasional radiculopathy. The L5 nerve root is most often involved, and symptoms are typically more severe in patients with more pronounced listhesis.

Spondylolisthesis is graded based upon the degree of subluxation. Grade I spondylolisthesis is defined as 0 to 25% anterior displacement of the involved vertebral body with respect to the segment below it. Grade II is defined as 25 to 50%; grade III is defined as 50 to 75%; and grade IV is defined as > 75%. Complete (100%) spondylolisthesis is referred to as spondyloptosis.

Most pars defects can be identified on plain radiographs, especially with associated listhesis. Occasionally, computed tomography (CT) may be necessary to identify the bony defects when subtle. On oblique views of the lumbar spine, pars defects characteristically present as a collar around a "Scottie dog's" neck between the pedicle (head) and articular facet (body/front leg).

Magnetic resonance imaging (MRI) is superior to both plain radiographs and CT in evaluating for nerve root compression. The pars defects may be identified as regions of bony disruption with or without edematous marrow signal changes on off-midline sagittal images. Axial images reveal pars defects that may initially be misinterpreted as facet joints; however, pars defects have a different orientation than the more vertically oriented lumbar facets and are located at the vertebral body level, rather than at the level of the intervertebral disc space. With associated subluxation, there is focal deformity and increased anteroposterior (AP) dimension of the spinal canal. Degenerative listhesis, on the other hand, narrows the spinal canal because both the ventral and dorsal portions of the vertebral body are displaced anteriorly.

Most patients with spondylolisthesis are either asymptomatic or treated conservatively with medical management. In more severe cases, progressive cases, or in those with failed medical management, surgical fixation may be required.

✓ Pearls

- Causes of spondylolisthesis include pars defects, degenerative, dysplastic, traumatic, and pathologic etiologies.
- Oblique radiographs demonstrate pars defects as the characteristic collar around a "Scottie dog's" neck.
- MRI is superior to both plain radiographs and CT in evaluating for nerve root compression.
- Axial images reveal pars defects at the vertebral body level with increased AP dimension of the spinal canal.

Suggested Reading

Ganju A. Isthmic spondylolisthesis. Neurosurg Focus 2002; 13(1):E1

Case 269

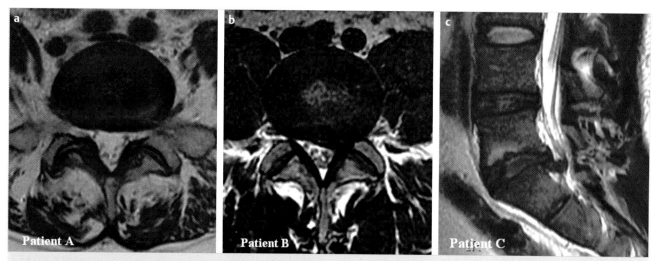

Fig. 269.1 Axial T2 magnetic resonance (MR) image through the lumbar spine (a) demonstrates disc dessication with a diffuse disc bulge, as well as bilateral facet and ligamentum flavum hypertrophy; there is mild right and minimal left lateral recess narrowing. Axial T2 MR image through the lumbar spine in a different patient (b) reveals a left central to subarticular disc protrusion with severe left lateral recess narrowing; there is displacement and compression of the descending nerve roots in the left lateral recess. Off-midline sagittal T2 MR image through the lumbar spine in a different patient (c) demonstrates a caudal and posterior disc extrusion that results in posterior displacement and impingement of the descending nerve roots. Edematous end plate marrow signal changes are seen along an inferior L5 Schmorl node.

▧ Clinical Presentation

Three adult patients with chronic low back pain and radiculopathy (► Fig. 269.1)

■ Key Imaging Finding

Degenerative disc disease involving the lumbar spine

■ Diagnosis

Disc terminology. Prior to the recommendations of a multispecialty task force, terminology used to describe lumbar spine degenerative disc disease was not standardized and subject to individual interpretation. This led to a degree of confusion, particularly for referring providers, because characterization of similar pathology would be described differently based upon where the study was performed and which radiologist provided the final interpretation. The combined task force alleviated the disparity in report terminology by providing accepted nomenclature for the classification of lumbar disc pathology.

As individuals age, the intervertebral disc undergoes degeneration with dessication of the central nucleus pulposis. Dessication results in loss of the normal T2 fluid signal intensity within the disc centrally. More acute disc injury may result in an annular tear or fissure that allows portions of the central nucleus to penetrate into and beyond the peripherally located annulus fibrosis. Annular fissures or tears are visualized as focal regions of increased T2 signal intensity within the peripheral annulus.

Degenerative disc disease is primarily broken down into disc bulges and herniations. A disc bulge is diffuse, affecting 50 to 100% of the disc circumference (180 to 360 degrees) with extension beyond the margin of the vertebral body. Herniated discs, on the other hand, refer to focal (< 25% or 90 degree) or broad-based (25 to 50% or 90 to 180 degree) extensions of disc material beyond the margin of the vertebral body. Herniations are further characterized into protrusions, in which the herniated material is no larger than its base in the same imaging plane, or extrusions, in which the herniated disc material exceeds the size of its base or neck in the same plane. Extrusions tend to migrate beyond the intervertebral disc space, often in a cephalad or caudad direction, due to the posterior restriction from the posterior longitudinal ligament. An extrusion that extends superiorly above the intervertebral disc space, for example, would be referred to as a cephalad disc extrusion. A sequestered disc is a subset of an extruded disc, which is characterized by a loss of contiguity with the parent disc. Typically, disc herniations are similar in signal characteristics compared with the parent disc, which allows for differentiation from other epidural processes.

The location of the disc pathology is as important as properly describing the disc disease. Accepted nomenclature includes central, right or left central, subarticular, foraminal, and extraforaminal or far lateral. The central zones primarily affect the central canal in terms of stenosis. The subarticular and portions of the right and left central zones affect the lateral recess, which contains the descending nerve roots for the level below. For example, the lateral recess at the L4–5 level contains the L5 nerve root. The foraminal zone affects the nerve root in the neural foramen, which is at the level of the intervertebral disc space. For example, the neural foramen at the L4–5 level contains the L4 nerve root.

Disc disease in combination with facet and ligamentum flavum hypertrophy/infolding and disc height loss often results in narrowing of the central canal, lateral recess, and/or neural foramina. The degree of narrowing is based upon a comparison with what is considered normal. Mild narrowing is defined as less than one-third narrowing; moderate is defined as between one- and two-thirds narrowing; and severe is defined as greater than two-thirds narrowing. As the degree of narrowing increases, there is increased likelihood of nerve root displacement or compression.

✓ Pearls

- A disc bulge is diffuse, affecting 50 to 100% of the disc circumference (180 to 360 degrees).
- Herniated discs, protrusions or extrusions, may be focal (< 25% or 90 degrees) or broad-based (25 to 50% or 90 to 180 degrees).
- Locations of disc disease include central, right or left central, subarticular, foraminal, and extraforaminal.
- The degree of central canal, lateral recess, or foraminal narrowing is based upon a comparison with normal.

Suggested Reading

Fardon DF, Milette PC Combined Task Forces of the North American Spine Society, American Society of Spine Radiology, and American Society of Neuroradiology. Nomenclature and classification of lumbar disc pathology: recommendations of the combined task force of the North American Spine Society, American Society of Spine Radiology, and American Society of Neuroradiology. Spine 2001; 26: E93–E113

Case 270

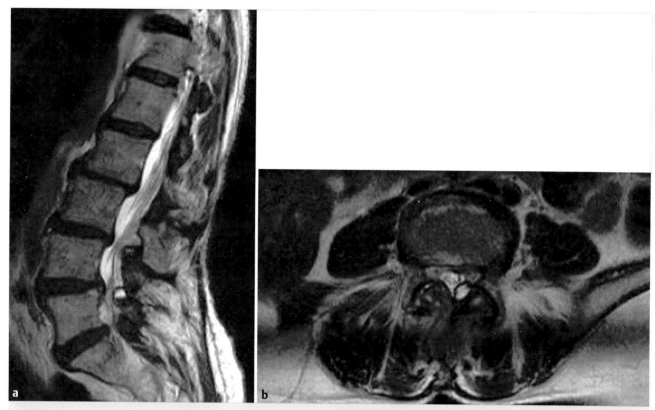

Fig. 270.1 Sagittal **(a)** and axial **(b)** T2-weighted sequences through the lumbar spine demonstrate a hyperintense epidural mass with a peripheral low signal margin along the left posterolateral aspect of the thecal sac at the L4–5 level adjacent to the articular facet. The mass effaces the dorsal aspect of the thecal sac. There are degenerative changes involving the facets and intervertebral disc spaces.

■ **Clinical Presentation**

A middle-aged adult man with back pain and radiculopathy (▶ Fig. 270.1)

▨ Key Imaging Finding

Extradural cystic mass adjacent to a degenerative facet

▪ Diagnosis

Synovial cyst. Synovial cysts are extradural lesions that result from facet degenerative arthropathy. They occur most frequently in middle-aged and older adults, are more common in women and in the setting of degenerative spondylolisthesis, and most often involve the lower lumbar spine.

The majority of synovial cysts are asymptomatic and incidental, especially when located along the posterior aspect of the facet joint. Anterior lesions may cause symptoms related to nerve root compression within the central canal, lateral recess, or neural foramen. The most common presenting symptom is painful radiculopathy.

Magnetic resonance imaging (MRI) is the modality of choice and demonstrates an extradural cystic lesion with a peripheral T2 hypointense rim in association with a degenerative facet joint. Increased protein content within the cyst may lead to slight increased signal intensity on T1 sequences. Peripheral inflammatory signal and enhancement may be seen, as can hemorrhage or calcification.

Treatment options include conservative management with analgesics, percutaneous steroid injection and/or drainage, and surgical resection in more severe cases.

✓ Pearls

- Synovial cysts are extradural lesions that result from facet degenerative arthropathy.
- The majority of synovial cysts are asymptomatic, although large lesions may cause nerve root compression.

- MRI demonstrates a cystic mass with peripheral T2 hypointensity in proximity to a degenerative facet joint.

Suggested Reading

Khan AM, Girardi F. Spinal lumbar synovial cysts. Diagnosis and management challenge. Eur Spine J 2006; 15: 1176–1182

Case 271

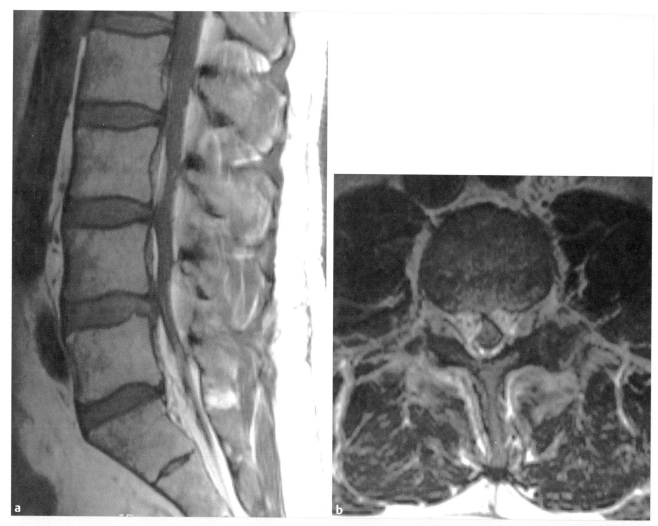

Fig. 271.1 Sagittal T1-weighted image **(a)** demonstrates increased proliferation of epidural fat throughout the lumbar spine with compression of the thecal sac. Prominence of subcutaneous fat is also noted posteriorly. Axial T2 image at the L4 level **(b)** reveals increased signal within the epidural space with compression of the thecal sac and central positioning of the descending nerve roots. The characteristic configuration of the thecal sac is due to underlying meningovertebral ligaments that anchor the dura to the overlying bony structures, best depicted midline anteriorly.

■ **Clinical Presentation**

A 43-year-old man with progressive back pain and radiculopathy (▶ Fig. 271.1)

Key Imaging Finding

Increased epidural fat with compression of thecal sac

Diagnosis

Epidural lipomatosis. Epidural lipomatosis refers to abnormal proliferation of epidural fat. It is most commonly seen in the thoracolumbar spine and is more common in men. Causative etiologies include excessive steroids (exogenous or endogenous) and obesity, although it may also be idiopathic. Patients may be asymptomatic or present with symptoms related to compressive neuropathy.

Magnetic resonance imaging (MRI) is the imaging modality of choice due to its superior evaluation of soft tissues. Findings include increased proliferation of fat signal intensity (increased signal on T1/T2 sequences and decreased signal on fat-suppressed sequences) within the epidural space with associated compression of the thecal sac. Axial images may demonstrate a characteristic Y-shaped or polygonal configuration due the presence of meningovertebral ligaments that serve as anchors for the dural sac.

Treatment is typically medical and geared toward weight reduction or cessation of the underlying cause of excessive steroids, when possible. Surgical decompression may be necessary in severe symptomatic cases where medical therapies are not viable or are unsuccessful.

✓ Pearls

- Lipomatosis refers to abnormal proliferation of epidural fat; etiologies include obesity and steroids but may also be idiopathic.
- MRI is the modality of choice, demonstrating increased proliferation of epidural fat and thecal sac compression.
- Axial images may show a characteristic Y-shaped or polygonal configuration due to meningovertebral ligaments.

Suggested Readings

Geers C, Lecouvet FE, Behets C, Malghem J, Cosnard G, Lengelé BG. Polygonal deformation of the dural sac in lumbar epidural lipomatosis: anatomic explanation by the presence of meningovertebral ligaments. Am J Neuroradiol 2003; 24: 1276–1282

Shaheen F, Singh M, Gojwari T et al. Idiopathic epidural lipomatosis. Appl Radiol 2008; 37: 40A–40B

Case 272

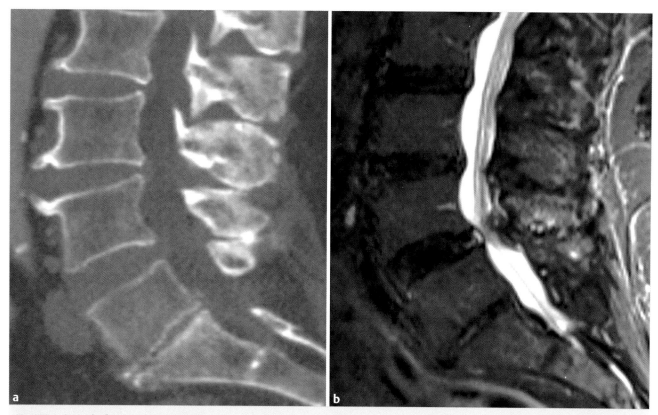

Fig. 272.1 Sagittal reformatted CT image **(a)** demonstrates multilevel degenerative changes of the lumbar spine, most pronounced at L5-S1, as well as abnormal bony enlargement, sclerosis, and apposition of the spinous processes. Sagittal short tau inversion recovery MR image **(b)** shows similar findings with increased signal intensity within the L4–5 interspinous ligament and subchondral cystic changes involving the spinous processes. Ligamentum flavum hypertrophy and an annular tear are seen at the same level.

■ Clinical Presentation

An 84-year-old man with low back pain, worse in extension and improved with flexion; no history of trauma (▶ Fig. 272.1)

■ **Key Imaging Finding**

Abnormal enlargement and apposition of the lumbar spinous processes

■ **Diagnosis**

Baastrup phenomenon. Baastrup phenomenon or disease, also referred to as "kissing spinous processes," refers to abnormal apposition and contact of contiguous vertebral spinous processes. There is an increased incidence with age and an association with low back pain, although that is somewhat controversial. Classic symptoms include back pain that is improved with flexion.

Plain radiographs and computed tomography (CT) demonstrate contact and enlargement of the involved spinous processes with intervening bony sclerosis. Magnetic resonance imaging (MRI) reveals similar findings, as well as mixed T2 signal intensity within the interspinous ligament; hypointensity is associated with ligamentous hypertrophy and hyperintensity is due to ligamentous degeneration. Adjacent T2 hyperintense cysts are commonly seen. Postcontrast sequences often demonstrate nonspecific inflammatory enhancement within and around the involved interspinous segment. Additional degenerative changes, including degenerative disc disease and facet/ligamentum flavum hypertrophy, are coexistent in nearly all cases.

Treatment options include medical pain management, percutaneous steroid injection, and surgical management.

✓ **Pearls**

• Baastrup phenomenon refers to abnormal apposition and contact of contiguous vertebral spinous processes.
• Classic clinical symptoms include low back pain in older patients that is improved with flexion.

• Plain films and CT demonstrate spinous process apposition and enlargement with intervening bony sclerosis.
• MRI reveals mixed T2 signal in the interspinous ligament (hypointense hypertrophy/hyperintense degeneration).

Suggested Reading

Jinkins JR. Acquired degenerative changes of the intervertebral segments at and suprajacent to the lumbosacral junction. A radioanatomic analysis of the nondiskal structures of the spinal column and perispinal soft tissues. Radiol Clin North Am 2001; 39: 73–99

Case 273

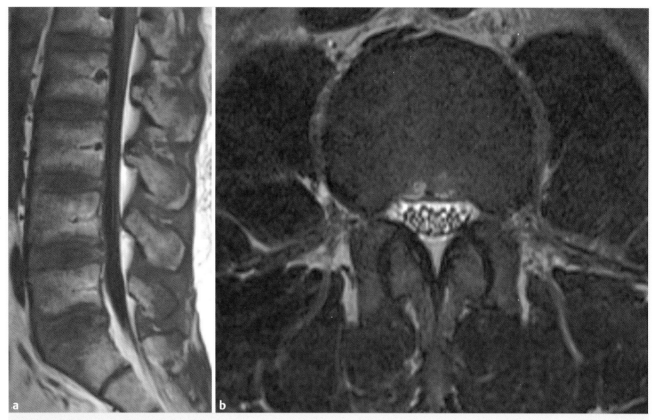

Fig. 273.1 Sagittal T1- **(a)** and axial T2-weighted image at the mid-L4 vertebral body level **(b)** demonstrate significant narrowing of the lumbar spinal canal secondary to shortened pedicles. The anteroposterior measurement was ~8 mm.

▨ Clinical Presentation

A 36-year-old man with chronic low back pain (▶ Fig. 273.1)

■ Key Imaging Finding

Narrowing of the lumbar spinal canal

■ Diagnosis

Congenital lumbar spinal stenosis. Spinal canal stenosis within the lumbar spine may be congenital or acquired. Acquired causes are far more common and result from degenerative disc and facet disease. Congenital causes, such as congenitally shortened pedicles, is less common but increases the likelihood of symptomatic degenerative disc disease in what may otherwise be asymptomatic in a patient with a normal-sized spinal canal.

Acquired stenosis occurs and is measured at the level of the intervertebral disc, which is where the pathology resides. Congenital spinal stenosis, on the other hand, is measured at the midvertebral level on sagittal views. There is much debate as to the cutoff measurement between a normal and congenitally narrowed lumbar spinal canal, mainly because of the types of studies used to determine a normative measurement. Early studies used anatomic specimens and plain radiographs, which based measurements on bony margins of the spinal canal. Later studies using myelography more accurately reflected the size of the cerebrospinal fluid (CSF)-lined thecal sac as opposed to the bony margins of the spinal canal. Magnetic resonance imaging (MRI) allows for optimal soft-tissue evaluation in determining the normal caliber of the spinal canal and thecal sac compared with overlying bony margins. In addition, the CSF-filled thecal sac naturally tapers as it descends and then terminates in the upper sacral region; this is optimally visualized on MRI.

Early studies based on anatomic specimens and plain radiographs listed a normal anteroposterior value of the lumbar spine somewhere between 12 and 15 mm. Using these cutoff values, the sensitivity would be relatively high and specificity would be relatively low. A more recent study using MRI and 2 standard deviations to determine the cutoff values for lumbar spinal stenosis recommends a value of 9 mm for calling congenital lumbar spinal stenosis; this cutoff value increases specificity but decreases sensitivity. A cutoff value of 10 mm for congenital central canal stenosis would likely optimize sensitivity and specificity.

✓ Pearls

- Acquired stenosis is measured at the level of the intervertebral disc, which is where the pathology resides.
- Congenital lumbar spinal stenosis is measured at the midvertebral level and is often due to shortened pedicles.
- There is much debate as to the cutoff for a congenitally narrowed lumbar spinal canal; 10 mm is reasonable.

Suggested Reading

Chatha DS, Schweitzer ME. MRI criteria of developmental lumbar spinal stenosis revisited. Bull NYU Hosp Jt Dis 2011; 69: 303–307

Case 274

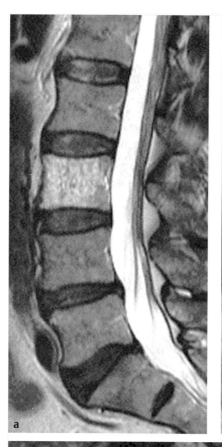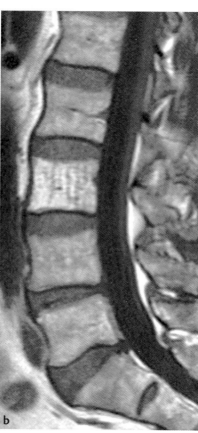

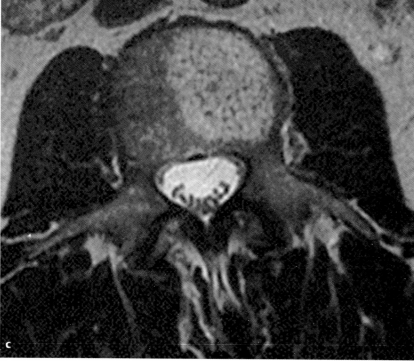

Fig. 274.1 Sagittal T2- **(a)** and T1-weighted **(b)** MR images demonstrate diffuse increased signal intensity within the L3 vertebral body with prominent vertical striations, which are isointense compared with marrow in adjacent vertebral segments. Axial T2 image through the L3 vertebral body **(c)** reveals a circumscribed region of increased T2 marrow signal intensity on the left with focal regions of isointense marrow centrally in a characteristic "polka dot" appearance.

■ Clinical Presentation

An adult man with chronic low back pain (▶ Fig. 274.1)

■ Key Imaging Finding

Increased T1 and T2 marrow signal intensity with a striated appearance

■ Diagnosis

Vertebral body hemangioma. Vertebral body hemangiomas are endothelial-lined vascular structures that are interspersed between the bony trabeculae of the spine. They may be solitary or multiple and are most commonly seen in the thoracic and lumbar spine. The vast majority of lesions are incidental and asymptomatic. Typically, hemangiomas are confined to the vertebral body, although they may occasionally extend into the posterior elements; aggressive or compressive hemangiomas are rare, more common in the thoracic spine, and may demonstrate extraspinal extension with compression of the thecal sac.

Plain radiographs and computed tomography (CT) demonstrate focal fat attenuation with prominence of vertical striations within the trabeculae. This leads to the characteristic "honeycomb" appearance best depicted on anteroposterior, lateral, sagittal, or coronal views, as well as the "polka dot" appearance on axial CT images. The magnetic resonance imaging (MRI) signal intensity may be more variable depending upon the fatty and vascular components within the lesion. Predominantly fatty lesions are hyperintense on T1- and T2-weighted sequences with loss of signal on fat-suppressed sequences. In the absence of characteristic vertical striations or polka dot appearance on axial sequences, these lesions may appear identical to focal fatty marrow. With increased vascularity, the signal characteristics are more variable and may demonstrate regions of decreased signal intensity on T1 and increased signal on fat-suppressed T2 sequences. Aggressive or compressive hemangiomas tend to be less well defined, have intermediate T1 signal intensity, and may demonstrate internal flow voids.

Typical hemangiomas do not require treatment or follow-up. Treatment options for aggressive or compressive hemangiomas include surgical decompression with or without preoperative transarterial embolization and radiation therapy.

✓ Pearls

- Vertebral body hemangiomas are endothelial-lined vascular structures interspersed between bony trabeculae.
- Radiographs and CT demonstrate a characteristic "honeycomb" or "polka dot" (axial CT) appearance.
- MRI signal characteristics depend on the composition of fat and vascular structures; most are T1/T2 bright.
- Compressive lesions are rare, have less characteristic imaging features, and may have extraspinal extension.

Suggested Reading

Rodallec MH, Feydy A, Larousserie F et al. Diagnostic imaging of solitary tumors of the spine: what to do and say. Radiographics 2008; 28: 1019–1041

Case 275

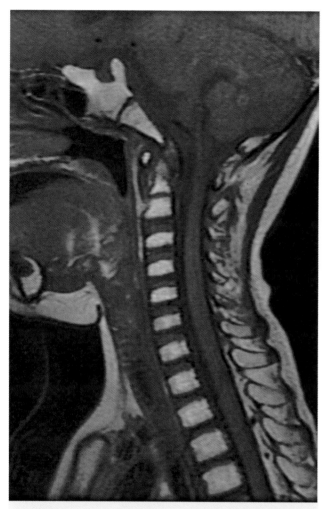

Fig. 275.1 Sagittal T1-weighted image demonstrates diffuse, pronounced, increased T1 marrow signal intensity throughout the visualized portions of the spine and skull base. The marrow signal intensity is equal to that of subcutaneous fat.

Clinical Presentation

A 6-year-old boy with prior treatment for medulloblastoma (▶ Fig. 275.1)

■ Key Imaging Finding

Diffuse, extensive fatty marrow infiltration

■ Diagnosis

Radiation marrow changes. The type and degree of post-treatment radiation changes of the spine are dependent upon the duration of treatment and radiation dose. Within the first few days of treatment, bone marrow edema may be seen, demonstrating decreased T1 and increased fat-suppressed T2 signal intensity with transient enhancement. The edema may be focal or diffuse but is typically confined to the radiation field. Although the edema normally evolves or resolves after the first 3 days or so post-treatment, in some cases it may persist for several weeks. After the marrow edema phase, the marrow signal intensity may initially show regions of T1 hyperintense hemorrhage, normalize, or begin to undergo fatty infiltration. Fatty infiltration may begin anytime as early as 10 days post-treatment or several months following therapy. Radiation-induced fatty marrow signal demonstrates pronounced T1 hyperintensity (similar to that of subcutaneous fat), is typically diffuse, and is confined to the field of radiation.

Complications of radiation therapy include insufficiency fractures, avascular necrosis (AVN), and regions of osteitis in adults, which manifest as focal marrow edema with narrow zones of transition and confinement to the radiation field. In children, radiation therapy may result in growth arrest and scoliosis. Potential long-term complications include neoplasm formation, both benign and malignant. Benign neoplasms occur more frequently in children who undergo radiation therapy. Osteochondroma is the most common radiation-induced benign tumor; aneurysmal bone cysts are less common. Malignant sarcomas include osteosarcomas (most common) and malignant fibrous histiocytomas.

✓ Pearls

- The type and degree of postradiation marrow changes are dependent upon treatment duration and dose.
- Within the first few days of treatment, bone marrow edema may be seen and subsequently evolves or resolves.
- Radiation-induced fatty marrow signal shows pronounced T1 hyperintensity confined to the treatment field.
- Potential radiation therapy complications include insufficiency fractures, AVN, osteitis, and tumor formation.

Suggested Reading

Daldrup-Link HE, Henning T, Link TM. MR imaging of therapy-induced changes of bone marrow. Eur Radiol 2007; 17: 743–761

Case 276

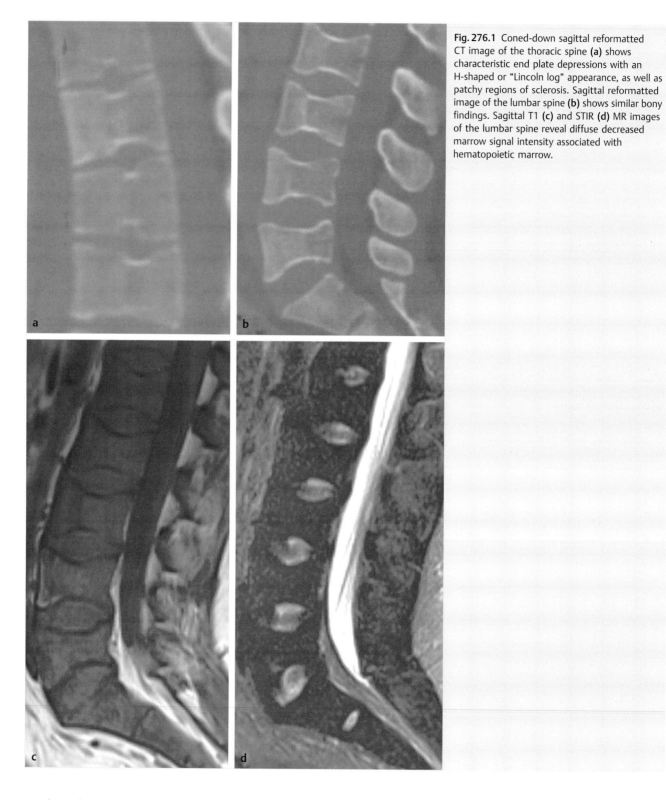

Fig. 276.1 Coned-down sagittal reformatted CT image of the thoracic spine **(a)** shows characteristic end plate depressions with an H-shaped or "Lincoln log" appearance, as well as patchy regions of sclerosis. Sagittal reformatted image of the lumbar spine **(b)** shows similar bony findings. Sagittal T1 **(c)** and STIR **(d)** MR images of the lumbar spine reveal diffuse decreased marrow signal intensity associated with hematopoietic marrow.

■ Clinical Presentation

A 22-year-old girl with chronic medical condition and back pain (▶ Fig. 276.1)

■ Key Imaging Finding

Multilevel end plate depressions with an H-shaped/"Lincoln log" appearance and diffuse hematopoietic marrow

■ Diagnosis

Sickle cell anemia (SCA). Sickle cell disease (SCD) is characterized by abnormally shaped hemoglobin/red blood cells, which may result in anemia due to increased red blood cell turnover and end-organ vascular occlusion due to luminal adhesion and aggregation. It is the most common genetic disorder in African Americans. With sickle cell trait, patients have one abnormal gene and the clinical course is relatively benign in terms of vascular occlusive disease. SCA refers to patients with two abnormal genes and their clinical course is far more severe in terms of end-organ ischemia due to vascular occlusion. Newborn screening for SCD is now commonplace in at-risk patient populations. Patients with SCA most often present in childhood with pain related to vascular occlusive disease. Nearly any organ may be affected; however, the lung/chest and musculoskeletal systems are most commonly involved.

Manifestations in the spine include marrow conversion, bone infarcts, and osteomyelitis. Normally, red or hematopoietic marrow converts to predominantly yellow or fatty marrow during childhood. Due to underlying anemia, patients with SCA not only have increased red marrow but also may demonstrate marrow expansion as a means of increased red blood cell production. On magnetic resonance imaging (MRI), this manifests as regions of decreased T1 marrow signal intensity compared with intervertebral discs and paraspinal musculature; decreased short tau inversion recovery (STIR) signal intensity helps differentiate red marrow from marrow infiltrative

processes such as leukemia or lymphoma, which typically demonstrate increased STIR signal.

Bone infarcts are common in patients with SCA. On plain radiographs and computed tomography (CT), infarcts initially present as regions of patchy lucency within the medullary cavity that progress to regions of patchy attenuation with a sclerotic rim. MRI is more sensitive, demonstrating regions of increased T2/STIR signal intensity with a thin, serpentine T1 hypointense rim which may demonstrate enhancement. The subchondral surfaces below the end plates are particularly susceptible to ischemia in the spine and result in a characteristic central depression referred to as H-shaped or "Lincoln log" vertebrae, which are essentially pathognomonic for SCA. This characteristic finding is seen in ~10% of patients with SCA.

Osteomyelitis is a dreaded complication of SCA. It occurs less frequently than bone infarcts and most often involves the diaphysis of long bones, although the spine may be involved as well. In addition to common bacteria, such as *Staphylococcus aureus*, patients with SCD are particularly susceptible to *Salmonella* colonization. Imaging typically demonstrates regions of lucency (plain radiographs and CT) or increased T2/STIR signal intensity (MRI) with periosteal reaction and enhancement. Prolonged infections may lead to subperiosteal and paraspinal abscesses. Chronic infections most often appear sclerotic.

Treatment of SCA is supportive with hydration and analgesics. Antibiotics are indicated in cases of bacterial infection.

✓ Pearls

- SCD is characterized by abnormally shaped red blood cells that result in anemia and vascular occlusion.
- Manifestations of SCA in the spine include marrow conversion and expansion, bone infarcts, and osteomyelitis.

- Subchondral ischemia within the spine results in characteristic H-shaped or "Lincoln log" vertebrae.

Suggested Reading

Lonergan GJ, Cline DB, Abbondanzo SL. Sickle cell anemia. Radiographics 2001; 21: 971–994

Case 277

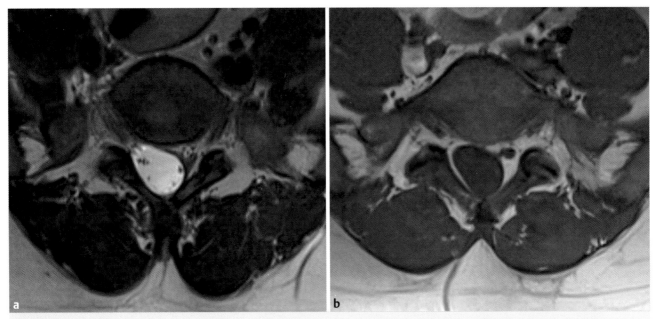

Fig. 277.1 Axial T2 MR image **(a)** shows asymmetric enlargement of the nerve root sleeve in the right neural foramen with two sets of exiting nerve roots. Axial T1 image **(b)** best depicts the asymmetric configuration of the thecal sac against the background of hyperintense epidural fat.

■ Clinical Presentation

A 42-year-old woman with back pain (▶ Fig. 277.1)

■ Key Imaging Finding

Paired nerve roots colocated in a single, enlarged nerve root sleeve

■ Diagnosis

Conjoined nerve roots. Conjoined nerve roots are paired nerve roots from adjacent levels that are colocated in a single nerve root sleeve. They may exit through the neural foramen at their expected levels or exit together through a single neural foramen. The anomaly typically occurs unilaterally and is most often incidental and asymptomatic; occasionally, conjoined nerve roots may be associated with radiculopathy. It is important to identify the presence of a conjoined nerve root prior to surgical intervention because the variant anatomy predisposes patients to inadvertent nerve injury.

Magnetic resonance imaging (MRI) is the noninvasive modality of choice in evaluating conjoined nerve roots. Findings on axial images include asymmetric enlargement of the nerve root sleeve on the involved side. The nerve root sleeve is typically located at the midpoint between the anticipated levels of the normal root sleeves, which makes the finding more conspicuous. Axial T1 images are particularly useful because the

hyperintense epidural fat outlines the enlarged hypointense cerebrospinal fluid–filled nerve root sleeve. The involved nerve roots may exit at their appropriate levels or at the same level. When exiting at the same level, they often have a parallel configuration and may remain separate or appear conglomerate, in which case they may mimic a nerve sheath tumor. Lack of visualization of nerve roots exiting at the adjacent spinal level and the characteristic configuration of the nerve root sleeve are useful discriminators in recognizing the presence of a conjoined nerve root. Mild foraminal enlargement is commonly seen.

Computed tomography (CT) myelography is utilized for confirmation of questionable cases on MRI or in patients with contraindications to MRI. Myelography provides exceptional detail of the thecal sac and nerve roots due to the differences in attenuation between the epidural fat and nerve roots compared with the contrast-filled thecal sac. Coronal reformatted images are particularly helpful. Findings are similar compared with MRI.

✓ Pearls

- Conjoined nerve roots are paired nerve roots from adjacent levels colocated in a single nerve root sleeve.
- MRI and CT myelography demonstrate paired nerve roots in an enlarged nerve root sleeve.

- Involved nerve roots may exit at their appropriate levels or at the same level.

Suggested Reading

Trimba R, Spivak JM, Bendo JA. Conjoined nerve roots of the lumbar spine. Spine J 2012; 12: 515–524

Case 278

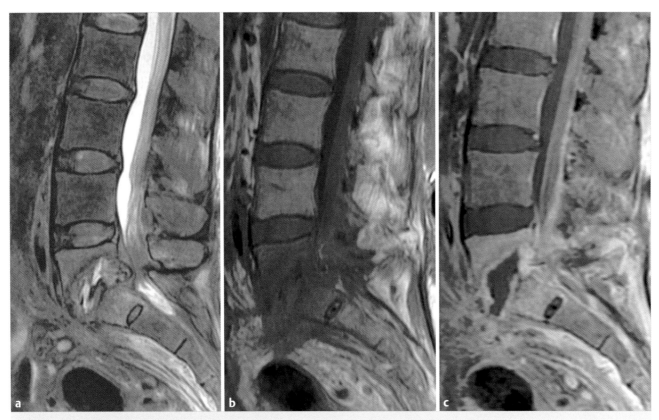

Fig. 278.1 1 Sagittal T2 MR image **(a)** demonstrates abnormal increased signal intensity within the L5-S1 disc space with extension into the L5 and S1 vertebral bodies; there is loss of the normal cortical margin, abnormal increased marrow signal intensity, and decreased height. Sagittal T1 images pre- **(b)** and postcontrast **(c)** administration reveal a rim-enhancing fluid collection centered at the disc space with abnormal enhancement extending into the L5 and S1 vertebral bodies, spinal canal, and surrounding paraspinal soft tissues. There is compression of the thecal sac at L5-S1 with both extra- and intradural inflammatory enhancement.

■ **Clinical Presentation**

An adult man with progressive back pain (▶ Fig. 278.1)

▧ Key Imaging Finding

Abnormal signal and enhancement centered at the disc space with extension into surrounding structures

▧ Diagnosis

Disc-osteomyelitis. Disc-osteomyelitis refers to infection involving two contiguous vertebral bodies and the intervening disc space. Most cases are the result of hematogenous spread from a distant infection; direct spread from a paravertebral source, surgical complication, or penetrating trauma are less common etiologies. The vast majority of cases are pyogenic. Tuberculosis spondylitis is less common. With pyogenic infections, organisms initially spread to the subchondral region of the vertebral body due to increased blood flow to this region and then spread throughout the vertebral body and across the disc space to involve the adjacent vertebral body.

Staphylococcus aureus constitutes the most common organism that results in pyogenic spondylitis. *Streptococcus*, *Enterococcus*, *Escherichia coli*, and *Pneumococcus* are less common. *Salmonella* is a subspecies that preferentially occurs in patients with sickle cell disease. Clinically, patients with pyogenic spondylitis typically present with insidious onset of constant, progressive back pain, with or without fever and elevated white blood cell count, erythrocyte sedimentation rate, or C-reactive protein, all of which are signs of infection or inflammation. The lumbar spine is most often involved, followed by the thoracic and cervical spine.

Plain radiographs and computed tomography (CT) may be normal during early stages of infection. As the infection progresses, there will be destruction of the endplates with loss of the sclerotic cortical margin and disc height loss. Chronic cases may demonstrate reactive bony sclerosis.

Magnetic resonance imaging (MRI) is the modality of choice for suspected cases of spondylitis. Pyogenic spondylitis demonstrates decreased T1 and increased T2 fluid signal within the affected disc spaces with extension into the adjacent vertebral bodies, as well as loss of the end plate cortical margins. Postcontrast imaging reveals enhancement of the vertebral bodies and intervening disc space; the enhancement pattern varies from homogeneous to patchy. Focal abscesses present as rim-enhancing fluid collections, whereas phlegmon demonstrates ill-defined or incomplete rim enhancement. There is often spread of the infectious process into the epidural space, neural foramina, and/or paraspinal soft tissues.

Most cases of pyogenic spondylitis may be treated successfully with intravenous antibiotics. Focal abscesses, however, typically require surgical or interventional drainage. Serial follow-up imaging is often performed to document improvement or resolution.

✓ Pearls

- Disc-osteomyelitis refers to infection involving two contiguous vertebral bodies and the intervening disc space.
- Most cases spread hematogenously and are pyogenic; *S. aureus* is the most common organism.

- Radiographs and CT may demonstrate loss of the sclerotic end plate cortical margin and disc height loss.
- MRI reveals fluid signal and enhancement of the vertebral bodies and disc; abscesses show rim enhancement.

Suggested Reading

Hong SH, Choi JY, Lee JW, Kim NR, Choi JA, Kang HS. MR imaging assessment of the spine: infection or an imitation? Radiographics 2009; 29: 599–612

Case 279

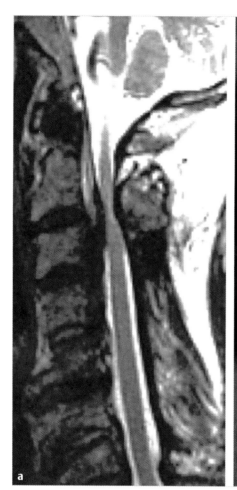 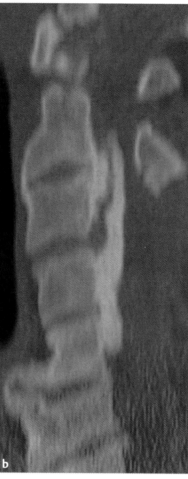

Fig. 279.1 Sagittal T2-weighted MR image **(a)** demonstrates a linear region of decreased signal intensity extending along the anterior epidural space with severe underlying cervical cord compression. Increased T2 signal intensity is noted within the compressed cord. Sagittal reformatted unenhanced CT image **(b)** shows increased density/ossification of the posterior longitudinal ligament, corresponding to the region of decreased T2 signal intensity. Remote dens and posterior element C2 fractures, as well as an anterior C5–6 osteophyte, are seen on both images. (Courtesy of Paul M. Sherman, MD.)

■ Clinical Presentation

An elderly man with long-standing neck pain and chronic, progressive myelopathy and remote history of trauma (▶ Fig. 279.1)

■ Key Imaging Finding

Increased attenuation/ossification of the posterior longitudinal ligament

■ Diagnosis

Ossification of the posterior longitudinal ligament (OPLL). As the name implies, OPLL refers to calcification or ossification of the posterior longitudinal ligament. It most often occurs in the cervical spine in adult patients and is more common in Asia. There is a fairly equal incidence in men and women. Although the pathogenesis is not entirely clear, there is an association with diffuse idiopathic skeletal hyperostosis (DISH) and spondyloarthropathies.

Patients may be asymptomatic or present with symptoms related to spinal canal stenosis and cord compression. Common symptoms include those related to myelopathy, radiculopathy, and occasionally bowel and bladder dysfunction; symptom onset is typically insidious.

OPPL is typically diagnosed on plain radiographs or computed tomography (CT); CT optimizes characterization of the regions of ligamentous calcification or ossification. Patterns of involvement include diffuse ossification of the posterior longitudinal ligament,

segmental involvement, mixed diffuse and segmental, and circumscribed, which refers to involvement at the level of a disc space. Ossification may extend along the dura. The thickness of calcification correlates with the degree of underlying spinal stenosis and cord compression.

Magnetic resonance imaging (MRI) is the modality of choice in evaluating the cord and neural foramina. The regions of OPLL are typically hypointense on all sequences, particularly gradient echo sequences. Intermediate signal intensity may be seen in more pronounced cases of ossification, as opposed to primarily calcification. Cord compression and foraminal stenosis is readily depicted. With more severe degrees of compression, underlying cord signal intensity may develop, typically corresponding clinically with myelopathy.

Treatment options for symptomatic and progressive cases include surgical decompression with or without fusion.

✓ Pearls

- OPLL most often occurs in the cervical spine in adult patients; there is an association with DISH.
- CT optimizes characterization of the degree and pattern of ligamentous and dural calcification/ossification.

- MRI best depicts cord compression and foraminal stenosis; OPLL is typically hypointense on all sequences.

Suggested Reading

Saetia K, Cho D, Lee S et al. Ossification of the poetrior longitudinal ligament: a review. Neurosurg Focus 2011; 30: 1–16

Case 280

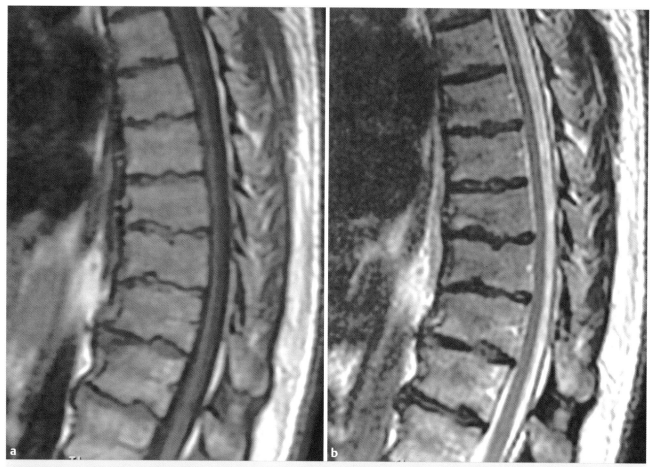

Fig. 280.1 Sagittal T1- **(a)** and T2-weighted **(b)** magnetic resonance images reveal multilevel Schmorl node deformities within the thoracic spine with anterior wedging of contiguous vertebral bodies and focal increased kyphosis. The involved disc spaces demonstrate irregularity and disc dessication. (Reprinted with permission: Tharin B, et al. J Am Osteopath Coll Radiol 2012;1(2):40.)

■ Clinical Presentation

A young adult man with chronic back pain (▶ Fig. 280.1)

▨ Key Imaging Finding

Multilevel Schmorl node deformities with anterior wedging and increased kyphosis

▨ Diagnosis

Scheuermann disease. Scheuermann disease is characterized by numerous Schmorl node deformities within contiguous vertebral segments with wedging of the vertebral bodies and focal increased kyphosis. It is thought to result from damage to the cartilaginous end plates in the skeletally immature spine and is a relatively common cause of chronic back pain in adolescents and young adults. Congenital end plate weakening or repetitive trauma are considered the most likely etiologies. The condition typically involves the thoracic spine and thoracolumbar junction. Pain is worsened by activity.

Diagnostic criteria on imaging include multiple Schmorl node deformities within at least three contiguous vertebral bodies (two disc spaces) and at least 5 degrees of anterior wedging at each level. Secondary findings include disc irregularity and dessication, scoliosis, focal thoracic kyphosis (>40 degrees is considered abnormal), and limbus vertebrae.

Treatment is typically conservative with analgesics, activity modification, physical therapy, and, occasionally, bracing. Surgical intervention is rare but may be necessary in severe cases with excessive kyphosis, intractable pain, or neurological deficits.

✓ Pearls

- Scheuermann disease is thought to result from congenital end plate weakening or repetitive trauma.
- Diagnostic criteria include Schmorl node deformities and anterior wedging of at least three contiguous vertebrae.

- Secondary findings include disc irregularity and dessication, scoliosis, focal kyphosis, and limbus vertebrae.

Suggested Reading

Swischuk LE, John SD, Allbery S. Disk degenerative disease in childhood: Scheuermann's disease, Schmorl's nodes, and the limbus vertebra: MRI findings in 12 patients. Pediatr Radiol 1998; 28: 334–338

Case 281

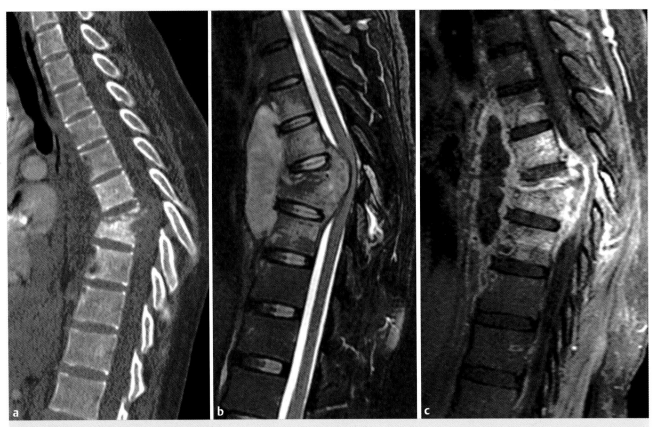

Fig. 281.1 Sagittal reformatted computed tomography image of the thoracic spine **(a)** demonstrates a wedge deformity of a mid-lower thoracic vertebra with focal gibbus deformity and a subchondral fracture subjacent to the superior end plate. Irregularity, expansion, and cortical disruption are noted along the posterior vertebral margin. Less conspicuous cortical irregularity is identified at multiple adjacent vertebral levels anteriorly. There are sclerotic changes of the primarily involved vertebra and adjacent vertebrae. Sagittal T2 **(b)** and postcontrast T1 with fat suppression **(c)** images show similar findings, as well as abnormal marrow signal intensity and enhancement within four contiguous vertebral segments. Subligamentous spread is identified with a large paraspinal abscess with rim enhancement seen within the anterior paraspinal soft tissues; a smaller epidural abscess is identified within the anterior epidural space. Inflammatory enhancement is seen along the dura, posterior elements, and dorsal paraspinal soft tissues. There is severe cord compression with abnormal cord signal intensity **(b)**. Of note, the intervertebral disc spaces and signal intensity are preserved **(b)**.

▦ Clinical Presentation

A middle-aged woman with fever, chronic cough, and back pain (▶ Fig. 281.1)

■ Key Imaging Finding

Abnormal marrow signal/enhancement and paraspinal abscesses with sparing of the disc spaces

■ Diagnosis

Tuberculosis (TB) spondylitis. TB spondylitis, or Pott disease, is caused by *Mycobacteruim tuberculosis*. It is more common in elderly or immunocompromised patients and may occur at any age in endemic regions; it preferentially involves the thoracic spine. Clinically, patients present with insidious onset of symptoms, typically back pain, due to the chronicity of the infection. In children, spinal infection may result in growth disturbances or arrest.

At times, the imaging appearance of pyogenic and TB spondylitis may be identical with abnormal signal and enhancement involving two contiguous vertebral segments and the intervening disc. Certain features on magnetic resonance imaging, however, are more characteristic and specific for TB spondylitis. In contrast to pyogenic infections, TB lacks destructive proteolytic enzymes, which often results in relative sparing of the intervertebral disc. TB spondylitis is also prone to subligamentous spread, resulting in multiple vertebral segment involvement and skip lesions, whereas pyogenic infections typically involve two contiguous segments. In terms of vertebral body signal abnormality and enhancement, pyogenic infections affect the subchondral regions along the end plates; TB spondylitis may have a similar appearance but is more likely to involve the entire vertebral body. A gibbus deformity is often seen with chronic TB spondylitis, characterized by focal wedging and kyphosis due to vertebral body collapse. An additional feature suggestive of TB spondylitis is the presence of large, well-defined, thin, rim-enhancing "cold" abscesses within the paraspinal soft tissues.

Treatment options include anti-TB medications and drainage of focal fluid collections. Surgical decompression and stabilization may be required for more severe cases with spinal compression or instability.

✓ Pearls

• In contrast to pyogenic infections, TB spondylitis often results in sparing of the intervertebral disc.
• TB spondylitis is prone to subligamentous spread with multiple vertebral-level involvement and skip lesions.

• The presence of a large, well-defined, thin, rim-enhancing paraspinal "cold" abscess is suggestive of TB.

Suggested Reading

Hong SH, Choi JY, Lee JW, Kim NR, Choi JA, Kang HS. MR imaging assessment of the spine: infection or an imitation? Radiographics 2009; 29: 599–612

Case 282

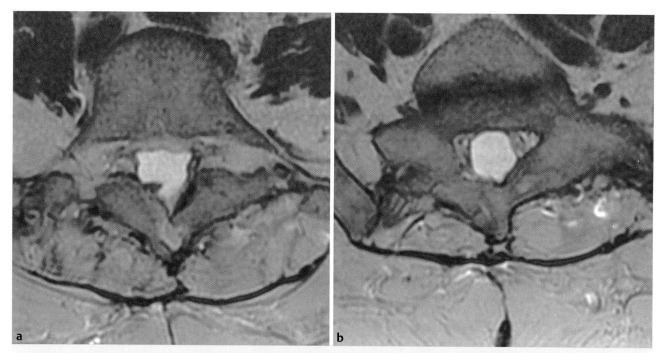

Fig. 282.1 Axial T2 image at the L4–5 level **(a)** demonstrates clumping of descending spinal nerve roots along the right posterolateral aspect of the thecal sac. Axial T2 image at L5-S1 **(b)** shows characteristic appearance of the "empty thecal sac" sign with lack of visualization of the descending nerve roots. There is severe fatty atrophy of the paraspinal musculature.

▨ Clinical Presentation

A 72-year-old woman with chronic back pain and a history of spinal surgery (▶ Fig. 282.1)

■ Key Imaging Finding

Peripheral and central adhesion of descending spinal nerve roots

■ Diagnosis

Arachnoiditis. Arachnoiditis refers to inflammation involving the cerebrospinal fluid (CSF) spaces. Common causes include infection, spinal surgery, hemorrhage, trauma, and intrathecal instrumentation for diagnostic or therapeutic purposes. Clinical presentation depends upon patient age, underlying etiology, and severity of the inflammatory process. Most patients suffer from chronic pain, which can be debilitating. The inflammatory process leads to adhesions, which account for the characteristic imaging findings.

Magnetic resonance imaging (MRI) is the modality of choice in evaluating patients with suspected arachnoiditis. Findings of adhesive arachnoiditis are characterized into three groups, one or all of which may be present in any given patient. Group 1 is characterized by central clumping of descending spinal nerve roots; group 2 is characterized by peripheral adhesion of nerve roots to the dural sac, resulting in the characteristic "empty thecal sac" sign; and group 3 is characterized by a soft-tissue mass replacing the subarachnoid space. Arachnoiditis is a dynamic rather than static process, so imaging findings may occur along a spectrum and may also change or evolve on subsequent examinations. Also, it is important to understand that a negative MRI exam does not entirely exclude arachnoiditis, especially early on in the disease process.

Some mimickers of arachnoiditis include CSF carcinomatosis, which may result in central clumping of descending nerve roots similar to group 1, and severe spinal stenosis, which may result in the appearance of a soft-tissue mass replacing the subarachnoid space similar to group 3.

✓ Pearls

- Arachnoiditis refers to inflammation of the CSF spaces; common causes include infection and iatrogenia.
- MRI is the imaging modality of choice in evaluating patients with suspected arachnoiditis.
- Arachnoiditis may result in central or peripheral ("empty thecal sac" sign) adhesion of descending nerve roots.

Suggested Reading

Ross JS, Masaryk TJ, Modic MT et al. MR imaging of lumbar arachnoiditis. Am J Roentgenol 1987; 149: 1025–1032

Case 283

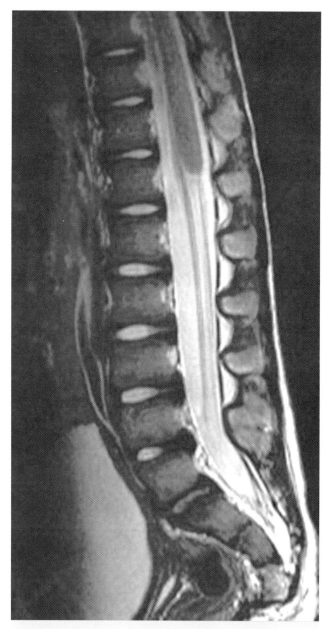

Fig. 283.1 Sagittal T2 image shows a blunted conus located at the mid-T12 level, as well as absence of the sacrum below the S2 level. A distended bladder is partially seen within the pelvis.

Clinical Presentation

A 3-year-old girl with scoliosis (▶ Fig. 283.1)

▦ Key Imaging Finding

High-riding, blunted conus with sacral dysgenesis

▦ Diagnosis

Caudal regression. Caudal regression syndrome (CRS) or caudal dysgenesis is a rare congenital malformation that primarily affects the distal neuroaxis and the lumbosacral spine. It is thought to result from some form of insult in the first 4 weeks of gestation. Associated genitourinary and anorectal malformations are common because there is a close association in terms of development of the distal neuroaxis and cloaca. Anomalies of the musculoskeletal system, particularly the lower extremities, may also be seen. Although the exact etiology remains uncertain, there is a strong association and increased incidence in infants of diabetic mothers.

There is a wide range of clinical manifestations and severity of CRS, ranging from relatively mild and asymptomatic to sirenomelia with severe malformations and fusion of the lower extremities (mermaid syndrome). Most patients present with some form of neurogenic bladder. Additional neurological and/or musculoskeletal defects are common at presentation.

There are two main types of CRS. Type 1 is characterized by a truncated or blunted, high-riding conus (L1 or above) with severe lumbosacral anomalies. Type 2 is characterized by an elongated, low-lying, tethered cord with less severe lumbosacral anomalies.

Type 1 has a higher association with additional developmental malformations and more severe clinical symptoms.

Prenatal ultrasound may identify CRS depending upon the severity and conspicuity of the findings. Magnetic resonance imaging is the modality of choice in characterizing the anomalies. Type 1 CRS reveals a blunted, high-riding conus and severe sacral dysgenesis. Prominence of the central canal within the distal cord is commonly seen. Type 2 presents with fetal elongation of the cord and less severe lumbosacral anomalies; the presence of lumbosacral anomalies is the key to distinguishing CRS from other causes of a tethered cord. Thickening of the filum and descending lumbosacral nerve roots are commonly seen. With both variants, it is important to evaluate the genitourinary, anorectal, and musculoskeletal systems (especially the lower extremities) to evaluate for coexistent anomalies.

Treatment includes surgical release for tethered cords, which often improves neurological outcomes. Surgical repair of genitourinary, anorectal, and musculoskeletal malformations is primarily based on the severity of anomalies and likelihood of improved function.

✓ Pearls

- CRS is a rare congenital malformation that primarily affects the distal neuroaxis and the lumbosacral spine.
- There is a strong association and increased incidence of CRS in infants of diabetic mothers.
- Type 1 CRS is characterized by a truncated or blunted, high-riding conus with severe lumbosacral anomalies.
- Type 2 CRS is characterized by an elongated, low-lying, tethered cord with less severe lumbosacral anomalies.

Suggested Reading

Rufener SL, Ibrahim M, Raybaud CA, Parmar HA. Congenital spine and spinal cord malformations—pictorial review. Am J Roentgenol 2010; 194 Suppl: S26–S37

Case 284

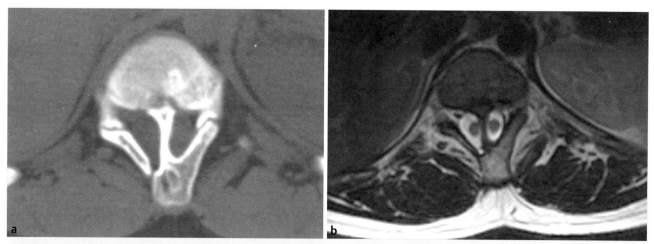

Fig. 284.1 Axial computed tomography image **(a)** reveals a bony septum separating the spinal canal into two segments. Axial T2 magnetic resonance image **(b)** demonstrates two hemicords, each with its own dural sac, separated by the central bony septum.

■ Clinical Presentation

An adolescent girl with spinal curvature and long-standing neurological deficits (▶ Fig. 284.1)

■ **Key Imaging Finding**

Two hemicords separated by an osseous septum

■ **Diagnosis**

Diastematomyelia. Diastematomyelia is characterized as a disorder of midline integration, which results in a sagittal cleft and formation of two hemicords of variable length, each with its own ventral and dorsal horns. There are two subsets with type 1 diastematomyelia consisting of two hemicords in separate dural sacs with an intervening cartilaginous or osseous septum; type 2 is characterized by two hemicords in the same dural sac with or without an intervening fibrous septum. The hemicords may be symmetric (more common) or asymmetric in size; asymmetry is more common in cases with separate dural sacs (type 1). Most cases occur in the upper lumber and lower thoracic region; upper thoracic or cervical lesions are rare. The hemicords unite proximal and distal to the cleft in the vast majority of cases. Associated vertebral segmentation anomalies and cord syrinx commonly coexist and are more severe with the type 1 variant.

Patients most often present clinically with scoliosis or a tethered cord. A tuft of hair, dimple, lipoma, or hemangioma is commonly seen at the level of diastematomyelia on physical examination.

✓ **Pearls**

- Diastematomyelia results in two hemicords of variable length, each with its own ventral and dorsal horns.
- Type 1 consists of two hemicords in separate dura with an intervening cartilaginous or osseous septum.
- Type 2 is characterized by two hemicords in the same dural sac with or without an intervening fibrous septum.
- Patients present with scoliosis or tethered cord; associated anomalies are more severe with the type 1 variant.

Suggested Reading

Rufener SL, Ibrahim M, Raybaud CA, Parmar HA. Congenital spine and spinal cord malformations—pictorial review. Am J Roentgenol 2010; 194 Suppl: S26–S37

Case 285

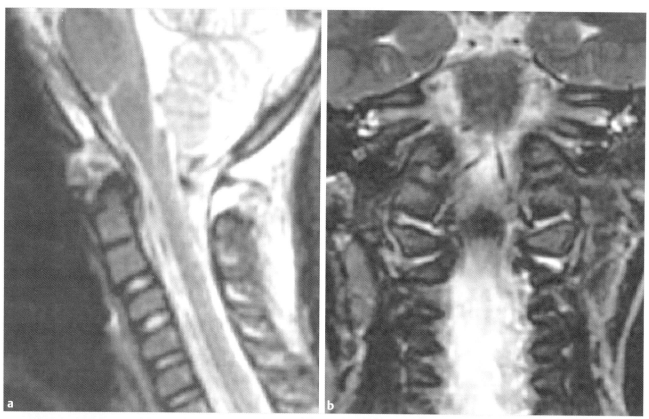

Fig. 285.1 Sagittal T2 image **(a)** demonstrates disruption of the stabilizing ligaments between the skull base/occiput and C1 with abnormal widening and increased signal intensity at the atlantooccipital junction. There is disruption of the apical ligament from the tip of the dens to the basion and uplifting of the tectorial membrane (continuation of the posterior longitudinal ligament) from the posterior margin of the clivus secondary to a retroclival hematoma. Coronal T2 image **(b)** reveals widening and intermediate T2 signal intensity between the occipital condyles and C1, more pronounced on the right. Increased T2 signal intensity is seen at the C1–2 and C2–3 levels.

■ **Clinical Presentation**

A young girl involved in a motor vehicle collision (MVC) (▶ Fig. 285.1)

▩ Key Imaging Finding

Post-traumatic ligamentous injury with widening of the atlantooccipital articulation

▩ Diagnosis

Atlantooccipital (AO) dislocation. AO dislocation is an uncommon injury of the craniocervical junction that typically results from significant trauma; MVCs are the leading cause. Children are more susceptible due to their relatively increased head size and underdeveloped stabilizing neck musculature. Prognosis is generally poor with associated intracranial and spinal injuries commonly seen. Although the majority of cases are fatal, early recognition and stabilization may improve chances of survival and meaningful recovery.

Plain films and computed tomography (CT) are the initial modalities in the setting of trauma. Common findings suggestive of AO dislocation include a distance ≥ 10 mm between the basion (anterior margin of the foramen magnum) and the odontoid and/or a distance ≥ 4 mm between the occipital condyles and C1 on the open-mouth odontoid view or coronal CT reformats. Associated traumatic findings include prevertebral and paraspinal soft-tissue swelling and vertebral body fractures.

Magnetic resonance imaging (MRI) is superior to plain films and CT in evaluating the stabilizing ligaments, cord, and soft-tissue structures. In addition to identifying widening of the AO articulation, it is important to evaluate the integrity of the stabilizing ligaments. Stabilizing ligaments include the tectorial membrane, apical ligament, alar ligaments, and anterior and posterior AO ligaments/membranes. The tectorial ligament is the primary stabilizer of the AO articulation and represents a continuation of the posterior longitudinal ligament; it attaches to the posterior margin of the clivus. The apical ligament extends from the tip of the dens superiorly to the inferior margin of the basion. The anterior AO ligament extends from the anterior arch of C1 to the anterior margin of the clivus, and the posterior AO membrane extends from the posterior arch of C1 to the opisthion (posterior margin of the foramen magnum). The presence of ligamentous injury or disruption, especially in the tectorial membrane, increases the likelihood of instability.

Cord and intracranial injuries are important to identify and describe and are also critical in determining the overall prognosis. CT and MRI play complimentary roles for the evaluation of bony and soft-tissue injuries.

When identified and amenable to therapy, AO dislocation is treated with immobilization and fixation.

✓ Pearls

- AO dislocation most often results from MVCs; children are more susceptible due to relatively large head size.
- Findings include ≥ 10 mm between the basion and odontoid or ≥ 4 mm between the occipital condyles and C1.

- Stabilizing ligaments include the tectorial membrane and the apical, alar, and anterior/posterior AO ligaments.

Suggested Readings

Benedetti PF, Fahr LM, Kuhns LR, Hayman LA. MR imaging findings in spinal ligamentous injury. Am J Roentgenol 2000; 175: 661–665

Hollingshead MC, Castillo M. MRI in acute spinal trauma. Appl Radiol 2007: 34–41

Case 286

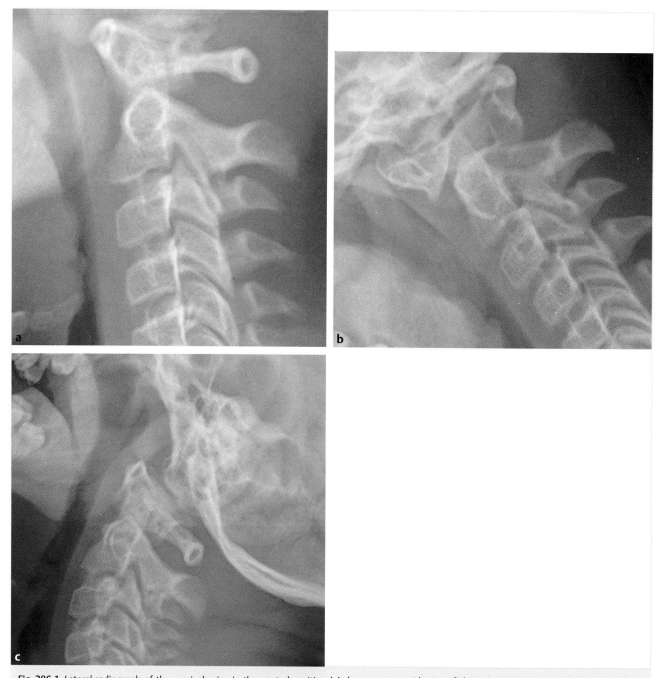

Fig. 286.1 Lateral radiograph of the cervical spine in the neutral position **(a)** demonstrates widening of the ADI, measuring approximately 6 mm. Lateral view in flexion **(b)** shows increase in the ADI. Lateral view in extension **(c)** reveals decrease in the ADI with the anterior arch of C1 contacting the dens.

▪ Clinical Presentation

A patient with intermittent neurological deficits; history otherwise withheld (▶ Fig. 286.1)

■ Key Imaging Finding

Increased atlantodental interval (ADI) that increases in flexion and decreases in extension

■ Diagnosis

Atlantoaxial instability (AAI). AAI refers to abnormal articulation and mobility between the atlas (C1) and the axis (C2). It may be congenital or acquired and the result of an underlying ligamentous (more common) or bony abnormality. Some of the more common causes of AAI include trauma, rheumatoid arthritis (RA), Down syndrome, an os odontoideum, and nonunion type II dens fracture. Additional causes include ankylosing spondylitis, osteogenesis imperfecta, neurofibromatosis type 1, mucopolysaccharidoses, and congenital atlantooccipital fusion anomalies. Patients may be asymptomatic or present with neurological deficits related to cord compression at the craniocervical junction as a result of the underlying instability.

The normal ADI is 3 mm in adults and 5 mm in children; it is measured from the posterior cortical margin of the anterior arch of C1 to the anterior cortical margin of the dens. In terms of stability, the transverse ligament is the primary stabilizer of the atlantoaxial articulation, preventing excessive anterior or posterior motion of the atlas with respect to the axis. Damage to or laxity of the transverse ligament is a leading cause of AAI. In the setting of an os odontoideum or type II odontoid fracture with nonunion, the transverse ligament remains intact; however, the atlas articulates with the os or fractured odontoid independent of the body of the axis, which may result in instability.

Imaging workup of AAI typically begins with plain radiographs. AAI is suggested by an increased ADI on the lateral, neutral projection. Confirmatory flexion and extension lateral views show increase of the ADI with flexion and decrease of the ADI with extension; a difference of 3 mm between flexion and extension views is indicative of instability. Computed tomography is useful in identifying a rotatory component of subluxation, as well as to better evaluate the bony structures. Erosions and pannus formation are seen in patients with RA. Patients with Down syndrome have a flat occiput and hypoplastic C1 arch. An os odontoideum or nonunion type II dens fracture presents as a corticated fragment that articulates with the C1 arch independent of the body of C2. Magnetic resonance imaging (MRI) is useful in both evaluating the atlantoaxial articulation, as well as for evaluating the cord for compression or injury. In setting of an inflammatory arthropathy, pannus, peridental effusions, and erosions are often seen at the atlantoaxial joint.

✓ Pearls

- AAI refers to abnormal articulation and mobility between the atlas (C1) and the axis (C2).
- Common causes of AAI include trauma, RA, Down syndrome, os odontoideum, or nonunion dens fracture.
- Plain radiographs show abnormal widening of the ADI that increases in flexion and decreases in extension.
- MRI is useful in evaluating for secondary findings, especially with RA, as well as for evaluating the cord.

Suggested Reading

Hung SC, Wu HM, Guo WY. Revisiting anterior atlantoaxial subluxation with overlooked information on MR images. Am J Neuroradiol 2010; 31: 838–843

Case 287

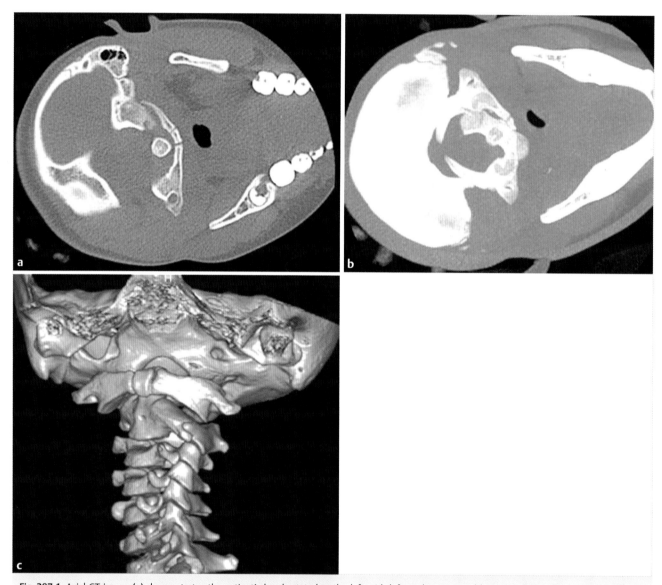

Fig. 287.1 Axial CT image **(a)** demonstrates the patient's head rotated to the left with leftward rotatory subluxation of C1 with respect to C2. The atlantodental interval or predental space is normal. Axial maximum intensity projection image **(b)** better depicts the rotation of C1 with respect to C2. Three-dimensional volume rendered image **(c)** again shows a rotatory component of C1 compared with the remainder of the cervical spine.

■ Clinical Presentation

A 6-year-old boy with torticollis post-trauma (▶ Fig. 287.1)

■ Key Imaging Finding

Abnormal rotation of C1 with respect to C2

■ Diagnosis

Atlantoaxial rotatory subluxation. The C1–2 articulation accounts for roughly half of the rotatory component of the entire cervical spine. Atlantoaxial rotatory subluxation refers to abnormal rotation of the C1–2 articulation at baseline, resulting in torticollis. Underlying etiologies include trauma, infectious or inflammatory processes, congenital abnormalities, and spontaneous or idiopathic causes. In the vast majority of cases, rotatory subluxation results in limited range of motion due to restriction or locking of the anterior C1 facet with respect to the C2 facet; rarely, fixation may occur. Underlying dislocation of C1–2 may or may not be present and manifests as anterior displacement of the C1 with respect to C2. There may also be widening of the atlantodental articulation or predental space. Atlantoaxial rotatory subluxation is classified based upon the presence or absence and degree of displacement of C1 compared with C2. Type I is the most common variant and demonstrates rotation without displacement.

Plain radiographs of the cervical spine demonstrate rotation of C1 on the lateral view and disparity of the C1 lateral masses with respect to midline on the frontal or open-mouth odontoid views. Dynamic computed tomography (CT) is helpful in distinguishing between atlantoaxial rotatory subluxation and fixation for cases that do not resolve or respond to conservative management. Images are first obtained with the patient at rest. Subsequently, imaging is performed with unassisted contralateral rotation of the head. With subluxation, there is some independent rotation of C1 with respect to C2 between the two examinations. In the setting of fixation, however, C1 and C2 maintain their alignment and do not rotate independently.

In the absence of known trauma, it is important to look for secondary findings that may identify an underlying cause of atlantoaxial rotatory subluxation, including congenital malformations or infectious processes of the head and neck (Grisel syndrome).

✓ Pearls

- Atlantoaxial rotatory subluxation refers to abnormal rotation of the C1–2 articulation, resulting in torticollis.
- Underlying etiologies include trauma, congenital abnormalities, inflammatory, and idiopathic causes.

- Plain radiographs demonstrate rotation of C1 and disparity of the C1 lateral masses with respect to midline.
- Dynamic CT is helpful in distinguishing between atlantoaxial rotatory subluxation and fixation.

Suggested Reading

Lustrin ES, Karakas SP, Ortiz AO et al. Pediatric cervical spine: normal anatomy, variants, and trauma. Radiographics 2003; 23: 539–560

Case 288

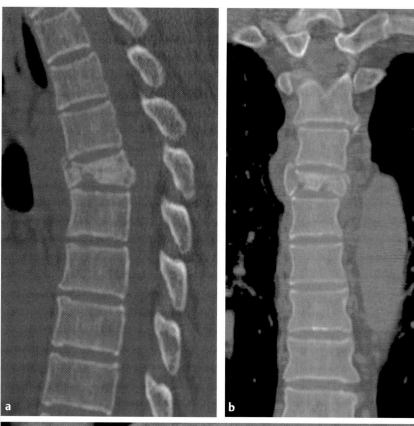

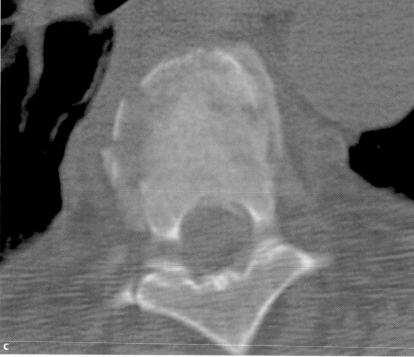

Fig. 288.1 Sagittal reformatted CT image **(a)** demonstrates a complex compression fracture of a midthoracic vertebral body with involvement of the anterior and middle vertebral columns. There is increased anteroposterior dimension of the involved vertebra with retropulsion of portions of the fracture into the spinal canal. Coronal reformatted CT image **(b)** reveals significant vertebral body height loss and lateral displacement of fracture fragments. Axial CT image **(c)** shows comminution of the complex fracture with fragment displacement in all directions, including a posterior component extending into the spinal canal. A paraspinal hematoma is identified on all images.

■ Clinical Presentation

A young adult man involved in a rollover motor vehicle collision, unrestrained (▶ Fig. 288.1)

■ Key Imaging Finding

Complex vertebral body fracture with height loss and disbursement of fracture fragments

■ Diagnosis

Burst fracture. A burst fracture refers to a complex, comminuted compression fracture of the vertebral body with disbursement of fracture fragments. It occurs in the setting of significant trauma, most often with an axial load (e.g., fall from height) and is most common at the thoracolumbar junction. Patients typically have neurological deficits corresponding to the level of injury. The degree of symptoms often correlates with the severity of injury, presence of instability, and extent of fragment displacement.

Plain radiographs and computed tomography (CT) demonstrate a compression fracture of the vertebral body that extends to the posterior cortical margin, thus involving at least two vertebral columns. There is associated vertebral body height loss and retropulsion of fracture fragments into the spinal canal. The involvement of the posterior cortical margin of the vertebral body differentiates a burst fracture from a simple wedge compression fracture. Fracture components may also involve the posterior column (pedicles, facets, lamina, spinous process and associated ligaments). In contrast to a Chance or seatbelt fracture, burst fractures are typically oriented in the sagittal plane, whereas Chance fractures are oriented in the axial plane due to the underlying mechanism of injury.

Anteroposterior plain films or coronal CT reformats may show widening of the interpedicular distance, which is indicative of underlying instability. With severe injury, there may also be malalignment of the vertebral column, as well as facet dislocation. Magnetic resonance imaging (MRI) is useful for evaluation of soft-tissue, ligamentous, and cord injury.

Treatment depends upon the clinical scenario and stability of the injury and includes both conservative and surgical options.

✓ Pearls

- Burst fracture refers to a comminuted vertebral body compression injury with disbursement of bony fragments.
- Imaging demonstrates a vertebral body compression fracture that extends to the posterior cortical margin.
- Widening of the interpedicular distance is indicative of instability; spinal malalignment may also be seen.
- MRI is useful for evaluation of soft-tissue, ligamentous, and cord injury.

Suggested Reading

Atlas SW, Regenbogen V, Rogers LF, Kim KS. The radiographic characterization of burst fractures of the spine. Am J Roentgenol 1986; 147: 575–582

Case 289

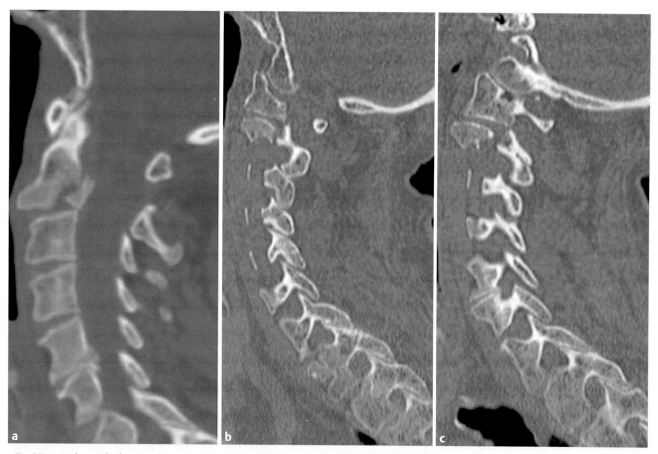

Fig. 289.1 Midsagittal reformatted CT image **(a)** demonstrates a fracture along the posteroinferior C2 vertebral body with anterior displacement of C2 with respect to C3, posterior displacement of the fracture fragment, and mild asymmetric widening of the anterior C2–3 disc space. Bilateral parasagittal images **(b,c)** reveal bilateral displaced pars fractures at C2.

■ **Clinical Presentation**

A 52-year-old man involved in a motor vehicle collision (▶ Fig. 289.1)

■ **Key Imaging Finding**

C2 fractures with listhesis

■ **Diagnosis**

Hanged man's fracture. Hyperextension injuries are most common in the cervical spine. When severe, they may result in fractures of the posterior elements and/or posterior vertebral body with widening of the anterior disc space. A hanged man's fracture refers to traumatic hyperextension injury of C2 with associated spondylolisthesis. It most often results from motor vehicle collisions and is considered an unstable injury.

The lateral view on plain radiographs demonstrates the C2 posterior element and/or vertebral body fractures with listhesis. Computed tomography (CT) is superior to plain films in characterizing the underlying bony injuries. Magnetic resonance imaging (MRI) is useful in evaluating for underlying ligamentous and cord injuries. Unlike hyperflexion injuries, the interlaminar line and interspinous articulations are typically maintained in the setting of hyperextension injury.

✓ **Pearls**

- Hyperextension injuries result in posterior element/vertebral body fractures with widened anterior disc space.
- A hanged man's fracture refers to traumatic hyperextension injury of C2 with associated spondylolisthesis.
- Lateral plain films demonstrate C2 posterior element and/or vertebral body fractures with listhesis.
- CT is superior to plain films in characterizing bony injuries; MRI best evaluates ligamentous and cord injuries.

Suggested Reading

Munera F, Rivas LA, Nunez DB, Jr, Quencer RM. Imaging evaluation of adult spinal injuries: emphasis on multidetector CT in cervical spine trauma. Radiology 2012; 263: 645–660

Case 290

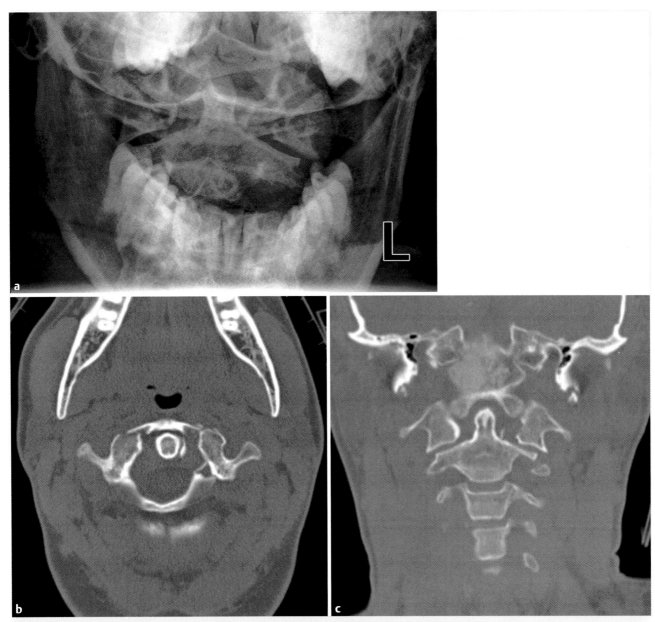

Fig. 290.1 Open-mouth odontoid view of the upper cervical spine **(a)** demonstrates bilateral but asymmetric widening of the interval between the dens and lateral mass of C1, more so on the left, with a small fracture fragment, as well as lateral displacement of the left C1 lateral mass with respect to C2. Axial CT image **(b)** shows bilateral fractures involving the anterior and posterior arches of C1 with regions of comminution and multiple fragments. Coronal reformatted CT image **(c)** shows similar findings compared with the open-mouth odontoid view with better depiction of the lateral displacement of the lateral mass of C1 on the right; "ground glass" attenuation of the skull base is incidentally noted. (Courtesy of Christopher Cerniglia, DO.)

■ Clinical Presentation

An adult man with high-velocity trauma (▶ Fig. 290.1)

▓ Key Imaging Finding

Fracture of C1 with displacement of the lateral masses

▓ Diagnosis

Jefferson fracture. Fractures of C1 most often result from axial loading or hyperextension injuries; diving accidents are a common etiology. Because the vertebral body acts as a ringlike structure, fractures occur in two places and may involve the anterior and/or posterior arches. With associated injury of the stabilizing ligaments, there may be instability with lateral displacement of the lateral masses of C1 with respect to C2.

On plain radiographs, the open-mouth odontoid view best evaluates C1 for appropriate alignment with respect to C2.

Instability is characterized by widening of the interval between the dens and the lateral mass of C1, which may be symmetric or asymmetric, as well as lateral displacement of the lateral mass of C1 beyond the lateral margin of C2. On computed tomography (CT), axial images readily identify the arch fractures, which often occur in an oblique sagittal plane; coronal reformats are ideal for evaluation of alignment and displacement of fracture components.

✓ Pearls

- Fractures of C1 result from axial loading or hyperextension injuries; diving accidents are a common etiology.
- Because C1 acts as a ring, fractures occur in two places and may involve the anterior and/or posterior arches.

- On plain films, the open-mouth odontoid view best evaluates C1 for appropriate alignment with respect to C2.
- On CT, axial images readily identify the fractures; coronal reformats are ideal for evaluation of alignment.

Suggested Reading

Munera F, Rivas LA, Nunez DB Jr Quencer RM. Imaging evaluation of adult spinal injuries: emphasis on multidetector CT in cervical spine trauma. Radiology 2012; 263: 645–660

Case 291

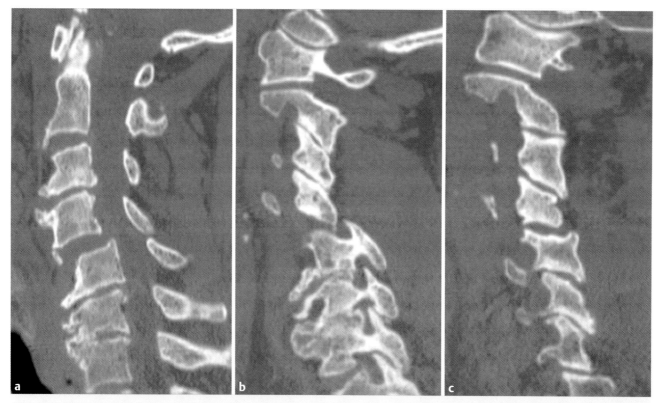

Fig. 291.1 Midline sagittal reformatted CT image of the cervical spine **(a)** demonstrates grade I anterolisthesis of C4 with respect to C5 with disruption of the anterior, posterior, and spinolaminar lines, as well as widening of the C4–5 disc space. Off-midline sagittal reformatted CT images through the facet joints **(b,c)** reveal a unilateral anteriorly displaced and locked facet **(b)**; contralateral facet alignment is maintained **(c)**. Degenerative changes are noted throughout the spine on all views.

▦ Clinical Presentation

An elderly man involved in a motor vehicle crash (▶ Fig. 291.1)

■ Key Imaging Finding

Cervical spine anterolisthesis with facet malalignment

■ Diagnosis

Facet dislocation. Flexion injuries commonly involve the cervical spine and include anterior teardrop fractures, facet dislocations (bilateral or unilateral), anterior wedge compression fractures, anterior subluxations, and the clay-shoveler fracture. Motor vehicle crashes are the most common underlying etiology. Anterior teardrop fractures and bilateral facet dislocations are considered unstable. Unilateral facet dislocation occurs in the setting of flexion with a rotatory component.

Bilateral facet dislocation occurs as a result of flexion injury with disruption of both the anterior and posterior longitudinal ligaments. The inferior facets at the involved segment are displaced superiorly and anteriorly compared with the superior facets of the subjacent inferior vertebra. The degree of subluxation ranges from partial with mild displacement, complete where the inferior facets at the involved level are perched on the superior facets of the lower level, and locked where the facet orientation is reversed with the inferior facets at the involved level positioned in front of the superior facets of the lower level. On lateral radiographs, there is disruption of the cervical lines with > 50% anterolisthesis at the involved level. Associated fractures may be identified. On axial computed tomography (CT) images, there is a naked facet sign in the setting of partial or complete (perched) subluxations, which refers to paired facets at the involved levels without articulation with the adjacent level. Locked facets demonstrate a reversal of the normal facet articulation. Secondary findings of flexion injury include focal kyphosis, widening of the posterior disc space, and widening of the interspinous distance.

Unilateral facet dislocations occur in the setting of flexion injury with rotation and commonly involve the mid to lower cervical spine. Although both facets are typically injured to some degree, the dislocation is unilateral. As with bilateral facet dislocation, the subluxation may be partial, complete (perched), or locked (reversed). Plain radiographs demonstrate loss of normal spinous process alignment on frontal views due to focal rotation at the involved level. Lateral views demonstrate focal loss of the normal cervical lines and varying degrees of anterolisthesis, measuring < 50%. Associated facet, vertebral body, and posterior element fractures may be seen. CT demonstrates similar findings compared with bilateral facet dislocation except that the findings are unilateral and there is a rotatory component at the involved level.

✓ Pearls

- Bilateral facet dislocation occurs with flexion injury and disruption of stabilizing longitudinal ligaments.
- Unilateral facet dislocation occurs in the setting of flexion injury with a rotatory component.
- Radiographs demonstrate > 50% anterolisthesis with bilateral and < 50% with unilateral facet dislocations.
- Naked facet sign is seen on CT with partial or complete (perched) dislocations; locked facets are reversed.

Suggested Readings

Lingawi SS. The naked facet sign. Radiology 2001; 219: 366–367

Pimentel L, Diegelmann L. Evaluation and management of acute cervical spine trauma. Emerg Med Clin North Am 2010; 28: 719–738

Case 292

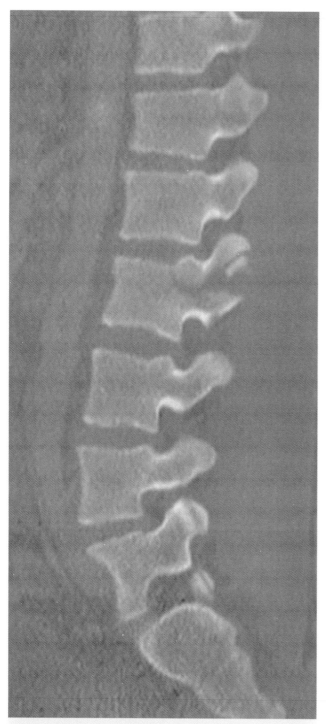

Fig. 292.1 Sagittal reformatted CT image reveals a displaced horizontal fracture extending through the posterior aspect of the L2 vertebral body and posterior elements, consistent with a flexion-distraction fracture.

■ Clinical Presentation

An adolescent girl who was a restrained passenger in a motor vehicle crash (▶ Fig. 292.1)

■ Key Imaging Finding

Horizontal displaced fracture through the lumbar posterior elements and vertebral body

■ Diagnosis

Chance fracture. A Chance or seatbelt fracture refers to a horizontal fracture of the neural arch due to flexion injury associated with rapid motor vehicle deceleration in patients wearing lap belts. Due to the location of the lap belts, the thoracolumbar junction is most commonly involved. There is a high incidence of associated visceral injuries that most often affect the small bowel and mesenteric vessels. Solid organ injuries of the pancreas, spleen, liver, kidneys, and uterus may also been seen. Interestingly, patients typically do not have neurological deficits despite the mechanism of fracture, which is generally considered unstable, especially when there is involvement of more than one vertebral column.

Chance fractures invariably involve the posterior elements with or without extension into the vertebral body. On frontal plain radiographs or coronal reformatted computed tomography (CT) images, the fractures are identified by horizontal lucencies through the pedicles, as well as displacement of fracture fragments of the spinous process, which results in the empty vertebral body sign. On the lateral or sagittal reformatted views, there may be distraction of the spinous process, and with severe injury, displacement of fracture components of the vertebral body. Instability results from disruption of the anterior and posterior longitudinal ligaments. The interspinous and posterior vertebral disc spaces may be widened, which is characteristic of flexion injuries.

Magnetic resonance imaging (MRI) is ideal for evaluation of ligamentous integrity and cord injury, as well as for evaluation of the intervertebral disc and paraspinal soft tissues. On both CT and MRI, it is important to evaluate visualized solid organs and hollow viscus.

✓ Pearls

- A Chance or seatbelt fracture refers to horizontal fracture of the neural arch due to flexion injury.
- Chance fractures involve the posterior elements with or without extension into the vertebral body.
- Frontal views often demonstrate transverse pedicle fractures and displacement of the spinous process.
- Lateral views show distraction of fracture fragments with interspinous and posterior disc space widening.

Suggested Reading

Bernstein MP, Mirvis SE, Shanmuganathan K. Chance-type fractures of the thoracolumbar spine: imaging analysis in 53 patients. Am J Roentgenol 2006; 187: 859–868

Case 293

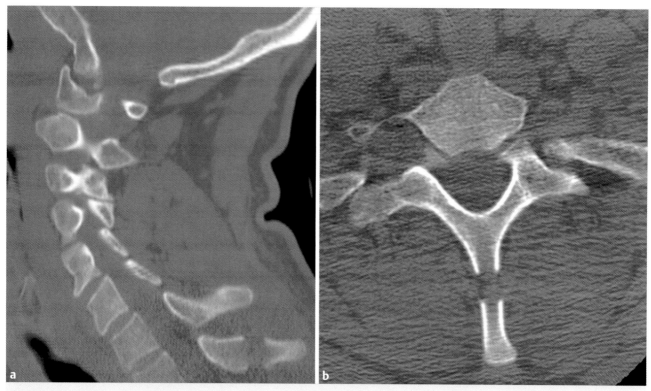

Fig. 293.1 Sagittal reformatted CT image **(a)** demonstrates a displaced spinous process fracture at the T1 level. Axial CT image **(b)** at the cervicothoracic junction shows the displaced spinous process fracture with a lack of corticated margins, confirming an acute fracture.

■ Clinical Presentation

An adult man involved in a motor vehicle crash (▶ Fig. 293.1)

▓ Key Imaging Finding

Displaced spinous process fracture at the cervicothoracic junction

▓ Diagnosis

Clay-shoveler fracture. A clay-shoveler fracture refers to a spinous process fracture at the cervicothoracic junction as a result of hyperflexion injury; C7 is the most commonly involved level. Historically, the fracture was named for an injury that occurred in workers shoveling clay where the clay would adhere to the shovel and cause abrupt flexion of the neck and spine. Nowadays, the most common mechanisms of injury include motor vehicle accidents and direct trauma.

Plain radiographs and computed tomography (CT) demonstrate a spinous process fracture involving the lower cervical or upper thoracic spine, often with some degree of displacement. Surrounding soft-tissue injury is commonly seen. In the acute setting, the fracture lacks corticated margins. Remote fractures with nonunion will demonstrate corticated margins, simulating an unfused apophysis.

✓ Pearls

- Clay-shoveler fracture refers to a lower cervical (usually C7) spinous process fracture due to hyperflexion.
- The most common present-day mechanisms of injury include motor vehicle accidents and direct trauma.

- Plain radiographs and CT demonstrate a spinous process fracture often with some degree of displacement.
- Remote fractures with nonunion will demonstrate corticated margins, simulating an unfused apophysis.

Suggested Reading

Lee P, Hunter TB, Taljanovic M. Musculoskeletal colloquialisms: how did we come up with these names? Radiographics 2004; 24: 1009–1027

Case 294

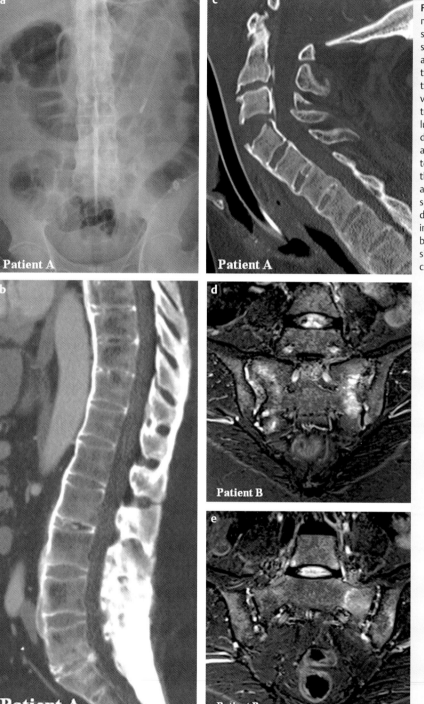

Fig. 294.1 KUB (kidney, ureter, and bladder) radiograph **(a)** demonstrates symmetric bilateral sacroiliitis with ankylosis of the SI joints, lateral spinal syndesmophytes with a "bamboo spine" appearance, and interspinous ligament ossification, resulting in the "dagger" sign throughout the midline spine; support tubes are partially visualized. Sagittal reformatted computed tomography (CT) image through the thoracolumbar spine in the same patient **(b)** better depicts the syndesmophyte formation anteriorly and ligamentous ossification and ankylosis posteriorly. Sagittal reformatted CT image through the cervical spine in the same patient **(c)** shows an acute unstable fracture through the C3–4 disc space with ligamentous and syndesmophyte disruption. Sagittal short tau inversion recovery images in a different patient **(d,e)** demonstrate bilateral sacroiliitis with focal regions of increased signal along the anteroinferior L5 end plate **(e)**, consistent with a "shiny corner" sign.

▨ Clinical Presentation

Two patients with chronic back pain; Patient A has a recent history of trauma (▶ Fig. 294.1)

Key Imaging Finding

Bilateral sacroiliitis with spinal syndesmophyte formation and ankylosis; acute spinal fracture in patient A

Diagnosis

Ankylosing spondylitis (AS). AS is a chronic, inflammatory, seronegative spondyloarthropathy that preferentially involves the sacroiliac (SI) joints and spine. It is thought to be an inherited syndrome with an increased incidence in patients with human leukocyte antigen (HLA)-B27, in conjunction with other spondyloarthropathies, such as psoriatic arthritis and reactive arthritis. Patients often present as adolescents or relatively young adults with chronic back pain and stiffness. Men are more commonly affected than women.

Imaging plays an important role in both the workup and management of patients with AS. The earliest radiographic manifestations involve the SI joints. The SI joints are typically involved in a bilateral symmetric fashion with early preferential involvement along the iliac side of the joints. Radiographic findings include bony erosions with regions of adjacent reactive bony sclerosis. As the disease progresses and becomes more severe, ankylosis or fusion occurs across the joint.

Early spinal involvement of AS results from an inflammatory enthesitis centered at the disc–end plate interface. Focal sclerosis (conventional radiographs or computed tomography) and bony edema (magnetic resonance imaging, MRI) are often seen along the anterior vertebral end plates, referred to as the "shiny corner" sign. Adjacent erosions may occur and incite reactive periosteal new bone formation, which results in "squaring" of the vertebral bodies due to loss of the normal vertebral concavity.

Syndesmophyte formation is commonly seen in patients with AS and results in calcification along the peripheral annulus fibrosis of the intervertebral discs, most pronounced along the anterior and lateral aspects of the spine. When extensive, the syndesmophyte formation leads to ankylosis of the spine and a characteristic "bamboo spine" appearance due to the undulating pattern of syndesmophytes. Enthesitis involving the interspinous ligaments may lead to ossification and ankylosis of the interspinous ligaments, producing the "dagger" sign on frontal radiographs (continuous midline ossification).

A fused or ankylosed spine is extremely susceptible to fracture, instability, and pseudoarthrosis. A high index of suspicion should be maintained in a known AS patient with trauma and new onset of pain or neurological deficits. In particular, spinal stabilization should be maximized during the clinical and imaging workup following trauma.

MRI has been shown to be useful in both documenting active disease and potentially establishing prognoses for disease progression. Active disease is suggested by the presence of inflammatory bone marrow edema or enhancement. A few studies have shown that the presence of active inflammatory disease correlates with subsequent development or progression of syndesmophytes in the spine.

✓ Pearls

- AS is an inflammatory seronegative spondyloarthropathy that preferentially involves the SI joints and spine.
- Spinal findings of AS on radiographs include vertebral body squaring, "bamboo spine," and the "dagger" sign.

- MRI shows marrow edema along the anterior vertebral body end plates, referred to as the "shiny corner" sign.
- A fused or ankylosed spine is extremely susceptible to fracture, instability, and pseudoarthrosis.

Suggested Reading

Ostergaard M, Lambert RGW. Imaging in ankylosing spondylitis. Ther Adv Musculoskelet Dis 2012; 4: 301–311

Case 295

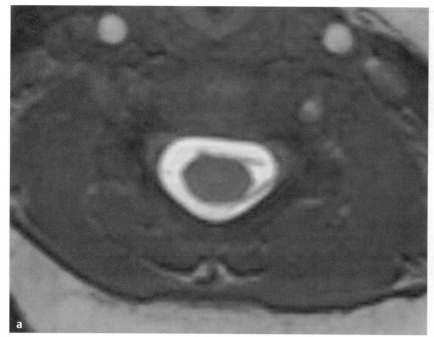

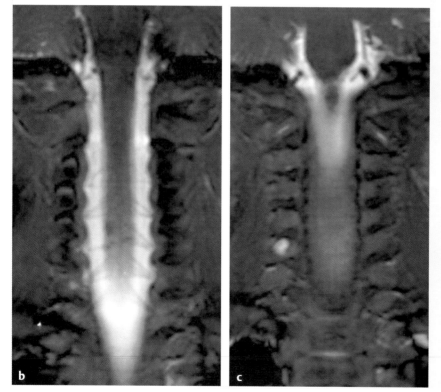

Fig. 295.1 Axial (**a**) and coronal (**b,c**) high-resolution T2-weighted images reveal avulsion of the right C6 nerve root (**a,b**) with a psuedo-meningocele in the corresponding neural foramen (**c**).

Clinical Presentation

A 12-week-old boy with birth-related right upper extremity neurological deficits (▶ Fig. 295.1)

■ Key Imaging Finding

Absence of cervical nerve roots with pseudomeningocele

■ Diagnosis

Nerve root avulsion. Brachial plexus nerve root injury results from excessive traction or stretching of the nerve roots. Common causes consist of birth injury or significant trauma, such as motor vehicle collisions (MVCs). Injury patterns are characterized as preganglionic or postganglionic and stretch injury versus avulsions. Although any level may be involved, the most common locations of injury include the upper brachial plexus at the C5 and C6 levels and lower plexus injuries at the C8 and T1 levels. Birth-related injuries include the more common upper plexus injury termed *Erb palsy* and the less common lower plexus injury termed *Klumpke palsy*. Upper plexus injuries result in motor deficits of the shoulder and upper arm; lower plexus injuries result in forearm, wrist, and hand weakness or paralysis.

Preganglionic avulsion injuries require nerve root transfers in order to regain nerve function. Postganglionic injuries may be treated conservatively or require nerve reconstruction, depending upon the specific nerve injury and clinical deficits.

Imaging evaluation of preganglionic brachial plexus injuries is best performed with computed tomography (CT) myelography and/or high-resolution magnetic resonance (MRI). Both allow for superior evaluation of ventral and dorsal nerve roots at each level. Imaging findings of avulsion injuries include discontinuity or absence of the nerve roots at the involved level. Pseudomeningocele or focal deformities of the nerve root sleeve are commonly seen due to dural tearing. Retracted portions of the nerve roots may be identified. MRI also allows for evaluation of postganglionic brachial plexus, soft-tissue, and focal cord injuries. Focal cord injuries include edema or hemorrhage in the acute phase; chronic cord injury may lead to regions of myelomalacia. Postganglionic stretch injuries may result in abnormal signal, thickening, and enhancement on MRI; these findings may represent postinjury neuroma formation or scarring.

✓ Pearls

- Brachial plexus injuries are most often caused by birth injury or significant trauma, such as MVCs.
- The most common locations of brachial plexus injury include the C5/C6 (upper) and C8/T1 (lower) levels.

- CT myelography and/or MRI are the modalities of choice in evaluating for preganglionic plexus injuries.
- Avulsions present with nerve root discontinuity, pseudomeningoceles, and/or nerve root sleeve deformities.

Suggested Readings

Smith AB, Gupta N, Strober J, Chin C. Magnetic resonance neurography in children with birth-related brachial plexus injury. Pediatr Radiol 2008; 38: 159–163

Yoshikawa T, Hayashi N, Yamamoto S et al. Brachial plexus injury: clinical manifestations, conventional imaging findings, and the latest imaging techniques. Radiographics 2006; 26 Suppl 1: S133–S143

Case 296

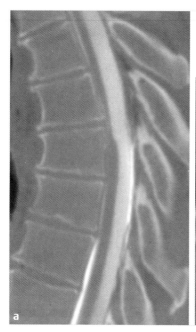 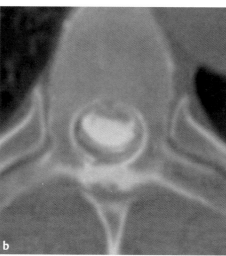

Fig. 296.1 Reformatted sagittal computed tomography (CT) myelogram image **(a)** demonstrates anterior displacement and a focal region of angulation and tethering involving the thoracic cord. The cord is atrophied at and above the level of angulation and normal in caliber below. Myelographic contrast is evenly distributed within the thecal sac without a visualized mass. The regions of relative increased attenuation along the dorsal and anterior aspect of the spinal canal represent extradural contrast. Axial CT image from the same study at the level of angulation **(b)** shows the degree of anterior cord displacement and volume loss, as well as soft tissue centrally extending beyond the dura anteriorly.

Clinical Presentation

A 63-year-old man with long-standing myelopathy (▶ Fig. 296.1)

▥ Key Imaging Finding

Displacement, focal angulation, and tethering of the cord

▥ Diagnosis

Spinal cord herniation. Spinal cord herniation is a rare entity characterized by herniation of portions of the cord through a dural defect. Common causes include trauma, iatrogenia, and unknown or idiopathic etiologies. The cord is most susceptible posteriorly within the cervical spine and anteriorly within the thoracic spine because spinal curvature in these regions results in approximation of the cord with the overlying dura. There is focal cord tethering at the level of the dural defect and associated cord injury. Patients often present with insidious onset of neurological deficits, which typically progress over the span of years.

Imaging reveals characteristic features with cord displacement and focal tethering with angulation. Visualization of cord material extending through a dural defect, when present, is diagnostic. The cord is often atrophic with or without signal abnormality on magnetic resonance imaging at and near the level of herniation.

The cord displacement results in prominence of cerebrospinal fluid (CSF) that is often mistaken as an intradural cyst causing cord displacement. Cross-sectional imaging, especially computed tomography myelogram, is helpful in excluding an underlying cyst. Meningeal cysts, even when in communication with the CSF, will typically demonstrate cyst walls and differing myelographic contrast attenuation compared with the surrounding CSF.

Treatment includes surgical release of the tethered cord with repair of the dural defect. Most often, patients show neurological improvement after surgical correction.

✓ Pearls

- Spinal cord herniation is characterized by focal herniation of portions of the cord through a dural defect.
- Imaging reveals characteristic features with cord displacement and focal tethering with angulation.

- Cord displacement results in prominence of CSF that may be mistaken for an intradural cyst.

Suggested Readings

Parmar H, Park P, Brahma B, Gandhi D. Imaging of idiopathic spinal cord herniation. Radiographics 2008; 28: 511–518

Watters MR, Stears JC, Osborn AG et al. Transdural spinal cord herniation: imaging and clinical spectra. Am J Neuroradiol 1998; 19: 1337–1344

Case 297

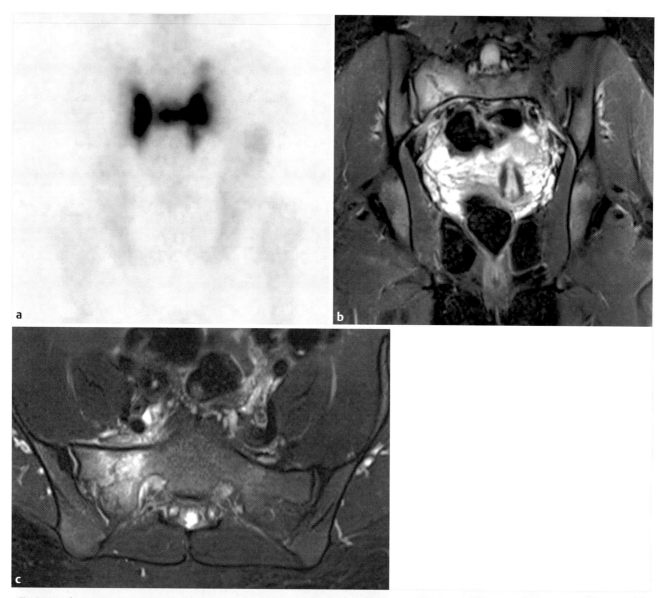

Fig. 297.1 Planar image over the pelvis from a technetium 99 m hydroxymethylene diphosphonate (HDP) bone scan **(a)** reveals intense uptake within the sacrum in an H-shaped configuration. Coronal **(b)** and axial **(c)** short tau inversion recovery MR images in a different patient demonstrate a vertically oriented hypointense fracture of the sacrum on the right with surrounding hyperintense marrow edema. (Image [a] courtesy of Jeffrey P. Tan, MD. and Kamal D. Singh, MD.)

■ Clinical Presentation

Patient A: 64-year-old woman with low back pain; Patient B: 19-year-old woman with back and hip pain after fall (▶ Fig. 297.1)

▦ Key Imaging Finding

Intense sacral uptake in an H-shaped configuration on bone scan and marrow edema on magnetic resonance imaging (MRI)

▦ Diagnosis

Sacral fracture. Sacral insufficiency fractures result from normal stresses on weakened bones, whereas traumatic sacral fractures result from abnormal stresses on normal bones. Insufficiency fractures most often occur in elderly women with osteoporosis; other predisposing factors include chronic corticosteroid use, rheumatoid arthritis, and pelvic radiation therapy. Clinical symptoms associated with sacral fractures include low back pain, which is exacerbated by movement, with radiation to the hip or groin. There may be point tenderness over the sacrum.

On nuclear medicine imaging, the classic findings include uptake vertically along the sacral ala bilaterally with an adjoining transverse line, resulting in an "H" configuration that resembles the Honda automotive symbol. It is therefore also referred to as the "Honda sign." Other variants include the "half butterfly" pattern where the superior aspects of the vertical lines are absent,

the bar pattern where the transverse line is thickened, and the tramline pattern where the transverse component of the "H" is absent.

Evaluation with conventional radiography may demonstrate the lucent fracture line through the sacral ala, cortical disruption, or sclerotic bands; however, evaluation is usually limited by overlying bowel gas. Computed tomography may demonstrate the fracture lines or sclerosis with greater sensitivity compared with conventional radiographs. MRI reveals a T1 hypointense fracture line with increased fat-suppressed T2 signal intensity within the marrow from underlying edema. In addition, MRI is useful to evaluate for an underlying pathological process.

Management of sacral insufficiency fractures consists of rest, analgesia, antiinflammatory therapy, limited weight-bearing, and physical therapy.

✓ Pearls

- Sacral insufficiency fractures result from normal stresses on weakened bones.
- Traumatic sacral fractures result from abnormal stresses on normal bones.

- On bone scan, there is typically a characteristic H-shaped configuration, known as the "Honda sign."
- MRI depicts the fracture line and marrow edema; it may also evaluate for an underlying pathological process.

Suggested Readings

Blake SP, Connors AM. Sacral insufficiency fracture. Br J Radiol 2004; 77: 891–896

Fujii M, Abe K, Hayashi K et al. Honda sign and variants in patients suspected of having a sacral insufficiency fracture. Clin Nucl Med 2005; 30: 165–169

White JH, Hague C, Nicolaou S, Gee R, Marchinkow LO, Munk PL. Imaging of sacral fractures. Clin Radiol 2003; 58: 914–921

Case 298

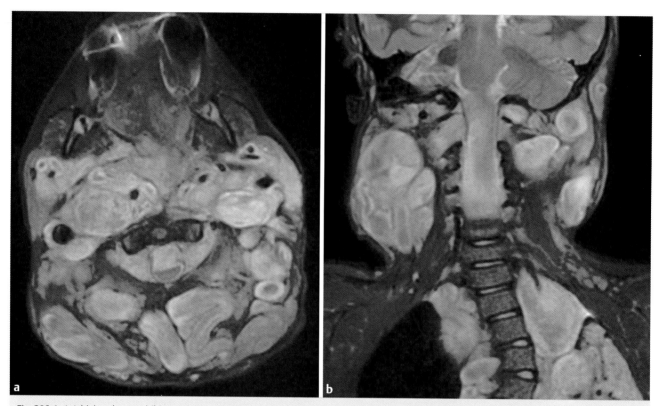

Fig. 298.1 Axial **(a)** and coronal **(b)** T2 images with fat suppression reveal multiple, large, lobulated, hyperintense paraspinal, extradural, and intradural extramedullary masses. Cord compression is seen at the C1–2 level **(a)**. The coronal image **(b)** shows focal scoliosis within the upper thoracic spine associated with numerous paraspinal masses, as well as foraminal extension and expansion within the upper cervical spine.

▓ Clinical Presentation

A 9-year-old girl with skin lesions, disfigurement, and scoliosis (▶ Fig. 298.1)

■ Key Imaging Finding

Multiple paraspinal, extradural, and intradural extramedullary masses

▩ Diagnosis

Neurofibromatosis type 1 (NF1). NF1, also known as von Reck-linghausen disease, is the most common of the neurocutaneous syndromes. It may occur sporadically or be inherited in an auto-somal dominant fashion. The genetic defect affects chromo-some 17q12 and results in decreased production of neurofibro-min, which acts as a tumor suppressor. The disease affects the brain, skull, orbits, spine, musculoskeletal system, and skin/integumentary system. Diagnostic criteria for NF1 include the presence of two or more of the following: first-degree relative with NF1, six or more café-au-lait spots, two or more neurofi-bromas (NFs) or one plexiform NF (PNF), optic pathway glioma, bony dysplasia, axillary or inguinal freckling, and two or more Lisch nodules.

Intracranial central nervous system (CNS) manifestations include characteristic NF "spots" and low-grade neoplasms. The NF spots may wax and wane for the first decade of life and then regress in both size and signal abnormality. The most common CNS neoplasms associated with NF1 are low-grade optic path-way gliomas (OPG). Bilateral optic nerve gliomas are pathogno-monic for NF1. Low-grade cerebellar, brain stem, tectal plate, and basal ganglia gliomas are also common in the setting of NF1. In addition to OPG, orbital findings include sphenoid wing dysplasia with pulsatile exophthalmos, buphthalmos (globe enlargement), and intraorbital extension of a PNF. Vascular abnormalities include regions of stenosis, moyamoya, and aneurysm formation. These are best visualized on magnetic res-onance angiography studies.

Spinal manifestations of NF1 include multiple bilateral NFs with extension through and expansion of the neuroformina. NFs are more likely than schwannomas to demonstrate the "tar-get sign," which refers to peripheral increased and central decreased T2 signal intensity. Large retroperitoneal PNFs are prone to malignant degeneration, which is best characterized by interval growth. Additional spinal manifestations include kyphoscoliosis, dural ectasia with posterior vertebral body scal-loping, and lateral thoracic meningoceles. Rarely, intramedul-lary lesions, typically low-grade astrocytomas, may present in patients with NF1.

Extra-CNS and spinal manifestations include cutaneous NFs, café-au-lait spots, extremity long-bone pseudoarthroses and bowing deformities, "ribbon" ribs, and hypertrophy or overgrowth of all or a portion of a limb. NF1 is associated with an increased incidence of several tumors, including phe-ochromocytoma, medullary thyroid carcinoma, gastro-intestinal stromal tumors, melanoma, Wilms tumor, leukemia, and lymphoma.

✓ Pearls

- NF1 is the most common neurocutaneous syndrome and results from a genetic defect affecting chromosome 17q12.
- Common spinal manifestations include multiple NFs with foraminal extension and bony remodeling.
- Scoliosis, dural ectasia with posterior vertebral body scallop-ing, and lateral meningoceles are common in NF1.

Suggested Readings

DiMario FJ, Jr, Ramsby G. Magnetic resonance imaging lesion analysis in neuro-fibromatosis type 1. Arch Neurol 1998; 55: 500–505

Egelhoff JC, Bates DJ, Ross JS, Rothner AD, Cohen BH. Spinal MR findings in neuro-fibromatosis types 1 and 2. Am J Neuroradiol 1992; 13: 1071–1077

Rodriguez D, Young Poussaint T. Neuroimaging findings in neurofibromatosis type 1 and 2. Neuroimaging Clin N Am 2004; 14: 149–170, vii

Case 299

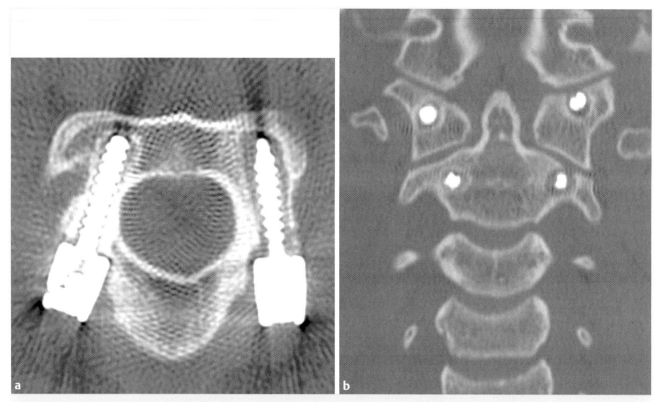

Fig. 299.1 Axial CT image through the C2 vertebral body **(a)** demonstrates abnormal lucency surrounding the entire fixation screw on the left and distal tip on the right. Coronal reformatted image **(b)** better depicts the lucency and also shows disruption of the cortex superiorly. Similar findings are noted on the left at C1. Fixations screws on the right reveal less pronounced lucency along the margins of the fixation hardware.

■ **Clinical Presentation**

A 13-year-old boy with neck pain (▶ Fig. 299.1)

▨ Key Imaging Finding

Lucency surrounding spinal fixation screw

▨ Diagnosis

Spinal hardware complication/loosening. Spinal stabilization and fusion is performed to correct and restore anatomic alignment and function secondary to underlying congenital, post-traumatic, neoplastic, or postinfectious/inflammatory defects. The surgical approach and hardware utilized depends upon both the underlying condition and the individual surgeon. Complications may arise in the immediate postoperative period or present years after the initial surgery.

Postoperative imaging typically consists of plain radiographs and computed tomography (CT) and is utilized to look for appropriate alignment, evidence of hardware complication, and to evaluate for bony fusion, when applicable. Pedicle screws are commonly used in the spine and require meticulous placement due to their proximity to critical neurovascular structures. Ideally, pedicle screws will traverse along the medial cortex of the pedicle because this location allows for maximal anchoring. Care must be taken not to disrupt the medial cortex because inadvertent penetration may result in narrowing of the spinal canal. With posterior fusion, the tip of the pedicle screw should approach but not extend through the anterior cortex of the vertebral body. Improper (or less than optimal) screw placement includes those that extend into the spinal canal, foramen transversarium, intervertebral disc space, or paraspinal soft tissues.

Properly placed screws may become fractured or loosened over time. Fractured hardware is not difficult to identify, but it is important to comment on the degree of displacement of the hardware components. Loosening is best evaluated on CT and presents as a rim of lucency surrounding the pedicle screw. Loosening allows for migration of the hardware that may result in instability.

✓ Pearls

- Spinal stabilization and fusion is performed to correct and restore anatomic alignment and function.
- Pedicle screws require meticulous placement due to their proximity to critical neurovascular structures.

- Less than optimal placement includes involvement of the spinal canal, foramen transversarium, and disc space.
- Hardware loosening is best evaluated on CT and presents as a rim of lucency surrounding the pedicle screw.

Suggested Reading

Young PM, Berquist TH, Bancroft LW, Peterson JJ. Complications of spinal instrumentation. Radiographics 2007; 27: 775–789

Case 300

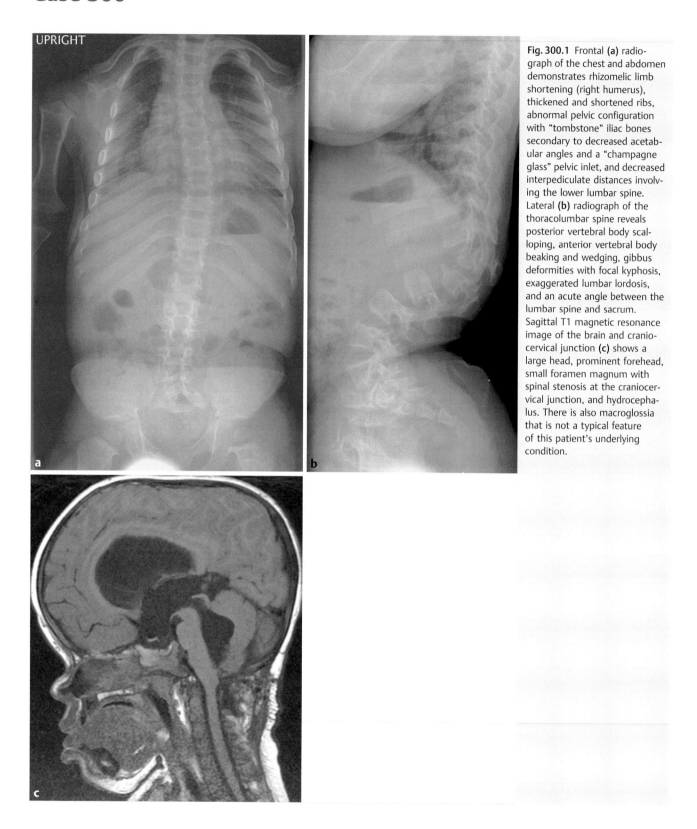

Fig. 300.1 Frontal **(a)** radiograph of the chest and abdomen demonstrates rhizomelic limb shortening (right humerus), thickened and shortened ribs, abnormal pelvic configuration with "tombstone" iliac bones secondary to decreased acetabular angles and a "champagne glass" pelvic inlet, and decreased interpediculate distances involving the lower lumbar spine. Lateral **(b)** radiograph of the thoracolumbar spine reveals posterior vertebral body scalloping, anterior vertebral body beaking and wedging, gibbus deformities with focal kyphosis, exaggerated lumbar lordosis, and an acute angle between the lumbar spine and sacrum. Sagittal T1 magnetic resonance image of the brain and craniocervical junction **(c)** shows a large head, prominent forehead, small foramen magnum with spinal stenosis at the craniocervical junction, and hydrocephalus. There is also macroglossia that is not a typical feature of this patient's underlying condition.

▪ Clinical Presentation

A young boy with short stature (▶ Fig. 300.1)

■ Key Imaging Finding

Rhizomelic dwarfism with spinal, craniocervical, thoracic, and pelvic anomalies

■ Diagnosis

Achondroplasia. The most common nonlethal skeletal dysplasia, achondroplasia is an autosomal dominant disease characterized by skeletal abnormalities attributable to decreased cartilage matrix production and endochondral ossification. Patients have predictable rhizomelic (proximal) limb shortening, enlarged head, midface hypoplasia, a long trunk, and spinal malformations. Cognitive function and development is normal.

Conventional radiographs of the extremities demonstrate proximal rhizomelic limb shortening with flared metaphyses. The hands and fingers are shortened with a trident appearance, especially during early bony development. Chest or thoracic spine radiographs show a long, narrow thorax with thick, shortened ribs.

Characteristic findings in the lumbar spine include decreased descending interpediculate distance within the lower lumbar, increased lumbar lordosis, anterior vertebral body beaking or wedging (most common at thoracolumbar junction), posterior vertebral body scalloping, and spinal stenosis. There is often an acute angle at the lumbosacral junction. The pelvis demonstrates shortened iliac bones with decreased (horizontal) acetabular angles and a "tombstone" appearance, as well as an inner pelvic contour with a "champagne glass" configuration.

Evaluation of the cranial vault and craniocervical junction demonstrates a disproportionately enlarged head, prominent forehead, depressed nasal bridge, and small skull base with stenosis at the foramen magnum. There is often brain stem/cord compression and instability at the craniocervical junction. In newborns and young children, there is often ventriculomegaly and enlargement of the extraaxial cerebrospinal (CSF) spaces. Hydrocephalus may result from impaired flow of CSF at the craniocervical junction and venous hypertension.

Patients often suffer from chronic otomastoiditis secondary to midface hypoplasia, which results in shortened eustachian tubes, a small pharynx, and relatively large adenoids and tonsils. Dental manifestations include a protruding jaw, and poorly aligned crowded teeth.

Hypochondroplasia is a less severe form of achondroplasia in which findings may be mild and limited to the spine.

✓ Pearls

- Achondroplasia is the most common nonlethal skeletal dysplasia and is autosomal dominant.
- Patients have rhizomelic limb shortening, a long trunk, enlarged head, and spinal/pelvic malformations.

- Hypoplasia of the skull base results in spinal stenosis and often instability at the craniocervical junction.
- Lumbar spine findings include decreased interpediculate distance, increased lordosis, and spinal stenosis.

Suggested Reading

Baujat G, Legeai-Mallet L, Finidori G, Cormier-Daire V, Le Merrer M. Achondroplasia. Best Pract Res Clin Rheumatol 2008; 22: 3–18

Index of Differential Diagnoses, by Case

Index of Key Findings and Roentgen Classics

Note: The index is ordered by case number within each section.